INFECTIOUS DISEASES

ALSO PUBLISHED BY OXFORD UNIVERSITY PRESS IN THE OXFORD GEOGRAPHICAL AND ENVIRONMENTAL STUDIES SERIES

The Globalized City
Economic Restructuring and Social Polarization in European Cities
Frank Moulaert, Arantxa Rodríguez, and Erik Swyngedouw

Of States and Cities
The Partitioning of Urban Space
Edited by Peter Marcuse and Ronald van Kempen

Globalization and Integrated Area Development in European Cities
Frank Moulaert

Globalization and Urban Change
Capital, Culture, and Pacific Rim Mega-Projects
Kris Olds

Sustainable Livelihoods in Kalahari Environments
Edited by Deborah Sporton and David S. G. Thomas

Conflict, Consensus, and Rationality in Environmental Planning
An Institutional Discourse Approach
Yvonne Rydin

Social Power and the Urbanization of Water
Flows of Power
Erik Swyngedouw

An Uncooperative Commodity
Privatizing Water in England and Wales
Karen J. Bakker

Manufacturing Culture
The Institutional Geography of Industrial Practice
Meric S. Gertler

Thailand at the Margins
Internationalization of the State and the Transformation of Labour
Jim Glassman

Industrial Transformation in the Developing World
Michael T. Rock and David P. Angel

Island Epidemics
Andrew Cliff, Peter Haggett, and Matthew Smallman-Raynor

War Epidemics
An Historical Geography of Infectious Diseases in Military Conflict and Civil Strife, 1850–2000
Matthew Smallman-Raynor and Andrew Cliff

Emergence and Re-Emergence

Infectious Diseases

A Geographical Analysis

A. D. Cliff, M. R. Smallman-Raynor,

P. Haggett, D. F. Stroup, S. B. Thacker

OXFORD
UNIVERSITY PRESS

OXFORD
UNIVERSITY PRESS

Great Clarendon Street, Oxford OX2 6DP

Oxford University Press is a department of the University of Oxford.
It furthers the University's objective of excellence in research, scholarship,
and education by publishing worldwide in

Oxford New York

Auckland Cape Town Dar es Salaam Hong Kong Karachi
Kuala Lumpur Madrid Melbourne Mexico City Nairobi
New Delhi Shanghai Taipei Toronto

With offices in

Argentina Austria Brazil Chile Czech Republic France Greece
Guatemala Hungary Italy Japan Poland Portugal Singapore
South Korea Switzerland Thailand Turkey Ukraine Vietnam

Published in the United States
by Oxford University Press Inc., New York

First published 2009

British Library Cataloguing in Publication Data
Data available

Library of Congress Cataloging in Publication Data
Library of Congress Control Number: 2009928980

Typeset by SPI Publisher Services, Pondicherry, India
Printed in Great Britain
on acid-free paper by
CPI Antony Rowe, Chippenham, Wiltshire

ISBN 978–0–19–924473–7

1 3 5 7 9 10 8 6 4 2

EDITORS' PREFACE

Even as processes of globalization expand in range and scale, the world remains marked by huge inequalities, social divisions and environmental degradation. We continue to live in a world marked by inequality and injustice; torn apart by poverty, war, and disputes over the right to own, control, and use resources, and by religious, ethnic, and racialized conflicts; and marked by differences in living standards and quality of life both within and between societies, based on class, gender, age, and other social distinctions. This series is driven by the desire to explore and explain these inequalities, a well as to investigate the possibilities of socio-spatial justice and environmental sustainability.

The key issues of our times are interwoven spatial issues. Climate change, global warming, the inequitable use of resources by the world's richest nations, the global movement of capital and labour, the development of new technologies, pandemics and new diseases that may jump the species gap, are transforming and remaking spatial divisions within and between power blocs, nation-states, regions, and communities.

New theoretical responses to these changes are also emerging both within and beyond geography as the practices, technologies, and significance of spatial difference are being addressed in a range of disciplines. The ubiquitous rhetoric of globalization and the uncritical division between the local and the global are being critically examined across disciplinary and academic borders and older versions of internationalism, social justice, and environmental management are being rethought by geographers and others in work that insists on the articulation of the local within larger frameworks as both an intellectual and an ethical project.

The Oxford Geography and Environmental Studies series aims to reflect these new approaches and interdisciplinary work, as well as to continue to publish the best original research in geography and environmental studies.

Gordon L. Clark
Diana Liverman
Linda McDowell
David Thomas
Sarah Whatmore

PREFACE

Over 50 churches worldwide, ranging eastwards from Bolivia to Hawaii, are dedicated to St Roche (San Rocco in Italy), the patron saint of plagues. Born in Montpellier in 1295, in his teens he travelled to Rome as a mendicant pilgrim, only to be caught up in the epidemic of plague just arriving in that city. The miraculous cures in several Italian cities attributed to him during his short life (he died in 1327) ensured that, when the trauma of the Black Death eventually swept Europe (1347–9), it was to St Roche—canonized in popular belief long before the Vatican caught up—that the afflicted first turned their intercessions.

If pestilence and prayer were thought of solely as quaint relics of medieval life, the late twentieth century came as a nasty shock. Since 1981, 25 million people have died from the AIDS pandemic, and Africa alone has 12 million AIDS orphans. The worldwide toll of HIV infection today has reached 33 million and, in some African countries, one-quarter of the adult population is infected. Worries over a new H5N1 strain of human influenza emerging rekindle memories of the devastating Spanish influenza pandemic of 1918–19. A brief outbreak of SARS in 2003 showed how rapidly pandemics can now race through the global urban network. All three are examples of what have come to be termed *emerging* infectious diseases.

The conventional concept of an emerging infectious disease has now become well established. The National Academy of Science's Institute of Medicine applies it to infectious diseases in humans that have increased over the past few decades or which threaten to increase in the near future. The World Health Organization adopts Stephen Morse's 1995 definition of emerging infectious diseases as 'diseases that have appeared in a population for the first time or that may have existed previously but are rapidly increasing in incidence or geographic range' (http://www.who.int/topics/emerging_diseases). This covers new infections resulting from changes in existing organisms (e.g. AIDS, SARS, H5N1 influenza), known infections spreading to new geographical areas or populations (e.g. West Nile), previously unrecognized infections appearing in areas undergoing ecological transformations (e.g. Lyme disease), and old infections re-emerging from antimicrobial quietude (e.g. tuberculosis) or a breakdown in public health measures (e.g. plague).

While this emphasis on current and recent threats is understandable, we argue in this book that disease emergence deserves to be set in a broader historical context. Study of the history of human disease over time shows that 'new' or 'renewed' infectious diseases are a constant theme rather than a recent episode. Very old diseases such as measles or cholera undergo periodic eruptions and invasions which share many of the features now associated with emerging diseases. This longer-run perspective helps to set the context within which recent events can be more firmly viewed, and enables the exceptional conditions which are forcing the present rapid pace of disease change to be more readily isolated.

The book is divided into three main sections: Part I looks at early disease emergence, Part II at the processes of disease emergence, and Part III at the future for emergent diseases. In writing this book, we have been acutely aware of the vast literature on emergent diseases. We have not attempted to be all-inclusive. Instead, we have concentrated on those papers which show a strong locational focus in the sense of reporting an epidemic or an outbreak in a particular country or region of the world, and we have woven these into a historical geography of disease emergence with examples that illustrate the broad causes of emergence.

Our research would not have been possible without the continuing support of a large number of institutions and individuals. The list will be a familiar one to readers of some of our other work on the geography of communicable diseases stretching back over three decades. Our first and greatest debt is to the Wellcome Trust. The work reported here is one of the outcomes of a seven-year programme grant entitled Historical Geography of Emerging and Re-emerging Epidemics: GIS (Geographical Information Systems) Programme. Without Wellcome's long-term support, the project could not have been completed. Peter Haggett has also had a further grant from Wellcome's History of Medicine panel for additional work on the Iceland records, while Matthew Smallman-Raynor was awarded a Philip Leverhulme Prize in 2001–3.

At the World Health Organization, Geneva, assistance was again provided by the staff of the WHO library. Here we have to thank especially Tomas Allen and Avril Reid. Librarians at the US Centers for Disease Control and Prevention (CDC) in Atlanta have also continued to give us full support. Especial thanks must also go to the directors and staff of the state archives in many Italian cities—Genoa, Naples, Palermo, Rome, Venice—for helping us with difficult seventeenth- and eighteenth-century manuscripts and cartographic material on the plague in Italy; similar thanks are extended to colleagues in the faculties of Classics and Medieval and Modern Languages in Cambridge. The Cartographic Unit in the Cambridge University Department of Geography undertook the enormous job of producing the maps and diagrams.

The origins of the group who together wrote this book go back a long way to a chance meeting in Evanston in 1966. The first Bristol–CDC link was established in 1982, just before a student's choice of a particular Cambridge college completed the pentagon of authors. Over the years during which this book and its predecessors have been researched, work on infectious diseases has taken one or more of us into some odd corners of the world from sub-Arctic countries to Pacific Ocean islands, and from Cotswold surgeries to Venetian archives. We hope this volume will help to explain to the many people not identified here, but who have encouraged and supported us in an infinity of ways, what motivated us to take what proved to be a longer journey than we had planned.

Venice
Feast of St Roche, 2008

CONTENTS

LIST OF FIGURES

LIST OF PLATES

LIST OF TABLES

LIST OF ABBREVIATIONS

ABLV	Australian bat lyssavirus
ACF	autocorrelation function
AHF	Argentine haemorrhagic fever
ARC	AIDS-related complex
ARV	Antiretroviral
ASF	Archivio di Stato di Firenze
ASN	Archivio di Stato di Napoli
ASP	Archivio di Stato di Palermo
ASR	Archivio di Stato di Roma
ASV	Archivio di Stato di Venezia
AVA	Agri-Food and Veterinary Authority
bp	before present
BRFSS	Behavioural Risk Factor Surveillance System
BSE	bovine spongiform encephalopathy
BTV	bluetongue virus
CASH	cancer and steroid hormone study
CCF	cross-correlation function
CCS	critical community size
CDC	Centers for Disease Control and Prevention, Atlanta, Georgia
CD-WGE	(WHO) Communicable Diseases Working Group on Emergencies
CJD	Creutzfeldt–Jakob disease
CNS	central nervous system
CSM	cerebrospinal meningitis
CSTE	(US) Council of State and Territorial Epidemiologists
CV	coefficient of variation
CWD	chronic wasting disease
DALY	disability-adjusted life year
DEFRA	Department for Environment, Food, and Rural Affairs
DOTS	directly observed treatment short course
DRC	Democratic Republic of Congo
EC	evacuation centre
EDA	Exploratory Data Analysis
EDR	excess death rate
EDT	(US) Eastern Daylight Time
EHEC	Enterohaemorrhagic *E. coli*
EHF	epidemic haemorrhagic fever
EIP	(CDC) Emerging Infections Program
EIS	Epidemic Intelligence Service
EM	erythema migrans
ENSO	El Niño–Southern Oscillation
Epi-Aids	(EIS) epidemic assistance investigations

EPR	(WHO) Epidemic and Pandemic Alert and Response
EV	enterovirus, Ebola virus
EWARN	early warning and response network
fCJD	familial Creutzfeldt–Jakob disease
FDA	(US) Food and Drug Administration
FFI	fatal familial insomnia
FMD	foot and mouth disease
FMDV	foot and mouth disease virus
FoodNet	(US) Foodborne Diseases Active Surveillance Network
FSE	feline spongiform encephalopathy
GCM	general circulation model
GIP	Great Indian Peninsular Railway
GIS	Geographical Information System
GNI	gross national income
GOARN	(WHO) Global Outbreak Alert and Response Network
GP	general practitioner
GSS	Gerstmann–Sträussler–Scheinker syndrome
HCH-dieldrin	hexachlorocyclohexane-dieldrin
HeV	Hendra virus
HEV	hepatitis E virus
HFRS	haemorrhagic fever with renal syndrome
HFV	hepatitis F virus
HGV	hepatitis G virus
HHV	human herpesvirus
HIV	human immunodeficiency virus
HPAI	highly pathogenic avian influenza
HPS	hantavirus pulmonary syndrome
HTLV-I	human T-cell lymphotropic virus type I
HUS	haemolytic uraemic syndrome
IAH	Institute for Animal Health
IATA	International Air Transport Association
ICD	*International Classification of Diseases*
iCJD	iatrogenic Creutzfeldt–Jakob disease
IDP	internally displaced persons
INS	(US Federal) Immigration and Naturalization Service
INSERM	Institut National de la Santé et de la Recherche Médicale
IPCC	Intergovernmental Panel on Climate Change
IPD	infectious and parasitic disease
IPV	inactivated poliovirus vaccine
IQR	interquartile range
IUATLD	International Union Against TB and Lung Disease
JEV	Japanese encephalitis virus
KHF	Korean haemorrhagic fever
LCMV	lymphocytic choriomeningitis virus
LPAI	low pathogenic avian influenza
MDR	multidrug-resistant
MEI	Multivariate ENSO Index

MenV	Menangle virus
MMR	measles, mumps, and rubella
MRC	(UK) Medical Research Council
MRSA	methicillin-resistant *Staphylococcus aureus*
MSF	Médecins sans Frontières
NARMS-EB	(US) National Antimicrobial Resistance Monitoring System for Enteric Bacteria
NATO	North Atlantic Treaty Organization
NEC	not elsewhere classified
NHS	(UK) National Health Service
NIS	newly independent states of the former Soviet Union
NNDSS	(US) National Notifiable Diseases Surveillance System
NOAA	(US) National Oceanic and Atmospheric Administration
OED	*Oxford English Dictionary*
OIE	World Organization for Animal Health (Organisation Mondiale de la Santé Animale)
OLS	ordinary least squares
ONUC	United Nations Operation in the Congo
PAHO	Pan American Health Organization
PFGE	pulsed-field gel electrophoresis
PHLIS	(US) Public Health Laboratory Information System
PTSD	Post-traumatic stress disorder
PZDI	Palmer 'Z' Drought Index
RR	relative risk
RT–PCR	reverse transcription–polymerase chain reaction
RVF	Rift Valley fever
SAM	service availability mapping
SARS	severe acute respiratory syndrome
sCJD	sporadic Creutzfeldt–Jakob disease
SENIC	Study of the Efficacy of Nosocomial Infection Control
SFI	sporadic fatal insomnia
SIR	standardized incidence ratio; susceptible–infective–removed (model)
SIV	simian immunodeficiency virus
SMR	standardized mortality ratio
SRSV	small round structures virus
SR TSE	small ruminants transmissible spongiform encephalopathy
SST	sea surface temperature
STARI	southern tick-associated rash illness
STD	sexually transmitted disease
TGV	Train à Grande Vitesse (high-speed train)
TME	transmissible mink encephalopathy
TSE	transmissible spongiform encephalopathy
TTP	thrombotic thrombocytopaenic purpura
TTV	transfusion-transmitted virus
UN	United Nations
UNAIDS	Joint United Nations Programme on HIV/AIDS

UNEP	United Nations Environment Programme
UNOSOM	United Nations Operation in Somalia
UNPROFOR	United Nations Protection Force
UNTAC	United Nations Transitional Authority in Cambodia
US	United States (of America)
USDA	US Department of Agriculture
VC/NVA	Viet Cong/North Vietnamese army
vCJD	new-variant Creutzfeldt–Jakob disease
VSP	(US) Vessel Sanitation Program
WAN	World Airline Network
WHO	World Health Organization
WMO	World Meteorological Organization
XDR	extensively drug-resistant

ACKNOWLEDGEMENTS

The authors and publisher are grateful for permission to reproduce the following material:

Scuola Grande di San Rocco, Venice. Reproduced by kind permission of the Guardian Grando (Dust Jacket)

Reprinted by permission from Macmillan Publishers Ltd (Figure 1.1 and Plate 7.1)

Rowman and Littlefield (Figure 2.7)

The American Association for the Advancement of Science (Figures 4.22 and 11.18, and Plate 8.2)

World Health Organization (Figures 4.23, 6.15, 7.14 and 11.21–11.27)

Reprinted, with permission, from the *Annual Review of Entomology*, Volume 17 ©1972 by Annual Reviews (www.annualreviews.org) (Figure 4.33)

Blackwell Publishing (Figure 4.34)

American College of Physicians (Figure 5.11)

Courtesy of the New York Academy of Medicine Library (Figure 5.12)

Elsevier (Figure 7.8)

The Editors, *Microbiology Australia* (Figure 9.28)

Wellcome Library, London (Plates 2.1 and 11.13)

American Geographical Society (Plate 8.1)

Although every effort has been made to trace and contact copyright holders, this has not always been successful. We apologise for any apparent negligence.

PART I

Early Disease Emergence: Pre-1850

1

Introduction

1.1 Introduction

This book is about the geography of emerging infectious diseases. The notion of emerging diseases goes back at least 150 years. Writing in 1861, two years after Charles Darwin had published his revolutionary *On the Origin of Species by Means of Natural Selection*, the great mid-Victorian statistician at the General Register Office of England and Wales, William Farr, turned evolution onto diseases to capture the idea of emergence:

> The types of diseases have probably undergone as many changes as the human species, which according to the great hypothesis of Darwin, is itself the crowning offshoot of simpler forms . . . Yet new species are generated by the same law; they are at first varieties confounded with old types, and are only recognized as distinct species when they have existed for some time, so it is impossible to fix on the precise point of origin. Diphtheria is an example. (Farr 1861: 183)

Farr developed these remarks a decade later:

> The zymotic [infectious] diseases replace each other; and when one is rooted out it is apt to be replaced by others which ravage the human race indifferently whenever the conditions of healthy life are wanting. They have this property in common with weeds and other forms of life; as one species recedes, another advances. (Farr 1874: 224)

The idea of disease emergence flitted in and out of the scientific literature over the next century, so that Daniel Thomson writing in 1955 felt it necessary to remake the case:

> it is clear that the epidemiological pattern of this country [England and Wales] has been in a constant state of flux, and it seems likely that the prevailing infections have not always been with us, nor have they existed in their present form for so very long. The responsible pathogens have undergone evolutionary changes, and some, of little present significance, may yet enter phases of great virulence, or deadly varieties may arise from the vastly greater number of viruses and bacteria which have not yet displayed pathogenic properties... (Thomson 1955: 116)

In the last 50 years, the pace of scientific discovery of new infections has quickened to such an extent that by 1995 a monthly journal, *Emerging Infectious Diseases*, was established devoted to the theme. And so it is now widely recognized that, down the generations, apparently wholly new conditions have periodically emerged to join familiar diseases which themselves have waxed and waned in their human impact. Examples are provided by the mysterious biblical plagues of Egypt described in Chapters 7–11 of Exodus, the sudden plagues, commonly war-related, of the Greeks and Romans, medieval plagues like the Black Death in fourteenth-century Europe, and, in our own times, a spectrum of infections first recognized from the late 1960s. They include such notorious conditions as acquired immunodeficiency syndrome (AIDS) caused by the human immunodeficiency virus (HIV), Marburg and Ebola fevers, hantavirus pulmonary syndrome, Legionnaires' disease, and, more recently, severe acute respiratory syndrome (SARS). Figure 1.1A shows the geographical distribution of some of the disease events caused by these and other newly recognized agents at the beginning of the twenty-first century.

In addition to apparently new conditions, an equally important strand in the idea of disease emergence is the periodic rise, from the epidemiological background, of known infectious agents to become cyclical killers. Influenza and cholera are the type examples. There have been four global pandemics of influenza since the late nineteenth century—in 1889, 1918, 1957, and 1968—and there is currently expectation of a new pandemic, possibly based on the highly pathogenic avian influenza strain H5N1. In a similar vein, classic Asiatic cholera has swept around the globe seven times since 1832. Figure 1.1B maps the geographical location of some of these re-emergent events around the millennium.

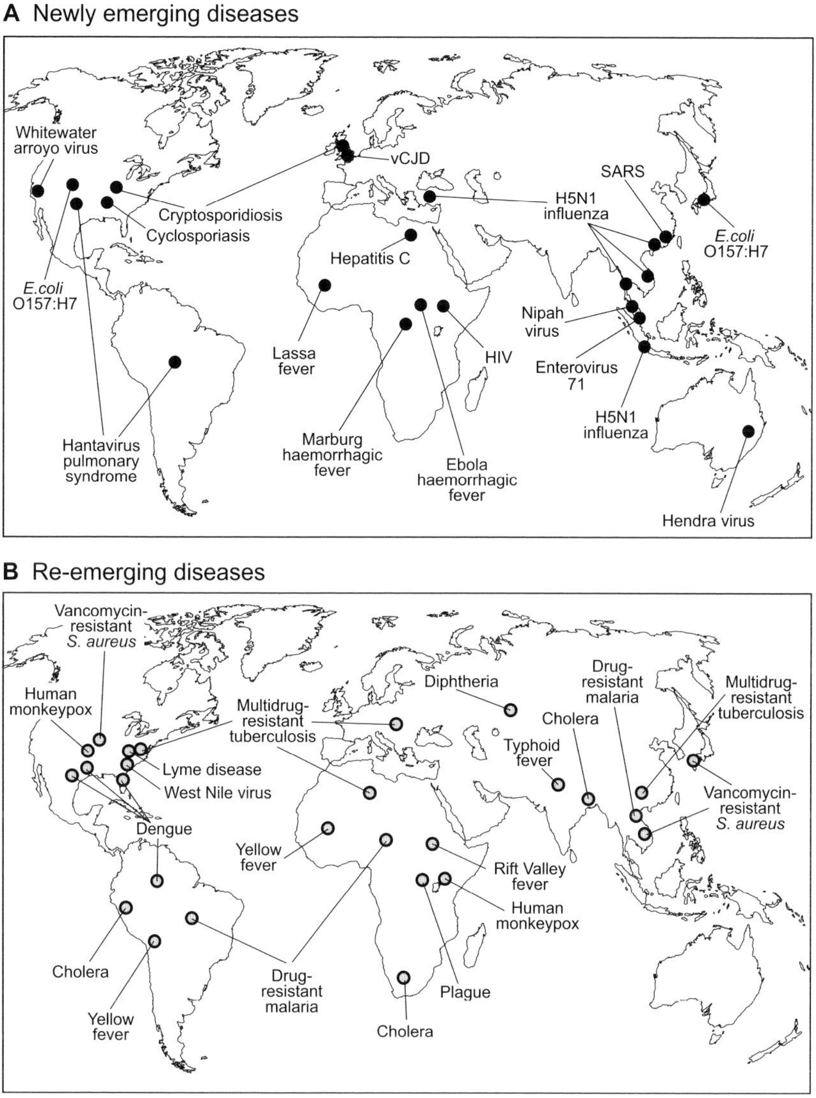

Fig. 1.1. Global distribution of sample emerging (A) and re-emerging (B) infectious diseases in the late twentieth and early twenty-first centuries

Source: Based on Morens *et al.* (2004, fig. 1, p. 243).

This book tackles the theme of disease emergence from a distinctive point of view—that of the geographer. In eleven chapters, we examine the geographical factors that underpin disease emergence and re-emergence. We conclude the book by addressing the fundamental question of how we might anticipate the emergence or re-emergence of a disease, and how emerging diseases might be controlled.

It has been with some trepidation that we have approached this subject. In selecting diseases, geographical regions, and time periods for study we have focused upon the intersection of these variables where quantitative data, capable of being analysed statistically, are available. In the time domain, this means that most of the work reported is post-1850. However, we do use some data for periods prior to the mid-nineteenth century to frame our in-depth studies. The analyses we describe are strongly spatial; we have been concerned to emphasize the locational variable both in discussing the factors underpinning disease emergence and re-emergence and in examining the dynamics by which emerging diseases have appeared in and moved from one geographical area to another. Our geographical focus has caused us to examine disease emergence at different spatial scales from the local to the global. Finally, geography has meant that we have looked at emerging diseases in different geographical environments.

1.2 Defining Emerging and Re-emerging Infections

In 1992 the US National Academy of Sciences' Institute of Medicine defined *emerging infectious diseases* as 'clinically distinct conditions whose incidence in humans has increased... Emergence may be due to the introduction of a new agent, to the recognition of an existing disease that has gone undetected, or to a change in the environment that provides an epidemiologic "bridge"' (Lederberg *et al.* 1992: 34). This definition—originally applied by Lederberg and colleagues to a two-decade period from the early 1970s—captures two important ideas, namely:

(1) Raised incidence in recent historical time or in the near future. The geographical scope—local, national, or international—of such raised incidence is not covered, nor is the temporal duration of the raised incidence.
(2) The notion of 'first time'. There are three strands to 'first time': (i) the disease is genuinely new in the population concerned, and this implies a need to articulate concepts of location, size of outbreak, and temporal duration; (ii) a disease which has been present in a population but which is newly detected because of changes or improvements in surveillance; (iii) identification through increased medical knowledge.

The National Institute of Medicine's definition is consistent with the *Oxford English Dictionary* (*OED*) definition of emergence when used in the context of diseases, i.e. (i) to become gradually visible or apparent. (ii) (of facts) become known. The *OED* goes on to define re-emergence as 'to emerge again'—as we have already noted, diseases may emerge, sink into the background, and re-emerge to significance in part of the human population at different points in time and in different geographical locations. Zinsser (1950: 301) has graphically described typhus in these terms:

> Typhus . . . will continue to break into the open whenever human stupidity and brutality give it a chance, as most likely they occasionally will. But its freedom of action is being restricted, and more and more it will be confined, like other savage creatures, in the zoological gardens of controlled diseases.

In the first issue of *Emerging Infectious Diseases*, Morse (1995: 7) recognized both the temporal and spatial dimensions to the concept of emergence in his definition of an emerging disease:

> Infectious diseases emerging throughout history have included some of the most feared plagues of the past. New infections continue to emerge today, while many of the old plagues are with us still . . . We can define as 'emerging' infections that have newly appeared in the population, or have existed but are rapidly increasing in incidence or geographic range . . .

Morse's definition does not include two features of that from the National Institute of Medicine—recognition that emergence may be a result of improved medical knowledge or surveillance.

In this book, we take a broad definition of emergence and re-emergence for infectious diseases, accepting as an emerging/re-emerging disease one which is characterized by raised incidence in time and space which can occur with: (i) an entirely new agent; (ii) a well-known agent ceasing to be a background disease for some reason; (iii) newness because of improved medical knowledge; or (iv) enhanced surveillance. As Morens *et al.* (2004: 242) note, some emerging and re-emerging diseases have been 'minor curiosities'—such as imported cases of monkeypox in the US in 2003. Others, such as SARS, had worldwide, if short-lived, impact. Yet others, such as the anthrax attacks in the US in 2001 fall within a third category—deliberately emerging diseases. On the basis of the available evidence, Morens and colleagues have proposed a threefold classification of diseases into *newly emerging*, *re-emerging and resurging*, and *deliberately emerging*, which they develop thus:

(i) *Newly emerging* diseases are 'those that have not previously been recognised in man' (Morens *et al.* 2004: 243). A large number of these are zoonotic, and their appearance in man represents dead-end transmission. Examples include the arenavirus haemorrhagic fevers (Argentine, Bolivian, Venezuelan, and Lassa fevers), hantavirus pulmonary syndrome, Nipah viral disease, and variant Creutzfeldt–Jakob Disease (vCJD). Other disease agents are environmentally persistent and may be transmitted from human to human, while, in yet other instances, old disease microbes may cause new diseases. One of the most challenging categories of newly emerging disease agents are those associated with chronic diseases and include hepatitis B and C (chronic liver damage and hepatocellular carcinoma), Epstein–Barr virus (Burkitt's lymphoma in Africa and nasopharyngeal carcinoma in China), and human herpesvirus (Kaposi's sarcoma).

(ii) *Re-emerging and resurging* diseases are 'those that have existed in the past but are now rapidly increasing in incidence or in geographical or human host range' (Morens *et al.* 2004: 245). Some of the factors associated with the emergence of new diseases have also played an important role in the process of re-emergence. Cyclical resurgences may also be climate-associated, as illustrated by the role of the El Niño–Southern Oscillation (ENSO) associated with resurgences of cholera and malaria.

(iii) *Deliberately emerging* diseases are those 'that have been developed by man, usually for nefarious use' (Morens *et al.* 2004: 247).

1.2.1 Index Medicus, *1879–2004*

A slightly different slant on the concepts of emerging and re-emerging diseases may be obtained by searching the records of *Index Medicus* to determine when and in association with which infections these terms have been used. The first issue of *Index Medicus* (Plate 1.1, left), the brainchild of Dr John Shaw Billings, a field surgeon in the Union army, appeared on 31 January 1879 with the aim of covering comprehensively the world's medical literature organized alphabetically by subject and author. The history of *Index Medicus* is outlined in Kunz (1979). With variations and now supported by electronic indexing via MEDLARS and MEDLINE, *Index Medicus* has appeared ever since to provide a priceless database to study temporal changes in disease emergence and re-emergence over the last 125 years as measured through citations.

Figure 1.2A plots the number of literature items on infectious diseases listed in *Index Medicus* which contain the word 'emerging/emergent' or 're-emerging' in their title. 'Emerging' was first used in 1961. The term appears to have passed into common usage during the 1970s and 1980s, with exponential growth in its deployment thereafter. 'Emerging' rather than variants like 'emergent' has been the dominant nomenclature, nearly always associated with 'disease' or 'virus'. The idea of re-emergence arrived much later on the scene, appearing for the first time in paper titles from 1995. Thereafter, and paralleling 'emerging', growth in use has been exponential.

Figure 1.2B plots the number of citations annually from 1949 in *Index Medicus* for several generally accepted new conditions. Consistent with Figure 1.2A, literature growth has been exponential. This contrasts

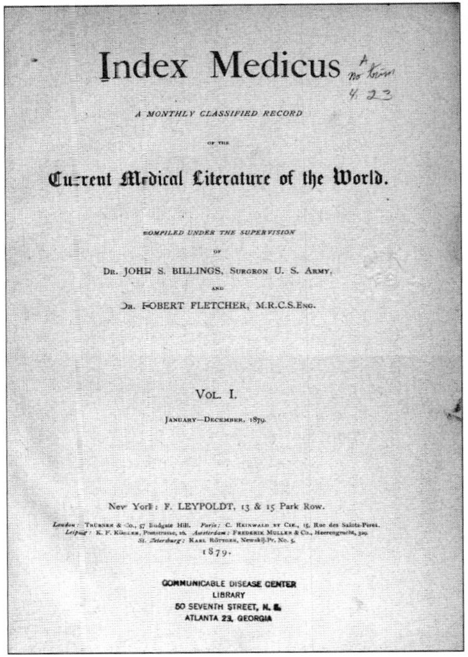

Index Medicus

A MONTHLY CLASSIFIED RECORD

OF THE

Current Medical Literature of the World.

COMPILED UNDER THE SUPERVISION

OF

DR. JOHN S. BILLINGS, SURGEON U. S. ARMY,

AND

DR. ROBERT FLETCHER, M.R.C.S.ENG.

VOL. I.

JANUARY—DECEMBER, 1879.

New York: F. LEYPOLDT, 13 & 15 Park Row.

1879.

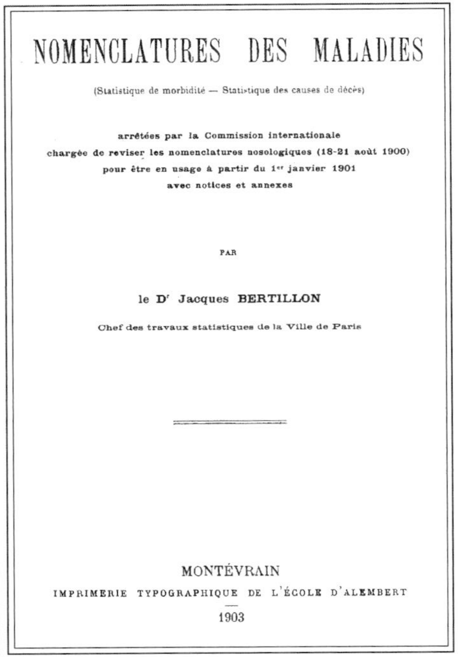

NOMENCLATURES DES MALADIES

(Statistique de morbidité — Statistique des causes de décès)

arrêtées par la Commission internationale
chargée de reviser les nomenclatures nosologiques (18-21 août 1900)
pour être en usage à partir du 1er janvier 1901
avec notices et annexes

PAR

le Dr Jacques BERTILLON

Chef des travaux statistiques de la Ville de Paris

MONTÉVRAIN
IMPRIMERIE TYPOGRAPHIQUE DE L'ÉCOLE D'ALEMBERT
1903

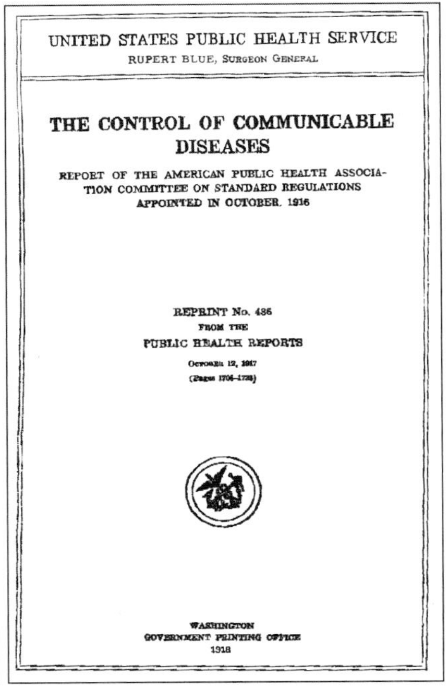

UNITED STATES PUBLIC HEALTH SERVICE
RUPERT BLUE, SURGEON GENERAL

THE CONTROL OF COMMUNICABLE DISEASES

REPORT OF THE AMERICAN PUBLIC HEALTH ASSOCIATION COMMITTEE ON STANDARD REGULATIONS APPOINTED IN OCTOBER, 1916

REPRINT No. 436
FROM THE
PUBLIC HEALTH REPORTS
OCTOBER 12, 1917
(Pages 1706–1728)

WASHINGTON
GOVERNMENT PRINTING OFFICE
1918

Pl. 1.1. Title pages from the first issues of (left) *Index Medicus*, (centre) *International Classification of Diseases*, and (right) *Control of Communicable Diseases Manual*

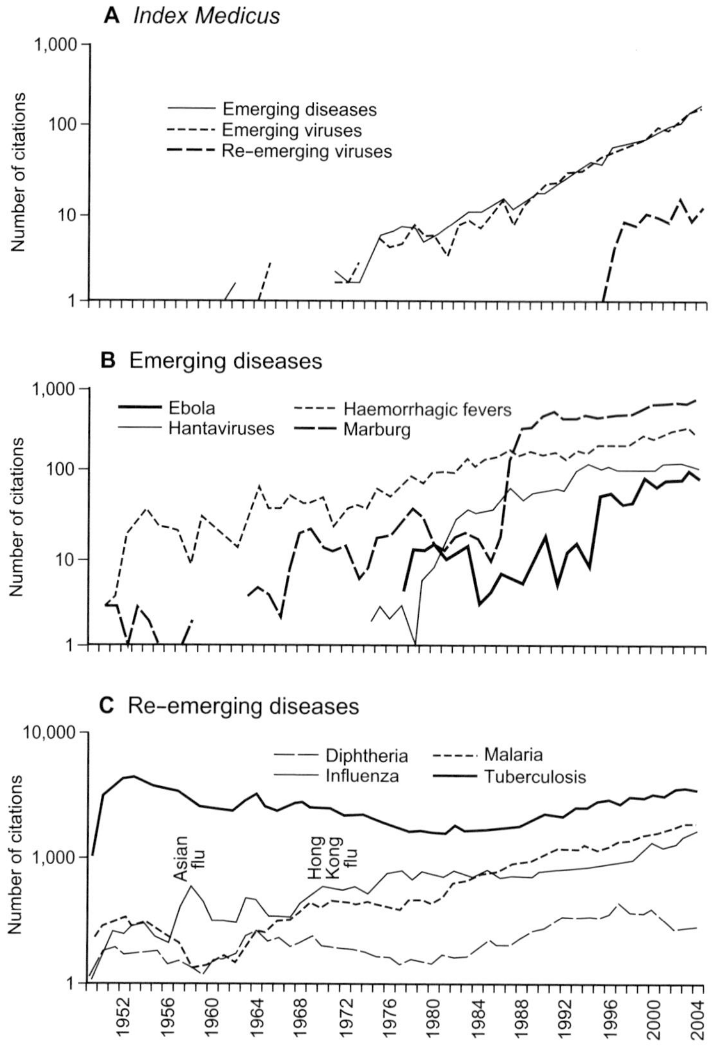

Fig. 1.2. *Index Medicus*: post-1949 time trends in 'emerging' and 're-emerging' infectious diseases.
(A) Annual use of 'emerging' and 're-emerging' as adjectives in article titles. (B) Annual citations in titles for four newly emergent diseases. (C) Annual citations in titles for four re-emerging diseases. All vertical axes are on logarithmic scales.

with the citation curves for re-emerging diseases, four of which (diphtheria, influenza, malaria, and tuberculosis) are plotted in Figure 1.2C. With these diseases, citation counts enable the regeneration of additional scientific interest caused by re-emergence to be tracked. For influenza, the literature spurts associated with the Asian (1957) and Hong Kong (1968–9) global pandemics are evident. With tuberculosis, interest waned as the disease yielded to new antibiotic treatments after World War II, only to start rising steadily from the mid-1980s as multidrug-resistant strains began to facilitate re-emergence of the disease, often in association with immunosuppression related to HIV infection. A parallel story can be told for diphtheria, while malaria's re-emergence can be tracked from the abandonment of the use of DDT for vector control from the 1970s.

It is with these various working concepts of 'emerging' and 're-emerging' in mind that we now turn in Sections 1.3–1.5 to consider models to explain disease emergence and re-emergence, beginning with the origins of human diseases.

1.3 The Origins of Human Diseases

1.3.1 Disease Agents: Equilibrium and Non-Equilibrium Paradigms

THE EQUILIBRIUM PARADIGM

Burnet's (1945) work on the virus as an organism provides a basis for understanding why infectious diseases emerge, retreat, and re-emerge. Continuous survival is ensured if the pathogen moves from one host to the next. A simple deterministic model is to assume that, for the pathogen to be successful, death of the host has to occur, while success for the patient is recovery from the illness induced by the pathogen and annihilation of the pathogen. But this naive explanation becomes untenable if we recognize that the parasite is a living organism that strives for continuous survival. Then, 'An acutely fatal infection is... disadvantageous for the survival of the parasite' (Burnet 1945: 26). Rather, a successful pathogen can be viewed as one that infects a host then maximizes the number of secondary cases arising from that host. This may require a balance between curtailing symptoms (so that the host remains alive and able to spread onward infections) and inducing symptoms that are associated with infectiousness. See the discussion in Burnet and White (1972) and Weiss (2001). Thus, the development of a more or less balanced interaction between the host and parasite appears to require the following:

(i) prolonged association;
(ii) opportunity for infection to involve a high proportion of the individuals of the host species; and,
(iii) no important means by which the pathogen can survive indefinitely in the absence of the host.

THE NON-EQUILIBRIUM PARADIGM

As Burnet (1945) notes, however, equilibrium is rarely found and a state of flux is the usual condition. Thus, contemporary ecological paradigms accept that natural systems are open, that episodic events are of great importance to the structure and functioning of ecosystems, and that process, as opposed to outcome, should be emphasized. Within epidemiology, oscillations in relationships are usually found even with a parasite in equilibrium with a host (for example, periods of epidemic prevalence occurring every few years). If we can accept that disturbance of equilibrium is a natural part of the cycle, then the emergence, re-emergence, and retreat of infectious diseases over time can be more readily understood.

DISTURBANCE AND REGENERATION

Once an equilibrium relationship between the host and the micro-organism has become established, it is unlikely to be disturbed unless an alteration occurs in the equation—to the host, to the micro-organism, or to both. These alterations may be triggered by external factors (for example, environmental triggers) but, if they result in a comparative advantage to either the host or the organism, the relationship between the two is likely to revert to an earlier stage of the trail to equilibrium—with, for example, failure of the pathogen to infect numerous hosts, perhaps due to some newly developed drugs or a vaccine, or, alternatively, fatal infections of the host caused by a shift in the strain of the micro-organism involved to which the host has no immunity.

The equilibrium relationship between the micro-organism and the host is effective only for the circumstances under which the equilibrium evolved. Any departure from this particular state is likely to disturb the equilibrium, usually resulting in high numbers of infections. As Corwin (1949: 35) has summarized: 'While on the one hand epidemic or epizootic diseases result from ecological imbalance in any of the triad—agent, host or environment—endemic or enzootic diseases often represent a climax or balanced state.' The possible cycle of emerging and re-emerging diseases is illustrated with reference to viral agents in Figure 1.3.

1.3.2 The 'Domestic-Origins Hypothesis': The McKeown Model

As Weiss (2001) observes, there are two possible origins of human microbial pathogens:

(1) co-evolution with human emergence from primate ancestors;
(2) the crossover of pathogens from animals to humans.

Co-evolving microbes typically exert a low mortality upon their hosts. Examples include members of the herpesvirus family, in which individual viruses in humans are genetically similar to those of host species that are

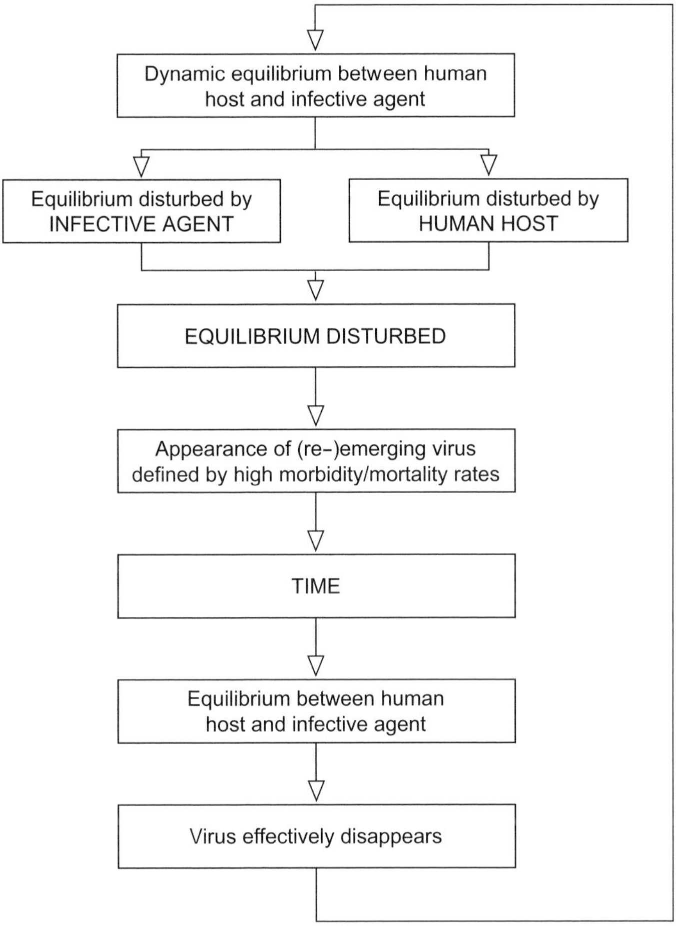

Fig. 1.3. Schematic diagram of infectious disease emergence and re-emergence in human populations

closest to us in evolution. Most human infections have, however, originated with an animal source and crossed the species to humans. Early examples of human infectious diseases of animal origins, with estimated dates of cross-over events, are provided in Table 1.1.

Animal-to-human infections can be categorized according to the pattern of infection. These are:

(i) *Animals as reservoirs; occasional human infection.* This category relates to zoonoses that may accidentally and sporadically arise in humans as a result of environmental contamination or as a consequence of direct contact with animals. Recent examples include Nipah viral disease, hantavirus pulmonary syndrome, and avian influenza A (H5N1).

Table 1.1. Examples of human infectious diseases of animal origin

Disease	Microbe	Animal source	Date of cross-over
Malaria	Protozoan	Non-human primate	*c.*8000 BC
Measles	Virus	Sheep, goat, or dog	*c.*6000 BC
Smallpox	Virus	Ruminant?	before 2000 BC
Tuberculosis	Mycobacterium	Ruminant?	before 1000 BC
Plague	Bacterium	Rodent	AD 541, AD 1347, AD 1665
Dengue	Virus	Non-human primate	*c.*AD 1000
Yellow fever	Virus	Non-human primate	AD 1641
Spanish influenza	Virus	Bird, pig	AD 1918
AIDS/HIV	Virus	Non-human primate	*c.*AD 1950

Source: Based on Weiss (2001, table 3, p. 962).

(ii) *Animal origin of human-to-human infections.* Much rarer than (i) are diseases which arise when a pathogen becomes adapted to humans and becomes epidemic or endemic. Examples include fully transmissible strains of influenza A, measles, and HIV.

(iii) *Animals as vectors.* This category relates to disease agents in which animals, usually an arthropod, cause transmission to humans. Examples include malaria, yellow fever, and dengue fever.

There has been a continuous exchange of infective organisms between man and other animals, with the outcome of the exchange being determined by climatic, social, and other conditions. Contact with animals increased under agriculture, both with domestic animals (for example, cattle, sheep, goats, pigs, and horses) and with intruders attracted to human settlements (for example, rats, mice, ticks, fleas, and mosquitoes). Owing to the species-specific nature of these infections, many of the pathogens to which humans were exposed did not result in infection. Occasionally, however, one would gain a foothold. Then, successful transmission between people would set the stage for the establishment of a human pathogen. For example, measles virus may have emerged from an infection of dogs (distemper) or ruminants (rinderpest), while the rhinoviruses which cause the common cold may have been derived from horses. It is possible that the human form of the tubercle bacillus derived from the bovine form, while the water buffalo may have been the original source of leprosy, the cow of diphtheria, and the monkey of syphilis. Plague may have arisen as an inapparent infection of gerbils in eastern Asia.

McKeown (1988) has argued that it was the growth of cities made possible by settled agriculture which was the primary early engine of the exchange of infections between animals and man. Early man was exposed to infectious diseases (especially zoonoses), but living in small groups, the disease agents could not be sustained by the susceptible population. Thus, in the early phase of human existence, from the Pleistocene up to about 8000 BC, infectious diseases due to micro-organisms that were specifically adapted to the human species—including the great herd diseases of the historical period—were non-existent. There were a few exceptions among the viral diseases (herpes simplex and chickenpox) and bacterial and protozoal diseases (tuberculosis, leprosy, and treponematosis), all of which are characterized by latency and recurrence.[1] The situation changed when humans began to live in large groups. The phase shift in community size began about 6,000 years ago, when large cities began to appear with the first great civilizations. This development was itself dependent upon improved farming techniques, especially irrigation. As McKeown (1988: 51) notes, 'Remarkably, we owe the origin of most serious infectious diseases to the conditions which led to our cultural heritage, the city states made possible by the planting of crops in the flood plains of Mesopotamia, Egypt and the Indus Valley.'

The massing of large populations served to facilitate the spread of airborne and other infections, while the hygienic conditions that followed the introduction of agriculture made it possible for new diseases to appear and existing diseases to become more serious. Hygienic conditions began to be important—especially those associated with the handling of food and water and the disposing of excreta and waste. Cholera, McKeown notes, emerged when villages and village water supplies were established, while malaria became serious when the size of human populations and the opportunities for breeding of vectors increased with advances in agriculture. Tuberculosis emerged as an important disease with the development of large cities, and its concomitant crowding, facilitating airborne spread, while intestinal infections (typhoid, dysentery, salmonella) resulted from the contamination of food and water.

McKeown (1988) notes that a further influence on infections (insufficient food) has proved the most controversial. It is evident that the state of health of an individual has a considerable bearing upon response to infection. The state of health of an individual is, in turn, closely linked to nutritional status. Measles provides the classic example, where infection and malnutrition enter into a synergistic relationship, resulting in severe disease. Notwithstanding the incomplete nature of the evidence (see, for example, Pearce-Duvet 2006), there is little doubt that, in the past, malnutrition and infectious diseases were frequently associated.

1.3.3 Palaeopathology and Infectious Disease Emergence

Palaeopathology is the study of ancient diseases of man and animals as inferred from skeletal and fossilized remains. Živanović (1982) notes that,

[1] The implied date of before 8000 BC for the emergence of tuberculosis as a human-adapted disease is consistent with the dates given by other authors, including before 1000 BC (Table 1.1) and <20,000 years ago (Table 1.3).

since the beginning of the twentieth century, palaeopathologists have studied more than 8,000 mummies in various locations around the world. The investigators have described a long series of diseases in these mummies, covering virtually every modern medical and surgical speciality. Traces of infectious diseases have been found, including scars resulting from smallpox, skin infections, and specific diseases such as tuberculosis and leprosy. Parasites, including lice and their nits, have also been found. However, as Wells (1964) notes, most of the specific infections that have spread in epidemic form over the past 3,000 years leave no imprint on bones, thereby ensuring the obscure history of these conditions.

Oxenham *et al.* (2004) have studied skeletal remains from northern Vietnam to determine the role of the transition from sedentary, foraging, coastally orientated economies to centralized chiefdoms (with attendant development and intensification of agriculture, trade, metal technologies, warfare, and population) in the emergence and increase in infectious diseases. Skeletal samples were dated to 6,000–*c.*1,700 years before present (BP). While skeletal evidence for infectious diseases was absent from the mid-Holocene period (6,000–5,000 years BP), more than 10 per cent of samples from the metal period (3,300–1,700 years BP) yielded evidence of lesions consistent with either infectious diseases or immune system disorders. Oxenham *et al.* suggest that a series of factors in the metal period may have contributed to the emergence of infectious diseases, including: (i) increased contact with bacterial or fungal pathogens, either directly or by way of vertebrate and/or arthropod vectors; (ii) higher levels of debilitation and decreased levels of immunocompetence; (iii) the development of increased virulence of pathogens that had already been present in the mid-Holocene period. Factors (i) and (ii) may be related to historically and archaeologically documented demographic (Han colonizing efforts) and economic (agricultural intensification) events in the region during the metal period.

More generally, Oxenham *et al.* (2004) note that numerous palaeopathological studies have presented evidence for an increase in the frequency of infectious diseases with changes in settlement patterns and the subsistence economy. There is evidence for such a phenomenon in eastern Europe, South Asia, Japan, Australia, and North, Central, and South America.

MOLECULAR PALAEOPATHOLOGY: PALAEOMICROBIOLOGY AND PALAEOVIROLOGY

As Zink, Reischl, *et al.* (2002) observe, the detection of ancient microbial DNA from skeletal and mummified tissue offers a new approach for the study of infectious disease agents in historic times. Beginning in the 1990s, the approach has resulted in the detection of a variety of bacterial, protozoal, and viral agents in ancient tissues. The earliest studies were undertaken on a Pre-Colombian South American mummy (*c.*AD 1000) and an Egyptian

Table 1.2. Sample infectious disease agents detected by molecular analysis of ancient human specimens

Disease agent	Human specimen			References
	Type	Location	Approximate date	
Trypanosoma cruzi	Mummified remains	Northern Chile & southern Peru	7050–3000 BC	Aufderheide *et al.* (2004)
Trypanosoma cruzi	Mummified remains	Northern Chile	2000 BC	Guhl *et al.* (1999)
Mycobacterium tuberculosis	Mummified body	Egypt	1550–1080 BC	Nerlich *et al.* (1997)
Corynebacterium spp.	Mummified head	Egypt	1550–1080 BC	Zink *et al.* (2001)
Eschericha coli	Bog body	North-west England	300 BC (2 BC–AD 119?)	Fricker *et al.* (1997)
HTLV-I	Mummified remains	Northern Chile	AD 500	Li *et al.* (1999)
Mycobacterium leprae	Bone sample	Bethany, Jordan	AD 600	Rafi *et al.* (1994)
Mycobacterium leprae	Skeletal remains	Hungary	10th century AD	Haas *et al.* (2000)
Mycobacterium tuberculosis	Mummified body	Southern Peru	AD 1000–1300	Salo *et al.* (1994)
Mycobacterium leprae	Skeletal remains	Seville, Spain	12th century AD	Montiel *et al.* (2003)
Human papillomavirus 18	Mummified body	Naples, Italy	AD 1503–68	Fornaciari *et al.* (2003)
Yersinia pestis	Skeletal remains of plague victims	France	AD 1590 & 1722	Drancourt *et al.* (1998)
Treponema pallidum	Skeletal specimen	Easter Island	AD 1760	Kolman *et al.* (1999)
Spanish influenza A	Tissues from influenza victims	US	AD 1918	Reid *et al.* (1999); Tumpey *et al.* (2005)

Table 1.3. Estimated time of emergence of some human pathogens

Pathogen	Estimated number of years since first major emergence
HIV-1	~70
Japanese encephalitis virus	~130
Mycobacterium tuberculosis	<20,000
Plasmodium falciparum	<50,000

Source: Conway and Roper (2000, table 2, p. 1426).

mummy from the New Kingdom (1550–1080 BC), both of which yielded evidence of infection with *Mycobacterium tuberculosis* (Salo *et al.* 1994; Nerlich *et al.* 1997). Subsequent studies have yielded evidence *of Mycobacterium leprae, Yersinia pestis, Plasmodium falciparum, Trypanosoma cruzi, Treponema pallidum, Escherichia coli,* and *Corynebacterium* spp. (Table 1.2).

Table 1.3 provides estimated times since the emergence of some major human pathogens in human hosts. The estimates are much shorter, and more precise, for viral than bacterial agents.

1.4 The Historical Record of (Re-)emerging Diseases

1.4.1 The Epidemiological Transition

Studies of the emergence, disappearance, and reappearance of infectious diseases often refer to the epidemiological transition. The basic principles of the transition and its relationship with the demographic transition are well known and have been outlined by authors such as Omran (1971, 1977), Caldwell (1982), and Phillips (1994). The epidemiological transition involves a one-way movement through a sequence of three stages. These start with an 'Age of Pestilence and Famine' (stage 1, persisting until the later eighteenth century in the developed world), through an 'Age of Receding Pandemics' (stage 2, nineteenth century through to the last quarter of the twentieth), to an 'Age of Degenerative and Man-Made Diseases' (stage 3, beginning in the last quarter of the twentieth century). Further changes in the mortality profile have been associated with a proposed fourth stage of the transition, in which the length of life expectancy increases (as the major killer diseases of earlier stages are better treated or detected)—but in which health status may deteriorate as the causes of chronic, non-fatal morbidity remain undefeated (Verbrugge 1984; Riley 1989; Riley and Alter 1989). An increasing incidence of mental disorders seems also to be characteristic of this fourth stage. Olshansky and Ault (1986) have called this the 'Age of Delayed Degenerative

Diseases'. The major degenerative causes of death that prevailed during stage 3 of the transition remain as major killers, but with relatively rapid improvements in survival concentrated among the older population. This stage is evident in a number of developed countries and in some middle- and higher-income newly industrializing countries, particularly in South-East and East Asia (Leete 1985).

An alternative fourth stage extension of Omran's model, the so-called 'Hybristic Stage', has been developed by Rogers and Hackenberg (1989). This model addresses factors of potential demographic importance which were not included in the original three-stage model including: an interplay between infectious and parasitic diseases, resulting in an increase in infectious and parasitic diseases with the rising prevalence of chronic diseases in an ageing population; the role of social pathologies (unintentional injuries, homicide, and suicide), especially among younger populations; individual behaviours in the timing of the expression of ageing-related mortality, including factors affecting longevity; and the negative effects of longevity upon economics and public policy.

1.4.2 The Fifth Stage of Epidemiological Transition: Re-emerging Infectious and Parasitic Diseases

So spectacular were the falls in mortality from infectious diseases during the first 75 years of the twentieth century that, in the developed world at least, plagues and epidemics began to be viewed as essentially historical phenomena, scourges that had devastated past human populations, but which had been largely eliminated with advances in medical knowledge and the advent of vaccines and antibiotics (Cairns 1975). However, epidemiological developments relating to infectious diseases since 1975 have thrown a radically new perspective upon this view and suggest that the countries of the developed world may now be on the brink of a unique phase in their epidemiological history (Olshansky *et al.* 1997). This new phase, which we tentatively refer to as the 'Age of Emergent and Re-emergent Infections', is associated with the resurgence of infectious and parasitic diseases (IPDs), both old and 'new', as a serious public health concern in developed countries. Olshansky *et al.* (1998: 213) have argued that the human immunodeficiency virus/acquired immunodeficiency syndrome (HIV/AIDS) in particular has 'created a dramatic and unprecedented impact on the rise and spread of IPDs'. HIV not only contributes directly to the IPD burden, but also, by weakening the immune system of HIV-infected patients, increases the likelihood of opportunistic infections by other IPDs. The spread of multidrug-resistant tuberculosis is an example of this development. This trend has prompted Olshansky and colleagues (1997: 12) to suggest that 'the unique attributes of this "new" trend in infectious disease mortality qualify it as a distinct stage in our epidemiologic history'. They observe (p. 213):

The re-emergence of IPDs during the last quarter of the 20th century is associated with demographic features that distinguish it from the Fourth or Hybristic stage of epidemiologic transition. A unique set of demographic and health circumstances in low mortality populations has contributed to a significant rise in IPDs, and to a pronounced shift toward older ages in the age groups of the population that are most affected by re-emergence. The uniqueness of the demographic features has led some researchers to hypothesize that some population subgroups have entered a Fifth stage of the epidemiologic transition—*The Re-emergence of Infectious and Parasitic Diseases* stage.

Support is added to this argument when we note the following:

(i) *The increased use of immunosuppressive agents*. Advances in medical treatment have resulted in increasing numbers of immunosuppressed patients (including those undergoing organ transplantation and cancer chemotherapy). Such patients may be at increased risk of infection with micro-organisms that are not usually associated with serious disease in healthy individuals. Many patients receiving chemotherapy or immunosuppressive drugs may also be treated with antimicrobial drugs, which, in turn, may have a pronounced effect on the bacterial flora of the intestinal tract. Such disturbances may predispose to colonization and infection with other micro-organisms, some of which may display increased virulence.

(ii) *Population ageing* also contributes to the re-emerging IPD burden. The population of many developed countries is rapidly ageing, with the elderly comprising 20–25 per cent of the total population. This represents a new and dramatic shift in the age structure of human populations. In addition to ageing-related diseases, the ageing population has weakening immune systems, rendering them particularly vulnerable to respiratory tract infections like pneumonia and influenza, and to intestinal infections such as salmonellosis (salmonella infections in the elderly are more likely to cause bacteraemia), and *Campylobacter* diarrhoea. The growth of the elderly population ensures that the number of immunologically compromised individuals will continue to grow. Population ageing also has a societal consequence that will contribute to the rise and spread of IPDs. As the population gets older, so the number living in elderly care homes increases and the dense population structure may enhance the possibility of transmission of IPDs. In such a population with fragile or compromised immune systems, acquired and nosocomial infections are frequently virulent, and they then occasionally escape into the general population.

(iii) *Malnutrition*. On a global scale, the leading cause of increased susceptibility to infection is malnutrition. The problems are accentuated in developing countries, especially in areas of famine and political unrest (Morris and Potter 1997).

A further feature of the fifth stage of epidemiologic transition is that 'new' diseases have emerged as a result of human action. Although not technically new, drug-resistant strains of bacteria and other micro-organisms that cause familiar diseases (for example, malaria, meningitis, pneumonia, and tuberculosis) have begun to appear.

Taking all these developments together, Olshansky *et al.* (1998: 214) summarize the position as follows:

> Large increases in the absolute size of the immunocompromised population resulting from global population ageing, a rise in the number of people living in nursing homes, and in prisons, medical treatments for cancer, and a growing number of people infected with HIV have together created an entirely new set of conditions that contribute to the rise of IPDs, and a shift in their age distribution to older ages. Other forces influencing today's unique characteristics of IPDs are permanent changes in the human age structure, forces that will have lasting and profound effects on future trends in IPDs.... All these forces combined represent a strong argument according to which the recent emergence of IPDs is a distinctly novel development in the history of human mortality. There are enough new attributes of this period of rising IPDs for it to be considered a Fifth stage in the epidemiologic transition. As is the case with Omran's original three-stage model, it is anticipated that the Fifth stage of the epidemiologic transition will occur at varying speeds, and for somewhat different reasons depending on the country.

OR THE RE-EMERGENCE OF THE FIRST STAGE OF EPIDEMIOLOGICAL TRANSITION?

As an alternative to seeing the current era as a fifth stage of epidemiological transition, Olshansky *et al.* (1998) suggest that the situation may be viewed as neither new nor novel, but rather as the continuation of a mortality pattern that was initially used to define the first stage of the transition. In support of this view, they note that, despite billions of people benefiting from modern developments in medicine, IPDs are still the leading killer globally. Much of the issue comes down to temporal scale. The vast majority of human history falls within the first stage of the transition—a volatile stage of mortality characterized by peaks and troughs. For those living in a trough that persists for several generations, it may appear that a new mortality pattern has emerged. Present developments may be nothing more than a temporal trend of favourable mortality. This is especially so when we view the long-term success of disease-causing micro-organisms:

> Academic scholars can identify stages of epidemiologic transition, but for infectious micro-organisms, the ebb and flow of their ecological and evolutionary success simply unfold. Trends toward emergence, re-emergence, or disappearance of IPDs are real short-term trends, but have little significance for the ongoing interactions between human beings and the microbes that cause human disease. (Olshansky *et al.* 1998: 215)

MODELS OF GLOBAL FUTURES, HEALTH SCENARIOS, AND THE FIFTH STAGE OF EPIDEMIOLOGICAL TRANSITION

Beginning from a platform of the original three stages of epidemiological transition, Martens and Huynen (2003) identify three stages beyond the age of chronic and degenerative diseases, namely: the age of emerging infectious diseases, the age of medical technology, and the age of sustained health. Integrating these possible health stages with current scenarios of global futures, Martens and Huynen suggest that, where a strong economic orientation prevails, health developments in developing counties will advance towards the 'age of emerging infectious diseases', while the developed world will advance to the age of 'medical technology' (comparable to the 'age of delayed degenerative diseases'). Conversely, scenarios that emphasize international cooperation (with a strong focus on meeting social and environmental sustainability goals) will be characterized by the advancement of developing and developed countries to an 'age of sustained health' (where investments in social services will lead to a sharp reduction in lifestyle-related diseases, and most environmentally related diseases will be eradicated).

1.5 Correlates of Disease Emergence

1.5.1 Emerging Diseases and the Zoonotic–Anthroponotic Spectrum

Morse (1995) has characterized the emergence of an infectious disease as a two-step process:

(i) introduction of the agent into a new host population;
(ii) establishment and further dissemination within the new host population.

The infection can be said to 'emerge' when it reaches the new population. Factors that promote steps (i) and (ii) can be viewed as precipitating the emergence process. Morse (1995: 9) comments:

> Most emerging infections appear to be caused by pathogens already present in the environment, brought out of obscurity or given a selective advantage by changing conditions and afforded an opportunity to infect new host populations... The process by which infectious agents may transfer from animals to humans or disseminate from isolated groups into new populations can be called 'microbial traffic'. A number of activities increase microbial traffic and as a result promote emergence and epidemics. In some cases, including many of the most novel infections, the agents are zoonotic, crossing from their natural hosts into the human population... In other cases, pathogens already present in geographically isolated populations are given an opportunity to disseminate further.

As McMichael (2004: 1051) observes, the first event in the emergence process for a new disease is novel physical contact between a potential pathogen and the human species. The contact may arise naturally, but, more commonly, it occurs as a consequence of social, cultural, behavioural, or technological change. Subsequent spread of the new disease will then depend on a series of environmental and social factors such as demographic characteristics, human mobility, land use, and consumption behaviours.

CATEGORIES OF EMERGING PATHOGEN

In a major survey, Taylor *et al.* (2001) identified a total of 1,415 species of human disease-causing pathogens. The distribution of these species by taxonomic division (viruses and prions, bacteria and rickettsiae, fungi, protozoa, and helminths) is shown in Figure 1.4A. The majority are bacteria (38 per cent), fungi (22 per cent), and helminths (20 per cent), with viruses (15 per cent) and protozoa (5 per cent) representing the balance. Of the 1,415 species, a review of the available evidence by Taylor and colleagues identified 175 as 'emerging' (Figure 1.4B), the majority of which are viruses and prions (44 per cent) and bacteria and rickettsiae (30 per cent). Some three-quarters of the emerging pathogens are zoonotic, with zoonotic viruses and prions, and bacteria and rickettsiae, representing 76 per cent of the subset (Figure 1.4C).

Relative Risk (RR) for Emergence

All pathogens. Figure 1.5A is based on the analysis of Taylor *et al.* (2001) and shows the relative risk (RR) for emergence of all pathogens. Here, RR is formed as the ratio of (1) the proportion of species in a given category which are emerging to (2) the proportion of species which are emerging and which are not in that category. Thus, a value of $RR > 1.00$ denotes a category that is over-represented among emerging species. For all pathogens, inspection of Figure 1.5A indicates that zoonotic diseases ($RR = 1.93$), viruses ($RR = 4.33$), protozoa ($RR = 2.49$), and diseases transmitted by direct contact ($RR = 1.47$) and by vectors ($RR = 2.35$) are over-represented among the emerging species.

Zoonotic pathogens. Recognizing that zoonotic pathogens are substantially over-represented among emerging species, Figure 1.5B shows the RR for categories of zoonotic species. For a given category, RR has been computed as the ratio of (1) the proportion of species emerging among zoonotic pathogens to (2) the proportion of species emerging among the non-zoonotic pathogens. The figure indicates that bacteria ($RR = 3.79$), fungi ($RR = 7.14$), and diseases transmitted by direct ($RR = 2.13$) and indirect ($RR = 2.60$) contact are over-represented among the zoonotic species.

The results suggest strong zoonotic status in the identification of risk factors for pathogen emergence. Although evidence is fragmentary, preliminary studies by Taylor and colleagues on a sample of diseases suggest a further risk factor for emergence: human-to-human transmissibility ($RR = 2.60$). As Taylor *et al.*

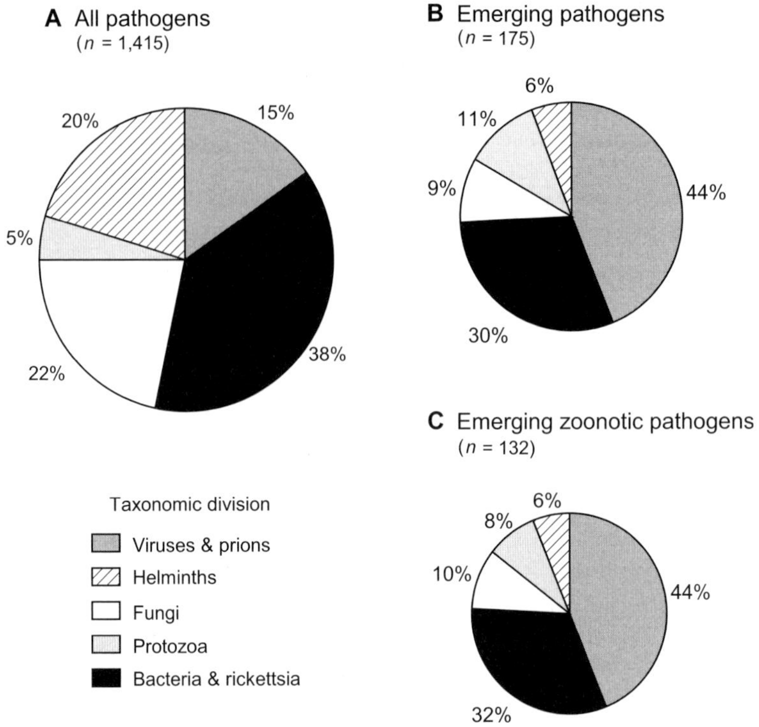

Fig. 1.4. Human disease-causing pathogens.
(A) Distribution of all pathogens by taxonomic division. (B) Distribution of emerging pathogens by taxonomic division. (C) Distribution of emerging zoonotic pathogens by taxonomic division.
Source: Based on Taylor *et al.* (2001).

(2001: 987) observe: 'The most important finding . . . is that emerging pathogens are not a random selection of all pathogens. The next challenge is to explain why some kinds of pathogen—such as zoonotic viruses and protozoa transmitted by indirect contact . . . —are likely to emerge while others are not.' Taylor's findings are also consistent with the view that diseases transmitted from animals to man (zoonoses), and those transmitted from one vertebrate to another by an arthropod (vector-borne diseases), rank among the most important of the newly emerging infectious diseases (Morens *et al.* 2004). An important related question is how a pathogen changes its position in the zoonotic–anthroponotic spectrum. Conway and Roper (2000) note the operation of two elements in this process: (i) pathogen adaptation to hosts; and (ii) extrinsic ecological changes in host populations.

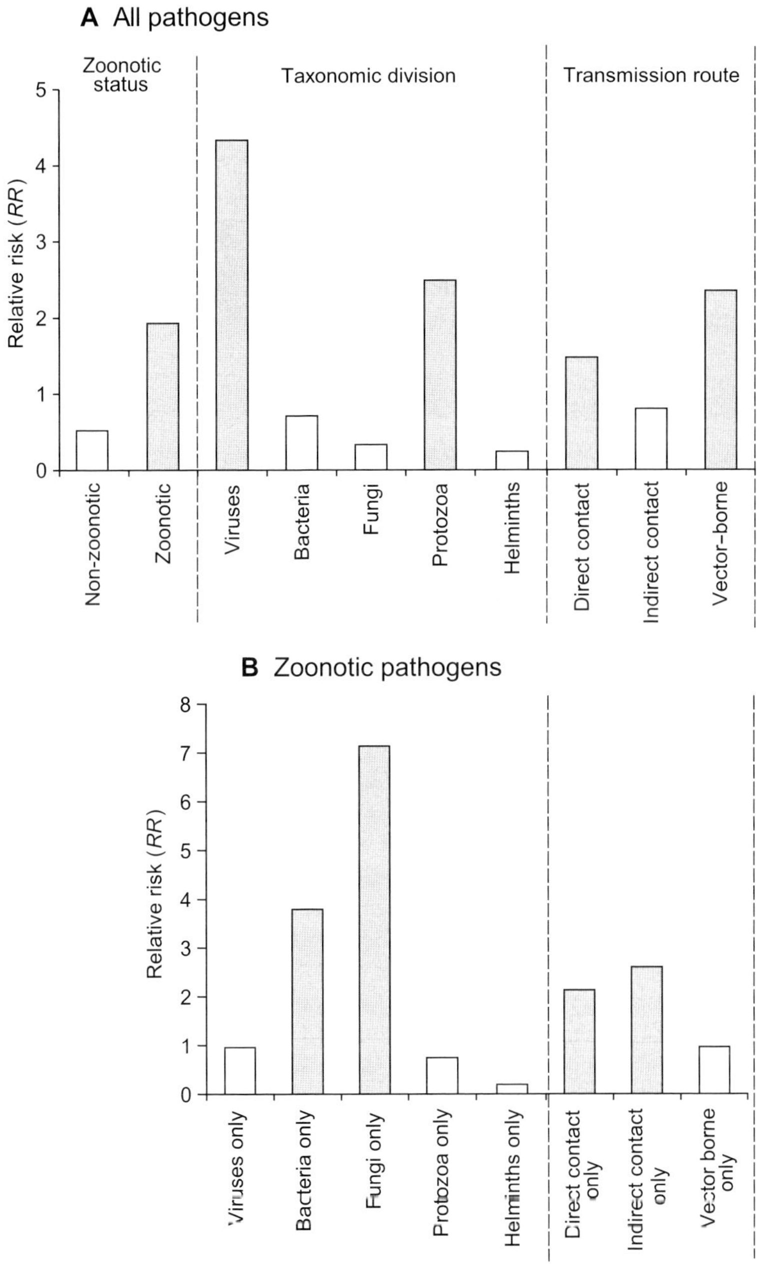

Fig. 1.5. Relative risk (*RR*) for emergence of human disease-causing pathogens. (A) All pathogens. (B) Zoonotic pathogens.

Source: Data from Taylor *et al.* (2001, table 1, p. 985).

1.5.2 Enabling Factors in Disease (Re-)emergence

Specific factors that have facilitated the emergence and re-emergence of infectious diseases in recent times are reviewed by Lederberg *et al.* (1992), Morse (1995), and Krause (1998). As Table 1.4 shows, 'emergence factors' encompass a complex of social, physical, and biological mechanisms, including human demographics and behaviour, technology and industry, economic development and land use change, international travel and commerce, microbial adaptation and change, and the breakdown of public health measures. These various factors operate at different stages of the emergence/re-emergence process (Figure 1.6), with several factors often working in combination or sequence to precipitate the (re)appearance of a disease agent in the human population (Table 1.4).

Adopting the categories developed by the Institute of Medicine report *Emerging Infections: Microbial Threats to Health in the United States* (Lederberg *et al.* 1992), with additional definitions from the US Centers for Disease Control and Prevention's (CDC's) emerging infections plan *Addressing Emerging Disease Threats: A Prevention Strategy for the United States* (Centers for Disease Control 1994*e*, 1998*d*), Morse (1995) has identified six factors that have contributed to the processes of disease emergence. With examples of the consequential disease developments, these are:

(1) *Ecological changes*, including those due to economic development and land use. These can precipitate the emergence of infectious diseases by placing people in contact with a natural reservoir or host of an unfamiliar (to humans) but already present infection. This contact may arise by increasing proximity or by changing conditions so that an increased microbe population results. Examples include schistosomiasis (dams), Rift Valley fever (dams, irrigation), Argentine haemorrhagic fever (agriculture), Korean haemorrhagic fever (agriculture), Lyme disease (deforestation/reforestation), and hantavirus pulmonary syndrome (weather anomalies in the US, 1993).

(2) *Human demographics and behaviour*, including societal events, population growth, migration, war and civil conflict, urban decay, sexual behaviour, and drug use. Example consequences include the introduction and spread of HIV and other sexually transmitted infections, and the spread of dengue. The United Nations estimates that, by 2025, 65 per cent of the world's population will live in cities. The process of urbanization, especially in developing countries, heightens the opportunity for the introduction of once-isolated infections in rural areas to large urban agglomerations. Thus, dengue haemorrhagic fever is common in some cities of Asia, where the high prevalence is attributed to the proliferation of open containers for water storage which provide breeding grounds for the mosquito vector.

Table 1.4. Factors involved in the emergence and re-emergence of infectious diseases

Emergence factor	Contributory factors	Disease examples
1. Human demographics and behaviour	Immunosuppression; population growth and density; rural–urban migration; sexual activity; substance abuse; urban decay	HIV (sexual activity, substance abuse); cryptosporidiosis (immunosuppression)
2. Technology and industry	Food processing and handling; globalization of food supply; modern medicine (organ and tissue transplantation, immunosuppressive drugs, nosocomial infections, use of antibiotics); water treatment	New-variant CJD (contaminated food products); BSE (contaminated cattle feed); hepatitis B and C (blood transfusions)
3. Economic development and land use change	Agricultural development; climate change/global warming; dam building; deforestation/reforestation; irrigation	Argentine haemorrhagic fever (agriculture); Rift Valley fever (dams; irrigation); HFRS (agriculture); HPS (weather anomalies); malaria (irrigation)
4. International travel and commerce	Air travel; commerce	'Airport' malaria; dissemination of O139 *V. cholerae*
5. Microbial adaptation and change	Natural variation/mutation; selective pressure and resistance	Multidrug-resistant tuberculosis; vector resistance (malaria, plague)
6. Breakdown of public health measures	Curtailment or reduction of disease prevention programmes; poor sanitation; war	Multidrug-resistant tuberculosis; louse-borne typhus and cholera among African refugees; diphtheria in former USSR

Notes: BSE = bovine spongiform encephalopathy; CJD = Creutzfeldt–Jakob disease; HFRS = haemorrhagic fever with renal syndrome; HIV = human immuno-deficiency virus; HPS = hantavirus pulmonary syndrome.
Source: Based on information in Lederberg *et al.* (1992: 49–112) and Morse (1995, table 2, p. 10).

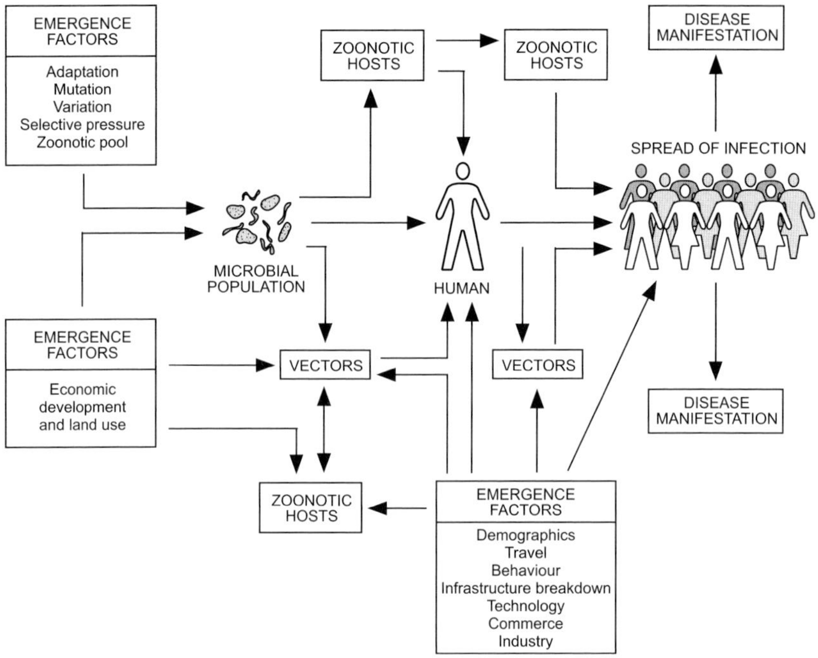

Fig. 1.6. Schematic diagram of infectious disease emergence by causal factors
Source: Adapted from Lederberg *et al.* (1992, fig. 2.1, p. 48).

(3) *International travel and commerce*, including the worldwide movement of goods and people. Examples include airport malaria, the dissemination of mosquito vectors, the introduction of cholera into South America, and the dissemination of *Vibrio cholerae* O139. Classic historical examples include the introduction of bubonic plague to Europe from Asia along the Silk Road in the fourteenth century, the carriage of yellow fever and its mosquito vector, *Aedes aegypti*, to the Americas in the sixteenth and seventeenth centuries associated with the importation of slaves from West Africa, and, in the nineteenth century, the dispersion of cholera around the world from its focus in the Ganges plain. Similar histories are being repeated. Rats have carried hantaviruses virtually worldwide, while, from 1982, the Asian tiger mosquito, *Aedes albopictus*, has been introduced to the US, Brazil, and parts of Africa with shipments of used tyres from Asia and has been associated with the spread of several viral diseases.

(4) *Technology and industry*, including the globalization of food supplies, changes in food processing, organ and tissue transplantation, immunosuppressive drugs, and widespread use of antibiotics. Examples

include *Escherichia coli* contamination of foodstuffs, bovine spongiform encephalopathy (BSE), and variant Creutzfeldt–Jakob disease (vCJD). The use of blood and tissue products has served to disseminate infections such as HIV and hepatitis B.

(5) *Microbial adaptation and change*, including microbial evolution and selection in the environment. Examples include antigenic drift in influenza virus, the emergence of antibiotic-resistant bacteria, and drug-resistant parasites. On rare occasions, the evolution of a fresh variant of a disease agent may result in the expression of a new clinical syndrome. One example is the epidemic of Brazilian purpuric fever in 1990, associated with a newly emerged variant of *Haemophilus influenzae*, biogroup *aegyptius*. Manifestations of Group A streptococcus, including necrotizing fasciitis, may also fall within this category.

(6) *Breakdown in public health measures*, including the curtailment or reduction in prevention programmes, inadequate sanitation, and vector control measures. Examples include the re-emergence of tuberculosis in the United States, cholera in refugee camps in Africa, and the resurgence of diphtheria in the former Soviet Union.

Similar and overlapping lists are given in Morens *et al.* (2004: 245) and McMichael (2004). Table 1.5 shows the multi-causal nature of disease emergence for many recently identified conditions by providing examples of emergent and re-emergent diseases and their associated disease agents.

1.5.3 Rates of Emergence

Table 1.6 is taken from Desselberger (2000) and provides examples of major aetiological agents of infectious diseases newly identified in the period 1971–2000, while the histogram in Figure 1.7 plots the number of agents by five-year period. Two features of the table and figure are noteworthy:

(1) the preponderance of viruses in the list of identified agents. Fewer bacteria and protozoa have been discovered, while, in recent times, unconventional diseases agents (prions) have also been identified;

(2) the marked increase in the number of discoveries, largely associated with viruses, in the 1990s. Examples are given in Table 1.6 and include several hepatitis viruses (HEV, HFV, HGV), herpesviruses (HHV-7, HHV-8) and influenza A viruses (H5N1, H9N2), as well as a range of severe viruses associated with meningitis and encephalitis (Hendra virus, Nipah virus).

The line trace in Figure 1.7 shows the average number of major aetiological agents identified per year. The upwards trend, from approximately 1.0 per year at the start of the series to 1.5 per year at the end of the series, is apparent.

Table 1.5. Examples of emergent and re-emergent diseases and disease agents in the late twentieth century

Disease agent	Related disease/symptoms	Mode of transmission	Cause(s) of emergence
	1. Bacteria, rickettsiae, and chlamydiae		
Borrelia burgdorferi	Lyme disease: rash, fever, neurologic and cardiac abnormalities, arthritis	Bite of infective *Ixodes* tick	Increase in deer and human populations in wooded areas
Escherichia coli O157:H7	Haemorrhagic colitis; thrombocytopaenia; haemolytic uraemic syndrome	Ingestion of contaminated food, especially undercooked beef and raw milk	Probably due to the development of a new pathogen; mass food processing technology allowing contamination of meat
Haemophilus influenzae biogroup *aegyptius*	Brazilian purpuric fever; purulent conjunctivitis, high fever, vomiting, and purpura	Contact with discharges of infected persons; eye flies are suspected vectors	Possibly an increase in virulence due to mutation; possibly new strain
Helicobacter pylori	Gastritis, peptic ulcer, possibly stomach cancer	Ingestion of contaminated food or water, especially unpasteurised milk; contact with infected pets	Increased recognition
Legionella pneumophila	Legionnaires' disease: malaise, myalgia, fever, headache, respiratory illness	Air-cooling systems, water supplies	Recognition in an epidemic situation
Mycobacterium tuberculosis	Tuberculosis: cough, weight loss, lung lesions	Exposure to sputum droplets	Immunosuppression; microbial adaptation and development of resistance
Orientia tsutsugamusghi	Scrub typhus: fever, headache, rash, enlargement of the lymph nodes	Exposure to infective larval trombiculid mites	Ecological changes associated with clearance of agricultural land, and hydroelectric and irrigation schemes
Vibrio cholerae	Cholera: severe diarrhoea, rapid dehydration	Ingestion of water contaminated with the faeces of infected persons; ingestion of food exposed to contaminated water	Poor sanitation/hygiene; possibly introduced via bilge-water from cargo ships
Yersinia pestis	Bubonic and pneumonic plague: fever, cough, ischaemic necrosis, haemorrhages, pneumonia, septicaemia	Bite of infective rat fleas	Breakdown in measures of disease control
	2. Viruses		
Crimean–Congo haemorrhagic fever	Haemorrhagic fever	Bite of an infected adult tick	Ecological changes favouring increased human exposure to ticks on sheep and small wild animals

Dengue	Haemorrhagic fever	Bite of an infected mosquito (primarily *Aedes aegypti*)	Poor mosquito control; increased urbanization in tropics; increased air travel
Filoviruses (Marburg, Ebola)	Fulminant high-mortality haemorrhagic fever	Direct contact with infected blood, organs, secretions, and semen	Unknown; in Europe and the US, virus-infected monkeys shipped from developing countries by air
Hantaan virus	Korean haemorrhagic fever: abdominal pain, vomiting, haemorrhagic fever	Inhalation of aerosolized rodent excreta	Human invasion of virus ecologic niche
Human immunodeficiency viruses (HIV-1 and HIV-2)	HIV disease and AIDS; severe immune system dysfunction, opportunistic infections	Sexual contact with or exposure to blood or tissues of an infected person; perinatal transmission	Urbanization; changes in lifestyles/mores; increased intravenous drug use; international travel; medical technology
Influenza A (pandemic)	Fever, headache, pneumonia	Airborne	Animal–human virus reassortment; antigenic shift
Japanese encephalitis	Encephalitis	Bite of an infective mosquito	Changing agricultural practices
Lassa fever	Fever, headache, sore throat, nausea	Contact with urine or faeces of infected rodents	Urbanization/conditions favouring infestation by rodents
Rift Valley fever	Febrile illness	Bite of an infective mosquito	Importation of infected mosquitoes and/or animals; development (dams, irrigation); possibly change in virulence or pathogenicity of virus
Venezuelan equine encephalitis	Encephalitis	Bite of an infective mosquito	Movement of mosquitoes and amplification hosts (horses)
Yellow fever	Fever, headache, muscle pain, nausea, vomiting	Bite of an infective *Aedes aegypti* mosquito	Lack of effective mosquito control and widespread vaccination; urbanization in tropics; increased air travel
	3. Protozoans, helminths, and fungi		
Babesia	Babesiosis; fever, fatigue, haemolytic anemia	Bite of *Ixodes* tick	Reforestation; increase in deer population; changes in outdoor recreational activity
Plasmodium	Malaria	Bite of an infective *Anopheles* mosquito	Urbanization; changing parasite biology; environmental changes; drug resistance; air travel
Toxoplasma gondii	Toxoplasmosis: fever, lymphadenopathy, lymphocytosis	Exposure to faeces of cats carrying the protozoan; sometimes food-borne	Immunosuppression; increase in cats as pets

Source: Abridged from Lederberg *et al.* (1992, table 2.1, pp. 36–41), with additional information from Morse (1995, table 1, p. 8), Lederberg (1998), and Chanteau *et al.* (1998).

Table 1.6. Sample aetiological agents of infectious diseases by year of discovery, 1971–2000

Year	Agent	Type of agent	Disease
1972	Small round structures viruses (SRSVs; caliciviruses)	Virus	Diarrhoea (outbreaks)
1973	Rotaviruses	Virus	Major cause of infantile diarrhoea worldwide
1975	Astroviruses	Virus	Diarrhoea (outbreaks)
	Parvovirus B19	Virus	Fifth disease
1976	*Cryptosporidium parvum*	Protozoan	Acute enterocolitis
1977	Ebola virus	Virus	Ebola viral disease
	Legionella pneumophilia	Bacterium	Legionnaires' disease
	Hantaan virus	Virus	Haemorrhagic fever with renal syndrome
	Campylobacter spp.	Bacterium	Diarrhoea
1980	Human T-cell lymphotropic virus type I (HTLV-I)	Virus	Adult T-cell leukaemia/ tropical spastic paraparesis
1982	Human T-cell lymphotropic virus type II (HTLV-II)	Virus	Hairy T-cell leukaemia
	Borrelia burgdorferi	Bacterium	Lyme disease
1983	Human immunodeficiency virus types 1 and 2 (HIV-1/HIV-2)	Virus	Acquired immunodeficiency syndrome (AIDS)
	Escherichia coli O157:H7	Bacterium	Haemorrhagic colitis; haemolytic uraemic syndrome
	Heliobacter pylori	Bacterium	Gastritis, gastric ulcers
1988	Human herpesvirus-6 (HHV-6)	Virus	Roseola infantum
1989	*Ehrlichia* spp.	Bacterium	Human ehrlichiosis
	Hepatitis C virus (HCV)	Virus	Parenterally transmitted non-A, non-B hepatitis
1990	Human herpesvirus-7 (HHV-7)	Virus	Exanthema subitum, pityriasis rosea
	Hepatitis E virus (HEV)	Virus	Enterically transmitted non-A, non-B hepatitis
1991	Hepatitis F virus (HFV)	Virus	Severe non-A, non-B hepatitis
1992	*Vibrio cholerae* O139:H7	Bacterium	Cholera
	Bartonella henselae	Bacterium	Cat-scratch disease, bacillary angiomatosis
1993	Sin Nombre virus	Virus	Hantavirus pulmonary syndrome
	Hepatitis G virus (HGV)	Virus	Non A–C hepatitis?
1994	Sabía virus	Virus	Brazilian haemorrhagic fever
	Human herpesvirus-8 (HHV-8)	Virus	Kaposi's sarcoma; body-cavity-based lymphoma
1995	Hendra virus	Virus	Meningitis, encephalitis
1996	Prion (BSE?)	Prion	New-variant Creutzfeldt–Jakob disease (vCJD)
1997	Influenza A (H5N1) virus	Virus	Influenza
	Transfusion-transmitted virus (TTV)	Virus	?
	Enterovirus 71 (EV71)	Virus	Epidemic encephalitis
1998	Nipah virus	Virus	Meningitis, encephalitis
1999	Influenza A (H9N2) virus	Virus	Influenza
	West Nile-like virus (lineage 1)	Virus	Encephalitis

Note: Year of discovery assigned on the basis of the year of isolation or identification of aetiological agent.
Source: Desselberger (2000, table I, p. 4).

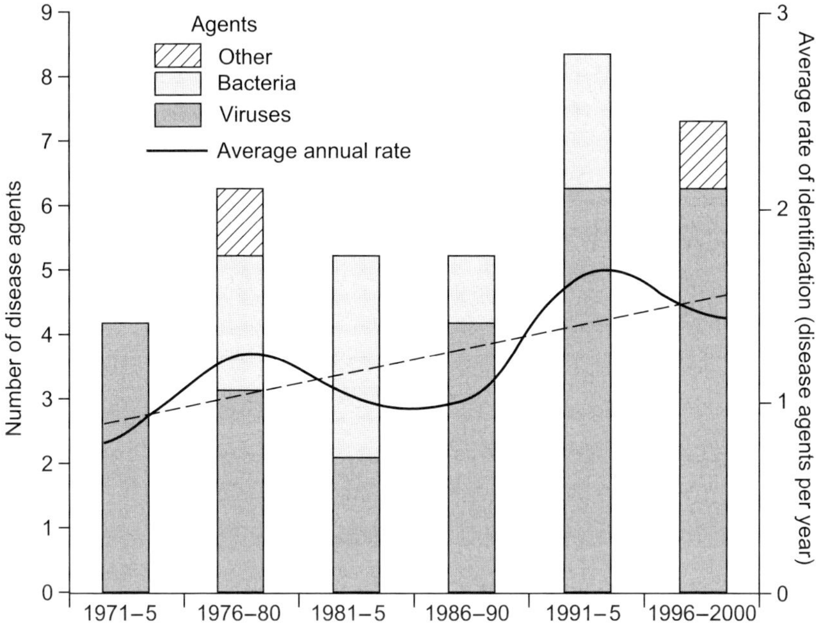

Fig. 1.7. Rate of identification of major aetiological agents of infectious disease, 1971–2000, by quinquennial periods

Source: Based on Desselberger (2000, table 1, p. 4).

Desselberger's work can be set within a century-long time-span which confirms his findings if we take a slightly different approach and use the *International Classification of Diseases*, 1900–1994, and *Control of Communicable Disease Manual*, 1917–2004, to construct frequency charts of the temporal occasions upon which different infectious conditions were recorded.

INTERNATIONAL CLASSIFICATION OF DISEASES, 1900–1994

The *International Classification of Diseases* (*ICD*) is the international standard diagnostic classification for all general epidemiological and many health management purposes. It is used to classify diseases and other health problems recorded on health and vital records including death certificates and hospital records. The idea of such a classification is to ensure comparability of data recording over space and time, thus facilitating the storage and retrieval of diagnostic information for clinical and epidemiological purposes. These records also provide the basis for the compilation of national mortality and morbidity statistics by country-level surveillance organizations. The list has gone through 10 versions since the first (*ICD*-1, Plate 1.1, centre) was endorsed

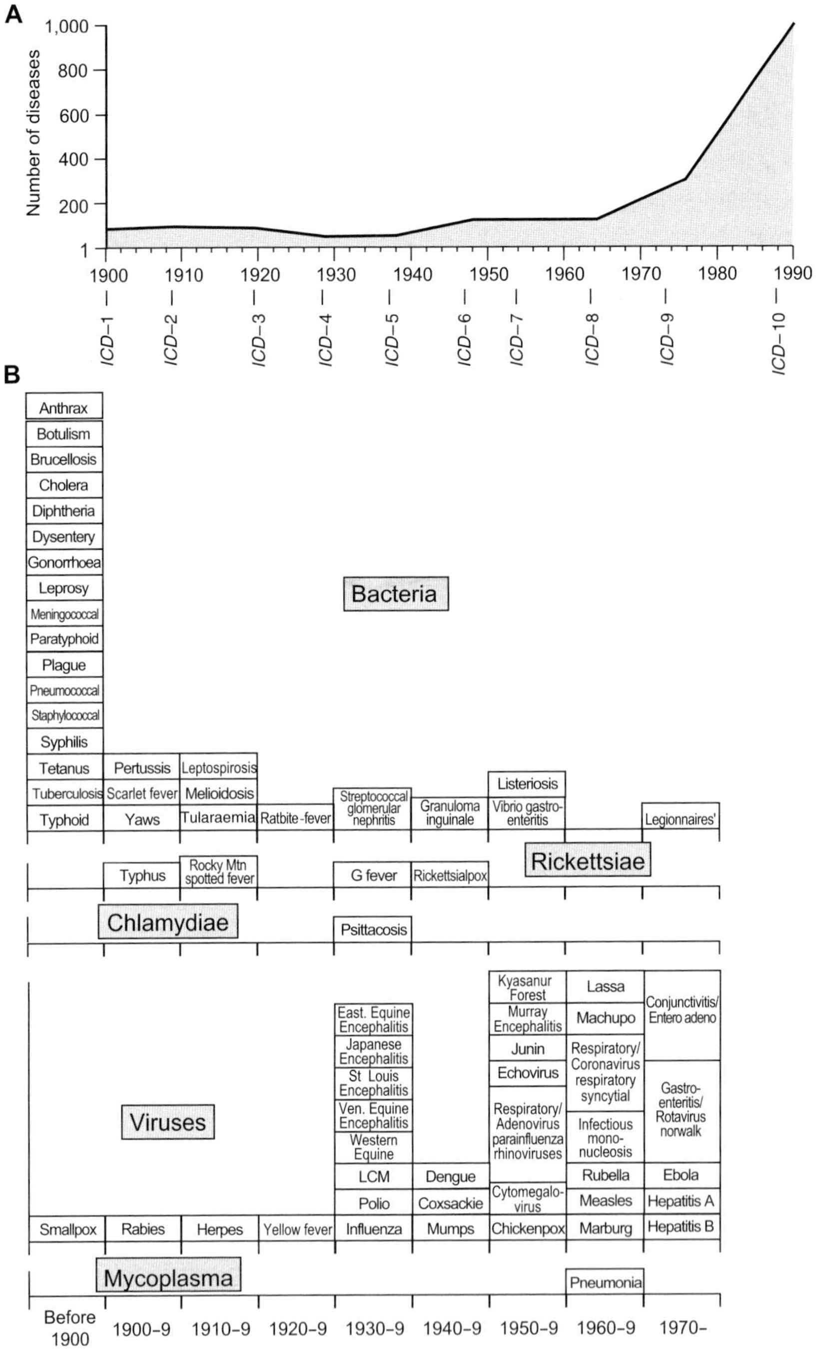

Fig. 1.8. *International Classification of Diseases*, 1900–1994. (A) Number of infectious diseases of humans recorded in *ICD*–1 to *ICD*–10. (B) Decade of discovery of principal infectious disease agents by taxonomic division of agents.

in 1900. The latest classification, *ICD*-10, came into use in WHO member states from 1994; see http://www.who.int/classifications/icd/en/ for a history.

Figure 1.8A shows the time series of the number of infectious diseases appearing in the *International Classification of Diseases* since its inception. The diseases included are those recorded in the so-called A and B lists. The number of diseases listed remained around 100 for the first 65 years of the *ICD*'s existence. In the Ninth and Tenth editions, however, the number rose sharply from around 350 (Ninth) to over 1,000 (Tenth). Figure 1.8B gives, on the same decennial basis, the dates of discovery of the main disease agents which have shaped this curve. Consistent with Desselbeger's work, the switch from bacterial to viral agents identified as the century progressed is evident.

CONTROL OF COMMUNICABLE DISEASES MANUAL, 1917–2004

Since the first edition of the *Control of Communicable Diseases Manual* (*CCDM*, Plate 1.1, right) appeared in 1917 as a 30-page booklet, it has evolved through 18 editions on a roughly 5–7-year cycle.[2] It provides a continuous record of infectious diseases of public health importance and, through its changing contents list, a window on the description and discovery of infectious diseases over the last century (Malloy and Marr 2001).

To analyse the time trends of recording in *CCDM*, the contents lists of all 18 editions were encoded, noting both edition in which each disease appeared and the causative agent (bacterium, virus, parasite, fungus, other). Figure 1.9A tracks the number of diseases by agent as a stacked line chart. The number of diseases recorded grew from 39 in 1917 to nearly 600 in the 2004 edition. Growth was rapid from the sixth edition (1945). The number of bacterial diseases recorded grew linearly over the period, and the rapid post-1943 growth is attributable mainly to new discoveries among virus and parasitic diseases. This interpretation is reinforced by Figure 1.9B. This plots the edition of first entry of each disease in *CCDM* by type of agent, expressing the number of entries by agent as a percentage of the total number of diseases in the edition. The graph shows the slow decline of bacterial diseases as a proportion of the total in each edition, and the rise in the share of viral and parasitic diseases.

Figure 1.9C plots the number of diseases by agent by the edition in which they first appeared. The new diseases appear to have been added in bursts, with major additions in 1935, 1945, 1955, 1965, 1981, and 1997. The period of greatest additions was for 40 years from the end of World War II. Since then, the rate of additions has declined.

[2] 1917, 1926, 1932, 1935, 1943, 1945, 1950, 1955, 1960, 1965, 1970, 1975, 1981, 1985, 1990, 1995, 2000, 2004.

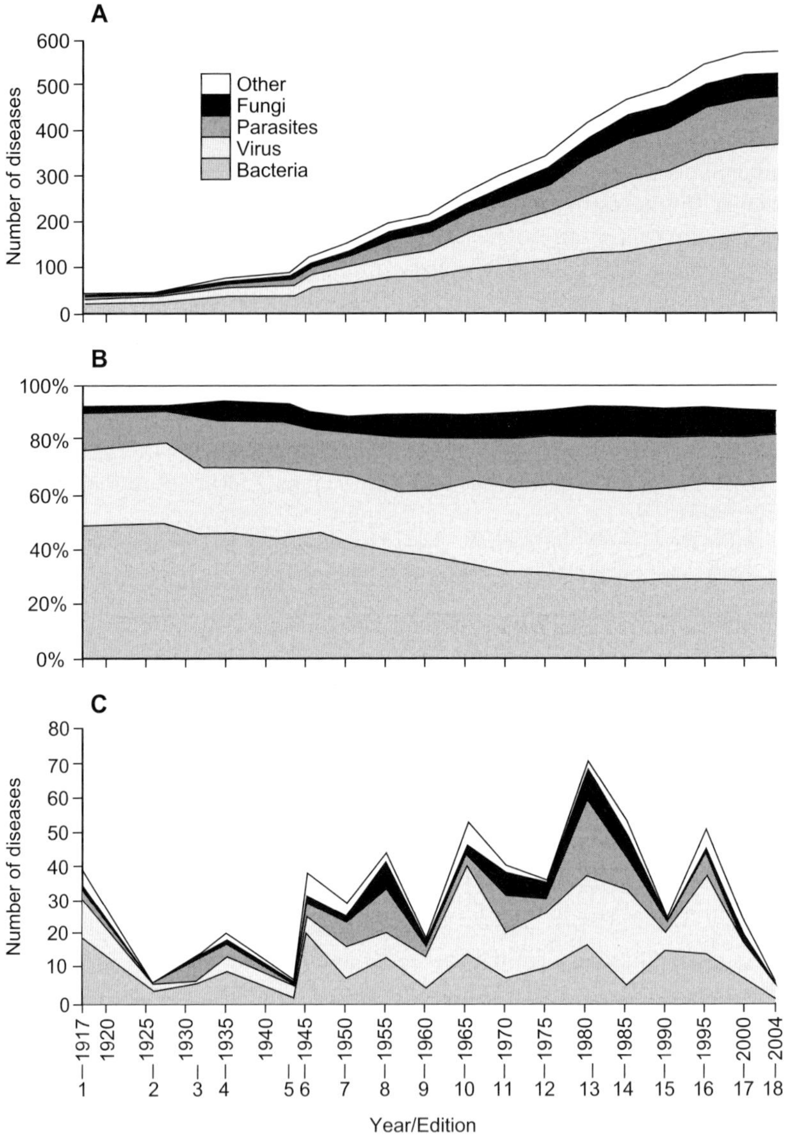

Fig. 1.9. *Control of Communicable Diseases Manual*, 1917–2004
(A) Number of infectious diseases recorded in each edition by taxonomic division of agents. (B) Percentage of diseases reported in each edition by taxonomic division of agents. (C) Number of diseases by type of agent and edition in which they first appeared.

1.6 Organization of the Book

This book is arranged in three parts (Figure 1.10). Chapter 2 of Part I, 'Early Disease Emergence: Pre-1850', looks at disease emergence and re-emergence up to the middle of the nineteenth century. Here the factors contributing to disease emergence and re-emergence outlined in Section 1.5 are used to illuminate a number of substantive case studies of emergence. Some of the great emergent diseases of history—leprosy, malaria, bubonic plague, measles, influenza, typhus, and cholera—are discussed. The chapter concludes with an analysis of the ebb and flow of infectious diseases in Britain between 1603 and 1849.

Part II, 'Processes of Disease Emergence: 1850–2006' (Chapters 3–9), examines disease emergence and re-emergence in the period of modern recording of morbidity and mortality data from about 1850. Particular emphasis is placed upon the twentieth century. Accordingly in Chapter 3, to guide our selection of diseases, locations, and time periods for study in later chapters, content analysis is undertaken of three information sources which span very different geographical scales—internationally, those generated by the communicable disease monitoring undertaken by the League of Nations/World Health Organization between 1923 and 1983; at regional and national scales in the CDC's landmark publication *Morbidity and Mortality Weekly Report* since its inception in 1952; and finally at a local scale in the epidemiological field investigations undertaken by CDC since 1946.

Using the regional–thematic matrix of diseases specified on the basis of Chapter 3, Chapters 4–9 look systematically at the factors identified in Section 1.5 as facilitating disease emergence. Chapter 4 examines evidence for agent change including microbial and vector adaptation, while Chapter 5 extends this work by considering the roles of technological and industrial developments in forcing the pace of microbial change. Chapters 6 and 7 focus upon changes in the human host and the environments within which human life is played out. In Chapter 6, the impact of population growth, the increasing tropicalization and urbanization of humans, and exponential increases in human mobility upon pathogenic micro-organisms are discussed. Environmental shifts also create possibilities for the emergence of new diseases by modifying the agent–human interface, and so it is to the disease consequences of environmental change that we turn in Chapter 7. One of the main topical concerns is the impact of global warming, which, by an extension of the tropical thermal range to mid-latitudes, greatly increases the potential for a spectrum of tropical arthropod-borne infections to spread broadly. Land use changes arising from changed agricultural practices, deforestation, and water management also facilitate disease emergence and re-emergence as illustrated by the haemorrhagic fevers.

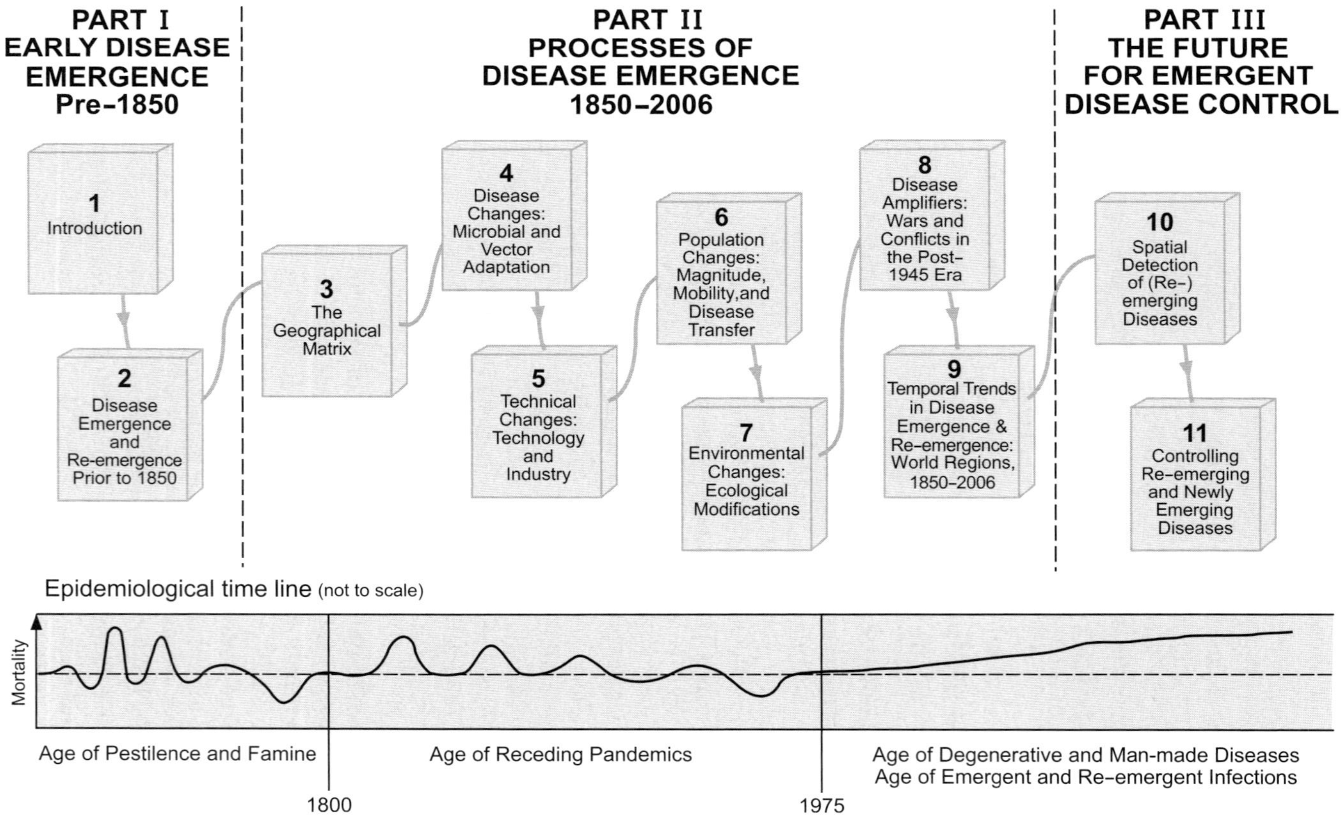

Fig. 1.10. Organization of the book.
The 11-chapter sequence of *EmergingDiseases*, arranged on a broadly historical basis. An emergence time line for a schematic epidemiological transition is shown.

Human history has been punctuated by wars and conflicts at all geographical scales. As summarized in Table 1.7, conflict is commonly associated with epidemic events. The threat of bioterrorism has added a new dimension and urgency to the role of conflict in disease emergence, and this forms the subject of Chapter 8. The emphasis of the chapter is on post-1945 conflicts where we explore the following themes: (i) disease emergence among military personnel fighting in epidemiologically 'new' environments; (ii) disease emergence in civil populations as a result of collapses in public health infrastructure; (iii) disease emergence in populations displaced by war; and (iv) bioterrorist potential and responses.

As we have noted, the emergence or re-emergence of a disease is rarely attributable to a single cause. In Chapter 9, we explore the multifactorial nature of disease emergence and re-emergence. The arrangement of material in this chapter is by geographical scale. At the world level, the plague and cholera pandemics which have circled the globe since the middle of the nineteenth century are discussed to show the surging nature of these cyclically re-emerging diseases. The newly emergent disease of HIV/AIDS has displayed a similar surging character since its emergence from the 1980s. At the regional level, we look at emerging diseases in the developed and developing economies. In the advanced economies, general trends in disease mortality in Europe and the South Pacific, 1901–75, are discussed. In the developing economies, we move from temperate to tropical latitudes to examine sample time sequences of disease emergence (Ebola–Marburg viral diseases) and cyclical re-emergence (meningococcal disease) in sub-Saharan Africa. The chapter is concluded at the local scale with a study of the long-term shape of epidemic mortality curves, epidemic wavelength, and epidemic magnitude in the city of London since 1850.

Because of the potentially high public health risk when a newly emergent disease appears in a community, or an existing condition returns after a long gap, a great deal of effort is being devoted nationally and internationally to ways of identifying likely new infections and devising appropriate strategies to control them. These topics are addressed in Part III, 'The Future for Emergent Disease Control' (Chapters 10 and 11). When a population encounters a new infection, or an existing condition reappears after a long absence, the herd immunity is likely to be low and, *ceteris paribus*, rapid geographical spread is likely to occur. Accordingly, in Chapter 10, we present a new model for estimating the velocity of spread and rate of recovery of geographical areas when attacked by either a single or recurrent epidemic waves. The model is illustrated by application to influenza as an example of a cyclically re-emerging disease caused by a rapidly evolving virus, and, as a contrast, to measles as an example of a disease caused by an unchanging virus. Use of the method in forecasting and early-warning systems is discussed. Chapter 11 concludes the book by examining strategies for controlling future outbreaks at different geographical scales from the global to the

Table 1.7. Sample epidemic events associated with war, 500 BC–AD 2000

Year	Conflict	Sample afflicted group and/or location	Disease	Estimated deaths
c.480 BC	Persian invasion of Greece (480–479 BC)	Persian army in Greece	Plague or dysentery?	>300,000?
430–425 BC	Great Peloponnesian War (431–404 BC)	Athens	Unknown	>100,000?
212 BC	Second Punic War (218–202 BC)	Roman army at Siege of Syracuse	Influenza?	?
88 BC	Social War (91–88 BC)	Army of Octavius in Rome	?	17,000
AD 125	Roman colonial wars, Africa	Roman army in Utica	?	≤30,000
251–66	Roman–Gothic War (249–70)	Africa, Europe, and Near East	Measles or smallpox?	≤5,000/day (Rome)
425	Hun raids on Roman empire (*c*.375–454)	Hun army (advance on Constantinople)	?	? (epidemic forced retreat)
569/571	Elephant War (569/571)	Abyssinian army at Siege of Mecca	Bubonic plague with smallpox?	60,000?
638–9	Muslim conquest of Persia (634–51)	Syrian army in Amwās	?	25,000 (in 639)
1010/1011	Later Viking raids in England (899–1016)	Danes in Kent	*Dolor viscerum* (dysentery)?	?
1148	Second Crusade (1147–9)	Army of Louis VII & civilians at Adalia	Typhoid, dysentery, or bubonic plague?	?
1218	Fifth Crusade (1217–21)	Crusader army at Damietta	Severe scurvy	? (15–20% of army)
1270	Eighth Crusade (1270)	Crusader army at Carthage	Dysentery	? ('many deaths')

1346	Siege of Kaffa	Tatar army at Kaffa	Bubonic plague	? ('infinite' numbers)
1485	Wars of the Roses (1455–85)	England	Sweating sickness	? ('most' students at Oxford)
1489–90	War of Granada (1482–92)	Spanish army in Granada	Typhus fever	? (up to 17,000 prior to 1490)
1495–	Italian Wars (1494–5)	Continental Europe	Syphilis	?
1518–20	Wars of Spanish conquest (1519–46)	Mexico	Smallpox	2–15 million
1552	Fifth War against Charles V (1552–9)	Army of Charles V at Metz	Typhus fever & dysentery	10,000
1596–1602	Anglo-Spanish War (1587–1604)	Spain	Bubonic plague	0.5–0.6 million
1632–3	Thirty Years War (1618–48)	Protestant population, Dresden	Bubonic plague	7,714
1643	English Civil War (1640–9)	Parliamentary army at Reading	Typhus fever	? ('great mortality')
1650	Cromwell's Irish campaign (1649–50)	Garrison at Kilkenny	Bubonic plague	900 (cavalry & footsoldiers)
1689	Irish War (1689–91)	Protestant army (near Dundalk)	Typhus fever	6,000
1709	Second Northern War (1700–21)	Danzig	Bubonic plague	32,599
1717	Austro-Turkish War (1716–18)	Austrian troops at Siege of Belgrade	Typhus & dysentery	4,000
1738	Russo-Austrian War (1735–39)	Russian troops	Bubonic plague	30,000
1761–2	Seven Years War	British forces at Siege of Habana	Yellow fever	8,000
1771–2	Russo-Turkish War (1768–72)	Moscow	Bubonic plague	52,300

(*continued*)

Table 1.7. (Continued)

Year	Conflict	Sample afflicted group and/or location	Disease	Estimated deaths
1781	Comuneros' uprising in New Granada (1781)	Socorro	Smallpox	6,000
1792–5	War of the First Coalition (1792–7)	Metz	Typhus fever	4,870
1801–3	Haitian-French War (1801–3)	French army in Haiti	Yellow fever	22,000
1808	Peninsular War (1808–14)	Besieged military and civilian population of Saragossa	Typhus fever	72,000
1809	Walcheren expedition (1809–10)	British army on Walcheren Island	Walcheren fever (malaria, typhus, typhoid, and/or dysentery)	3,960
1812–13	Napoleon's Russian expedition (1812–13)	French soldiers and civilians at Vilna	Typhus fever	55,000
1831	Polish Insurrection (1830–1)	Warsaw province	Cholera	13,103
1854–6	Crimean War (1853–6)	British & French Armies, Black Sea	Cholera	*c.*18,000
1866	Austro-Prussian War (1866)	Austrian crownlands	Cholera	165,000
1870–1	Franco-Prussian War (1870–1)	France & Germany	Smallpox	*c.*300,000
1877–8	Russo-Turkish War (1877–8)	Russian army	Typhoid & typhus fevers	*c.*33,000
1898	Spanish-American War (1898)	US Volunteer Army	Typhoid fever	*c.*1,500

1902–4	Philippine-American War (1899–1902)	Philippines	Cholera	*c*.200,000
1914–15	World War I (1914–18)	Serbian soldiers/ Austrian prisoners of war, Serbia	Typhus & relapsing fevers	30,000
1917–22	Revolution & Civil War, Russia (1917–21)	Russia	Typhus fever	2.5–3.0 million
1918–19	World War I (1914–18)	Global pandemic	Influenza	20–40 million
1942–5	World War II (1939–45)	Allied forces in Pacific and South-East Asia	Scrub typhus	636
1942–3	World War II (1939–42)	Servicemen and civilians, Malta	Poliomyelitis	37
1965–5	Vietnam War (1964–73)	Vietnam	Bubonic/pneumonic plague	838 (1966–70)
1971	Pakistan Civil War (1971)	East Pakistan refugees in India	Cholera	*c*.10,000
1980s	Mozambican Civil War (1976–92)	War-displaced persons, Mozambique	HIV/AIDS	?
1984–94	Sudanese Civil War (1956–)	Upper Nile, southern Sudan	Visceral leishmaniasis	95,000–112,000
1984–7	Salvadorean (1977–92) and Nicaraguan (1982–90) civil wars	Nicaraguan and Salvadorean refugees in Honduras	Measles	454
1995–7	Burundian Civil War (1993–)	Internally displaced persons	Louse-borne typhus	?
1999	Angolan Civil War (1975–)	Luanda and other provinces	Poliomyelitis	*c*.80

Source: Smallman-Raynor and Cliff (2004*b*, table 1.1, pp. 6–7).

local. Linked to appropriate surveillance technology, quarantine and vaccination are likely to remain the front line of defence. The ways in which these approaches will have to be integrated and deployed to contain future disease patterns as the twenty-first century unrolls will change, but it is certain that continued vigilance and application of early-warning systems will be at the leading edge of global preparedness.

2

Disease Emergence and Re-emergence Prior to 1850

2.1 Introduction

Infectious diseases have been evolving since the dawn of humankind. In Section 1.3, we noted some of the palaeopathological studies that have extended our knowledge of the occurrence of human infections back into pre-history, while recent genetic studies have indicated that the agents of diseases such as malaria (*Plasmodium* spp.) and leprosy (*Mycobacterium leprae*) first emerged in the human species many thousands of years ago (Carter and Mendis 2002; Monot *et al.* 2005). For the most part, however, our knowledge of the long history of disease emergence is based on the written record of earlier ages. In the present chapter, in so far as the historical evidence allows, we provide a brief and necessarily highly selective overview of disease emergence and cyclical re-emergence from the beginning of the written record to the mid-nineteenth century.

HISTORICAL PERSPECTIVES ON DISEASE EMERGENCE PROCESSES

McMichael (2004) identifies four great historical transitions in the relationship of humans and microbes that, since the initial advent of agriculture and livestock herding, have promoted the emergence and re-emergence diseases. These four transitions, each associated with a progressive increase in the geographical scale of operation (local → continental → intercontinental → global), are:

(i) *First historic transition (5,000–10,000 years ago).* A local transition when early agrarian-based settlements brought humans into contact with sylvatic enzootic pathogens. As described under the 'domestic-origins hypothesis' in Section 1.3.2, close and prolonged exposure to domesticated animals and urban pests (for example, rodents and flies) resulted in the cross-species transmission of the ancestral agents of many modern-day human infectious diseases, including influenza, measles, smallpox, tuberculosis, and typhoid.

(ii) *Second historic transition (1,500–3,000 years ago).* A continental-level transition fuelled by the military and trade contacts of early Eurasian civilizations which resulted in the cross-civilization transmission of infectious agents. In the wake of this historical transition, a trans-European 'equilibration' of infectious agents occurred and the diseases became endemic to the population.

(iii) *Third historic transition (200–500 years ago).* An intercontinental transition associated with European expansion, resulting in the trans-oceanic spread of infectious agents. This transition began with the discovery of the Americas and continued for some three centuries or more with the transatlantic slave trade and European explorations of the Asia–Pacific region.

(iv) *Fourth historic transition (present day).* A global transition in which demographic, environmental, behavioural, and technological factors have led to the appearance of apparently new diseases.

For each of the four transition periods, (i)–(iv), Figure 2.1 provides an indication of the relative importance of six principal social and environmental factors in the disease emergence complex. Reading from the bottom of the diagram, the most important influencing factors (ranks 1 and 2) shifted over the millennia from (*a*) a local focus on human–animal relations and demographic and social conditions at 5,000–10,000 years BP, through (*b*) continental and intercontinental trade, travel, migration, war, and conquest at 1,500–3,000 and 200–500 years BP, to (*c*) the global environmental change and demographic and social conditions of the present day.

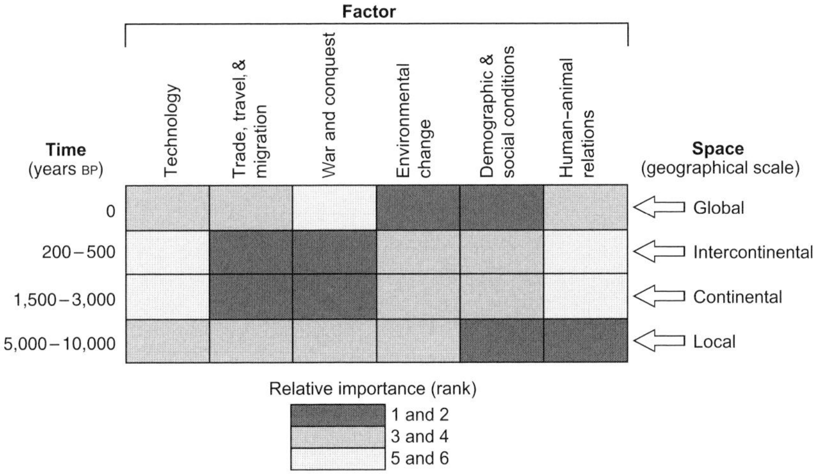

Fig. 2.1. Rank importance of six principal environmental and social factors on the emergence of infectious diseases by historical period
Principal environmental and social factors are grouped by rank of importance (rank 1 = most important). Time periods relate to each of four historic transitions in disease emergence as defined by McMichael (2004): (i) first historic transition (5,000–10,000 years BP); (ii) second historic transition (1,500–3,000 years BP); (iiii) third historic transition (200–500 years BP); and (iv) fourth historic transition (present day). Note the sequential increase in the geographical scale of developments from the first (local) to the fourth (global) transition.
Source: Based on McMichael (2004, fig. 1, p. 1053).

LAYOUT OF CHAPTER

Framed by Figure 2.1, our examination of the history of disease emergence begins in Section 2.2 with a review of the plagues and pestilences of ancient times (2000 BC–AD 500)—a period that overlaps with the military and commercial contacts encompassed by McMichael's 'second historic transition'. In Section 2.3, we take a sample of the major infectious diseases of humans included in August Hirsch's renowned *Handbook of Geographical and Historical Pathology* (1883–6) and trace the evidence for their relative antiquity in the epidemiological record. Special attention here is paid to three diseases (plague, influenza, and Asiatic cholera) which, by virtue of their cyclical re-emergence as pandemic events, are treated in subsequent parts of the book. Finally, for the period embraced by McMichael's 'third historic transition' (200–500 years BP), Section 2.4 draws on two classic data sources (the London *Bills of Mortality* and the General Register Office's cause-of-death statistics) to analyse the ebb and flow of infectious diseases at the local level of London, 1603–1849. The chapter is concluded in Section 2.5.

2.2 Ancient Epidemics (2000 BC–AD 500)

It is generally held that many of the ancient epidemics recorded from the second millennium BC were related to warfare, mass migrations, and the consequent breakdown of public health (Adamson 1980; Wiseman 1986). They were frequently spatially emergent, appearing for the first time in new locations. Table 2.1 lists a sample of such epidemics, along with summary information on the possible nature of the associated disease(s) and the principal afflicted populations. Our survey of the biblical and Egyptian (Section 2.2.1) and classical (Section 2.2.2) evidence draws on the account of Smallman-Raynor and Cliff (2004*b*: 66–73).

2.2.1 Biblical and Ancient Egyptian Evidence

The prophets and compilers of the Old Testament frequently portrayed the Lord's wrath in terms of apocalyptic visitations of war, famine, and disease. The boils and blains of man and beast described in Plague Six of the Ten Plagues of Egypt (Exodus 7–11)—variously interpreted in the literature as anthrax, ecthyma, or glanders, among other conditions—are cited by Marr and Malloy (1996) as one of the earliest examples of an 'emerging disease' in the written record.[1] Elsewhere, in considering Joshua's account of the sacking of Jericho in the fourteenth century BC (Joshua 6), Hulse (1971) attributes the abandonment of the city to the contamination of the main water supply (Elisha's Well) with the agent of urino-genital schistosomiasis (*Schistosoma haematobium*). In a similar vein, the Plague of Ashdod (1 Samuel 5) which afflicted the Philistines at Ashdod during the Hebrew–Philistine War, *c.*1190 BC, has been interpreted as bubonic plague (Simpson 1905; Wilson and Miles 1946; Hirst 1953; Rendle Short 1955), bacillary dysentery (Shrewsbury 1964), and, more recently, tularaemia (Trevisanato 2007*a*).

Other Ancient References

Trevisanato (2004) draws attention to an unusual epidemic, mentioned in both the Hearst Papyrus and the London Medical Papyrus, that spread in Egypt in the middle of the Bronze Age, *c.*1715 BC. Both texts characterize the disease as 'the one of the Asiatics'—an apparent reference to the people of the Syria–Canaan–Transjordan area. Trevisanato (2004) rejects earlier suggestions that the disease was plague or typhus and proposes it to have been tularaemia, probably introduced to Egypt by caravan or ship from the east. The same disease may also account for the prolonged epidemic ('Hittite plague') that spread in the eastern Mediterranean in the fourteenth century BC (Trevisanato 2007*b*).

[1] For an alternative perspective on the causes of the Ten Plagues of Egypt, see Trevisanato (2006*a*,*b*).

Table 2.1. Sample epidemics in antiquity, 2000 BC–AD 500

Year	Epidemic/disease	Afflicted population/area
Biblical and ancient Egyptian references		
*c.*1715 BC	*t3nt '3mw* (plague? typhus? tularaemia?)	Eastern Nile delta
*c.*1492–1425 BC (?)	Ten Plagues of Egypt: Plague 6 (anthrax? ecthyma? glanders?)	Egyptian empire
*c.*1335–1295 BC	The 'Hittite plague' (tularaemia?)	Eastern Mediterranean
*c.*1190 BC	Plague of Ashdod (bubonic plague? dysentery? tularaemia?)	Philistines at Ashdod, Gath, and Ekron
*c.*701 BC	Plague of the Assyrian army (bubonic plague? dysentery?)	Assyrian army at Jerusalem or Pelusium
*c.*588–587 BC	Starvation (accompanied by disease?)	Jerusalem
Ancient Greece		
*c.*1200 BC	Literary reference to undetermined disease	Greek army outside Troy
480 BC	Plague of Xerxes (bubonic plague? dysentery?)	Persian army
430–425 BC	Plague of Athens (multiple hypotheses on aetiology)	Athens and southern Greece
*c.*410 BC	Thasian epidemic (mumps)	Thasos
*c.*400 BC	'Cough of Perinthus' (diphtheria? influenza? whooping cough?)	Perinthus
396 BC	Smallpox?	Carthaginian army at Syracuse
Rome and the Roman empire		
451 BC	Roman Pestilence (anthrax? tuberculosis?)	Romans and Aequians
390 BC	?	Gaul army besieging Rome
212 BC	Influenza?	Carthaginian, Roman, and Sicilian armies at Syracuse
88 BC	?	Army of Octavius at Rome
*c.*AD 125	Plague of Orosius	Roman army at Utica
AD 165–80	Plague of the Antonines/ Galen (smallpox? measles?)	Roman empire (and beyond)
251–66	Plague of Cyprian (smallpox? measles?)	Roman empire (and beyond)
425	?	Hun army advancing on Constantinople

Sources: Adapted from Smallman-Raynor and Cliff (2004*b*, table 2.2, p. 69), with additional information from Marr and Malloy (1996), Kohn (1998), and Trevisanato (2004, 2007*a*,*b*).

2.2.2 The Graeco-Roman Period

While the physicians and medical writers of classical Greece and Rome provide ample evidence of the circulation of infectious and other diseases of varying severity, modern scientific understanding of the nature of many of the conditions alluded to in the ancient texts is incomplete. As Stannard (1993: 262) comments:

> Our knowledge of the diseases of classical antiquity stands somewhere between demonstrative certainty and complete ignorance. There is, after all, a sizable body of Greek and Latin texts, and it, in turn, has generated an even larger body of secondary literature. But for all that, our knowledge of the diseases of classical antiquity is far from complete. There are several reasons for its incompleteness, but it is important to keep in mind the enormous differences between the conceptual bases of the modern medical sciences and those of antiquity. These differences have important consequences in any attempt to identify the diseases of classical antiquity and to understand their effects.

Among the infectious diseases for which we find reasonably clear accounts in the early classical literature, Hippocrates provides a seemingly evident description of a mumps epidemic at Thasos in *c*.410 BC (Kim-Farley 1993*b*). The same source describes the periodicity of intermittent fevers (quotidian, tertian, quartan) and notes the enlargement of the spleens of those inhabiting low, marshy districts, suggestive of the establishment of malaria in ancient Greece (Dunn 1993). Later, in the first century AD, clinical descriptions of bubonic plague and diphtheria can be deciphered in the writings of Rufus of Ephesus and Aretaeus (Stannard 1993).

EPIDEMICS IN ANCIENT GREECE

Ancient Greek historians such as Herodotus, Thucydides, and Diodorus Siculus provide classical accounts of the devastation wrought by epidemic pestilences that spread with the wars of the time (Table 2.1). During the Persian invasion of Greece (480–479 BC), for example, Herodotus describes an epidemic (*λοιμός*) which attacked the 800,000-strong Persian army under Xerxes in 480 BC. With failing supplies and with undernourishment lowering the resistance of the army, *λοιμός* (possibly plague and/or dysentery) spread widely in the Persian ranks, reputedly claiming many tens of thousands of lives and forcing the Persian retreat from Thessalia (Zinsser 1950).

The Plague of Athens

One of the great epidemics of classical times was the Plague of Athens, described by Thucydides (460?–395? BC) in book 2 of his celebrated *History of the Peloponnesian War* (431–404 BC). See Figure 2.2.

> The disease is said to have begun south of Egypt in Aethiopia; thence it descended into Egypt and Libya, and after spreading over the greater part of the Persian empire,

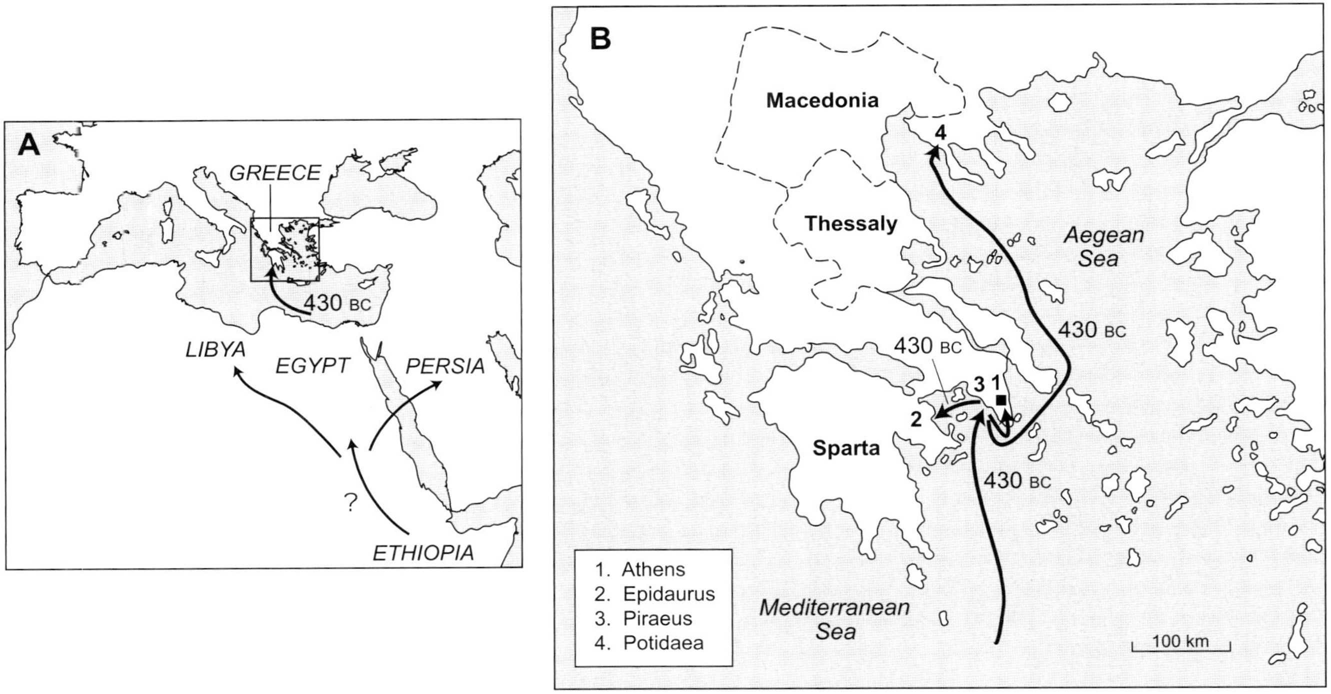

Fig. 2.2. Spread of the Plague of Athens (430–425 BC)
Vectors show the documented routes of disease transmission in the period up to 430 BC. According to the celebrated account of Thucydides, the epidemic appeared in Athens during the invasion of Attica by the Peloponnesian (Spartan) army in the summer of 430 BC. Thereafter, the disease followed Athenian military excursions to Potidaea and Epidaurus. Having spread in Athens as two waves, the epidemic was finally extinguished in the winter of 426–425 BC.

Source: Redrawn from Smallman-Raynor and Cliff (2004*b*, fig. 2.2, p. 71).

suddenly fell upon Athens. It first attacked the inhabitants of Piraeus . . . It afterwards reached the upper city, and then the mortality became far greater. (Thucydides 2. 48, trans. Jowett 1900: 135)

The 200,000 or so refugees who had fled the Athenian countryside for the relative safety of the city appear to have suffered most. 'For, having no houses of their own, but inhabiting in the height of summer stifling huts,' Thucydides noted, 'the mortality among them was dreadful, and they perished in wild disorder. The dead lay as they had died, one upon another, while others hardly alive wallowed in the streets and crawled about every fountain craving for water' (Thucydides 2. 52, trans. Jowett 1900: 138–9).

From Athens, military operations served to spread the pestilence to other parts of Greece. In the summer of 430 BC, the disease followed the Athenian troops who were sent as reinforcements in the blockade of Potidaea. Elsewhere, Plutarch (AD 46?–120?) records that a second Athenian expedition—to Epidaurus—suffered a similar fate in the summer of 430 BC (see Major 1940: 15).

The initial outbreak of the plague is said to have lasted for some two years, abating in the summer of 428 BC. Thereafter, the disease lingered on in southern Greece, recrudescing in the early winter of 427–426 BC. By the following winter, the epidemic was finally spent (Thucydides 2. 87, trans. Jowett 1900: 246–7). Exactly how costly the epidemic was in terms of human lives is not known. Pericles, the Athenian strategus, was one of many notables to succumb during the first wave of the visitation, while the second wave is said to have claimed the lives of 4,400 hoplites, 300 horsemen, and an unknown number of 'common people' (Thucydides 2. 87, trans. Jowett 1900: 246–7). More generally, the Athenian mortality rate is estimated to have been of the order of 25 per cent (Carmichael 1993*c*) in a population that, at a maximum in 430 BC, had been swelled by refugees from 100,000 to 300,000–400,000 (Morens and Littman 1992).

Identifying the cause of the Plague of Athens has given rise to a lively academic debate. Most recently Olson *et al.* (1996) have speculatively added Ebola fever to an already existing list of 30 or so contending diseases ranging from typhus fever, smallpox, typhoid fever, and bubonic plague through to measles and influenza. Others have argued that the disease may have been 'antique plague' or some other malady which no longer occurs (Prinzing 1916; Holladay 1986).

EPIDEMICS IN ROME AND THE ROMAN EMPIRE

While Table 2.1 traces the epidemic record for Rome and the Roman empire back to at least 451 BC, when the so-called 'Roman Pestilence' of that year forced the Aequians to forgo a planned attack on the Eternal City, the available evidence suggests that epidemics were relatively geographically contained in the pre-Christian era. In the early Christian era, events changed for the worse when military operations associated with the maintenance and control of the Roman empire fuelled two of the major pandemics of early European history: the Antonine Plague (AD 165–80) and the Plague of Cyprian (AD 251–66).

The Antonine Plague (AD 165–180)

The origins and course of the Antonine Plague (sometimes referred to as the Plague of Galen from the medical description of the disease given in Galen's *Methodus Medendi*) is summarized by Major (1940: 17–21). Descriptions of symptoms suggest smallpox, possibly spreading in a virgin soil population, but others have viewed the disease as typhus fever, measles, a form of 'antique plague', or a mixture of diseases (see, for example, Crawfurd 1914: 72; Prinzing 1916: 12). Whatever the exact nature of the epidemic, its effects were severe and wide-ranging. The disease was first carried to Rome by returning soldiers, where the subsequent spread within the civil population is said to have resulted in tens of thousands of victims. From Rome it spread throughout the rest of Italy, resulting in large-scale depopulation. North of Italy, the plague advanced as far as the Rhine, while, to the west, it is said to have reached the shores of the Atlantic. The epidemic continued for some 15 years until AD 180, during which time it claimed the lives of two Roman emperors: Lucius Verus (d. AD 169) and his co-regent, Marcus Aurelius Antoninus (d. AD 180) (Major 1940; Kohn 1998).

The Plague of Cyprian (AD 251–266)

The Plague of Cyprian gravely affected the entire Mediterranean basin during the period of instability associated with the Roman–Gothic Wars (AD 249–68). The epidemic spread throughout much of North Africa, the Near East, and Europe. At its height, it is documented to have claimed 5,000 victims a day in Rome. The pestilence devastated the Roman legions. It disrupted supply lines and the means of revenue collection, thereby contributing further to the military and political instability of the empire. As described by St Cyprian, the Bishop of Carthage, symptoms of the disease included reddened eyes, an inflamed throat, vomiting, and diarrhoea, with loss of senses (hearing and sight) in survivors. The disease may have been measles or smallpox; bubonic plague has largely been ruled out as contemporary accounts fail to mention swellings (Castiglioni 1947; McNeill 1976; Kohn 1998).

2.3 Historical Sample

As we noted in Chapter 1, many infectious diseases due to micro-organisms that are specifically adapted to the human species (including the great herd diseases of the historical period) are unlikely to have existed much before 5,000–10,000 years ago—an evolutionary development that was contingent on the environmental changes associated with McMichael's 'first historic transition' (Section 2.1). In the present section, we review the epidemiological record to see what clues it can provide regarding the emergence and re-emergence of major human infectious diseases down the ages. Our examination begins in Section 2.3.1 by examining the evidence for the relative antiquity of sample infectious diseases covered in August Hirsch's *Handbook of Geographical and Historical Pathology* (1883–6). In subsequent sections, we briefly consider the historical geography of three major human diseases that, by virtue of their cyclical re-emergence as pandemic events, are treated in later parts of the book: plague (Section 2.3.2); influenza (Section 2.3.3); and cholera (Section 2.3.4). While these diseases are well known to modern science, the historical record is replete with examples of the sudden emergence, and the equally sudden disappearance, of mysterious and unidentified diseases. Two such examples from the late Middle Ages onwards (the sweating sicknesses of Europe, and the haemorrhagic fevers, or *cocoliztli*, of colonial Mexico) are considered in Section 2.3.5.

2.3.1 Overview

In the sixth decade of the nineteenth century, August Hirsch (Plate 2.1), Professor of Special Pathology and Therapeutics and of the History of

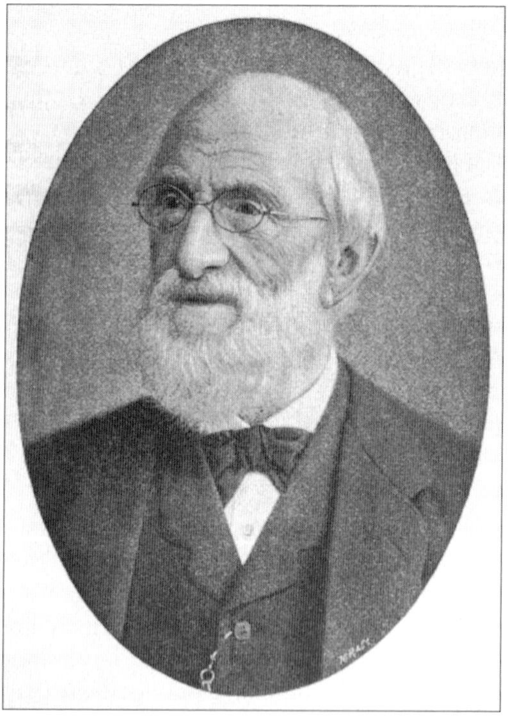

Pl. 2.1. August Hirsch (1817–1894)
Professor of Special Pathology and Therapeutics and of the History of Medicine at the University of Berlin. Hirsch's great work was his *Handbuch Historisch-Geographischen Pathologie*, the second edition of which was published in English under the title *Handbook of Geographical and Historical Pathology* in 1883–6.

Medicine at the University of Berlin, began the assembly of his seminal work *Handbook of Geographical and Historical Pathology*. The second edition of the *Handbook*, published in three volumes, reviews the early history and geography of the (then recognized) major infectious and other diseases of humans (Hirsch 1883–6). The work was based not only upon clinical experience and library research, but also upon a voluminous correspondence with colleagues and medical authorities around the world. For the infectious diseases covered by Hirsch, the *Handbook* remains one of the definitive surveys of the early history and world distribution of these conditions.

Table 2.2 is based on the evidence included in Hirsch's *Handbook* and gives, for a sample of 21 infectious diseases, summary information on their relative antiquity. The diseases are grouped by era (antiquity, prior to AD 500; the Middle Ages, AD 500–1500; and the modern period, AD 1500–1850), with sample dates of early (actual or possible) epidemics indicated for reference. The evidence is supplemented by perspectives on the longevity of the diseases from Hirsch (1883–6) and other authoritative sources. Finally, for six of the sample diseases in Table 2.2, Figure 2.3 summarizes the historical sequence of recognized pandemics, major epidemic periods, and periods of raised incidence as documented by Hirsch and others.

In interpreting the evidence in Table 2.2, we recognize that any attempt to classify diseases by the era of their apparent appearance in the epidemiological record is fraught with difficulties. As we have seen in Section 2.2, our knowledge of the early record is fragmentary and there are many and conflicting views regarding the causes of ancient plagues and epidemics. Some diseases, such as measles and smallpox, were not clearly differentiated in medical writings until the Middle Ages, although the weight of evidence indicates that both conditions existed in much earlier times (Cliff, Haggett, and Smallman-Raynor 1993). For yet other apparently ancient diseases, such as Asiatic cholera, references to their epidemic character are lacking until relatively late in the disease record (see, for example, Macpherson 1884), thereby instilling a degree of ambiguity in the temporal classification of Table 2.2.

Accepting these and similar difficulties, the evidence in Table 2.2 is consistent with the biological arguments in Section 1.3.2 and leads us to conclude that a number of the great infectious diseases of humans (including Asiatic cholera, diphtheria, dysentery, influenza, leprosy, malaria, measles, mumps, plague, smallpox, and pulmonary tuberculosis) extend back to ancient times. In more recent centuries, Table 2.2 traces the first epidemic accounts of the mysterious English sweating sickness, along with venereal syphilis and epidemic louse-borne typhus fever, to the late Middle Ages. In the modern era, a raft of familiar (dengue, meningococcal meningitis, relapsing fever, scarlet

Table 2.2. The earliest records of sample infectious diseases

Disease	Agent(s)	Earliest recorded epidemics	Notes/perspectives
Antiquity (to AD 500)			
Asiatic cholera	Bacterium (*Vibrio cholerae*)	AD 1629, Indonesia; AD 1638, Goa; AD 1689, Indonesia; AD 1781–3, India; AD 1782, Ceylon (MacNamara 1876; Hirsch 1883–6: i)	'The accounts of . . . cholera (Asiatic) in India reach back to the remotest times' (Hirsch 1883–6: i. 432).
			'. . . it must be admitted that in 1817 a new epoch in the history of cholera began, because that year marks the onset of the first of a series of pandemics during which the infection, after having gained impetus in India through a particularly severe and widely-spread incidence, extended its sway to other parts of the world, paying heed neither to distances and natural obstacles nor to the vain attempts at warding off its attacks through cordons and other quarantine measures. One may claim, therefore, that cholera which, as far as is known, had hitherto been of more or less localized importance only, began to become a most serious concern of the world in 1817' (Pollitzer 1959: 17).

Diphtheria	Bacterium (*Corynebacterium diphtheriae*)	*c*.400 BC, Perinthus, Turkey (?); AD 856, Rome (?); AD 1039, Byzantine empire (?); AD 1389, England (?); AD 1517, Rhine districts (?); AD 1544–5, Lower Germany (?); AD 1576, Paris; AD 1583, Spain (Hirsch 1883–6, iii; Kohn 1998)	'The history of malignant sore-throat (diphtheria) may be followed up into antiquity with a high degree of certainty . . . [I]n the writings of some of the later Greek physicians, particularly Aretæus and Aetius, we meet with descriptions of an affection of the throat, as to the identity of which there can be hardly any doubt' (Hirsch 1883–6: iii. 73).
			'The first absolutely trustworthy epidemiological information . . . dates from the end of the sixteenth and beginning of the seventeenth century. It comes from Spain, where the disease . . . was epidemic year after year for full thirty years (1583–1618)' (Hirsch 1883–6: iii. 76).
			'It is impossible to determine whether diphtheria was at any point a 'new' disease in recorded human history, though it is so described during the early modern period' (Carmichael 1993*b*: 682).

(*Continued*)

Table 2.2. (Continued)

Disease	Agent(s)	Earliest recorded epidemics	Notes/perspectives
Dysentery	Protozoan (*Entamoeba histolytica*); bacteria (*Shigella* spp.)	*c.*1190 BC, Plague of Ashdod (?); 480 BC, Plague of Xerxes (?); AD 1081–3, army of Henry IV at Rome (Kohn 1998)	'Our information on the history of dysentery goes back to the remotest periods accessible to historical enquiry at all. Dysentery . . . is often mentioned in the Hippocratic collection, and is accurately described along with diarrhoea . . . The excellent descriptions of dysentery given by Aretaeus, Celsus and Archigenes more particularly, and next in order by Galen, Caelius Aurelianus and other writers of antiquity, together with the references to it in the medical compendiums of the Arabians and the mediaeval practitioners, serve to show that in all those periods dysentery was an important thing in medical practice and well known to the profession' (Hirsch 1883–6: iii. 285).

Influenza	Virus		415 BC, Athenian army in Sicily (?); AD 591, Tours and Nîmes, France (?); AD 877, France, Germany (?); AD 927, France, Germany (?); AD 1173, England, Germany, Italy; AD 1323, France, Italy; AD 1328, Italy; AD 1387, France, Italy; AD 1580, Italy (Hirsch 1883–6: i; Clemow 1889–90; Kohn 1998)	'. . . the history of the disease may be followed into the remotest periods from which we have any epidemiological record at all, and its geographical distribution . . . extends over the whole habitable globe . . . Beyond the year 1173 the epidemiological data, although they certainly relate to influenza, bear a stamp too little characteristic to make them likely to be useful for . . . inquiry' (Hirsch 1883–6: i. 7).
				'When there exists an account of a pest which attacked nearly everyone, with fever, cough, catarrh, pain in the head and limbs, but of which few died, it would seem only rational to conclude that this was an influenza' (Clemow 1889–90: 359).
				'Although influenza could be among the older diseases of civilization, . . . there is no clear evidence of its spread among humans until Europe's Middle Ages, and no undeniable evidence until the fifteenth and sixteenth centuries' (Crosby 1993*a*: 808).

(*Continued*)

Table 2.2. (Continued)

Disease	Agent(s)	Earliest recorded epidemics	Notes/perspectives
Leprosy	Mycobacterium (*Mycobacterium leprae*)		'The earliest accounts, that are at all reliable, of the occurrence of the disease on extra-European soil date from the time of the Exodus of the Israelites from Egypt, the wanderings in the Desert, and the establishment of their power in Palestine . . . An antiquity hardly inferior to this appears to belong to the leprosy of India and perhaps also to that of China' (Hirsch 1883–6: ii. 2).
Malaria	Protozoa (*Plasmodium* spp.)	AD 1081–3, army of Henry IV at Rome; AD 1557–8, European pandemic; AD 1678–82, European pandemic (Hirsch 1883–6: i; Kohn 1998)	'Not many of the forms of people's sickness can be followed with so certain a clue as the malarial, through all intermediate periods up to the first beginnings of scientific medicine, although the ancient and mediaeval chronicles, medical and other, do not enable us to estimate the extent of their epidemic and endemic prevalence. It is, indeed, with the epidemiological

			records of the sixteenth century that the historical research begins' (Hirsch 1883–6: i. 197). 'Since at least the mid-Pleistocene, many thousands of generations of humans have been parasitized by the plasmodia' (Dunn 1993: 860).
Measles	Virus (measles)	AD 165–80, Antonine Plague (?); AD 251–66, Plague of Cyprian (?); AD 998–1025, Japan (Kohn 1998)	'. . . we may conclude so much at least as to the history of measles in past centuries, that the disease was in all probability widely diffused over Asiatic and European soil during the middle ages; and it has retained that position as a sickness of the people in the centuries following' (Hirsch 1883–6: i. 155). '. . . Rhazes is generally credited with the first authentic written record of measles by differentiating the two diseases [smallpox and measles] in approximately AD 910' (Kim-Farley 1993*a*: 873).

(*Continued*)

Table 2.2. (Continued)

Disease	Agent(s)	Earliest recorded epidemics	Notes/perspectives
Mumps	Virus (mumps)	*c.*410 BC, Thasos, Greece (Hirsch 1883–6: iii)	'Epidemics of inflammation of the parotid gland, known under various colloquial names such as mumps . . . were long ago described in a masterly fashion by Hippocrates, who also pointed to the fact observed by himself in an epidemic on the island of Thasos, that swelling of the testicle may occur in the course of the disease . . . But . . . it is not until the beginning of the eighteenth century that it receives more consideration in the history of epidemic sickness (Hirsch 1883–6: iii. 277).
Plague	Bacterium (*Yersinia pestis*)	*c.*1190 BC, Plague of Ashdod (?); 430–425 BC, Plague of Athens (?); first century AD, Egypt, Libya, Syria; AD 542, Plague of Justinian (Hirsch 1883–6: i; Kohn 1998)	'The history of plague may be followed into remote antiquity, and, with a certain measure of certainty, even as far as the end of the third or beginning of the second century of the pre-Christian era . . . It is not until the sixth century [AD] that we meet with authentic descriptions of the bubo-plague . . . which spread over the whole Roman Empire of the East and West, and even

			far beyond the limits of the empire, in the time of Justinian' (Hirsch 1883–6: i. 494–5). 'The first known cycle of widespread human plague occurred during late Greco-Roman antiquity' (Carmichael 1993*a*: 630).
Smallpox	Virus (smallpox)	430–425 BC, Plague of Athens (?); 396 BC, Carthaginian Plague (?); AD 165–80, Roman empire (?); AD 251–66, Roman empire (?); AD 569–71, Saudi Arabia (Kohn 1998)	'The first unambiguous statements about the disease from a medical source occur in the well-known treatise of the tenth century [AD] by Rhazes . . . in which it is established that Galen was acquainted with the disease . . . Rhazes speaks of the smallpox as a disease generally known over the East' (Hirsch 1883–6: i. 123). Smallpox may well have circulated among the ancient Egyptians. The face, neck, and shoulders of Pharaoh Ramses V, who died in 1157 BC, are disfigured by a rash of elevated pustules like those of smallpox (Crosby 1993*b*: 1009).

(Continued)

Table 2.2. (Continued)

Disease	Agent(s)	Earliest recorded epidemics	Notes/perspectives
Tuberculosis, pulmonary	Mycobacterium (*Mycobacterium tuberculosis*)		'Consumption of the lungs may be traced with certainty in the writings of every period as far back as the earliest attempts of the ancient world to deal with medicine according to a method . . . there can be no question that pulmonary consumption has held at all times and among all civilised peoples a foremost place among the national diseases' (Hirsch 1883–6: iii. 169).
			'Archaeological evidence indicates that tuberculosis afflicted prehistoric men and women in Eurasia and Africa at least from the Neolithic period' (Johnston 1993: 1062).
Middle Ages (AD 500–1500)			
English sweating sickness	?	AD 1485, England; AD 1508, England; AD 1517, England; AD 1528–9, northern Europe; AD 1551, England (Creighton 1891–4: i)	'Just as it appeared suddenly . . . as a malady quite unknown to doctors or to the public, a hitherto unheard of phenomenon, so in 1551 it went clean away from the earth and from men's memories, leaving no trace' (Hirsch 1883–6: i. 85).

Syphilis, venereal	Bacterium (*Treponema pallidum*)	AD 1494–5, French army at Naples; AD 1512, Japan (Kohn 1998)	'If . . . [the] facts . . . justify us in concluding that the venereal diseases, and particularly syphilis, had not only occurred during antiquity and the Middle Ages, but were even by no means uncommon, the fact that syphilis broke out in the form of a wide-spread and malignant epidemic towards the end of the fifteenth century is still a very remarkable episode in its history' (Hirsch 1883–6: ii. 63).
Typhus fever	Rickettsia (*Rickettsia prowazekii*)	AD 1083, Cava, Italy; AD 1096, Bohemia; AD 1489, Granada, Spain; AD 1497, Italy; AD 1502–4, Germany (Hirsch 1883–6: i)	'The earliest references to typhus epidemics, having a degree of definiteness, date from the eleventh century . . . Especially towards the end of the fifteenth century, typhus appears to have been widely spread in many countries of Europe' (Hirsch 1883–6: i. 546). 'Although it has been speculated that certain ancient plagues were probably typhus, the first contemporary accounts of a disease that may well have been typhus appeared near the end of the fifteenth century [AD]' (Harden 1993: 1082).

(*Continued*)

Table 2.2. (Continued)

Disease	Agent(s)	Earliest recorded epidemics	Notes/perspectives
Modern period (AD 1500–1850)			
Dengue	Virus (dengue)	AD 1779, Cairo; AD 1826–8, Caribbean and US (Hirsch 1883–6: i; Kohn 1998)	Not until the great epidemic of dengue which overran the West Indies and part of the North and South American continents in 1827 and 1828, was the attention of physicians drawn to the peculiar characters of the disease . . . and thus the record of dengue, so far as historical research can make use of it, begins really with the third decade of the present [nineteenth] century (Hirsch 1883–6: i. 60). 'There can be no doubt that . . . the disease has been much more common and more widely spread in past centuries . . . than we have any knowledge of from the scanty epidemiological records' (Hirsch 1883–6: i. 59).
Meningococcal meningitis	Bacterium (*Neisseria meningitidis*)	AD 1805, Geneva; AD 1815, Albenga, Italy (Hirsch 1883–6: iii; Kohn 1998)	'The historical research which was set on foot whenever the disease became known, has resulted in showing that there had been previous epidemics of it in the early years of this century

			[nineteenth] . . . but so far as concerns former centuries, there is no trustworthy information of its existence; and at all events the general diffusion . . . is an affair of recent date' (Hirsch 1883–6: iii. 547). '. . . although the first clinical description was of cases in Geneva in 1805, it seems highly unlikely that meningitis of meningococcal or other etiology is really such a new infection in humans' (Patterson 1993: 877).
Miliary fever	?	AD 1718, northern France; AD 1723, northern France; AD 1726, northern France (Hirsch 1883–6: i)	'The history of miliary fever does not extend beyond the beginning of the eighteenth century. The first unambiguous information about the disease dates from 1718, in which year, according to the statements of chroniclers, it was observed for the first time in various parts of Picardy' (Hirsch 1883–6: i. 88).
Relapsing fever	Bacterium (*Borrelia recurrentis*)	AD 1739, Dublin, Ireland; AD 1741, Scotland; AD 1742–3, Sweden (?); AD 1745, Ireland; AD 1748, Ireland; AD 1764–5, Ireland (Hirsch 1883–6: i; Kohn 1998)	'The history of relapsing fever . . . does not permit of being followed back beyond the eighteenth century, so far as epidemiography is our guide; although it is probable that the disease . . . had occurred before, and had been confounded with other diseases allied to it in symptoms, especially with malarial fever and other so-called typhus fevers' (Hirsch 1883–6: i. 593).

(Continued)

Table 2.2. (Continued)

Disease	Agent(s)	Earliest recorded epidemics	Notes/perspectives
Scarlet fever	Bacterium (*Streptococcus pyogenes*)	AD 1543, Sicily; AD 1627, Germany; AD 1642, Germany; AD 1652, Germany; AD 1661, England and Wales (Hirsch 1883–6: i)	'The earliest information about scarlet fever, to which any historical certainty appertains, goes hand in hand . . . with the information about measles. Both morbid processes were discussed in common . . . by the mediaeval physicians as well as those of the earlier centuries of the modern period; and as late as the 17th century, after the special features of the scarlatinal process had come to be recognised, many physicians clung to the opinion that it was only a modification of measles. It was not until the middle of the eighteenth century that a perfectly clear understanding of this point was arrived at' (Hirsch 1883–6: i. 171). 'It is possible that outbreaks [of scarlet fever] were observed by Near Eastern practitioners of

			the Arabian school, but the first undoubted account of a disease with a fiery rash as a characteristic was provided by Filippo Ingrassia of Palermo in 1553' (Hardy 1993*a*: 991).
Whooping cough	Bacterium (*Bordetella pertussis*)	AD 1578, Paris; AD 1749–64, Sweden; AD 1778, Faeroe Isles; AD 1804, St Bartholomew, West Indies (Hirsch 1883–6: iii)	'The history of whooping-cough cannot be followed farther back than the middle of the 16th century. There are, it is true, historians who believe that they have found indications of the disease in the medical writings of antiquity and of the Arabian period, as well as in the physicians and chroniclers of the middle ages. But all these statements rest . . . upon arbitrary interpretations of the text or upon errors of diagnosis, such as the confounding of whooping-cough with influenza' (Hirsch 1883–6: iii. 28). 'The first undoubted information about whooping-cough dates from 1578 . . . It is not until the 18th century that we meet with a succession of accounts of whooping-cough epidemics' (Hirsch 1883–6: iii. 29).

(*Continued*)

Table 2.2. (Continued)

Disease	Agent(s)	Earliest recorded epidemics	Notes/perspectives
			'The history of whooping cough before the twentieth century is obscure. It cannot with certainty be traced back further than the mid-sixteenth century and it was almost certainly unknown to the ancient world' (Hardy 1993*b*: 1095).
Yellow fever	Virus (yellow fever)	AD 1635, Guadeloupe; AD 1640, Guadeloupe; AD 1647, Barbados; AD 1648, Guadeloupe (Hirsch 1883–6: i)	'The earliest history of yellow fever in . . . [the Americas] is enveloped in an obscurity which we cannot now enlighten . . . It is not only the defectiveness of the records from these earliest times of our intercourse with the Western Hemisphere, that renders all historical research on the subject illusory; a still more serious impediment . . . is the frequent confounding of yellow fever with bilious remittent malaria fevers' (Hirsch 1883–6: i. 316). 'The first reliable accounts of yellow fever date from the middle of the seventeenth century' (Hirsch 1883–6: i. 317).

fever, whooping cough, and yellow fever) and not so familiar (miliary fever) diseases emerge to prominence in the historical record.

2.3.2 Plague

Plague (ICD-10 A20) is a zoonosis caused by the bacillus *Yersinia pestis*. The natural vertebrate reservoirs of *Y. pestis* are wild rodents. The disease in humans occurs as a result of (i) intrusion into the zoonotic (sylvatic) cycle, or (ii) by the entry of sylvatic rodents or their infected fleas into human habitats. The most frequent source of exposure resulting in human disease worldwide has been the bite of infected fleas (especially *Xenopsylla cheopis*, the oriental rat flea). Plague occurs in two major forms. Bubonic plague is caused by the bite of an infected flea and manifests as a painful swelling of the lymph glands ('buboes'). Bacteraemia and septicaemia often follow, as may secondary pneumonia. Primary pneumonic plague (contracted through exposure to the airborne exhalations of patients with primary pneumonic plague or the secondary pneumonia of bubonic plague) manifests as severe malaise, frequent cough with mucoid sputum, severe chest pains, and rapidly increasing respiratory distress. The incubation period is usually 1–7 days (bubonic plague) and 1–4 days (primary pneumonic plague). Untreated bubonic plague has a case-fatality rate of 50–60 per cent; untreated primary pneumonic plague is almost invariably fatal (Poland and Dennis 1998; Heymann 2004: 406–12).

ORIGINS AND EARLY HISTORY

Human plague is a disease of considerable antiquity. References to plague-like diseases can be traced back to the twelfth century BC (Table 2.2), while Jean-Pierre Papon (1800), cited in Simpson (1905), provides a chronological list of 41 possible plague epidemics in the empires and nations of the Mediterranean basin in the pre-Christian era. In later times, the forty-fourth book of the *Collectanea* of Oribasius, dating from the fourth century AD, includes an excerpt from the writings of Rufus of Ephesus (*fl.* first century AD) that makes mention of a certain disease as 'pestilentes bubones maxime letales et acuti, qui maxime circa Libyam et Ægyptum et Syriam observantur' (cited in Hirsch 1883–6: i. 494). The accompanying clinical description leaves no doubt that the malady was bubonic plague, prompting Simpson (1905: 5) to conclude that:

> The evidence is sufficient to establish the fact that plague is of great antiquity and that it prevailed in Libya, Egypt, and Syria at an early period of the world's history when these countries on the southern and eastern shores of the Mediterranean played a leading part in the civilisation of the day and their towns were important centres of commerce.

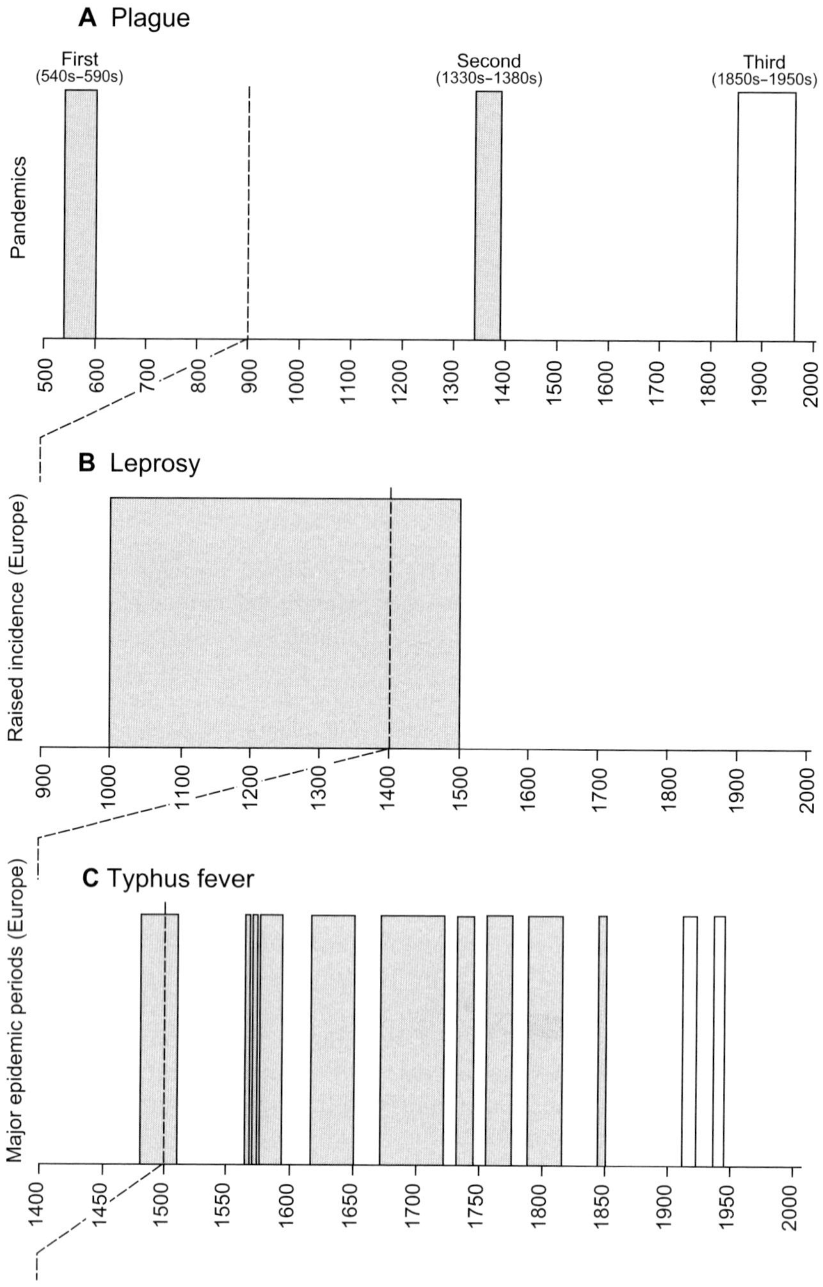

Fig. 2.3. Historical sequence of six sample infectious diseases

Charts identify the timing of recognized pandemics, major epidemic periods, and periods of raised incidence for each of six sample diseases in Table 2.2. (A) Plague pandemics, AD 500–2005. (B) Leprosy, raised incidence in Europe, AD 900–2005. (C) Typhus fever, major epidemic periods in Europe, AD 1400–2005. (D) Malaria, pandemics and major epidemics in Europe, AD 1500–2005. (E) Influenza pandemics and possible pandemics in Europe, AD 1500–2005. (F) Cholera pandemics, AD 1800–2005. Epidemiological events with onset prior to 1850 are represented by the shaded portions of the charts.

Sources: Based primarily on information in Hirsch (1883–6), Pollitzer (1954, 1959), and Kohn (1998), with supplementary information from WHO sources.

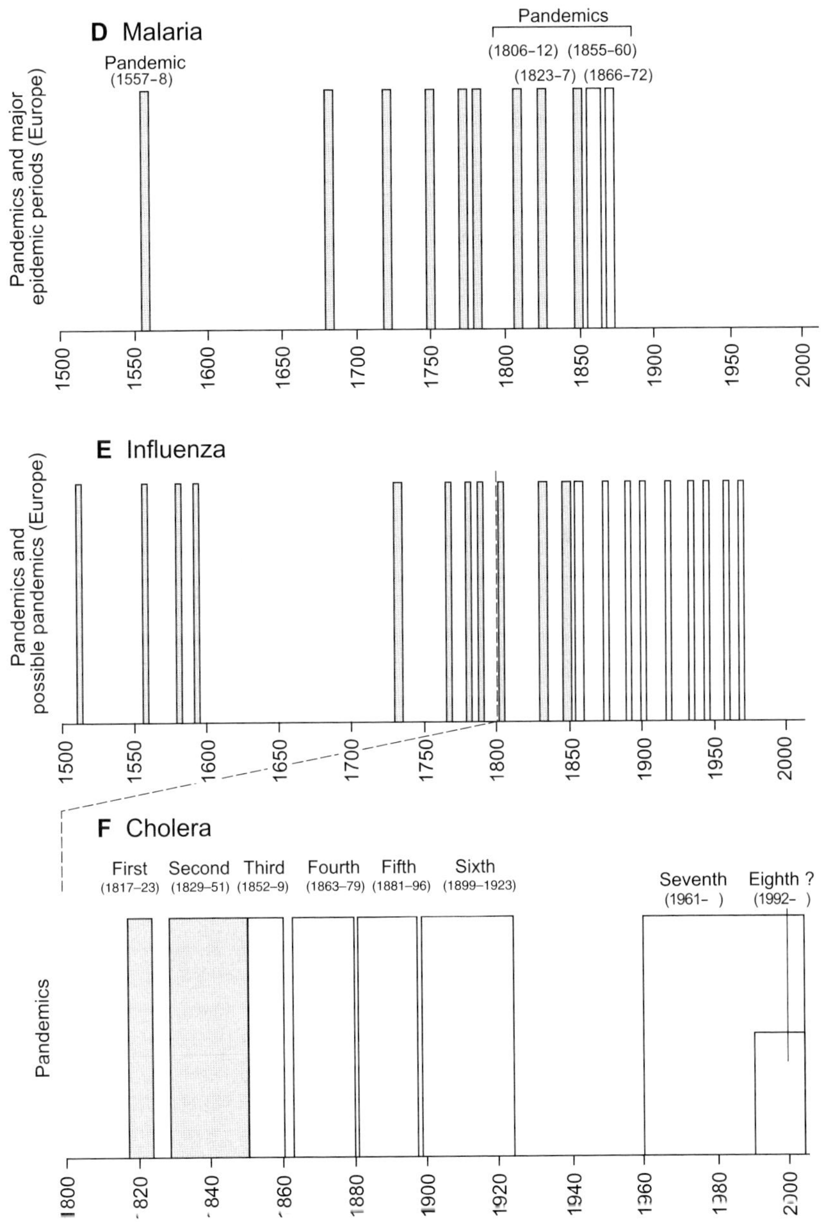

Fig. 2.3 (Continued)

Consistent with these observations, an examination of the archaeoentomological, archaeozoological, and biogeographical evidence leads Panagiotakopulu (2004) to hypothesize that Pharaonic Egypt was the most probable place of origin of bubonic plague as an epidemic disease.

THE PANDEMIC SPREAD OF PLAGUE

While the plague epidemics of antiquity appear to have been relatively geographically confined, the history of the disease from the early Middle Ages is dominated by three great pandemic cycles, each of 50–100 years' duration and each resulting in the spread of *Y. pestis* across much of the civilized world (Figure 2.3A). Here, we examine the diffusion of the First (530s–590s) and Second (1330s–1380s) Plague Pandemics. Our review draws on the accounts of Smallman-Raynor and Cliff (2004*b*: 74–5) and Cliff, Haggett, and Smallman-Raynor (2004: 21–5). The course of the Third Plague Pandemic (1850s–1950s) is treated in Section 9.2.1.

The First Plague Pandemic: The Plague of Justinian (540s–590s)

The sixth century AD is generally recognized as marking the first pandemic cycle of human bubonic plague. An eyewitness account of the emergence and initial spread of the pandemic and its particular coincidence with Byzantine military operations during Emperor Justinian's wars with the Goths and the Persians is provided by the Byzantine historian Procopius (b. *c.*AD 500). According to Procopius, plague first came to light among the Egyptians at Pelusium in 541. From there, the disease

> divided and moved in one direction towards Alexandria and the rest of Aegypt, and in the other direction it came to Palestine on the borders of Aegypt; and from there it spread over the whole world... And this disease always took its start from the coast, and from there went up to the interior. (Procopius 2. 22, trans. Dewing 1914: 455)

Plague reached Byzantium in the spring of 542, where, during the height of the four-month visitation, 'the tale of the dead reached five thousand each day, and again it even came to ten thousand and still more than that' (Procopius 2. 23, trans. Dewing 1914: 465).

It seems reasonable to infer that the epidemic spread outwards from Byzantium with the movements of soldiers who were deployed in operations against the Italian Goths to the west and the Persians to the east; see Kohn (1998). We learn from Procopius that plague 'fell... upon the land of the Persians and visited all the other barbarians besides' (Procopius 2. 23, trans. Dewing 1914: 473). The same source (2. 24) cites the appearance of the disease among the former peoples both as a precipitating factor in Persian efforts to treat for peace in 543 and as an immediate spur for the Roman Byzantine forces to invade Persarmenia. More generally, Russell (1972) suggests that the epidemic resulted in a contraction of the European–Mediterranean population by some 25 per cent. With later recrudescences, the pandemic caused a regional population decline of some 50–60 per cent in the period to 570 and it has been viewed as a major contributor to the political and military decline of the classical Mediterranean civilizations.

The Second Plague Pandemic: The Black Death (1330s–1380s)

In terms of its grip on the public imagination, the Black Death remains one of the most visible symbols of the power and influence of epidemic disease. In 1346 Europe, northern Africa, and the Levant (the westward parts of the Middle East) had a population of the order of 100 million (McEvedy 1988). Within a decade, nearly a quarter of them had died and the population rise that had marked the evolution of medieval society had come to an abrupt end. Although not all historians agree, the cause of what was known as the Great Dying or the Great Pestilence (it was only later that the term 'Black Death' emerged) is generally accepted to have been *Y. pestis*, which, a full eight centuries after its first pandemic cycle in the human population, again spread across the Eurasian landmass.[2]

The spatial origins and full geographical extent of the Black Death still remain to be determined. There are two main competitors for the dubious honour of being the source: (i) an origin east of the Caspian, possibly in eastern Mongolia, Yunnan, or Tibet, and (ii) an origin south of the Caspian in Kurdistan or Iraq. The first is suggested by Arabic sources and by the fact that plague is still enzootic there in various populations of wild rodents. From either of these sources, plague might have spread along the Mongol trade routes east to China, south to India, and west to the Black Sea ports.

Whatever the dispute about the origins, the westward trajectory of the pandemic into and across Europe is well established (Figure 2.4). It reached the Crimea from Central Asia in the winter of 1346–7 and Constantinople by early spring 1347. From there, it moved in two directions: (i) counter-clockwise into the eastern Mediterranean and the Levant; and (ii) clockwise through the western Mediterranean and Europe. As the time-contours on Figure 2.4 indicate, most of Europe was affected before the main wave of the pandemic finally subsided in 1352.

EUROPE: LATER EPIDEMIC CYCLES AND THE RETREAT OF PLAGUE

Cycles of plague continued to visit Europe at intervals over a 450-year period up to the end of the eighteenth century. Mortality in these later epidemics remained high, although the overall devastation of the fourteenth-century pandemic wave was never repeated. Figure 2.5 graphs plague deaths in one London parish (London was then Europe's largest city) for 60 years in the

[2] For evidence of *Y. pestis* as the cause of the Black Death, see Raoult, Aboudharam, *et al.* (2000). For a consideration of alternative aetiologies, see Paterson (2002).

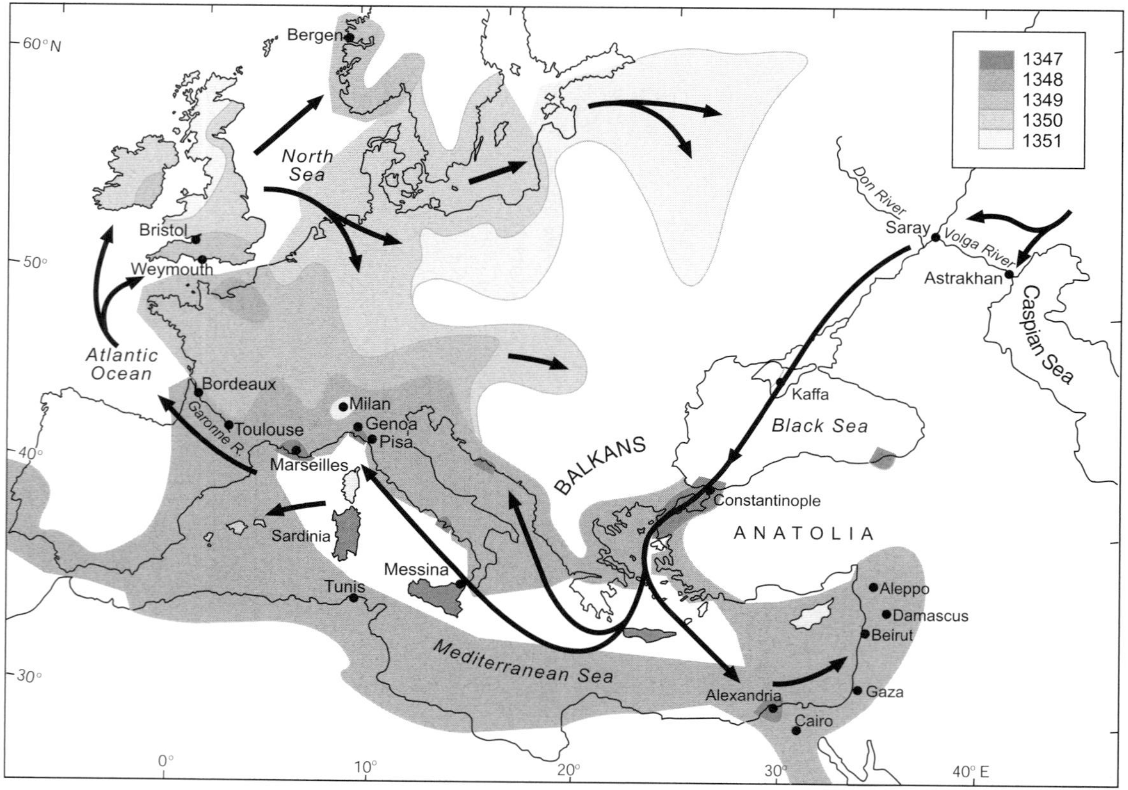

Fig. 2.4. Spread of the Black Death, 1347–1352
Vectors show the main routes by which bubonic plague diffused from Central Asia, via the Ukrainian city of Kaffa, to the Mediterranean and northern Europe. The Mongol–Italian conflict of the mid-1340s, centred on the Genoese occupation of Kaffa, facilitated the spread of the disease from the Black Sea to the Mediterranean ports of Genoa, Venice, and elsewhere.

Sources: Redrawn from Cliff, Haggett, and Smallman-Raynor (1998, fig. 1.3, p. 15), originally from Brock (1990, fig. 1, p. 5).

sixteenth century. Over this time-span some six epidemic episodes were recorded and their effect upon the overall pattern of burials is evident. Later, in 1665, the Great Plague of London was associated with almost 69,000 recorded deaths in a population then estimated at 439,000 (see Section 2.4.2).

The Retreat of Plague

As Hirsch (1883–6: i) observes, the latter part of the seventeenth century marked a turning point in the epidemic history of plague in Europe. The epidemics that had become a more or less permanent epidemiological feature for 300 years began to subside, and the disease began to recede from western and central areas of the continent (Table 2.3). By the mid-eighteenth century, south-eastern Europe remained the only seat of the disease, and, from there, *Y. pestis* occasionally spread northwards—but rarely beyond the Balkan

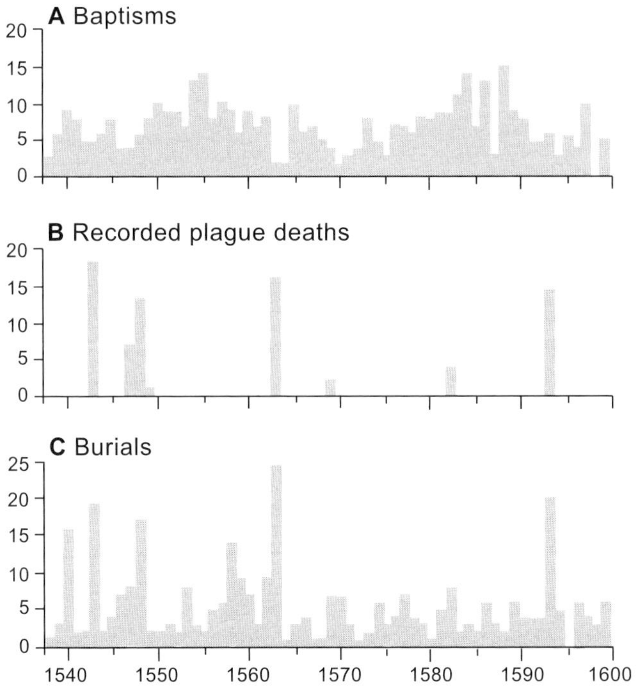

Fig. 2.5. Medieval plague deaths in relation to overall demography
Sixty years of records from a London parish, St Pancras, Soper Lane, from 1538 to 1599. (A) Baptisms. (B) Recorded plague deaths. (C) Burials. Note the lower number of baptisms (bearing in mind the duration of pregnancy) and greater number of burials around plague years.

Sources: Redrawn from Cliff, Haggett, and Smallman-Raynor (2004, fig. 2.9, p. 23), originally based on data in Shrewsbury (1970, fig. 22, p. 175).

Table 2.3. Last recorded epidemics of plague in sample European countries, 1650–1849

Year	Country
1650	Ireland
1654[1]	Denmark
1657[1]	Sweden
1657[2]	Italy
1664–6	Netherlands
1665	England
1667–8[3]	France
1667–8	Switzerland
1669	Belgium
1677–81	Spain
1707–14	Germany
1841	Turkey

Notes: [1] Hirsch (1883–6: i. 501) observes, however, that the disease attacked 'several' places in Denmark and Sweden in the course of 1707–14.[2] An importation of the disease occurred in the province of Bari in 1691.[3] Plague reappeared in Provence in 1720.

Source: Based on information in Hirsch (1883–6: i. 500–4).

peninsula and neighbouring countries. The last epidemic of plague in Turkey was recorded in Constantinople in 1841. Thereafter, no further outbreaks of any size were recorded in Europe until the Third Plague Pandemic of the 1850s–1950s (Raettig *et al.* 1954–61*b*) (Section 9.2.1).

The cause of the retreat of plague from Europe has been a rich source of scholarly debate; see Simpson (1905); Lien-Teh (1936); Pollitzer (1954); Appleby (1980); and Eckert (2000). Improvements in sanitation and hygiene, changing patterns of commerce and trade, the development of resistance to *Y. pestis* in human and/or rodent populations, climate change, the use of arsenical compounds in rodent control, and, as discussed in Section 11.2.1, the development of quarantine control methods have all been advanced to account for the retreat. As Appleby (1980: 173) observes of the available evidence, 'No single explanation seems to fit satisfactorily all the facts drawn from all the geographical regions affected at one time or another,' and the debate over the mechanisms of the retreat is set to continue.

GLOBAL STATUS OF PLAGUE *C.*1850

By the mid-nineteenth century, plague had retreated to permanent enzootic foci in Central Asia and East Africa (see Figure 9.2). As described in Section 9.2.1, it was from the eastern reaches of the vast Central Asian focus that the third great cycle of plague erupted in the 1850s.

2.3.3 *Influenza*

Influenza (ICD-10 J10, J11) is a highly contagious respiratory disease caused by influenza A, B, and C viruses. Epidemic events are restricted to influenza A and B viruses, while pandemic events are associated with the genetically mutable A virus. In human populations, the predominant route of virus transmission is via exposure to droplet emissions from the respiratory tract. Clinically, a short incubation period (typically 1–3 days) is followed by the sudden onset of sore throat, cough, headache, fever, generalized muscle pain, lassitude, and prostration. In mild cases, symptoms may subside in 1–2 weeks, although lethargy and depression may persist for 3–4 weeks. Secondary complications involve the organs of the lower respiratory tract, the cardiovascular system, and the central nervous system (Glezen and Couch 1997; Heymann 2004: 281–7).

INFLUENZA BEFORE AD 1500

Perspectives on the early history of influenza are provided by Hirsch (1883–6: i. 7–54), Clemow (1889–90), and Crosby (1993*a*); see Table 2.2. While the origins of influenza are unknown, biological inference leads Crosby (1993*a*) to suggest that the disease was unlikely to have been common in the period prior to the developments in agriculture, nucleated settlements, and human–animal relations engendered by McMichael's (2004) first historic transition around 5,000–10,000 years ago (Section 2.1). Even then, Clemow (1889–90: 359) submits that it is 'almost impossible' to verify the occurrence of influenza in the pre-Christian era. Hippocrates records an epidemic in 400 BC or thereabouts ('Cough of Perinthus') that could have been influenza (Table 2.1). Several years earlier, in 415 BC, the epidemic that struck the Athenian army during its campaign in Sicily has been adduced by some as influenza. In the Christian era, Clemow (1889–90) provides several instances of influenza-like epidemics in the sixth to

Table 2.4. Epidemics of influenza identified by August Hirsch, 1173–1499

Year	Month	Area of epidemic prevalence
1173	Dec.	England, Germany, Italy
1323	Aug.	France, Italy
1328	Mar.	Italy
1387	Jan.	France (Montpellier), Italy
	Mar.	Germany
1404	—	Germany (Saxony and Thuringia), Netherlands (Flanders)
1411	—	France (Paris)
1414	Jan.	Italy (Bologna, Florence, Forli, and Venice)
	Feb.	France (Paris)
1427	Sept.	France (Paris)

Source: Hirsch (1883–6: i. 7–17).

eleventh centuries, although Hirsch (1883–6: i. 7) argues that many such early references 'bear a stamp too little characteristic' of the disease, and his own survey of influenza begins in AD 1173 (Table 2.4).

THE MODERN PERIOD (AD 1500–1849)

Figure 2.6 is based on the global review of Hirsch (1883–86: i. 7–17) and plots, by year, the number of epidemic outbreaks of influenza documented in the literature from AD 1501. Beginning with the sparse records of the sixteenth and seventeenth centuries, the graph depicts a marked increase in the number and frequency of documented epidemics from the 1720s, reaching a peak in the 1830s.

Cyclical Re-Emergence: The Pandemic Record

Alongside the routine inter-annual upswings in epidemic activity, the influenza record in Figure 2.6 includes events associated with the episodic emergence of novel subtypes of influenza A virus for which the human population has little or no existing immunity. These events, which impart the special character of a cyclically re-emerging disease, underpin the great influenza pandemics that have periodically rolled around the world. Section 4.2.2 reviews the mechanisms

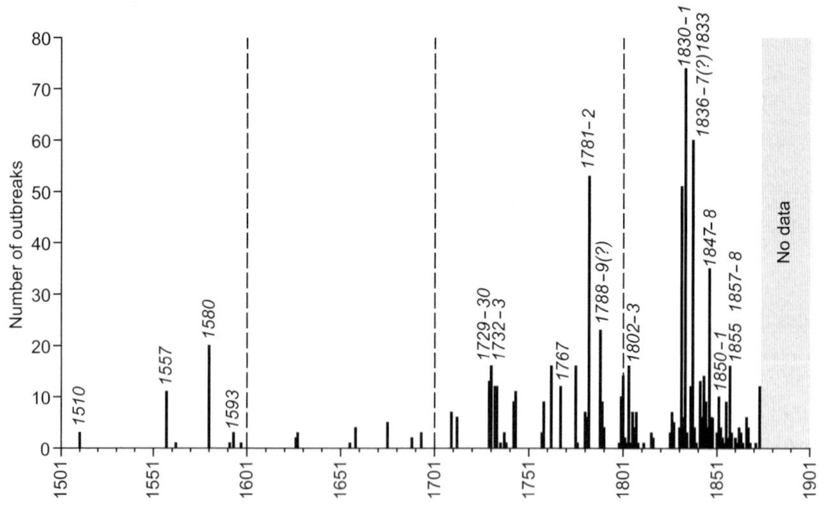

Fig. 2.6. The historical record of influenza outbreaks, 1501–1873
The bar chart plots, by year, the global count of influenza outbreaks as documented in the second edition of August Hirsch's *Handbook of Geographical and Historical Pathology*. The dates of pandemic and probable pandemic events as reported by Hirsch (1883–6) and Patterson (1986) are indicated (see Table 2.5).
Source: Based on Hirsch (1883–6: i. 7–17).

involved in the emergence of pandemic strains of influenza A virus, while Table 2.5 is based on the combined evidence of Hirsch (1883–6: i) and Patterson (1986) and provides summary details of influenza pandemics and probable pandemics in the period 1500–1849. The available evidence points to 13 pandemic events in the 350-year observation period. These events occurred on a highly irregular basis, with an average spacing of 27 years (range 2–136 years) and with a noteworthy absence of evidence of any pandemic activity in the 1600s (Table 2.5).

The maps in Figure 2.7 are based on the analysis of Patterson (1986) and reconstruct the spatial diffusion of five influenza pandemics in the European continent, 1700–1849. Each pandemic wave spread in a characteristic east–west direction, beginning in European Russia and diffusing across the continent as a well-defined wave-front, eventually to reach Iberia after an average interval of 6–8 months. As for the geographical source of the novel influenza A viruses that underpinned these events, Patterson (1986) discounts an origin in southern China (Section 4.2.2) and suggests that the broad area encompassed by south-western Siberia, northern Kazakhstan, and the steppe country between the Volga and the Urals better fits the pre-twentieth-century evidence.

We continue our examination of the pandemic transmission of influenza A viruses, with special reference to the period from 1850, in Sections 4.2 and 10.3.

2.3.4 Asiatic Cholera

Classic Asiatic cholera (ICD-10 A00) is a severe, often rapidly fatal, diarrhoeal disease produced by the bacterium *Vibrio cholerae*. Transmission of the bacterium usually occurs via the ingestion of faecally contaminated water and, less commonly, food. As regards its clinical course, an incubation period of 2–5 days is usually followed by the sudden onset of diarrhoea and vomiting, giving rise to massive fluid loss and dehydration. Consequent symptoms include cramps, a reduction in body temperature, and blood pressure leading to shock and, ultimately, death within a few hours or days of symptom onset. Mortality is typically witnessed in 40–60 per cent of untreated cases (Tauxe 1998; Heymann 2004: 103–11).

The alkaline soils and water of the Ganges–Brahmaputra delta region of north-eastern India form the natural locus of *Vibrio cholerae*, an area whose fertility has ensured historically high population densities. As Tauxe (1998) observes, the bacterium is well adapted to the estuarine environment of the delta region and is likely to have been endemically established for many centuries prior to the sequence of pandemic upwellings depicted in Figure 2.3F.

PRE-PANDEMIC HISTORY: ASIATIC CHOLERA PRIOR TO 1817

The early (pre-pandemic) history of cholera is reviewed by MacNamara (1876), Hirsch (1883–6: i), Macpherson (1884), Pollitzer (1959), and Barua

Table 2.5. Pandemics and probable pandemics of influenza, 1500–1849

Year(s)	Source of information: Hirsch (1883–6)[1,2]	Source of information: Patterson (1986)[3]	Interval since previous pandemic (years)	Notes
1510	[4]	No information	?	'General diffusion in Europe' (Hirsch 1883–6: i. 8)
1557	[4]	No information	47	'General diffusion in Europe' (Hirsch 1883–6: i. 8)
1580	[4]	No information	23	'General diffusion over the East, in Africa and in Europe' (Hirsch 1883–6: i. 8)
1593	[4]	No information	13	'General diffusion' (Hirsch 1883–6: i. 8)
1729–30		[4]	136	Pandemic 'may have become truly worldwide' (Patterson 1986: 14)
1732–3	[4]	[4]	2	'Seemingly a general diffusion over the globe' (Hirsch 1883–6: i. 9)
1767	[4]		34	'Widely diffused over North America and Europe' (Hirsch 1883–6: i. 10)
1781–2	[4]	[4]	14	'General diffusion over the Eastern Hemisphere' (Hirsch 1883–6: i. 11)
1788–9		[4,5]	6	'General diffusion over the Western Hemisphere [1789–90]' (Hirsch 1883–6: i. 11)
1802–3	[4]		13	No information
1830–3	[4]	[4,6]	27	'General diffusion over the Eastern and Western Hemispheres' (Hirsch 1883–6: i. 13)
1836–7	[4]	[4,5]	3	'Considerable diffusion in the Eastern Hemisphere' (Hirsch 1883–6: i. 14)
1847–8	[4]		10	'Generally diffused over the Eastern Hemisphere' (Hirsch 1883–6: i. 16)

Notes: [1] Years 1500–1849.[2] Excludes 'pandemics' listed by Hirsch (1883–6: i. 19) as exclusive to the Western Hemisphere (1647, 1737–8, 1757–8, 1761–2, 1789–90, 1798, 1807, 1815–16, 1824–6, and 1843).[3] Years 1700–1849.[4] Pandemics and probable pandemics. Table 4.1 provides a summary of pandemics and probable pandemics in the period 1850–2005.[5] 'Probable' pandemic.[6] Patterson (1986) defines separate pandemics in the years 1830–1 and 1833.

Sources: Abstracted from Smallman-Raynor and Cliff (2008, table 1, p. 555), originally based on information in Hirsch (1883–6: i. 7–54) and Patterson (1986, table 5.1, p. 83).

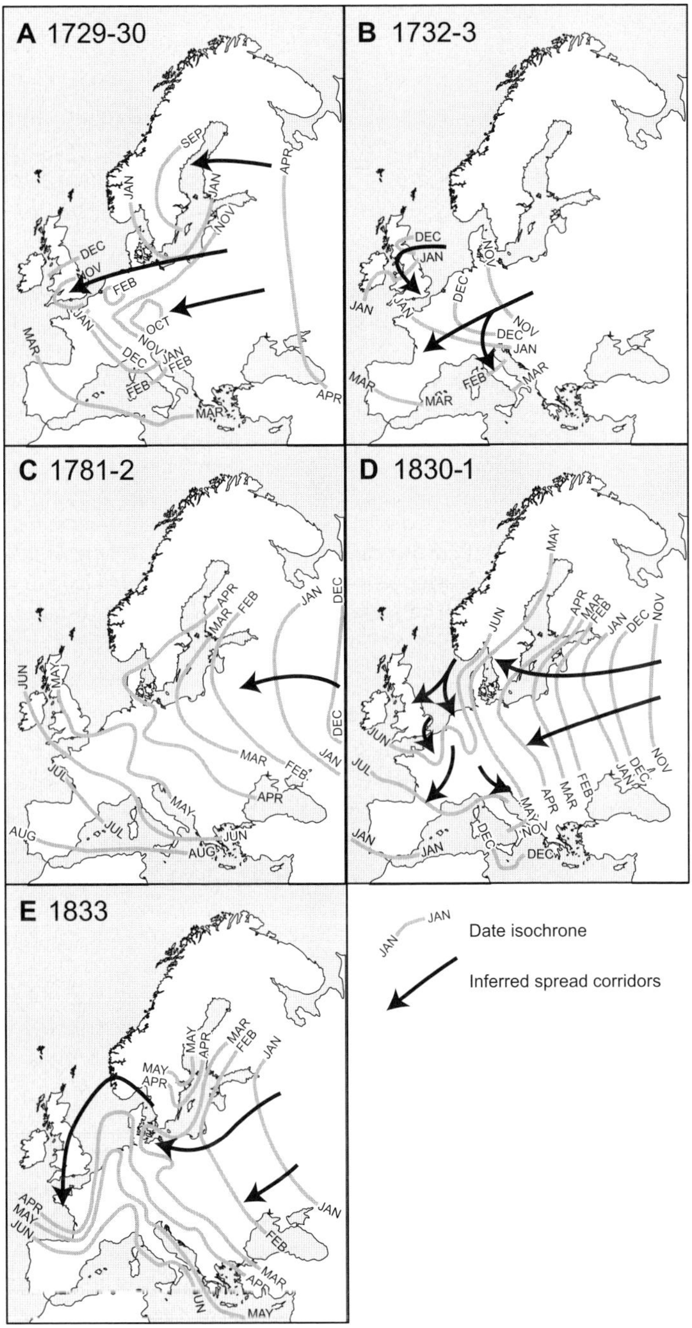

Fig. 2.7. Diffusion of pandemic influenza in Europe, 1700–1849
Maps plot the diffusion of five definite pandemics of influenza identified by Patterson (1986) in the interval 1700–1849 (see Table 2.5). (A) 1729–30. (B) 1732–3. (C) 1781–2. (D) 1830–1. (E) 1833.

Source: Redrawn from Patterson (1986, maps 2.1, 2.2, 2.4, 3.3, 3.4, pp. 14, 16, 21, 34, 37).

(1992), among others. While Sanskrit accounts of cholera or cholera-like illnesses can be deciphered in the writings of Hindu medicine, these and other ancient and medieval notices fail to mention the epidemic character of the disease. Beginning in the early sixteenth century, however, European visitors provide evidence of epidemic cholera over much of India:

> Chronicles describing the spread of cholera epidemics in India... have been left by European travellers, but during the sixteenth century these travellers had little knowledge of any part of India except its Western coast, and the records mainly refer to Calicut, Goa and neighbouring places. In the following century, however, the references extend over a much wider area. Correa described cholera near Calicut in 1503, A'Costa in Kanara in 1577, LeBlanc and LinSchott in Goa in 1580 and 1589, Mandelsloe in Goa in 1639, DeThevenot between Surat and Berhampur in 1666 and Dellon in Goa and Western India in 1676. Later, Thenrhyne mentions outbreaks along the coasts of India in 1679; Colonel Tod gives details of an epidemic of cholera in Goa and Surat in 1683–84; Père Martin in Madura in 1703; Grose in Malabar coast and Bombay in 1750–64; and Orme an epidemic in Tinnevelly in 1757. In the latter half of the eighteenth century the disease seems to have frequently broken out with epidemic violence along the Madras coast, and by the end of the century it had been observed in almost every part of India. (Russell 1929: 1)

'Incomplete or even fragmentary though the evidence... often is,' Pollitzer (1959: 16) observes, 'it leaves no room for doubt that cholera, present in India since ancient times, not only continued to exist but was apt to manifest itself periodically in widespread conflagrations.' Even then, the weight of evidence adduced by Hirsch (1883–6: i) and Pollitzer (1959) indicates that true Asiatic cholera remained largely confined to India and proximal countries prior to 1817.

THE PANDEMIC EMERGENCE OF CHOLERA

The year 1817 marked 'a new epoch in the history of cholera' (Pollitzer 1959: 17). In that year, cholera began to spread as the first in a series of great pandemic waves that, in the ensuing decades, would extend across much of the inhabited world (Figure 2.3F). The reasons why these pandemic outpourings occurred are not known for certain, but they have been linked to the steady improvements throughout the nineteenth century in travel and transport facilities. Cholera became in this way one of the most important modern pandemic diseases and, apart from influenza and HIV/AIDS, it has covered larger areas of the globe than any other infectious disease.

Authorities are divided on the exact number and timings of cholera pandemics in the nineteenth and early twentieth centuries. In the post-war literature, Pollitzer's (1959) account of six pandemics in the period 1817–1923 is probably the best known, and we follow his historical sequence in the present analysis (Table 2.6).[3] For the two pandemic events with onset in the period prior to 1850,

[3] For perspectives on the pandemic timings of Pollitzer (1959), see Tauxe (1998: 224) and Speck (1993: 647).

Table 2.6. Dates of occurrence of cholera pandemics, 1817–2005

	Authority						
Pandemic	Haeser (1882)	Hirsch (1883–6)	Sticker (1912)	Kolle and Prigge (1928)	Pollitzer (1959)	Wilson and Miles (1975)	Kaper *et al.* (1995)
First	1816–23/ 1826–37	1817–23	1817–38		1817–23	1817–23	
Second	1840–50	1826–37	1840–64		1829–51	1826–37	
Third	1852–60		1863–75		1852–9	1846–62	
Fourth	1863–73	1865–75	1881–96		1863–79	1864–75	
Fifth			1899–	1883–96;	1881–96	1883–96	
Sixth				1902–23	1899–1923	1899–1923	
Seventh							1961–present
Eighth?							1992–present

Sources: Adapted from Pollitzer (1959, table 1, p. 17), Barua and Greenough (1992, table 1, p. 8), and Kaper *et al.* (1995, table 8, p. 68).

Figure 2.8 traces the diffusion corridors of the First Cholera Pandemic (1817–23; map A) and the two major phases of the Second Cholera Pandemic (1829–36, 1840–51; maps B, C). We briefly consider each pandemic in turn.

The First Cholera Pandemic (1817–1823) (Figure 2.8A)

Details of the course of the First Cholera Pandemic are provided by Hirsch (1883–6: i. 394–7) and Pollitzer (1959: 17–21), and we draw on their accounts here. The earliest reliable information relating to the spread of the pandemic can be traced to the Ganges–Brahmaputra delta region of India, where the disease had attained epidemic proportions by the late summer of 1817. Cholera diffused over the 'greater part' of India in the course of the following year (MacNamara 1876: 52) with onwards transmission, across the borders of indigenous territory, for Ceylon, Burma, Siam, Mauritius, and Réunion by 1819. Thereafter, the disease penetrated East Africa, Arabia, Persia, and, by way of the latter, Astrakhan in non-European Russia. The actions of the authorities at Astrakhan served to halt the further advance of cholera towards European soil and, with the onset of the winter of 1823–4, the pandemic finally retreated from Central Asia and other extra-Indian locations.

The Second Cholera Pandemic (1829–1851) (Figure 2.8B,C)

Following an epidemiological lull of some six years, cholera re-emerged with pandemic force in the late 1820s. The pandemic was characterized by two major phases of transmission (1829–36 and 1840–51), each phase presaged by an increased level of cholera activity in north-eastern India, and with each associated with the extensive spread of the disease in Arabia, North Africa, Central Asia, and on for Europe and the Americas in 1832 (Figure 2.8B) and 1849 (Figure 2.8C). Inasmuch as the two phases differed substantially in their geographical reach, the second was marked out by a major visitation of the

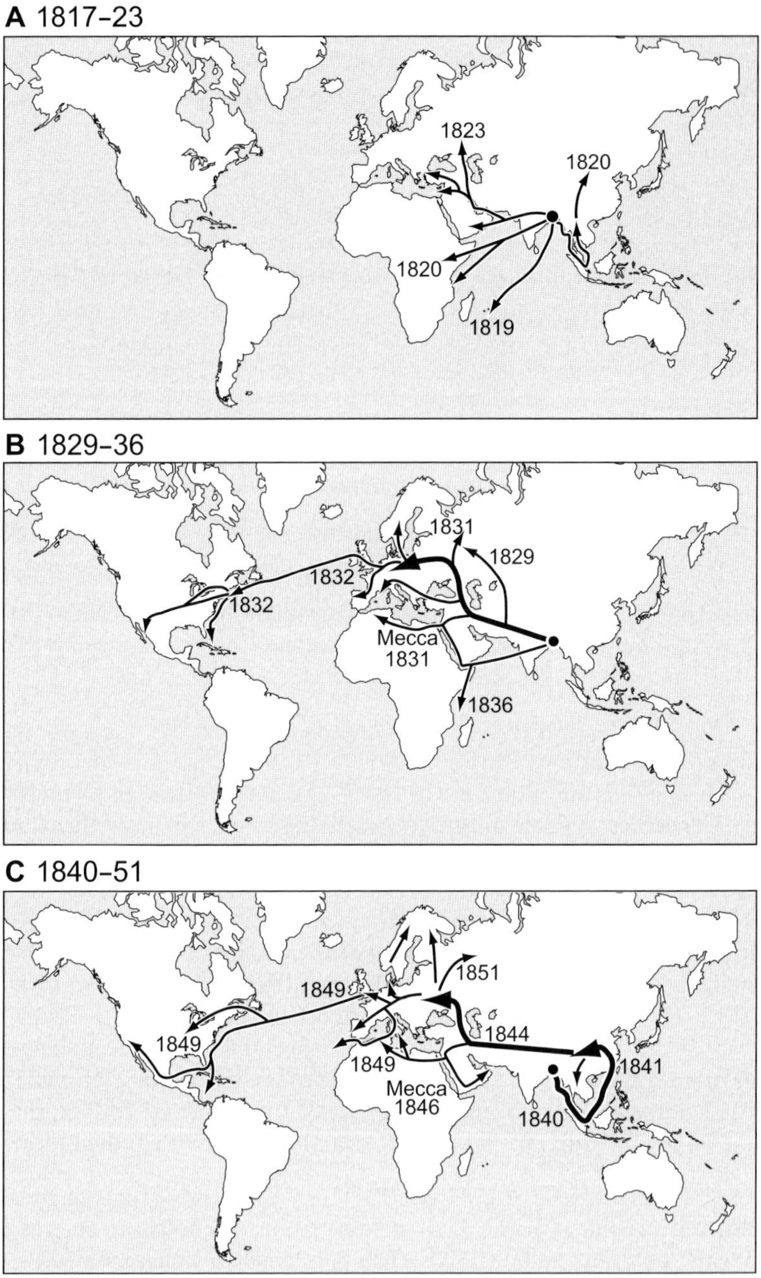

Fig. 2.8. Global diffusion routes of the First (1817–1823) and Second (1829–1851) Cholera Pandemics

Vectors show the diffusion of cholera associated with the first pandemic (1817–23; map A) and the two major phases of the second pandemic (1829–36, 1840–51; maps B, C). Pandemic timings are based on Pollitzer (1959); see Table 2.6.

Source: Redrawn from Cliff and Haggett (1988, fig. 1.1D, p. 5).

disease in China and other parts of South-East Asia (Hirsch 1883–6: i. 397–413; Pollitzer 1959: 21–30).

GLOBAL STATUS OF CHOLERA *C*.1850

Vibrio cholerae appears to have lingered in at least some of the places touched by the second pandemic, leading Pollitzer (1959: 30) to describe the succeeding pandemic (1852–9) as 'the combined result of local recrudescences due to a temporary encroachment of the infection and of repeated importations of the disease'. We return to the historical sequence of cholera pandemics, with special reference to the period from 1850, in Section 9.2.2.

2.3.5 Mysterious and Undetermined Conditions

Epidemic history is littered with examples of mysterious and unidentified diseases that have suddenly appeared, and spread for greater or lesser periods of time, before retreating into obscurity. In this subsection, we briefly examine two such examples from the late Middle Ages onwards: the sweating sicknesses of Europe and the haemorrhagic fevers (*cocoliztli*) of colonial Mexico.

SWEATING SICKNESSES IN EUROPE

English Sweating Sickness

In the midsummer of 1485—just as the English Wars of the Roses (1455–85) were about to reach their conclusion at Bosworth Field—a previously unknown, and rapidly fatal, infection began to extend across England. As described by T. Forrestier in 1490, the disease had an acute onset with 'a sudden great sweating and stinking with redness of the face and of all the body' (T. Forrestier, cited in Hunter 1991: 303)—symptoms from which the name 'English sweating sickness' was derived. Other manifestations included fever, headache, lethargy, pulmonary involvement, and delirium. The course of the disease was generally swift, often with fatal outcome (probably due to dehydration, circulatory shock, and electrolyte loss) within a day of clinical onset; for those who did not succumb, there was usually complete recovery in 1–2 weeks (Hecker 1859).

The English sweating sickness of 1485 appears to have been an entirely novel disease; it spread in epidemic form on just four subsequent occasions (Table 2.7),[4] before apparently disappearing from the epidemiological scene.

[4] There is some discrepancy in the literature regarding the exact dates of the five recorded outbreaks of English sweating sickness. Hecker (1859) follows the epidemic timings in John Caius' treatise of 1552, giving the dates as 1485, 1506, 1517, 1528, and 1551. Hirsch (1883–6: i. 82–4) gives the dates as 1486, 1507, 1518, 1529, and 1551, and Creighton (1891–4: i. 237–81) gives the dates as 1485, 1508, 1517, 1528–9, and 1551. Hirsch's date for the first outbreak, which coincided with the Battle of Bosworth Field (1485), is clearly in error, while Creighton (1891–4: i. 244 n. 1) notes that Hecker's date for the second visitation is also erroneous. Under these circumstances, we follow Creighton's authoritative *History* in the timings of the outbreaks given in Table 2.7.

Table 2.7. Summary details of recorded outbreaks of English sweating sickness, 1485–1551

Year(s)	Dates: Onset	Dates: End	Place of first report	Infected locations
1485	Sept.	Early winter	London	England (Bristol, London, Oxford)
1508	*c.*July	Aug.?	London	England (London, Oxford?)
1517	*c.*July	Dec.?	London	England (London, Oxford), France (Calais)
1528–9	May/June 1528	*c.*Dec. 1529	London	England, Denmark, France (Calais), Germany, Livonia, Lithuania, Netherlands, Poland, Russia, Sweden, Switzerland
1551	Apr.	Sept.	Shrewsbury	England

Source: Based on information in Creighton (1891–4: i. 237–81).

The exact nature of the disease is uncertain. Medieval and early modern observers appear to have distinguished it from influenza, malaria, plague, and typhus fever (Thwaites *et al.* 1997), while Vergil states that it was 'a new kind of disease, from which no former age had suffered, as all agree' (cited in Creighton 1891–4: i. 240). Among modern assessments of aetiology, Wylie and Collier (1981) suggest that the disease was probably caused by an arbovirus. Hunter (1991) favours an enterovirus, while Thwaites *et al.* (1997) and Taviner *et al.* (1998) postulate a viral agent with a marked pulmonary component and a rodent reservoir. In a further contribution to the debate, Carlson and Hammond (1999) contend that the epidemiological and clinical profile corresponds to one of the haemorrhagic fevers, of which only Crimean Congo haemorrhagic fever had the potential to establish itself in enzootic form in England during the medieval period. Most recently, McSweegan (2004) has suggested that the disease may have been inhalational anthrax.

Miliary Fever ('Picardy Sweat')

Well over a century and a half after the last documented outbreak of English sweating sickness, a clinically similar acute infective illness appeared in France. Known as 'miliary fever', 'Suette des Picards', or the 'Picardy sweat', the disease was characterized by the sudden onset of profuse sweating with a penetrating odour, the sensation of a severe constriction in the pit of the stomach, shortness of breath, palpitations, gastric symptoms, and a characteristic papular and vesicular rash. Beginning with the first unambiguous outbreaks of the disease, centred on Abbeville and Amiens in Picardy, northern France, in the summer of 1718, Hirsch (1883–6: i. 88–95) documents a total of 194 outbreaks of miliary fever in France to 1874. These outbreaks were largely concentrated in the periods 1730–85 and 1820–70 (Figure 2.9) and were associated with a progressive extension of the disease from

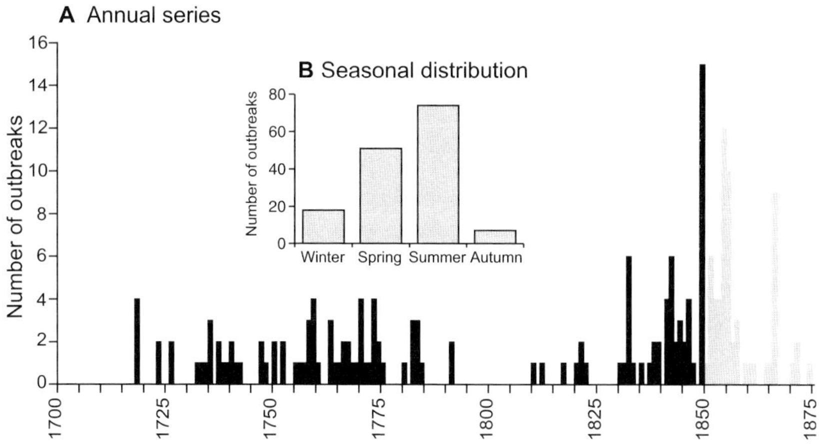

Fig. 2.9. Outbreaks of miliary fever in France, 1700–1874
(A) Number of documented outbreaks by year, 1700–1849 (black bars) and 1850–74 (grey bars). The inset graph (B) shows the seasonal distribution of documented outbreaks, with a characteristic peak of disease activity in the spring and summer months.
Source: Drawn from Hirsch (1883–6: i. 89–93).

a primary focus in northern *départements* to include parts of central and southern France in later years (Figure 2.10). Most of the outbreaks are said to have remained limited to a single village or a few localities, although Hirsch (1883–6: i. 94) observes that the outbreaks of 1832, 1842, 1853, and 1854 were more widespread and 'imparted a pandemic character to the disease'.

Miliary fever was by no means restricted to France. Reports of the disease began to accumulate in Italy from the mid-eighteenth century, Germany from the start of the nineteenth century, and, to a lesser extent, Belgium from the late 1830s (Hirsch 1883–6: i. 95–9).[5] The disease continued to occur through the nineteenth century, with the last significant outbreak recorded in France in 1926 (Kohn 1998). As to the nature of miliary fever, Hecker (1859) differentiates it from the earlier English sweating sickness on account of the presence of a characteristic rash and the longer duration of febrile symptoms. Hirsch (1883–6: i. 110), however, has 'no doubt . . . of the close relations between the two diseases' and cites the 1802 outbreak of a malignant sweating illness at Röttingen, Bavaria, as evidence of a malady that shared characteristics of both miliary fever and the English sweat.[6]

[5] The early history of miliary fever in Germany is unclear. Hecker (1859) traces the disease back to Leipzig in 1652, with further outbreaks in Germany throughout the second half of the 17th century. Hirsch (1883–6: i), however, points to the confusion of miliary fever with other conditions in German medical writings (pp. 86–7) and suggests that the first reasonably clear records of the disease in the country date to about 1801 (p. 97).

[6] We note here that Hecker (1859) distinguishes the Röttingen sweating sickness of 1802 from miliary fever and claims it to have been a reappearance of the English sweating sickness of earlier times.

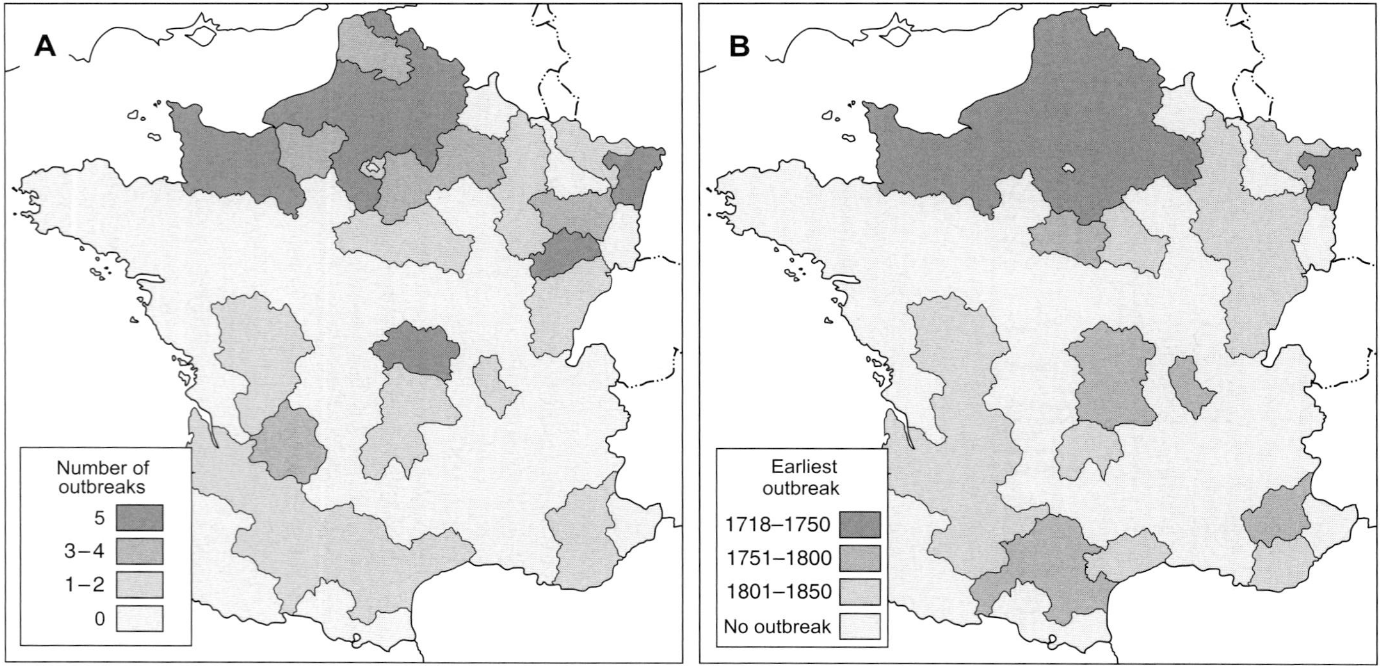

Fig. 2.10. Miliary fever outbreaks in the *départements* of France, 1718–1850
(A) Documented number of outbreaks by *département*, showing a primary focus of outbreak activity in northern France. (B) Date of earliest documented outbreak in each *département*, showing a progressive extension of the disease from northern France to other parts of the country from the mid-18th century.

Source: Drawn from Hirsch (1883–6: i. 89–93).

EMERGENT HAEMORRHAGIC FEVERS: *COCOLIZTLI* IN MEXICO (1545–1815)

Acuna-Soto, Romero, *et al.* (2000) and Acuna-Soto, Stahle, Cleaveland, *et al.* (2004) record how, in 1545–8, a previously unrecognized haemorrhagic disease with high fatality spread in the native Indian population of highland Mexico. The illness was characterized by the acute onset of fever, with vertigo, headache, bleeding from the nose, ears, and mouth, jaundice, severe abdominal and thoracic pain, and acute neurological manifestations. The epidemic lasted for four years, extending across the country and coinciding with the loss of some 80 per cent of the native Indian population. The disease was termed *cocoliztli* (Nahuatl for 'pestilence') and both Aztec and Spanish physicians differentiated it from such Old World infections as smallpox, measles, typhus fever, pertussis, and malaria. Further major epidemics of clinically similar haemorrhagic fevers (later termed *matlazahuatl*) were recorded in 1576, 1736, and 1813, with a number of lesser outbreaks in the intervening years.[7]

As to the nature of *cocoliztli*, Acuna-Soto, Romero, *et al.* (2000) suggest that the course of the disease is reminiscent of the viral haemorrhagic fevers. Marr and Kiracofe (2000) concur, and propose that agricultural and other ecological changes in Post-Colombian Mexico may have precipitated as yet unidentified pathogenic arenaviruses of the type responsible for such rodent-borne conditions as Argentine, Bolivian, and Venezuelan haemorrhagic fevers (Section 7.2.1). Consistent with the possible rodent-borne nature of the disease, evidence is accumulating that sixteenth-century outbreaks of *cocoliztli* responded to the precipitation regime of Mexico in a manner reminiscent of that described for hantavirus pulmonary syndrome (HPS) in Section 7.5.3 (Acuna-Soto, Stahle, Cleaveland, *et al.* 2002, 2004).[8]

2.4 Long-Term Trends: The London Mortality Series, 1603–1849

2.4.1 Background: The Ebb and Flow of Infection in Britain

Well over a century has passed since the first publication of Charles Creighton's *A History of Epidemics in Britain* (Creighton 1891–4). Endorsed at the time by *The Lancet* as 'a great work—great in conception, in learning, in industry, in philosophic insight' (Anonymous 1894: 1543), Creighton's *History* provides a

[7] Outbreak years include: 1555, 1559, 1566, 1587–8, 1592–3, 1601–2, 1604–7, 1613, 1624–31, 1633–4, and 1641–2. See Acuna-Soto, Romero, *et al.* (2000) for further details.

[8] The ideas are developed further by Acuna-Soto, Stahle, Therrell, *et al.* (2005), who hypothesize that, in much earlier centuries, 'the massive population loss of the Terminal Classic Period in Mesoamerica (AD 750–950) may have been due in part to epidemics of hemorrhagic fevers during the megadroughts of the eighth, ninth and tenth centuries' (p. 407).

singular and unrivalled account of epidemic-prone diseases in the British Isles, AD 664–1894. Beginning with the spread of a mysterious pestilence (*pestis ictericia*) in southern England in AD 664, and ending with an appended note on the emergence of a seemingly new disease ('cerebrospinal fever' or meningococcal meningitis) in mid-nineteenth-century Britain, Creighton's narrative is imbued with a sense of the historical ebb and flow of infection:

In the long period covered by this history we have seen much coming and going among the epidemic infections, in some cases a dramatic and abrupt entrance or exit, in other cases a gradual and unperceived substitution. Some of the greatest of those changes have fallen within the two hundred years since Sydenham kept notes of the prevalent epidemics of London. We are that posterity, or a generation of it, which he expected would have its own proper experiences of epidemics and at the same time would know all that had passed meanwhile . . . (Creighton 1891–4: ii. 631)

Daniel Thomson (1955: 106) follows Creighton by pointing to the rise and fall of a long succession of infectious diseases that 'became fatalistically accepted . . . in the inevitable order of things' by the people of the British Isles. Elements of that succession are captured in Figure 2.11, where plague, followed by typhus fever, smallpox, measles, scarlet fever, cholera, typhoid fever, diphtheria, and influenza, are each shown to have emerged as prominent epidemiological forces at various times from the seventeenth to the twentieth centuries.

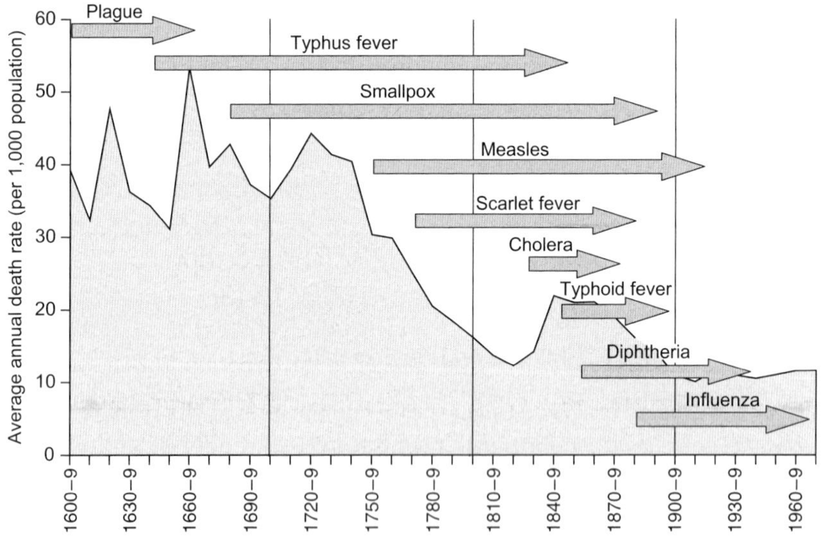

Fig. 2.11. The ebb and flow of infectious diseases in Britain
Vectors are based on information included in Thomson (1955) and Creighton (1891–4: i and ii) and depict major periods of activity associated with sample infectious diseases, 1600–1979. The line trace plots, by 10-year period, the average annual death rate per 1,000 population for the city of London.

2.4.2 The London Mortality Series

To examine long-term trends in the ebb and flow of infectious diseases, we draw on two classic sources in historical epidemiology (the London *Bills of Mortality* and the General Register Office's cause-of-death statistics) to construct annual series of cause-specific mortality for London, 1603–1849. Our examination of these series is framed by a substantial literature on historical patterns of mortality in London, including the major studies and overviews of Creighton (1891–4), Matossian (1985), Landers (1993), and, beyond the immediate time-frame of the present section, Hardy (1993*c*).

THE DATABASE

Information relating to the annual count of deaths for all causes and 12 sample infectious diseases was abstracted for London from the *Bills of Mortality* (1603–1836) and the Registrar General's *Annual Report* (1837–1920) and *Statistical Review* (1921–73) to yield a 13 (cause) × 371 (year) matrix of deaths, 1603–1973. Here, the time brackets of the matrix extend from the onset of the regular publication of the *Bills of Mortality* (1603) to the cessation of the routine publication of London mortality statistics with the termination of the *Statistical Review* (1973). The original matrix of deaths was then scaled by annual population estimates, generated by linear interpolation from the 50- and 10-year population estimates for London included in Mitchell (2007), to form a further 13 × 371 matrix of deaths per 1,000 population. In the present section, we use the matrices of annual deaths and death rates to examine long-term trends in mortality in the

Table 2.8. Average annual mortality due to sample infectious diseases, London, 1600s–1800s

	Average annual count of deaths[1]		
Cause of death	1603–99	1700–99	1800–49
Cholera	0 (0.00)	0 (0.00)	1,202 (0.12)
Diphtheria	0 (0.00)	0 (0.00)	0 (0.00)
Influenza	0 (0.00)	0 (0.00)	72 (0.03)
Leprosy	1 (0.00)	2 (0.00)	0 (0.00)
Measles	79 (0.21)	194 (0.30)	808 (0.46)
Meningococcal disease[2]	0 (0.00)	0 (0.00)	0 (0.00)
Plague	1,885 (5.03)	0 (0.00)	0 (0.00)
Scarlet fever	0 (0.00)	3 (0.00)	1,811 (0.20)
Smallpox	1,012 (2.70)	1,945 (2.99)	928 (0.61)
Syphilis[3]	56 (0.15)	70 (0.11)	36 (0.02)
Tuberculosis (pulmonary)[4]	3,094 (8.25)	4,056 (6.24)	5,195 (3.11)
Whooping cough	0 (0.00)	174 (0.27)	962 (0.51)
All causes	15,686 (41.83)	22,858 (35.17)	27,991 (15.69)

Notes: [1] Average annual death rate per 1,000 population in parentheses. [2] Cerebrospinal meningitis. [3] Classified under 'French pox' in the London *Bills*. [4] Classified under 'consumption' in the London *Bills*.

period to 1849. For reference, Table 2.8 gives average annual counts of mortality associated with the 13 causes of death, along with the corresponding death rates per 1,000 population, for intervals in the period under observation. The corresponding data for the period 1850–1973 are analysed in Section 9.5.

Data Quality

Reviews of data quality are provided for the *Bills of Mortality* by Landers (1993: 91–3, 193–4) and for the Registrar General's cause of death statistics by Hardy (1994). For the centuries covered by the *Bills*, the accuracy of the available data cannot be established with any degree of certainty, although substantial levels of under-recording are generally suspected. Officially, the *Bills* only include information relating to burials within Anglican grounds. Even then, it seems doubtful that the records are entirely accurate, and both systematic and random elements impinge on the confidence that can be placed in the available data. By the end of the eighteenth century, the geographical limits of London as a functioning urban unit extended well beyond the limits of the parishes covered by the *Bills*, thereby ensuring the omission of deaths in areas that, at one time or another, constituted the outer reaches of the metropolitan sprawl. Difficulties also arise in the interpretation of specific causes of death. In the context of the present analysis, the term 'consumption' was used not exclusively for deaths arising from pulmonary tuberculosis, but also as a catchall category for wasting, marasmus, and other ill-defined conditions. Confusion between smallpox, measles, and other diseases is a perennial problem in early mortality records, while a number of major infectious conditions (including influenza and scarlet fever) were not differentiated as distinct clinical entities in the *Bills* until the late eighteenth and nineteenth centuries. While vital registration ushered in a more precise set of diagnostic categories, Matossian (1985: 185) observes that, as late as 1860, almost 20 per cent of all deaths were uncertified and that registration 'was not reasonably complete until after 1861'. Under these circumstances, all results to be presented are subject to the caveat of data quality.

MORTALITY CURVES

The black section of the histogram in Figure 2.12 plots the estimated annual death rate per 1,000 population for London, 1603–1849. Consistent with the early stages of Omran's epidemiological transition model (Section 1.4.1), the first 150 years of the mortality curve are characterized by high background death rates (30–50 deaths per 1,000 population), punctuated by a series of plague-related 'mortality crises' in 1603, 1609, 1625, 1636, and 1665. From the mid-eighteenth century, levels of mortality begin a secular decline that continues until the statistical hiatus associated with the introduction of national vital registration in 1837.[9] Beyond the time-frame of the current

[9] The statistical hiatus associated with the introduction of vital registration in 1837 can be accounted for by the more complete recording of deaths, including the enumeration of Dissenters and those buried in non-Anglican lands.

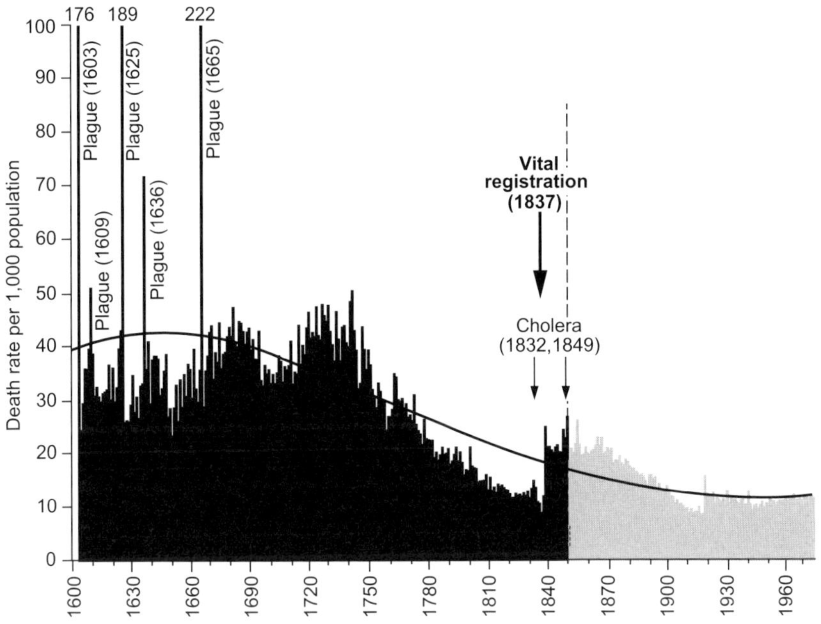

Fig. 2.12. Estimated annual death rate per 1,000 population, London, 1603–1849
The graph plots, as the black section of the histogram, the estimated annual death rate for 1603–1849. The equivalent information for the interval 1850–1973 is plotted in grey. The overall trend in the death rate, 1603–1973, is depicted by a polynomial regression line fitted to the data by ordinary least squares. The last of the major plague epidemics (1603–65) and the first of the major cholera epidemics (1832–49) to strike London are indicated.

discussion, the grey section of the histogram shows a resumption of the downward trend in mortality in subsequent years (see Section 9.5.1).

Infectious Diseases

Mortality curves for each of the 12 sample diseases in Table 2.8 are given in Figure 2.13. The shaded sections of the curves plot, by 10-year period, the average annual death rate per 1,000 population, 1600–1849.[10] For reference, the unshaded sections of the curves plot the corresponding information for later decennial periods. Subject to the limitations of the available data, the graphs underscore the locally complex pattern of disease succession in the period prior to 1850. While the 1670s marked the final extinction of plague in the city (Figure 2.13G), other diseases were in the ascendancy. Smallpox, which is said to have begun to attain significance as a cause of death in the reign of James

[10] Note that, with the exception of plague, no data are available for the decennial periods 1600–9 and 1610–19. For plague, the average annual death rate for 1600–9 has been computed on the basis of the seven observation points for which data are available (1603, . . . , 1609).

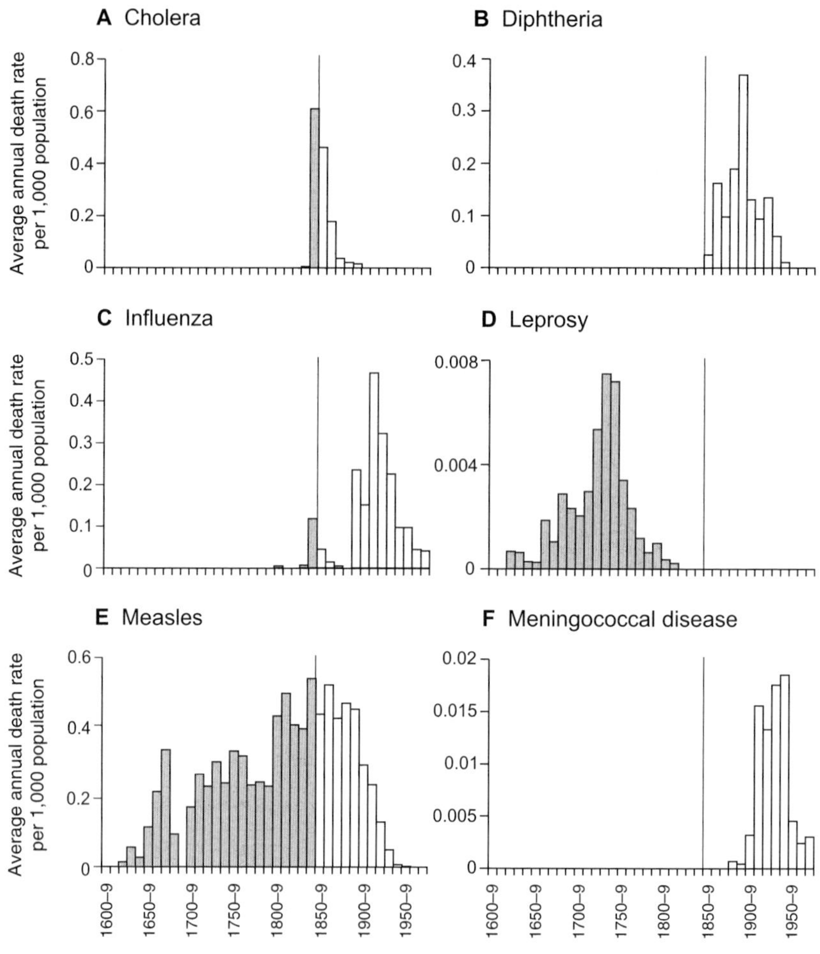

Fig. 2.13. Time series of reported mortality for sample infectious diseases in London Histograms plot, by 10-year period, the average annual death rate per 1,000 population for 1600–1849 (shaded bars); the corresponding information for later periods is shown for reference (unshaded bars). (A) Cholera. (B) Diphtheria. (C) Influenza. (D) Leprosy. (E) Measles. (F) Meningococcal disease (cerebrospinal meningitis). (G) Plague. (H) Scarlet fever. (I) Smallpox. (J) Syphilis. (K) Tuberculosis (pulmonary). (L) Whooping cough. Note that, with the exception of plague, no data are available for the decennial periods 1600–9 and 1610–19. For plague, the average annual rate for 1600–9 has been computed on the basis of the seven observation points for which data are available (1603, . . . , 1609).

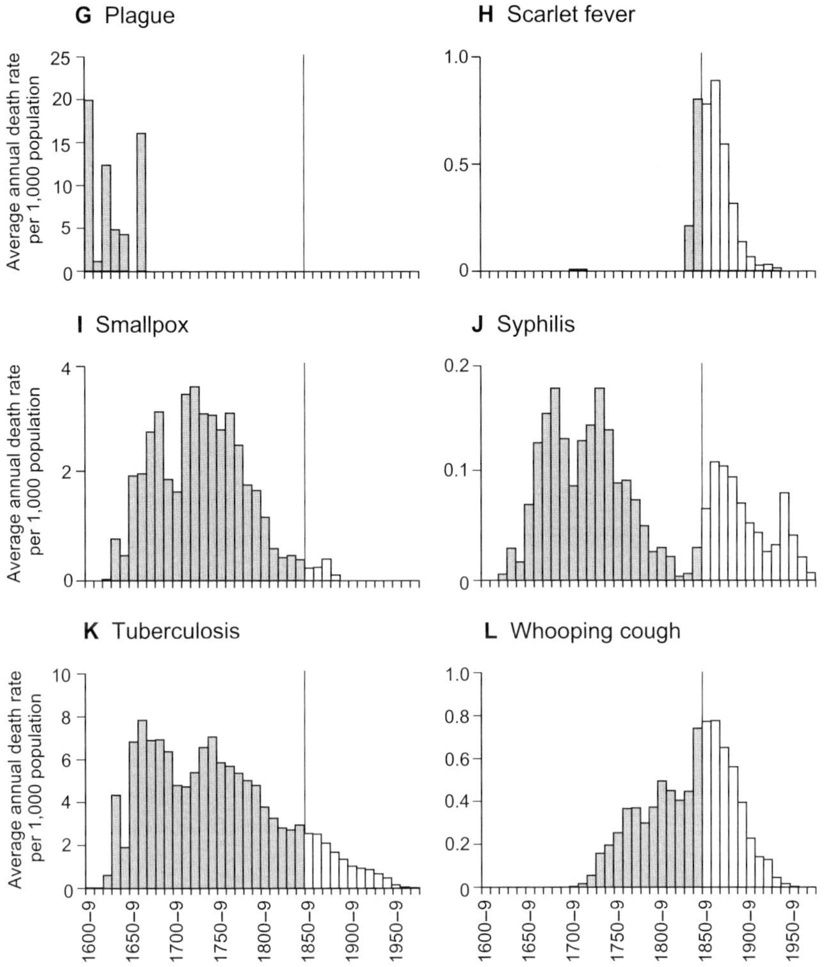

Fig. 2.13 (Continued)

I (1603–25), had achieved the status of an 'alarming disease' in London by the mid-seventeenth century (Figure 2.13I) (Creighton 1891–4: ii. 436)[11]—a situation that was gradually quelled by inoculation, among other factors, from the late eighteenth century (Hardy 1983). As smallpox retreated, mortality due to two other long-term incumbents of the city—measles (Figure 2.13E) and whooping cough (Figure 2.13L)—was increasing, with the great measles epidemic of 1807–8 marked out as 'the first of a series of epidemics in which the disease established not only its equality with smallpox as a cause of infantile

[11] Hardy (1983) notes that the 'native strain' of smallpox virus in Britain was probably of a mild form and that the introduction of more virulent strains from abroad would account for the documented increase in smallpox mortality during the 17th and 18th centuries.

deaths but even its supremacy over the latter' (Creighton 1891–4: ii. 650). Shortly thereafter, cholera exploded onto the epidemiological scene in the 1830s and 1840s (Figure 2.13A).

Some of the other conditions in Figure 2.13 were long present in the city, but not formally recorded as separate disease categories until relatively recent times—an indicator of growing medical awareness of the conditions. Influenza emerged from the 'epidemic agues' as a distinct clinical entity in the *Bills* at the end of the eighteenth century (Figure 2.13C), while scarlet fever was formally differentiated from fevers, measles, and other causes of death in the 1830s—'long after it had become an important factor in ... mortality' (Figure 2.13H) (Creighton 1891–4: ii. 719). The remaining graphs in Figure 2.13 chart the rise and fall of leprosy (D), syphilis (J), and tuberculosis (K) at various times during the seventeenth to nineteenth centuries, while the emergence of diphtheria (B) and meningococcal disease (F) as distinct clinical entities in the post-1849 period is examined in Section 9.5.

EPIDEMIC WAVELENGTH

The population of London grew exponentially over the period embraced by the shaded sections of the histograms in Figure 2.13, increasing from an estimated 200,000 (1600) to 2,600,000 (1849). Here, we examine whether this order of magnitude growth in the urban population reservoir was associated with changes in the epidemic frequency or *wavelength* of the diseases in Table 2.8.

Method: Autocorrelation Functions (ACFs)

One standard approach to the identification of cyclical components in a time series is to compute the autocorrelation function (ACF). The theory involved is discussed in Box *et al.* (1994: 21–45). In brief, the ACF computes the degree of correlation between all pairs of observations in a series which are 1, 2, 3, ..., T time intervals apart. Let y_t denote the value of some variable (in the present analysis, death rates per 1,000 population) at time t and y_{t-k} denote its value at a time period k lags removed from t. Then, the kth lag autocorrelation, r_k, can be computed from

$$r_k = \left[\sum_{t=1}^{T-k} (y_t - \bar{y})(y_{t+k} - \bar{y}) \right] / \sum_{t=1}^{T} (y_t - \bar{y})^2, \qquad (2.1)$$

where $\bar{y}$ is the mean of the T-element time series. The greater the degree of association between all pairs of observations k lags apart, the bigger will be the correlation. Perfect positive association yields a value of 1.0, a perfect inverse relationship a value of–1.0, while no association yields a value of zero. The number of time periods separating any pair of observations is termed the lag. This is plotted on the horizontal axis of an ACF, while the correlation, r_k for lag k, is plotted on the vertical axis.

For each of the 12 sample diseases in Table 2.8, ACFs were computed on the basis of the annual series of death rates per 1,000 population for seven discrete time periods: 1650–99, 1700–49, 1750–99, 1800–49, 1850–99, 1900–49, and 1950–73. To meet the basic assumption of time-stationarity in the ACF methodology, all analysis was undertaken on data that had been detrended by the technique of first differencing (Chatfield 2003: 19–20). In the discussion to follow, we examine the resulting ACFs for the time intervals 1650–99, 1700–49, 1750–99, and 1800–49. The ACFs for later time periods are examined in Section 9.5.2.

Results

To illustrate the analysis undertaken, the ACFs for one disease (measles) are plotted as graphs A–D in Figure 2.14. Reading across the set of ACFs, the changing value of lag k at which the maximum correlation r_k occurs is indicative of a reduction in the wavelength of the dominant epidemic cycle from four (1650–99) to three (1700–49, 1750–99) to two (1800–49) years. The combined results of the ACF analysis are summarized in Figure 2.14E by plotting, as the black circles, epidemic wavelength (vertical axis) against time period (horizontal axis); the corresponding information for later time periods (see Section 9.5.2) is plotted as the white circles, while, for reference, the heavy line trace depicts the population growth of London.

The graphs in Figure 2.15 parallel Figure 2.14E and plot the dominant epidemic wavelengths for six further diseases: (A) influenza, (B) scarlet fever, (C) smallpox, (D) syphilis, (E) tuberculosis (pulmonary), and (F) whooping cough.[12] Two features of Figure 2.15 are apparent. First, consistent with epidemiological expectation, the diseases differ widely in terms of their epidemic wavelength in any given time period. Second, notwithstanding these differences, the general pattern in the period 1650–1849 is for approximately stable (syphilis and whooping cough) or reducing (smallpox and tuberculosis) epidemic wavelengths. Insufficient data are available to draw conclusions for two further diseases (influenza and scarlet fever).

Discussion

C. J. Duncan *et al.* (1996*a*,*b*, 1997) have suggested how, during the seventeenth to the nineteenth centuries, the epidemic wavelengths of measles, smallpox, and whooping cough in London shifted in response to both (i) long-term population growth and (ii) malnutrition associated with fluctuating patterns of food scarcity in the city (Table 2.9). Accepting differences in methodology and the time periods for which the evidence is presented, the

[12] Evidence for five additional diseases in Table 2.8 has been excluded from Fig. 2.15 on the grounds of lack of data in the period 1650–1849 (cholera, diphtheria, meningococcal disease, and plague) or lack of evidence of clearly defined epidemic cycles (leprosy).

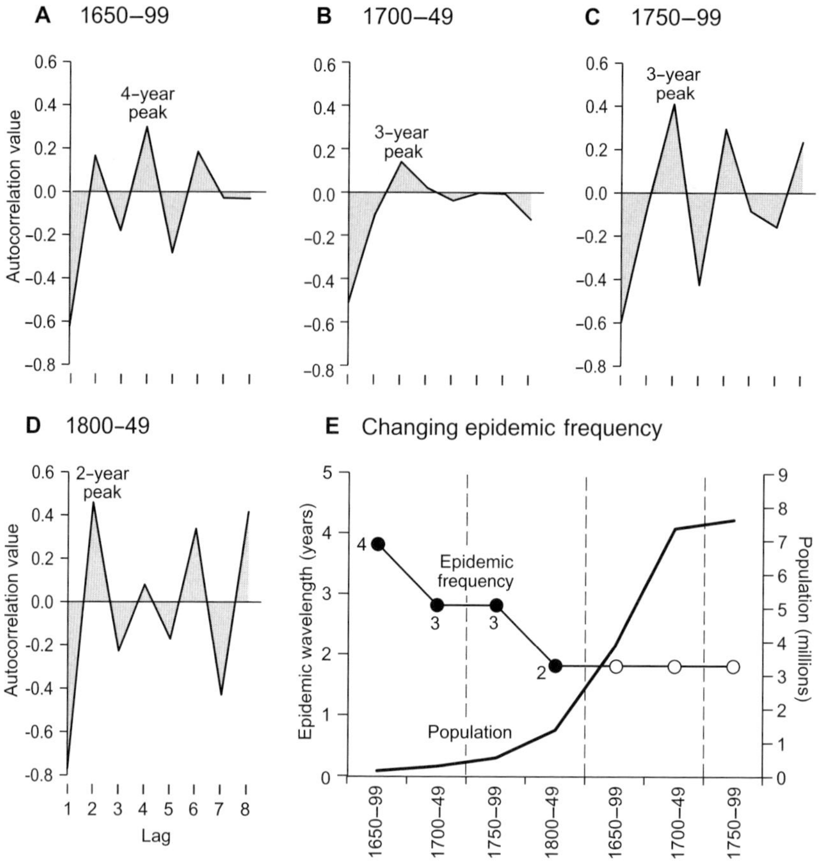

Fig. 2.14. Changing wavelength of measles epidemics in London, 1650–1849 Autocorrelation functions (ACFs) of the detrended series of annual measles death rates per 1,000 population are plotted for four time periods in graphs A–D. Graph E plots, in years, the shift in the dominant epidemic wavelength for 1650–1849 (black circles), along with the corresponding information for 1850–1973 (white circles). The population growth of London is plotted on graph E as the heavy line trace. Evidence for the period 1850–1973 is examined in Section 9.5.2.

reduction in epidemic wavelength (≡ increase in epidemic frequency) identified here for measles (Figure 2.14E) and smallpox (Figure 2.15C) corresponds closely with Duncan *et al.*'s assessment for the two diseases in Table 2.9. While the present analysis identifies a broadly similar response of increasing epidemic frequency for tuberculosis (Figure 2.15E), other diseases for which pre-1850 trends can be detected are associated with stable epidemic frequencies for most of the period under examination. The analysis highlights the apparently differential impact of such factors as population growth

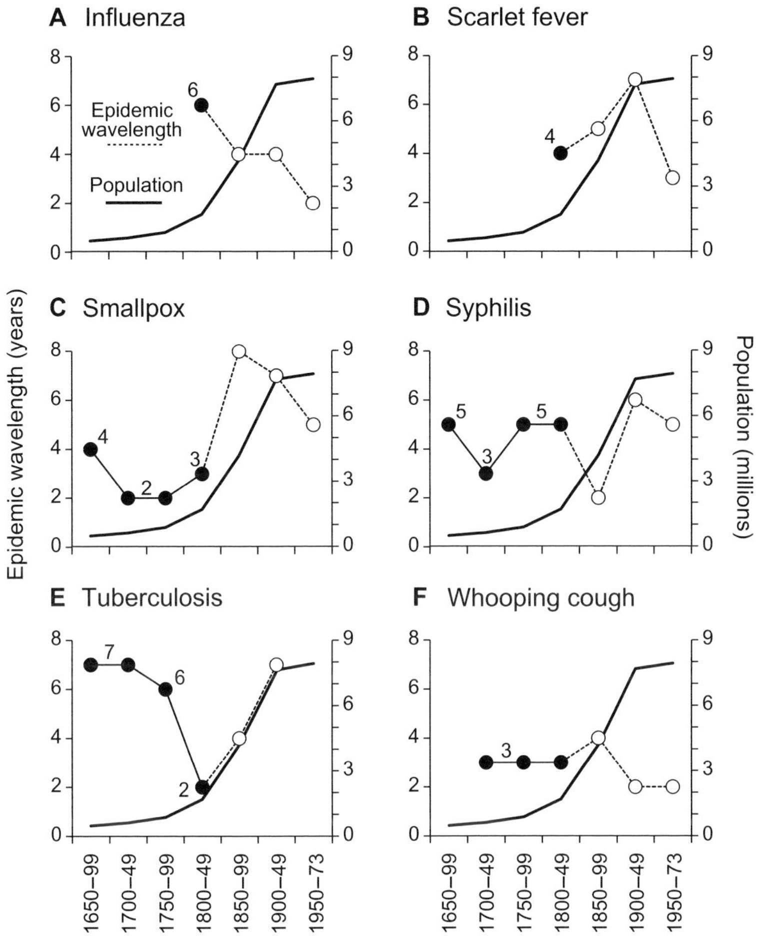

Fig. 2.15. Changing wavelength of epidemics for six sample infectious diseases, London, 1650–1849

Graphs plot the dominant epidemic wavelength in years for sample time periods in the interval 1650–1849 (black circles), along with the corresponding information for 1850–1973 (white circles). (A) Influenza. (B) Scarlet fever. (C) Smallpox. (D) Syphilis. (E) Tuberculosis (pulmonary). (F) Whooping cough. The population growth of London is plotted on each graph as the heavy line trace. Evidence for the period 1850–1973 is examined in Section 9.5.2.

Table 2.9. Duncan and colleagues' estimates of epidemic wavelengths for sample infectious diseases in London, 1600s–1800s

Measles		Smallpox		Whooping cough	
Time period	Wavelength (years)	Time period	Wavelength (years)	Time period	Wavelength (years)
1700–20	5/4	1659–1707	4/3		
1720–50	4/3	1708–50	3/2	1720–50	5
1750–85	3	1751–1800	3	1750–85	3
1785–1837	3/2	1801–35	2/3	1785–1812	5
		1835–70	4		

Sources: Duncan *et al.* (1996*a*, table 1, p. 450; 1996*b*; 1997, table 1, p. 160).

and food scarcity on the epidemic frequency of different infectious diseases in London, 1650–1849.

EPIDEMIC MAGNITUDE

To test for long-term changes in the epidemic magnitude of a given disease, the detrended (first differenced) time series of annual death rates per 1,000 population was examined to determine the largest (maximum) and smallest (minimum) annual rate in each 10-year period from 1630–9 to 1840–9; earlier time periods were excluded from the analysis owing to lack of data. The resulting series of decennial maxima (peaks) and minima (troughs) are plotted for six sample diseases in Figure 2.16. To capture the underpinning trends, linear regression models were fitted to each series of maxima/minima by ordinary least squares. The model used was

$$y_t = \beta_0 + \beta_1 t + e_t, \tag{2.2}$$

where y_t is the value of the maximum/minimum death rate in decennial period t, β_0 and β_1 are parameters to be estimated, and e_t is an error term. The fitted regression lines are plotted in Figure 2.16, while Table 2.10 gives the slope (β_1) coefficients, along with the associated Student's t-statistics, the coefficients of determination (R^2), and the F-ratios. Statistically significant slope coefficients at the $p = 0.05$ level (one-tailed test) are used to classify the trends as 'rising' (positive slope coefficient) or 'falling' (negative slope coefficient); trends associated with non-significant slope coefficients are classified as 'stable'.

Inspection of Figure 2.16 and Table 2.10 reveals a complex pattern of rising, stable, and falling trends for the six diseases. Whooping cough is distinguished from the other diseases by rising peaks and falling troughs, implying that the secular increase in death rates depicted in Figure 2.13L was associated with epidemic events of increasing amplitude from the early eighteenth century. In contrast, smallpox and syphilis share a common

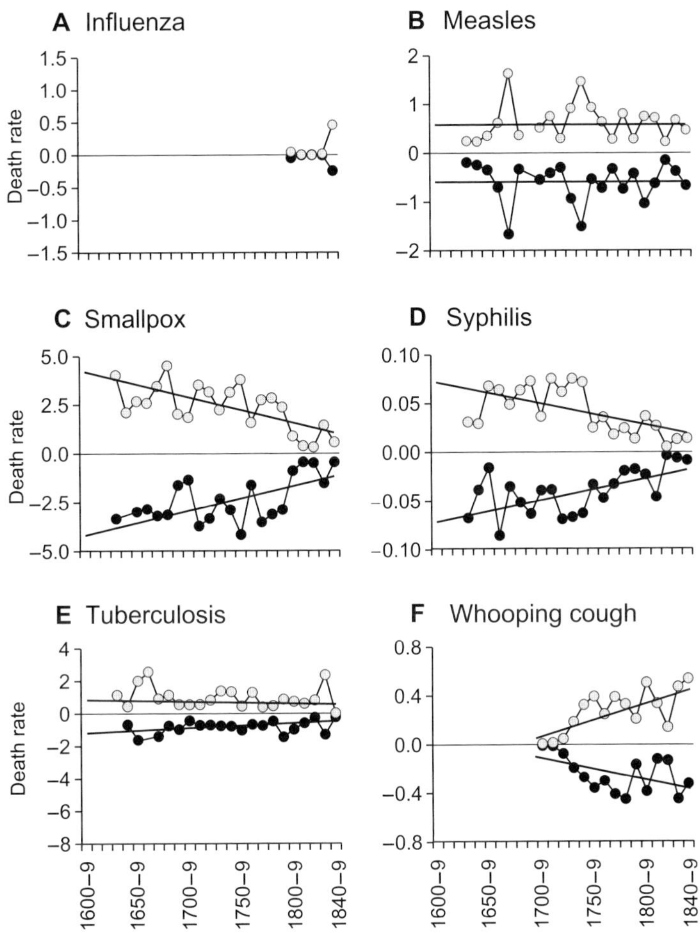

Fig. 2.16. Changing epidemic magnitude, London, 1630–1849
Graphs plot, by 10-year period, the series of maximum (shaded circles) and minimum (solid circles) annual death rates for each of six diseases. (A) Influenza. (B) Measles. (C) Smallpox. (D) Syphilis. (E) Tuberculosis (pulmonary). (F) Whooping cough. Trends are depicted by the linear regression lines, fitted to the series of maxima and minima by ordinary least squares. The slope coefficients of the fitted regression models are given in Table 2.10.

pattern of falling peaks and rising troughs, consistent with a progressive decline in epidemic amplitude as the death rates in Figures 2.13I (smallpox) and 2.13J (syphilis) waxed and waned over the observation period. Of the remaining diseases, the approximately flat trend lines for measles and tuberculosis imply a basic stability in the magnitude of epidemic swings, while interpretation of the evidence for influenza is limited by the few data points available for analysis.

Table 2.10. Regression slope coefficient values for OLS trend lines fitted to maximum (peaks) and minimum (troughs) annual death rates by 10-year period, London, 1630–1849

Disease	Peaks			Troughs		
	Slope coefficient (t-statistic)	R^2 (F-ratio)	Direction of trend	Slope coefficient (t-statistic)	R^2 (F-ratio)	Direction of trend
Influenza	0.08 (1.56)	0.45 (2.43)	Stable	−0.04 (−1.31)	0.36 (1.71)	Stable
Measles	0.00 (0.30)	0.00 (0.09)	Stable	−0.00 (−0.13)	0.00 (0.02)	Stable
Smallpox	−0.12 (−3.82**)	0.42 (14.63**)	Falling	0.11 (3.01**)	0.32 (9.06**)	Rising
Syphilis	−0.00 (−3.38**)	0.36 (11.40**)	Falling	0.00 (3.28**)	0.35 (10.74**)	Rising
Tuberculosis[1]	−0.02 (−1.09)	0.06 (1.19)	Stable	0.01 (1.33)	0.09 (1.76)	Stable
Whooping cough	0.03 (3.74**)	0.52 (13.96**)	Rising	−0.02 (−2.14*)	0.26 (4.57*)	Falling

Notes: [1] Extreme outliers omitted. * Significant at the $p = 0.05$ level (one-tailed test). ** Significant at the $p = 0.01$ level (one-tailed test).

CONCLUSION

In his comprehensive review of the mortality regime of London from the later seventeenth to the early nineteenth centuries, Landers (1993: 353) expresses the view that 'only typhus fever has any claim to be considered a "new disease" '. 'The remaining infections', Landers adds, 'are likely to have been relatively long established by the early eighteenth century'—a perspective that does not exclude the possible appearance of new and more virulent strains of established pathogens, as may have been the case with smallpox (Hardy 1983). For the diseases examined in the present section, the ebb and flow of infection in London can be characterized as a complex amalgam of old and newly recorded/classified scourges that waxed and waned in terms of their overall mortality, epidemic frequency, and epidemic magnitude in the period 1603–1849. These developments occurred in a rapidly increasing, and increasingly impoverished, industrial population reservoir that—bar contemporary developments in inoculation against smallpox—lacked modern methods of infectious disease control. We continue our examination of the changing epidemic profile of London through to the late twentieth century in Section 9.5.

2.5 Conclusion

Drawing on a small sample of a vast historical literature, this chapter has traced the record of disease emergence from the earliest days of the written word to the brink of the statistical period. Our primary focus has been on the major infectious diseases of humans, some of which can be traced back—with variable certainty—to ancient times. Other infections, such as venereal syphilis and typhus fever, gain prominence in the epidemiological record of the late Middle Ages. Yet others, such as meningococcal meningitis and miliary fever, do not attract the attention of physicians and medical writers until the modern era. The extent to which these developments represent the true emergence of 'new' diseases or merely clinical distinction can only remain conjecture. In that they gain recognition at a particular period in history, for whatever reason, this justifies their classification as 'emerging diseases'.

In the next chapter, we begin our study of emerging diseases for the period of consolidated statistical data post-1850 by identifying, from a content analysis of three major sources of epidemiological information, the diseases, areas, and time windows upon which we focus in the remainder of the book.

PART II

Processes of Disease Emergence: 1850–2006

Introduction to Part II

In Part II of this book, we turn to an examination of the factors that have facilitated the emergence and re-emergence of infectious diseases in the period since 1850. Particular emphasis is placed on developments in the twentieth and early twenty-first centuries. From the list of enabling factors identified in the scientific literature over the last 10–15 years (see Section 1.5.2), we have selected the five overarching themes shown in Figure II.1 for close examination in Chapters 4–8: 'Disease Changes: Microbial and Vector Adaptation' (Chapter 4); 'Technical Changes: Technology and Industry' (Chapter 5); 'Population Changes: Magnitude, Mobility, and Disease Transfer' (Chapter 6); 'Environmental Changes: Ecological Modifications' (Chapter 7); and 'Disease Amplifiers: Wars and Conflicts' (Chapter 8). In selecting the five themes, we emphasize that the associated processes are not discrete but often operate in combination or sequence to precipitate the (re)appearance of a disease agent in the human population. To round off our discussion of processes in Part II, Chapter 9 examines temporal trends in disease emergence and re-emergence at the spatial scales of world, region, country, and city.

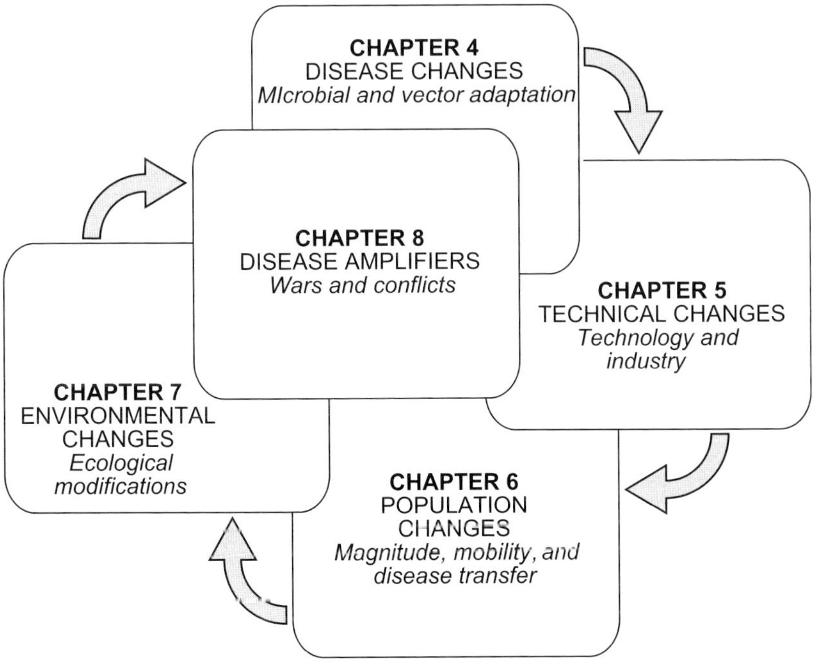

Fig. II.1. Diagram showing themes for analysis in Chapters 4–8

As a prelude to Part II, Chapter 3 undertakes a content analysis of three major sources of epidemiological information—the annual statistical reports of the League of Nations/World Health Organization (1923–83), the US Centers for Disease Control and Prevention's (CDC's) *Morbidity and Mortality Weekly Report* (1952–2005), and the inventory of epidemic assistance investigations undertaken by CDC's Epidemic Intelligence Service (1946–2005)—to identify patterns in the recognition and recording of communicable diseases of public health importance. We use the analysis presented here to guide our selection of diseases and locations for study in subsequent chapters.

3

The Geographical Matrix

3.1 Introduction

A historical–geographical exploration of disease emergence is confronted by a series of fundamental questions: Which diseases have emerged? When? And where? For some high-profile diseases, such as Legionnaires' disease, Ebola viral disease, and severe acute respiratory syndrome (SARS), the first recognized outbreaks are well documented in the scientific literature and the space–time coordinates of these early events can be fixed with a high degree of certainty. But, for some other diseases—especially those that, over the decades, have periodically resurfaced as significant public health problems—the times and places of their rise to prominence can be harder to specify. Accordingly, in this chapter we undertake a content analysis of three major epidemiological sources to identify patterns in the recognition and recording of communicable diseases of public health significance in the twentieth and early twenty-first centuries.

Our analysis begins, in Section 3.2, with an examination of global and world regional patterns of communicable disease surveillance as documented in the annual statistical reports of the League of Nations/World Health Organization, 1923–83. In Section 3.3, we turn to the US Centers for Disease Control and Prevention's (CDC's) landmark publication *Morbidity and Mortality Weekly Report* (*MMWR*) to identify 'headline trends' in the national and international coverage of communicable diseases, 1952–2005. Finally, in Section 3.4, the inventory of epidemic assistance investigations (Epi-Aids) undertaken by CDC's Epidemic Intelligence Service (EIS), 1946–2005, provides a unique series of insights from the front line of epidemic investigative research. Informed by the evidence presented in these sections, Section 3.5 concludes by specifying the regional–thematic matrix of diseases for analysis in Chapters 4–9.

3.2 International Patterns of Communicable Disease Surveillance, 1923–1983

3.2.1 The League of Nations/World Health Organization Data Set

The systematic international recording of information about morbidity and mortality from disease begins with the Health Organization of the League of Nations,[1] established in the aftermath of the Great War. The first meeting of the Health Committee of the Health Section of the League took place in August 1921 to consider 'the question of organising means of more rapid interchange of epidemiological information' (Health Section of the League of Nations 1922: 3). To meet this need, several publications were instituted and these are described in Cliff, Haggett, and Smallman-Raynor (1998: 389–95). Among the publications, the *Annual Epidemiological Report* and its successors are the main source of published international data by country on morbidity and mortality from 1921 until 1983. The series titles are as follows:

(i) *Annual Epidemiological Report* (1921–38), published by the Health Section of the League of Nations, Geneva; this was succeeded by

[1] The Health Organization of the League of Nations consisted of a Health Committee, an Advisory Council and the Health Section, the latter operating as an executive organ and forming an integral part of the League Secretariat (Health Organization of the League of Nations, 1931, p. 4).

MALADIES A DÉCLARATION OBLIGATOIRE DANS DIFFÉRENTS PAYS EN 1930.
NOTIFIABLE DISEASES IN VARIOUS COUNTRIES IN 1930.

Le signe ◆ indique que la déclaration de la maladie est obligatoire. — The sign ◆ indicates that the disease is notifiable.

Maladies / Diseases	Actinomycose / Actinomycosis	Angine fuso-spirillaire de Vincent / Vincent's angina	Angine à streptocoques / Septic sore-throat	Angine tonsillaire / Angina tonsillaris	Ankylostomiase / Ankylostomiasis	Béribéri / Beri-beri	Bilharziose / Bilharziasis	Blennorragie / Gonorrhœa	Botulisme / Botulism	Bronchite aiguë / Acute bronchitis	Broncho-pneumonie / Broncho-pneumonia	Cancer / Cancer	Chancre mou / Soft chancre	Charbon / Anthrax	Choléra asiatique / Cholera
Numéros de la nomenclature internat. détaillée revisée en 1929 / Detailed International List Nos., as revised in 1929	43 B	115 B	115 B	115 B	40	61	42	35	177	106 a	107	53	35	20	12
Afrique / Africa:															
Afrique-Occidentale française / French West Africa	—	—	—	—	—	—	—	—	—	—	—	—	—	—	◆
Algérie / Algeria	—	—	—	—	—	—	—	—	—	—	◆	—	—	—	◆
Angola / Angola	◆	—	—	—	◆	◆	◆	◆	—	—	—	—	—	◆	◆
Bassoutoland / Basutoland	—	—	—	—	—	—	—	—	—	—	—	—	—	—	◆
Cameroun (mandat français) / Cameroons (French Mand.)	—	—	—	—	—	—	—	—	—	—	—	—	—	—	◆
Congo belge / Belgian Congo	—	—	—	—	—	—	—	◆	—	—	—	—	◆	◆	◆
Côte de l'Or / Gold Coast	—	—	—	—	—	—	—	—	—	—	—	—	—	◆	◆
Cyrénaïque / Cyrenaica	—	—	—	—	—	—	—	—	—	—	—	—	—	◆	◆
Egypte / Egypt	—	—	—	—	—	—	—	—	—	—	—	—	—	◆	◆
Erythrée / Eritrea	—	—	—	—	—	—	—	—	—	—	—	—	—	—	◆
Kénia / Kenya	—	—	—	—	—	◆	—	—	—	—	—	—	—	◆	◆
Madagascar / Madagascar	—	—	—	—	—	—	—	—	—	—	—	—	—	—	◆
Maroc, Protectorat français / French Protectorate of Morocco	—	—	—	—	—	—	—	—	—	—	—	—	—	—	◆
Maurice, Ile / Mauritius	—	—	—	—	—	—	—	—	—	—	—	—	—	◆	◆
Mozambique / Mozambique	—	—	—	—	—	—	—	—	—	—	—	—	—	—	◆
Nigéria / Nigeria	—	—	—	—	—	—	—	—	—	—	—	—	—	—	◆
Nyassaland, Prot. / Nyasaland Protect.	—	—	—	—	—	—	—	—	—	—	—	—	—	—	◆
Ouganda / Uganda	—	—	—	—	—	—	—	—	—	—	—	—	—	—	◆
Réunion / Reunion	—	—	—	—	—	—	—	—	—	—	—	—	—	—	◆
Rhodésie du Nord / Northern Rhodesia	—	—	—	—	—	—	—	—	—	—	—	—	—	◆	◆
Rhodésie du Sud / Southern Rhodesia	—	—	—	—	—	—	—	—	—	—	—	—	—	◆	◆
Sierra-Leone / Sierra Leone	—	—	—	—	—	◆	—	—	—	—	—	—	—	—	◆
Somalie britann. / British Somaliland	—	—	—	—	—	—	—	—	—	—	—	—	—	—	◆
Somalie française / French Somaliland	—	—	—	—	—	—	—	—	—	—	—	—	—	—	◆
Soudan anglo-égyptien / Anglo-Egyptian Sudan	—	—	—	—	—	—	—	—	—	—	—	—	—	—	◆
Tanganyika, Territoire du (mandat britannique) / Tanganyika Territory (British Mandate)	—	—	—	—	—	◆	—	—	—	—	—	—	—	◆	◆
Togo (mandat français) / Togo (French Mandate)	—	—	—	—	—	—	—	—	—	—	—	—	—	—	◆
Tripolitaine / Tripolitania	—	—	—	—	—	—	—	—	—	—	—	—	—	◆	◆
Tunisie / Tunis	—	—	—	—	—	—	—	—	—	—	—	—	—	—	◆
Union de l'Afrique du Sud / Union of South Africa	—	—	—	—	—	—	—	—	—	—	—	—	—	◆	◆
Zanzibar / Zanzibar	—	—	—	—	—	◆	—	—	—	—	—	—	—	◆	◆

Maladies / Diseases	Coqueluche / Whooping-cough	Delirium tremens / Delirium tremens	Dengue / Dengue fever	Diarrhée et entérite, 0-2 ans / Diarrhœa and enteritis, 0-2 years	Diarrhée et entérite, 2 ans et plus / Diarrhœa and enteritis, 2 years and over	Diphtérie et croup / Diphtheria and croup	**Dysenterie, non spécifiée / Dysentery, unspecified	Dysenterie amibienne / Dysentery, amœbic	Dysenterie bacillaire / Dysentery, bacillary	Echinococcose / Hydatid disease	Empoisonnement chronique par le phosphore / Chronic phosphorus poisoning	Empoisonnement chronique par le plomb / Chronic lead poisoning	Encéphalite léthargique / Encephalitis lethargica	Erysipèle / Erysipelas	Favus / Favus
Numéros de la nomenclature internat. détaillée revisée en 1929 / Detailed International List Nos., as revised in 1929	9	75	44	119	120	10	13	13 a	13 b	41 a	77	77	17	15	43
Afrique / Africa:															
Afrique-Occidentale française / French West Africa	—	—	—	—	—	◆	◆	—	—	—	—	—	—	—	—
Algérie / Algeria	◆	—	—	—	—	◆	◆	—	—	—	—	—	◆	◆	—
Angola / Angola	◆	—	◆	—	—	◆	◆	—	—	—	—	—	◆	◆	—
Bassoutoland / Basutoland	—	—	—	—	—	—	—	—	—	—	—	—	—	—	—
Cameroun (mandat français) / Cameroons (French Mand.)	—	—	—	—	—	◆	◆	—	—	—	—	—	—	—	—
Congo belge / Belgian Congo	—	—	◆	—	—	◆	—	◆	◆	—	—	—	◆	◆	—
Côte de l'Or / Gold Coast	—	—	—	—	—	—	—	—	—	—	—	—	◆	—	—
Cyrénaïque / Cyrenaica	—	—	—	—	—	◆	—	◆	◆	—	—	—	◆	—	—
Egypte / Egypt	◆	—	◆	—	—	◆	◆	—	—	—	—	—	◆	◆	—
Erythrée / Eritrea	—	—	—	—	—	—	—	—	—	—	—	—	—	—	—
Kénia / Kenya	◆	—	—	—	—	◆	—	—	—	—	—	—	◆	◆	—
Madagascar / Madagascar	—	—	—	—	—	◆	◆	—	—	—	—	—	—	—	—
Maroc, Protectorat français / French Protectorate of Morocco	—	—	—	—	—	◆	—	◆	◆	—	—	—	◆	—	—
Maurice, Ile / Mauritius	—	—	—	—	—	◆	—	—	—	—	—	—	◆	◆	—
Mozambique / Mozambique	◆	—	—	—	—	—	—	◆	◆	—	—	—	—	◆	—
Nigéria / Nigeria	—	—	—	—	—	◆	—	—	—	—	—	—	—	—	—
Nyassaland, Prot. / Nyasaland Protect.	◆	—	—	—	—	◆	—	—	—	—	—	—	—	—	—
Ouganda / Uganda	◆	—	—	—	—	◆	—	—	—	—	—	—	—	◆	—
Réunion / Reunion	—	—	—	—	—	◆	◆	—	—	—	—	—	—	—	—
Rhodésie du Nord / Northern Rhodesia	◆	—	—	—	—	◆	◆	—	—	—	—	—	—	◆	—
Rhodésie du Sud / Southern Rhodesia	—	—	—	—	—	◆	—	—	—	—	—	—	—	◆	—
Sierra-Leone / Sierra Leone	—	—	—	—	—	◆	◆	—	—	—	—	—	—	◆	—
Somalie britann. / British Somaliland	—	—	—	—	—	◆	—	—	—	—	—	—	—	—	—
Somalie française / French Somaliland	—	—	—	—	—	◆	◆	—	—	—	—	—	—	—	—
Soudan anglo-égyptien / Anglo-Egyptian Sudan	—	—	—	—	—	◆	—	—	—	—	—	—	—	—	—
Tanganyika, Territoire du (mandat britannique) / Tanganyika Territory (British Mandate)	—	—	—	—	—	◆	—	—	—	—	—	—	◆	—	—
Togo (mandat français) / Togo (French Mandate)	—	—	—	—	—	◆	◆	—	—	—	—	—	—	—	—
Tripolitaine / Tripolitania	—	—	—	—	—	◆	—	◆	◆	—	—	—	◆	—	—
Tunisie / Tunis	—	—	—	—	—	◆	—	◆	◆	—	—	—	—	—	—
Union de l'Afrique du Sud / Union of South Africa	—	—	—	—	—	◆	—	—	—	—	—	—	◆	◆	—
Zanzibar / Zanzibar	◆	—	—	—	—	◆	◆	—	—	—	—	◆	◆	◆	—

Maladies / Diseases	Fièvre bilieuse hémoglobinurique / Blackwater fever	Fièvre continue / Continued fever	Fièvre des tranchées / Trench fever	Fièvre jaune / Yellow fever	Fièvre ondulante / Undulant fever	Fièvres paratyphoïdes / Paratyphoid fevers	Fièvre puerpérale / Puerperal fever	Fièvres récurrentes / Relapsing fevers	Fièvre tachetée des Montagnes Rocheuses / Rocky Mountain spotted fever	Fièvre typhoïde / Typhoid fever	Filariose / Filariasis	Gale / Scabies	Gingivite nécrosante / Necrotic gingivitis (Trench mouth)	Goitre / Goitre	Grippe / Influenza
Numéros de la nomenclature internat. détaillée revisée en 1929 / Detailed International List Nos., as revised in 1929	44	200	44	37	5	2	145 a	4	44	1	42	153 b	115 A	66 a	11
Afrique / Africa:															
Afrique-Occidentale française / French West Africa	—	—	—	◆	—	—	—	◆	—	◆	—	—	—	—	—
Algérie / Algeria	—	—	—	◆	◆	◆	—	◆	—	◆	—	—	—	—	◆
Angola / Angola	◆	—	—	◆	◆	◆	◆	◆	—	◆	—	◆	—	—	◆
Bassoutoland / Basutoland	—	—	—	◆	—	—	—	—	—	—	—	—	—	—	—
Cameroun (mandat français) / Cameroons (French Mand.)	—	—	—	◆	—	—	—	◆	—	◆	—	—	—	—	—
Congo belge / Belgian Congo	—	—	—	◆	◆	◆	◆	◆	—	◆	—	—	—	—	◆
Côte de l'Or / Gold Coast	—	—	—	◆	—	—	—	—	—	—	—	—	—	—	◆
Cyrénaïque / Cyrenaica	—	—	—	◆	—	◆	—	—	—	◆	—	—	—	—	—
Egypte / Egypt	—	—	—	—	◆	—	◆	◆	—	◆	—	—	—	—	◆
Erythrée / Eritrea	—	—	—	◆	—	—	—	—	—	—	—	—	—	—	—
Kénia / Kenya	—	—	—	◆	◆	◆	◆	—	—	◆	—	—	—	—	—
Madagascar / Madagascar	—	—	—	◆	—	—	—	◆	—	◆	—	—	—	—	—
Maroc, Protectorat français / French Protectorate of Morocco	—	—	—	◆	◆	◆	◆	◆	—	◆	—	—	—	—	—
Maurice, Ile / Mauritius	—	—	—	◆	◆	◆	◆	—	—	◆	—	—	—	—	—
Mozambique / Mozambique	◆	—	—	◆	—	◆	—	—	—	◆	—	—	—	—	◆
Nigéria / Nigeria	—	—	—	◆	—	◆	—	—	—	◆	—	—	—	—	—
Nyassaland, Prot. / Nyasaland Protect.	—	—	—	◆	—	◆	—	—	—	◆	—	—	—	—	—
Ouganda / Uganda	—	—	—	◆	—	◆	◆	◆	—	◆	—	—	—	—	—
Réunion / Reunion	—	—	—	◆	—	—	—	◆	—	◆	—	—	—	—	—
Rhodésie du Nord / Northern Rhodesia	◆	—	—	◆	◆	◆	◆	◆	—	◆	—	—	—	—	—
Rhodésie du Sud / Southern Rhodesia	—	—	—	—	◆	◆	◆	—	—	◆	—	—	—	—	—
Sierra-Leone / Sierra Leone	—	—	—	◆	—	◆	◆	◆	—	◆	—	—	—	—	◆
Somalie britann. / British Somaliland	—	—	—	◆	—	◆	—	—	—	◆	—	—	—	—	—
Somalie française / French Somaliland	—	—	—	◆	—	—	—	◆	—	◆	—	—	—	—	—
Soudan anglo-égyptien / Anglo-Egyptian Sudan	—	—	—	—	—	◆	—	◆	—	◆	—	—	—	—	—
Tanganyika, Territoire du (mandat britannique) / Tanganyika Territory (British Mandate)	—	◆	—	◆	—	◆	—	◆	—	◆	—	—	—	—	◆
Togo (mandat français) / Togo (French Mandate)	—	—	—	◆	—	—	—	◆	—	◆	—	—	—	—	—
Tripolitaine / Tripolitania	—	—	—	◆	—	◆	—	—	—	◆	—	—	—	—	—
Tunisie / Tunis	—	—	—	◆	◆	◆	—	◆	—	◆	—	—	—	—	—
Union de l'Afrique du Sud / Union of South Africa	—	—	—	◆	◆	◆	◆	—	—	◆	—	—	—	—	—
Zanzibar / Zanzibar	—	—	—	◆	◆	◆	◆	◆	—	◆	—	—	—	—	—

Pl. 3.1. Health Organization of the League of Nations: disease matrix

Detail of a country-by-disease matrix, showing those countries of Africa (rows) in which specified diseases (columns) were subject to mandatory notification in the sample year of 1930. Diseases subject to mandatory notification are identified by the diamond-shaped pips.

(ii) *Annual Epidemiological and Vital Statistics* (1939–61), published by the World Health Organization (WHO), Geneva; this was retitled as
(iii) *World Health Statistics Annual* (1962–83).[2]

In sources (i) and (ii) for the years 1923–37, 1946, 1949–55, and 1958, a chart or table was published which recorded in matrix format (diseases × countries) which diseases were *notifiable*. Plate 3.1 shows a detail of the chart for 1930.

Between 1959 and 1983, the country matrices of notifiable diseases were not published, but equivalent matrices of *reported* diseases by country can be constructed from the raw returns of recorded mortality and morbidity published by the WHO in sources (ii) and (iii). Such matrices were built for the years 1963, 1965, 1970, 1975, 1980, and 1983. In this list, 1963 and 1965 were selected because these years spanned the shift in the recording of morbidity and mortality from hand returns to computer-processed (1964 for mortality by cause and 1965 for morbidity from infectious diseases). The year 1983 was included because it was the last in which data on morbidity from communicable diseases were routinely published in *World Health Statistics Annual*. The years 1970, 1975, and 1980 served as intermediate quinquennial sampling points.

From 1983, the systematic recording of morbidity data by the WHO ceased as publications were progressively modified to reflect the launching of the Global Strategy for Health for All by the Year 2000 by the 32nd World Health Assembly in 1979. The adoption of the global strategy resulted in changed priorities for information support and the need to reflect progress in implementing Health for All by monitoring and evaluating specific programmes in health systems, health care, health resources, and patterns and trends in health status. As a result, from the mid-1980s, morbidity data became scattered piecemeal through other WHO publications that dealt with epidemiological information, and systematic reporting was left to national agencies.

FORMATION OF THE DATABASE

For each of the 29 sample years (1923–37, 1946, 1949–55, 1958, 1963, 1965, 1970, 1975, 1980, and 1983), information for a total of 237 diseases and 193 WHO member states was abstracted from sources (i)–(iii) above to yield a 29 (years) × 237 (diseases) × 193 (member states) 1/0 matrix of diseases subject/not subject to globally documented surveillance. For the reasons outlined in the foregoing discussion, the operation of national surveillance activities for a given disease was assessed according to (*a*) the notifiable status of the disease (1923–58) or (*b*) the publication of reported cases of the disease by the WHO (1963–83). The geographical sample included 100 per cent of WHO member states (2008 status), distributed according to the six standard WHO regions as illustrated in Figure 3.1. All analysis to follow

[2] Although the printed version of the *World Health Statistics Annual* continued until 1996, the time bracket 1962–83 encompasses the period for which national morbidity data were systematically published in the *Annual*.

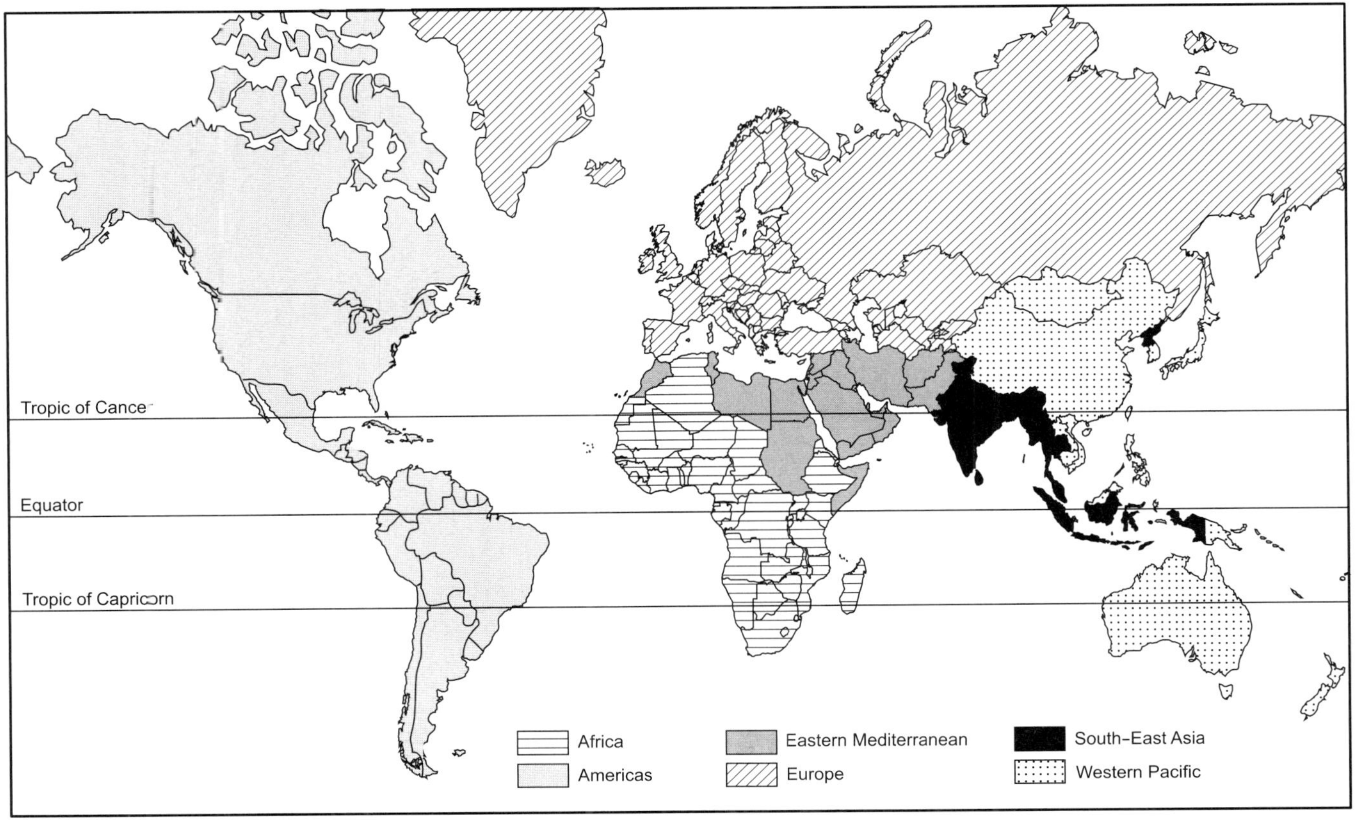

Fig. 3.1. Standard regions of the World Health Organization (WHO)

is based on the record of disease surveillance (notifiable status, 1923–58, and case reporting, 1963–83) for the 29 annual periods and 193 WHO member states, with the analysis restricted to 123 sample disease categories that fall within Chapter I ('Certain Infectious and Parasitic Diseases, A00–B99') of the Tenth Revision of the WHO's *International Classification of Diseases* (*ICD*-10); see Section 1.5.3. The 123 sample disease categories are given by *ICD*-10 code in Table 3.1.

Table 3.1. Sample disease categories for analysis: Certain Infectious and Parasitic Diseases (*ICD*-10 A00–B99)

ICD-10 code	Title of category	Diseases[1]
A00–A09	Intestinal infectious diseases	Cholera (A00); typhoid and paratyphoid fevers (A01); other salmonella infections (A02); shigellosis (A03); other bacterial intestinal infections (A04); botulism (A05); other bacterial foodborne intoxications (A05); amoebiasis (A06); other protozoal intestinal diseases (A07); viral and other specified intestinal infections (A08); diarrhoea and gastroenteritis (A09)
A15–A19	Tuberculosis	Respiratory tuberculosis (A15–A16); tuberculosis, non-respiratory (A17–A19)
A20–A28	Certain zoonotic bacterial diseases	Plague (A20); tularaemia (A21); anthrax (A22); brucellosis (A23); glanders (A24); rat-bite fevers (A25); leptospirosis (A27); other zoonotic bacterial diseases, not elsewhere classified (A28)
A30–A49	Other bacterial diseases	Leprosy (A30); infection due to other mycobacteria (A31); tetanus (A33–A35); other tetanus (A35); diphtheria (A36); whooping cough (A37); scarlet fever (A38); meningococcal infection (A39); other septicaemia (A41); actinomycosis (A42); bartonellosis (A44); erysipelas (A46); gas gangrene (A48); rhinoscleroma (A48); colibacillosis (A49)
A50–A64	Infections with a predominantly sexual mode of transmission	Congenital syphilis (A50); syphilis (A50–A53); early syphilis (A51); late syphilis (A52); other and unspecified syphilis (A53); gonococcal infection (A54); chlamydial lymphogranuloma (venereum) (A55); chancroid (A57); granuloma inguinale (A58); trichomoniasis (A59); unspecified sexually transmitted disease (A64)
A65–A69	Other spirochaetal diseases	Yaws (A66); relapsing fever, tick-borne (A68); relapsing fever, unspecified (A68); other spirochaetal infections (A69)
A70–A74	Other diseases caused by chlamydiae	Psittacosis (A70); trachoma (A71)
A75–A79	Rickettsioses	Typhus fever (A75); Brill's disease (A75); typhus, endemic (murine typhus) (A75); spotted fever (A77); Boutonneuse fever

		(A77); Q fever (A78); other rickettsioses (A79); trench fever (A79)
A80–A89	Viral infections of the central nervous system	Poliomyelitis (A80); atypical virus infections of central nervous system (A81); rabies (A82); mosquito-borne viral encephalitis (A83); tick-borne viral encephalitis (A84); encephalitis lethargica (A85); unspecified viral encephalitis (A86); viral meningitis (A87); other viral infections of central nervous system, not elsewhere classified (A88); unspecified viral infection of central nervous system (A89)
A90–A99	Arthropod-borne viral fevers and viral haemorrhagic fevers	Dengue fever (A90); other arthropod-borne viral fevers, not elsewhere classified (A93); sandfly fever (A93); unspecified arthropod-borne viral fever (A94); yellow fever (A95); arenaviral haemorrhagic fever (A96); other viral haemorrhagic fevers, not elsewhere classified (A98); unspecified viral haemorrhagic fever (A99)
B00–B09	Viral infections characterized by skin and mucous membrane lesions	Chickenpox (B01); zoster (B02); smallpox (B03); measles (B05); rubella (B06); foot and mouth disease (B08)
B15–B19	Viral hepatitis	Viral hepatitis (B15–B19); acute hepatitis B (B16); other acute viral hepatitis (B17); chronic viral hepatitis (B18)
B25–B34	Other viral diseases	Mumps (B26); infectious mononucleosis (B27); viral conjunctivitis (B30); other viral diseases, not elsewhere classified (B33)
B35–B49	Mycoses	Dermatophytosis (B35); candidiasis (B37); coccidioidomycosis (B38); histoplasmosis (B39); blastomycosis (B40); other mycoses, not elsewhere classified (B48); unspecified mycosis (B49)
B50–B64	Protozoal diseases	Malaria (B50–B54); unspecified malaria (B54); leishmaniasis (B55); African trypanosomiasis (B56); Chagas' disease (B57); toxoplasmosis (B58); other predominantly sexually transmitted diseases, not elsewhere classified (B63); unspecified protozoal disease (B64)
B65–B83	Helminthiases	Schistosomiasis (B65); other fluke infections (B66); echinococcosis (B67); other cestode infections (B71); filariasis (B74); trichinellosis (B75); ancylostomiasis (B76); ascariasis (B77); other intestinal helminthiases, not elsewhere classified (B81); unspecified intestinal parasitism (B82); other helminthiases (B83)
B85–B89	Pediculosis, acariasis, and other infestations	Pediculosis (B85); scabies (B86); unspecified parasitic disease (B89)
B99	Other infectious diseases	Other and unspecified infectious diseases (B99)

Note: [1] Three-character *ICD*-10 codes in parentheses.

3.2.2 Global Trends

AGGREGATE TRENDS

Figure 3.2 plots, by annual period, the number of sample infectious and parasitic disease categories (lower line trace) and the associated number of WHO member states (upper line trace) for which surveillance activities were documented in the League of Nations/WHO data set. Trends are depicted by linear regression lines fitted by ordinary least squares; the hinge period associated with the change of data type, from notifiable status (1923–58) to published disease reports (1963–83), is indicated for reference. As the graph shows, the number of disease categories under surveillance by WHO member states varied between 40 and 60 per annum for much of the observation period, but with a rapid increase to >80 in the early 1980s. The same interval was associated with a steady and progressive increase in the number of WHO member states for which surveillance activities for the sample disease categories were documented, from 85 (44 per cent of WHO member states) at the start of the observation period to a peak of 160 (83 per cent of WHO member states) in the early 1970s.

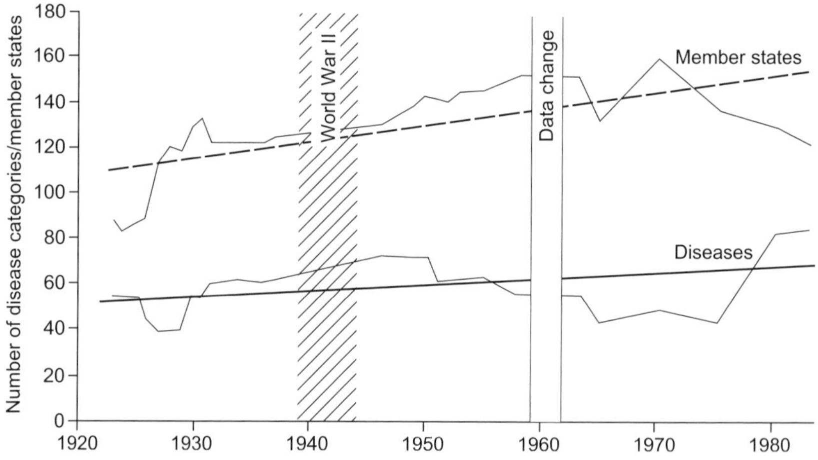

Fig. 3.2. Trends in global surveillance for 123 sample infectious and parasitic disease categories, 1923–1983. I: Total counts

For sample years, the graph plots the number of disease categories (lower line trace) and the associated number of WHO member states (upper line trace) for which surveillance activities were documented in the League of Nations/WHO data set. Surveillance activities have been assessed on the basis of the notifiable status of diseases (1923–58) and published disease reports (1963–83); the hinge period marking the change in data type is indicated. Trends are depicted by linear regression lines fitted to the data by ordinary least squares. The 123 sample disease categories (ICD-10 codes A00–B99) are listed in Table 3.1.

Diseases

As noted, the time series of diseases in Figure 3.2 is based on the count of different disease categories across the set of member states. Over the time series the number of member states also varied in terms of the number of diseases for which surveillance activities were documented. To capture this variability, Figure 3.3A plots the median number of sample infectious and parasitic disease categories per WHO member state for which surveillance activities were documented (heavy line trace), along with the inter-quartile range (Q1 and Q3; shaded envelope) and maximum and minimum (broken line traces) counts. The first four decades of the observation period were associated with a steady increase in the median number of disease categories, rising from 15 (1923) to 30 (1963), but with a sharp reduction thereafter. As judged by the inter-quartile range in Figure 3.3A, many WHO member states approximated this general surveillance pattern.

WHO Member States

Paralleling Figure 3.3A, Figure 3.3B plots the median, inter-quartile range and maximum and minimum count of WHO member states in which surveillance activities were documented for each of the disease categories in Table 3.1. As judged by the median line trace, the post-war period was associated with a pronounced increase in the number of WHO member states, rising from <25 states in the 1930s and 1940s to >80 in the early 1960s. Consequent upon the change in data available for examination, the median line trace fell sharply from the mid-1960s, to pre-war levels by the early 1980s. Although the broad trend of post-war increase and decline is mimicked by the inter-quartile range, disease categories varied widely in terms of the number of member states for which surveillance activities were documented, from >100 (maximum line trace) to <5 (minimum line trace) member states.

CLUSTER ANALYSIS

To classify the 123 infectious and parasitic disease categories (Table 3.1) in terms of surveillance trends, the annual time series of the number of WHO member states in which each category was monitored, 1923–83, were subjected to complete linkage cluster analysis. The analysis yielded the five clearly defined groups of disease categories (groups 1–5) in Table 3.2. Group 1 is especially noteworthy for the inclusion of, among other conditions, the great quarantine diseases (cholera, plague, relapsing fever, smallpox, typhus fever, and yellow fever) subject to notification to the WHO under the 1951 International Sanitary Regulations. The remaining groups, 2–5, include a diverse set of infectious and parasitic diseases that, in the first instance, appear to defy any simple categorization on aetiological or epidemiological grounds.

To examine the temporal trends that underpin the group-wise classification in Table 3.2, Figure 3.4 plots the average number of WHO member states with

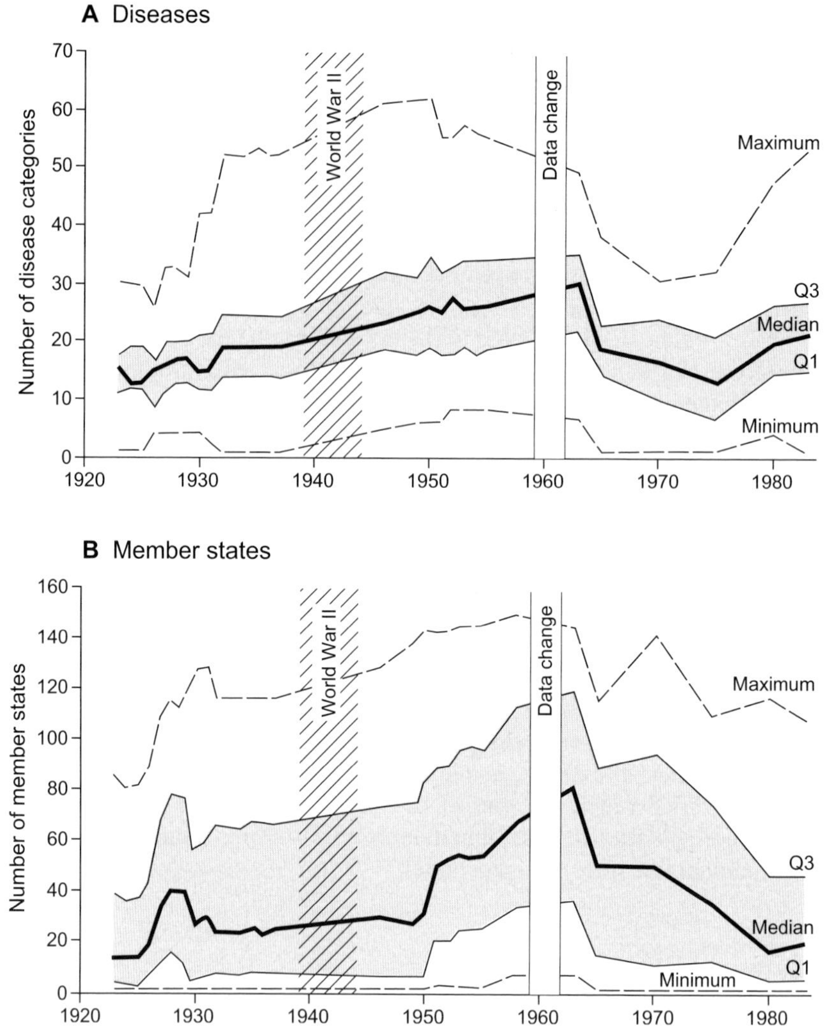

Fig. 3.3. Trends in global surveillance for 123 sample infectious and parasitic disease categories, 1923–1983. II: Summary statistics

(A) Number of disease categories per WHO member state for which surveillance activities were documented in the League of Nations/WHO data set. (B) Number of WHO member states in which surveillance activities for the diseases were documented in the League of Nations/WHO data set. Graphs plot the median (heavy line trace), inter-quartile range (Q1, Q3; shaded envelope) and maximum and minimum counts (broken line traces) of disease categories (graph A) and member states (graph B) for sample years. Surveillance activities have been assessed on the basis of the notifiable status of diseases (1923–58) and published disease reports (1963–83); the hinge period marking the change in data type is indicated. The 123 sample disease categories (*ICD-10* codes A00–B99) are listed in Table 3.1.

Table 3.2. Disease groups as determined by complete linkage cluster analysis

Group[1]	Disease (*ICD*-10 code)[1]
1	Cholera (A00); botulism (A05); diarrhoea and gastroenteritis (A09); plague (A20); glanders (A24); rat-bite fevers (A25); tetanus (A33–A35); actinomycosis (A42); bartonellosis (A44); colibacillosis (A49); syphilis (A50–A53); chancroid (A57); yaws (A66); relapsing fever, unspecified (A68); other spirochaetal infections (A69); typhus fever (A75); rabies (A82); dengue fever (A90); other arthropod-borne viral fevers, not elsewhere classified (A93); yellow fever (A95); zoster (B02); smallpox (B03); rubella (B06); foot and mouth disease (B08); malaria (B50–B54); leishmaniasis (B55); Chagas' disease (B57); trichinellosis (B75); ancylostomiasis (B76); ascariasis (B77); scabies (B86)
2	Typhoid and paratyphoid fevers (A01); shigellosis (A03); amoebiasis (A06); tularaemia (A21); anthrax (A22); brucellosis (A23); leptospirosis (A27); leprosy (A30); diphtheria (A36); scarlet fever (A38); meningococcal infection (A39); erysipelas (A46); gas gangrene (A48); chlamydial lymphogranuloma (venereum) (A55); granuloma inguinale (A58); psittacosis (A70); trachoma (A71); typhus, endemic (murine typhus) (A75); other rickettsioses (A79); poliomyelitis (A80); unspecified viral encephalitis (A86); unspecified mycosis (B49); African trypanosomiasis (B56)
3	Other salmonella infections (A02); other bacterial intestinal infections (A04); other bacterial foodborne intoxications (A05); other protozoal intestinal diseases (A07); viral and other specified intestinal infections (A08); infection due to other mycobacteria (A31); other septicaemia (A41); late syphilis (A52); trichomoniasis (A59); unspecified sexually transmitted disease (A64); spotted fever (A77); atypical virus infections of central nervous system (A81); mosquito-borne viral encephalitis (A83); tick-borne viral encephalitis (A84); viral meningitis (A87); other viral infections of central nervous system, not elsewhere classified (A88); unspecified viral infection of central nervous system (A89); sandfly fever (A93); unspecified arthropod-borne viral fever (A94); arenaviral haemorrhagic fever (A96); other viral haemorrhagic fevers, not elsewhere classified (A98); unspecified viral haemorrhagic fever (A99); other acute viral hepatitis (B17); chronic viral hepatitis (B18); infectious mononucleosis (B27); viral conjunctivitis (B30); candidiasis (B37); histoplasmosis (B39); blastomycosis (B40); other mycoses, not elsewhere classified (B48); toxoplasmosis (B58); other predominantly sexually transmitted diseases, not elsewhere classified (B63); unspecified protozoal disease (B64); schistosomiasis (B65); echinococcosis (B67); other cestode infections (B71); filariasis (B74); other intestinal helminthiases, not elsewhere classified (B81); unspecified intestinal parasitism (B82); other helminthiases (B83); unspecified parasitic disease (B89)
4	Respiratory tuberculosis (A15–A16); tuberculosis, non-respiratory (A17–A19); other zoonotic bacterial diseases, not elsewhere classified (A28); other tetanus (A35); whooping cough (A37); congenital syphilis (A50); early syphilis (A51); other and unspecified syphilis (A53); gonococcal infection (A54); relapsing fever, tick-borne (A68); Brill's disease (A75); Boutonneuse fever (A77); Q fever (A78); chickenpox (B01); measles (B05); viral hepatitis (B15–B19); acute hepatitis B (B16); mumps (B26); unspecified malaria (B54); pediculosis (B85); other and unspecified infectious diseases (B99)
5	Rhinoscleroma (A48); trench fever (A79); encephalitis lethargica (A85); other viral diseases, not elsewhere classified (B33); dermatophytosis (B35); coccidioidomycosis (B38); other fluke infections (B66)

Note: [1] Three-character *ICD*-10 codes in parentheses.

documented surveillance activities for the disease categories in each of the five groups. A striking feature of the graph is the sustained increase in the time series for group 4 diseases (heavy line trace)—a group of diseases that, in addition to such high-profile conditions as gonococcal infection, measles, viral hepatitis, syphilis, tuberculosis, and whooping cough, includes the *ICD*-10 classifications A28 (other zoonotic bacterial diseases, not elsewhere classified) and B99 (other and unspecified infectious diseases); see Table 3.2. Recognizing the temporal shift in the nature of the available data on which to monitor trends in Figure 3.4, the graph shows that, by the early 1970s, group 4 had surpassed all other groups in terms of the average number of member states for which surveillance activities were documented. Among the remaining disease groups, three features of Figure 3.4 are especially noteworthy:

(1) *Groups 1 and 2*. International concern with the monitoring of diseases in these groups, which include a number of the great infectious and parasitic killers of earlier times (Table 3.2), expanded during the first 40 years of the observation period. Thereafter, the sharp reduction in the time series—which is especially pronounced for group 1—reflects the relatively few WHO member states that reported cases of many of the constituent diseases during the last two decades of the observation period.

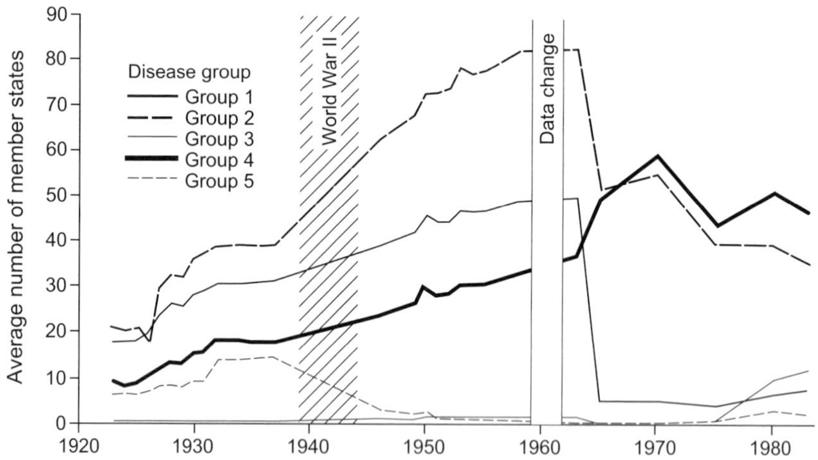

Fig. 3.4. Temporal trends in global surveillance for each group of disease categories in Table 3.2, 1923–1983
Line traces plot the average number of WHO member states with documented surveillance activities for the disease categories in each of groups 1–5 of Table 3.2. Surveillance activities have been assessed on the basis of the notifiable status of diseases (1923–58) and published disease reports (1963–83); the hinge period marking the change in data type is indicated.

(2) *Group 3*. International concern with the monitoring of diseases in this large group was at minimal levels until the latter years of the observation period, when a small but noteworthy increase in the average number of WHO member states that reported cases was registered. As we note below, this development reflected an extension of the *ICD* recording classes and the first-time inclusion of many of the diseases in the WHO surveillance records in the 1980s.

(3) *Group 5*. International concern with the monitoring of the small number of diseases in this group fell to near-zero levels in the post-1945 period.

EMERGING DISEASES IN THE GLOBAL SURVEILLANCE RECORD

Of the 123 disease categories in Table 3.1, 53 were included in the League of Nations/WHO records for the 1920s. For the remaining 70, Figure 3.5 shows

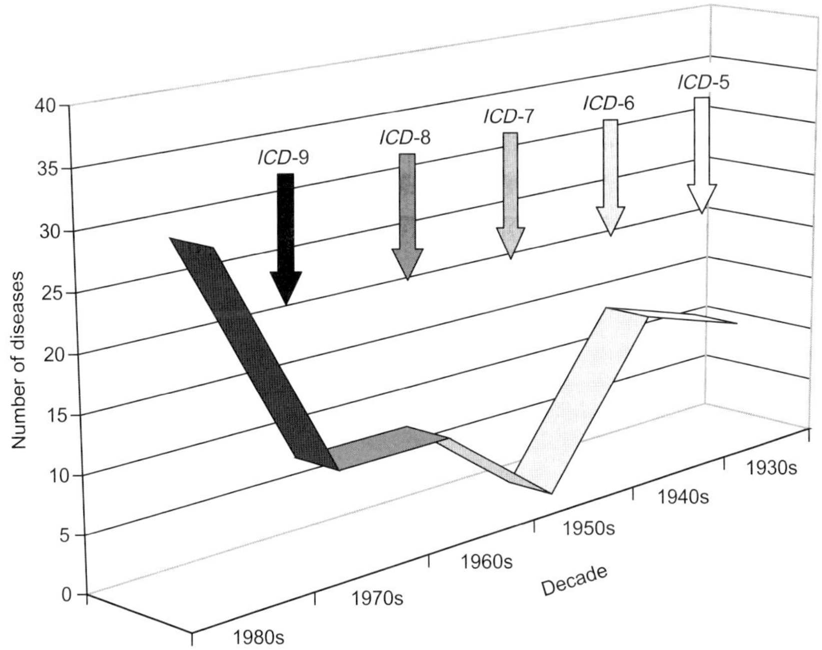

Fig. 3.5. Emergence of sample infectious and parasitic diseases in the global surveillance record. I. Newly recorded disease categories by decade, 1930s–1980s
The graph plots the number of disease categories first included in the League of Nations/WHO data set in a given decade, 1930s, . . . , 1980s. The disease categories are listed in Table 3.3. The timings of successive revisions of the *International Classification of Diseases* (*ICD*), described in Section 1.5.3, are indicated for reference.

Table 3.3. League of Nations/WHO: disease categories included for the first time in global surveillance records, 1930s–1980s

Decade of first inclusion	Disease category (*ICD*-10 code)
1930s	Shigellosis (A03); amoebiasis (A06); tularaemia (A21); rat-bite fevers (A25); rhinoscleroma (A48); other spirochaetal infections (A69); psittacosis (A70); foot and mouth disease (B08); coccidioidomycosis (B38); other fluke infections (B66); other helminthiases (B83)
1940s	Bartonellosis (A44); gas gangrene (A48); colibacillosis (A49); chlamydial lymphogranuloma (venereum) (A55); typhus, endemic (murine typhus) (A75); Q fever (A78); trench fever (A79); unspecified viral encephalitis (A86); other arthropod-borne viral fevers, not elsewhere classified (A93); zoster (B02); viral hepatitis (B15–B19); infectious mononucleosis (B27); Chagas' disease (B57); ascariasis (B77)
1950s	None
1960s	Other tetanus (A35); congenital syphilis (A50); early syphilis (A51); late syphilis (A52); other and unspecified syphilis (A53); relapsing fever, tick-borne (A68); Brill's disease (A75); unspecified malaria (B54)
1970s	Other zoonotic bacterial diseases, not elsewhere classified (A28); infection due to other mycobacteria (A31); Boutonneuse fever (A77); tick-borne viral encephalitis (A84); acute hepatitis B (B16); other acute viral hepatitis (B17); chronic viral hepatitis (B18); other and unspecified infectious diseases (B99)
1980s	Other salmonella infections (A02); other bacterial intestinal infections (A04); other bacterial foodborne intoxications (A05); other protozoal intestinal diseases (A07); viral and other specified intestinal infections (A08); trichomoniasis (A59); unspecified sexually transmitted disease (A64); atypical virus infections of central nervous system (A81); mosquito-borne viral encephalitis (A83); viral meningitis (A87); other viral infections of central nervous system, not elsewhere classified (A88); unspecified viral infection of central nervous system (A89); sandfly fever (A93); unspecified arthropod-borne viral fever (A94); arenaviral haemorrhagic fever (A96); other viral haemorrhagic fevers, not elsewhere classified (A98); unspecified viral haemorrhagic fever (A99); viral conjunctivitis (B30); candidiasis (B37); histoplasmosis (B39); blastomycosis (B40); other mycoses, not elsewhere classified (B48); toxoplasmosis (B58); other predominantly sexually transmitted diseases, not elsewhere classified (B63); unspecified protozoal disease (B64); other cestode infections (B71); other intestinal helminthiases, not elsewhere classified (B81); unspecified intestinal parasitism (B82); unspecified parasitic disease (B89)

the number first included in the surveillance records by decadal period, 1930s, . . . , 1980s; the associated diseases are given in Table 3.3. While 'new' disease categories were added to the surveillance records at various stages during the six-decade interval, some 25 per cent of the 123 categories included in the analysis were recorded for the first time in the 1980s. As a rule, this latter development reflected the extension of *ICD* recording classes, graphed in Figure 1.8, to include 'other', 'unspecified', and 'not elsewhere classified' disease categories associated with a broad range of bacterial, fungal, helminthic, protozoal, and viral diseases (Table 3.3).

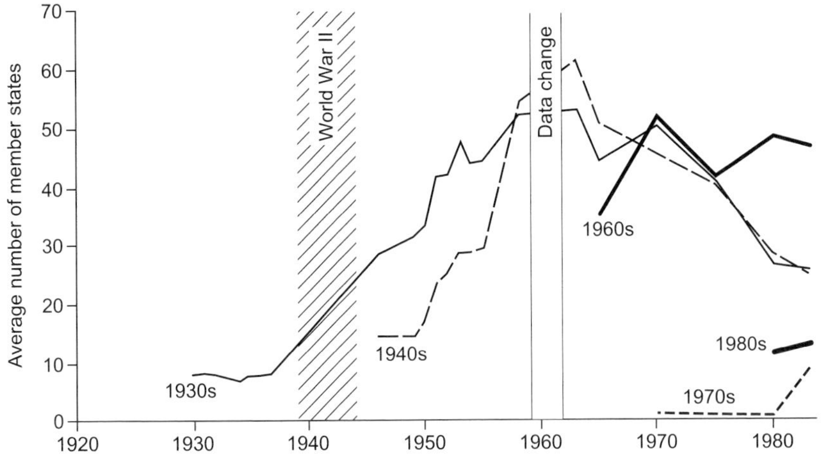

Fig. 3.6. Emergence of sample infectious and parasitic diseases in the global surveillance record. II: Trends in national surveillance, 1930s–1980s
For each decade-specific set of newly recorded disease categories in Table 3.3, the line traces plot the average number of WHO member states for which surveillance activities were documented in the League of Nations/WHO data set. Surveillance activities have been assessed on the basis of the notifiable status of diseases (1923–58) and published disease reports (1963–83); the hinge period marking the change in data type is indicated.

The Evolution of Surveillance for 'New' Diseases

Some impression of the evolution of surveillance for disease categories that were incorporated into the League of Nations/WHO records in the post-1920s period can be gained from Figure 3.6. For diseases first recorded in a given decadal period, the line traces plot the average number of WHO member states in which the diseases were notifiable (1930–58) or for which cases were published by WHO (1963–83). Beginning at relatively low levels, the average number of WHO member states that undertook surveillance for disease categories first included in surveillance records in the 1930s and 1940s grew rapidly to a peak of >50 states (1930s diseases) and >60 states (1940s diseases) in the early 1960s. Thereafter, the number of member states associated with both groups reduced rapidly, to <30 by the end of the series. The reporting of disease categories first introduced in the 1960s (including the categories of 'congenital', 'early', 'late', and 'other and unspecified' syphilis; Table 3.3) was adopted from the outset by a substantial proportion of WHO member states. Finally, the reporting of categories first introduced in the 1970s and 1980s was, on average, associated with few WHO member states over the time period for which data are available.

3.2.3 World Regional Patterns

Based on the set of 123 sample disease categories and 193 WHO member states, Figure 3.7 plots the number of disease categories monitored by longitude and latitude in the period 1923–83. Although the varying global distribution of land and water produces an irregular surface, peaks in the number of diseases are clearly identified in the regions of the Americas, Europe, and South-East Asia. With the notable exception of West Africa, which stands as a prominent peak to the south of Europe, troughs in the monitoring surface are identified in the Africa and Eastern Mediterranean regions.

REGIONAL DISEASE PATTERNS

One important geographical question that can be asked of the data set relates to the regional specificity of disease surveillance activities. More particularly, is it possible to identify distinctive regional concentrations of disease

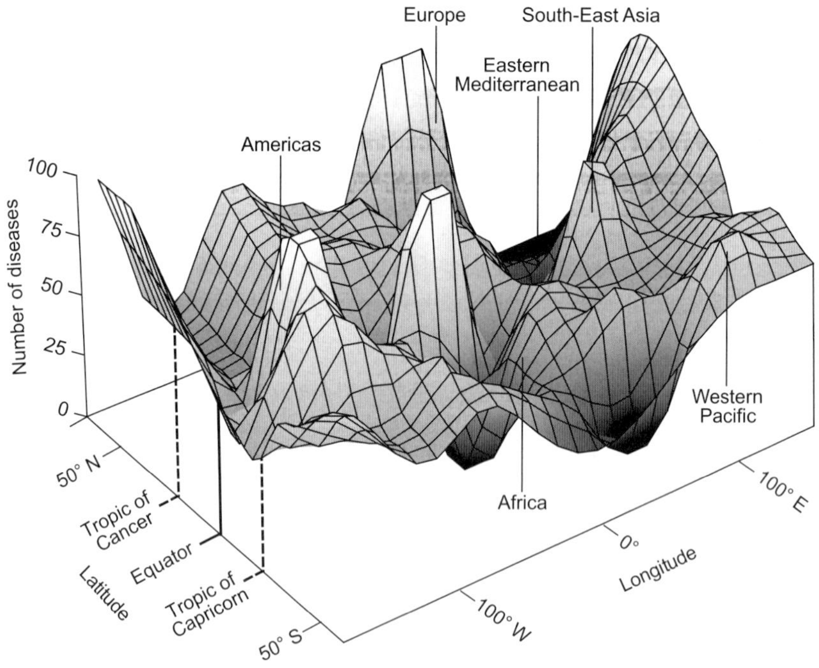

Fig. 3.7. Global surface of infectious and parasitic disease surveillance, 1920s–1980s The surface shows global variations in the number of disease categories in Table 3.1 for which surveillance activities were documented in WHO member states, 1923–83. Standard WHO regions are indicated for reference.

categories for which surveillance was undertaken and, if so, did these regional concentrations change over time? To examine the issue, let P_{Rt} represent the proportion of WHO member states in each of the six standard WHO regions R for which a given disease category was notifiable (1923–58) or for which cases were published by WHO (1963–83) in decadal period t. The regional concentration of documented surveillance activities for a given disease category and time period is then given by the ratio

$$P_{Rt}/P_{Gt}, \tag{3.1}$$

where P_{Gt} is the proportion of all WHO member states with documented surveillance activities for the disease category in the specified decade. Here, ratio values >1.00 mark a regional surfeit of documented surveillance activities for a given disease category relative to the global level, while values <1.00 mark a regional deficit.

Results

Table 3.4 gives, for each of the six WHO regions and seven decadal periods, the disease categories with the five highest ratios (ranks 1–5) in terms of equation 3.1. For the purposes of clarity, entries are limited to disease categories with ratio values >1.50, while, to highlight the pattern of disease emergence in the global surveillance record, categories first included in the data set in the specified decade are identified (see note 2 in the table).

Table 3.4 identifies a series of distinctive marker diseases for several of the world regions. In Africa, for example, African trypanosomiasis (1920s–1980s), schistosomiasis (1920s–1960s), and relapsing fever (1940s–1970s) feature in the list in three or more decadal periods. Likewise, spotted fever (1920s–1970s), coccidioidomycosis (1930s–1950s), and yellow fever (1960s–1980s) are prominent in the Americas, as are trench fever (1920s–1950s), tularaemia (1950s–1970s), and Brill's disease (1960s–1980s) in Europe, and echinococcosis (1920s–1940s) and diarrhoea and gastroenteritis (1940s–1960s) in the Western Pacific. Only in relatively rare instances, however, does a single disease category remain important throughout the entire observation period. Rather, the general tendency is for a disease category newly to enter the list for a given region and remain for one, two, or three decades, to be succeeded by other disease categories in subsequent periods. Two further features of Table 3.4 are also evident.

(1) During the 1930s and 1940s, the regional lead in the monitoring of 'new' disease categories was taken by the Americas (coccidioidomycosis, colibacillosis, gas gangrene, Q fever, and rat-bite fevers), Europe (infectious mononucleosis), and the Western Pacific (other helminthiases, chlamydial lymphogranuloma, and viral hepatitis). These regions were joined, in the 1960s and 1970s, by Africa (certain

Table 3.4. Regional specificity of infectious and parasitic disease categories most commonly subject to monitoring in WHO member states, 1920s–1980s

		Disease[1]				
World region	Decade	Rank 1	Rank 2	Rank 3	Rank 4	Rank 5
Africa	1920s	African trypanosomiasis (B56) [3.60][2]	Schistosomiasis (B65) [1.68][2]	Brucellosis (A23) [1.60][2]	—	—
	1930s	African trypanosomiasis (B56) [3.60]	Yaws (A66) [3.10]	—	—	—
	1940s	African trypanosomiasis (B56) [2.78]	Yaws (A66) [1.82]	Relapsing fever, unspecified (A68) [1.72]	Schistosomiasis (B65) [1.54]	—
	1950s	African trypanosomiasis (B56) [2.78]	Leishmaniasis (B55) [1.63]	—	—	—
	1960s	African trypanosomiasis (B56) [2.66]	Relapsing fever, tick-borne (A68) [2.10][2]	Smallpox (B03) [2.00]	Schistosomiasis (B65) [1.68]	Leishmaniasis (B55) [1.66]
	1970s	Tick-borne viral encephalitis (A84) [4.20][2]	Rubella (B06) [4.20]	Chronic viral hepatitis (B18) [4.20][2]	Relapsing fever, tick-borne (A68) [3.50]	Pediculosis (B85) [3.36]
	1980s	Unspecified viral infection of the CNS (A89) [4.2][2]	Unspecified arthropod-borne viral fever (A94) [4.20][2]	Coccidioidomycosis (B38) [4.20]	Histoplasmosis (B39) [4.20][2]	African trypanosomiasis (B56) [3.24]
Americas	1920s	Filariasis (B74) [5.51][2]	Spotted fever (A77) [5.51][2]	Dengue fever (A90) [2.28][2]	Syphilis (A50–A53) [2.19][2]	Leptospirosis (A27) [2.10][2]
	1930s	Rat-bite fevers (A25) [5.51][2]	Coccidioidomycosis (B38) [5.51][2]	Spotted fever (A77) [5.51]	Pediculosis (B85) [4.60]	Tularaemia (A21) [4.40]
	1940s	Rat-bite fevers (A25) [5.51]	Gas gangrene (A48) [5.51][2]	Colibacillosis (A49) [5.51][2]	Q fever (A78) [5.51][2]	Coccidioidomycosis (B38) [5.51]
	1950s	Spotted fever (A77) [5.51]	Q fever (A78) [5.51]	Coccidioidomycosis (B38) [5.51]	Other fluke infections (B66) [5.51]	Ascariasis (B77) [5.51]

	1960s	Spotted fever (A77) [5.51]	Granuloma inguinale (A58) [2.83]	Other spirochaetal infections (A69) [2.76]	Unspecified mycosis (B49) [2.76]	Yellow fever (A95) [2.74]
	1970s	Diarrhoea and gastroenteritis (A09) [5.51]	Infection due to other mycobacteria (A31) [5.51][2]	Spotted fever (A77) [4.14]	Other and unspecified infectious diseases (B99) [2.76][2]	Yellow fever (A95) [2.34]
	1980s	Yellow fever (A95) [3.90]	Erysipelas (A46) [3.31]	Dengue fever (A90) [2.65]	Plague (A20) [1.79]	Viral hepatitis (B15–B19) [1.64]
Eastern Mediterranean	1920s	Dermatophytosis (B35) [2.92][2]	—	—	—	—
	1930s	—	—	—	—	—
	1940s	Schistosomiasis (B65) [1.63]	Echinococcosis (B67) [1.60]	—	—	—
	1950s	Pediculosis (B85) [1.54]	Echinococcosis (B67) [1.52]	—	—	—
	1960s	Congenital syphilis (A50) [8.77][2]	Cholera (A00) [1.55]	—	—	—
	1970s	Typhus, endemic (murine typhus) (A75) [5.26]	Acute hepatitis B (B16) [4.39]	Other acute viral hepatitis (B17) [4.39][2]	Pediculosis (B85) [1.75]	Malaria (B50–B54) [1.63]
	1980s	Unspecified protozoal disease (B64) [8.77][2]	Blastomycosis (B40) [4.39][2]	Leishmaniasis (B55) [2.96]	Other intestinal helminthiases, NEC (B81) [2.30][2]	Other fluke infections (B66) [2.19]
Europe	1920s	Trench fever (A79) [3.71][2]	Unspecified mycosis (B49) [3.71][2]	Pediculosis (B85) [3.71][2]	Scabies (B86) [3.71][2]	Other viral diseases, NEC (B33) [3.71][2]
	1930s	Other specified bacterial diseases (A48) [3.71]	Trench fever (A79) [3.71]	Other viral diseases, NEC (B33) [3.71]	Leptospirosis (A27) [2.81]	Glanders (A24) [2.43]
	1940s	Other specified bacterial diseases (A48) [3.71]	Other rickettsioses (A79) [3.71]	Trench fever (A79) [3.71]	Sandfly fever (A93) [3.09]	Infectious mononucleosis (B27) [2.78][2]
	1950s	Trench fever (A79) [3.71]	Other arthropod-borne diseases, NEC (A93) [3.71]	Botulism (A05) [2.23]	Tularaemia (A21) [2.19]	Infectious mononucleosis (B27) [1.86]
	1960s	Late syphilis (A52) [3.71][2]	Brill's disease (A75) [3.71][2]	Q fever (A78) [2.86]	Tularaemia (A21) [2.50]	Echinococcosis (B67) [2.12]
	1970s	Other zoonotic bacterial diseases, NEC (A28) [3.71][2]	Brill's disease (A75) [3.71]	Boutonneuse fever (A77) [3.71][2]	Tularaemia (A21) [3.25]	Psittacosis (A70) [3.09]

(Continued)

Table 3.4. (Continued)

World region	Decade	Disease[1]				
		Rank 1	Rank 2	Rank 3	Rank 4	Rank 5
	1980s	Brill's disease (A75) [3.71]	Infection due to other mycobacteria (A31) [3.71]	Unspecified sexually transmitted disease (A64) [3.71][2]	Q fever (A78) [3.71]	Zoster (B02) [3.71]
South-East Asia	1920s	Leishmaniasis (B55) [2.51][2]	Diarrhoea and gastroenteritis (A09) [1.74][2]	—	—	—
	1930s	Diarrhoea and gastroenteritis (A09) [3.76]	Filariasis (B74) [1.75]	—	—	—
	1940s	—	—	—	—	—
	1950s	—	—	—	—	—
	1960s	Cholera (A00) [2.61]	Plague (A20) [1.77]	—	—	—
	1970s	Smallpox (B03) [2.35]	—	—	—	—
	1980s	Relapsing fever, tick-borne (A68) [17.54]	Atypical virus infections of the CNS (A81) [8.77][2]	Arenaviral haemorrhagic fever (A96) [5.85][2]	Other mycoses, NEC (B48) [5.85][2]	Unspecified viral haemorrhagic fever (A99) [5.85][2]
Western Pacific	1920s	Echinococcosis (B67) [7.15][2]	Dermatophytosis (B35) [4.77][2]	Botulism (A05) [3.57][2]	Actinomycosis (A42) [3.57][2]	Granuloma inguinale (A58) [3.57][2]
	1930s	Other helminthiases (B83) [7.15][2]	Echinococcosis (B67) [3.91]	Other fluke infections (B66) [3.57]	Schistosomiasis (B65) [3.18]	Other septicaemia (A41) [2.38]
	1940s	Chlamydial lymphogranuloma (venereum) (A55) [2.10][2]	Echinococcosis (B67) [1.82]	Diarrhoea and gastroenteritis (A09) [1.80]	Viral hepatitis (B15–B19) [1.68][2]	Filariasis (B74) [1.62]
	1950s	Diarrhoea and gastroenteritis (A09) [2.17]	Filariasis (B74) [2.12]	Rubella (B06) [2.03]	Dengue fever (A90) [1.93]	Viral hepatitis (B15–B19) [1.76]
	1960s		Cholera (A00) [1.76]	Yaws (A66) [1.74]	Dengue fever (A90) [1.69]	Filariasis (B74) [1.62]

	Diarrhoea and gastroenteritis (A09) [1.98]				
1970s	Other acute viral hepatitis (B17) [3.57]	Leptospirosis (A27) [2.90]	Syphilis (A50–A53) [1.98]	Unspecified viral encephalitis (A86) [1.69]	Gonococcal infection (A54) [1.56]
1980s	Unspecified parasitic disease (B89) [7.15][2]	Mosquito-borne viral encephalitis (A83) [4.86][2]	Arenaviral haemorrhagic fever (A96) [3.57][2]	Candidiasis (B37) [3.57][2]	Other acute viral hepatitis (B17) [3.43]

Notes: [1] Rank importance of disease category as determined by equation 3.1. The top five ranked disease categories (rank 1 = highest ratio) are given, along with their associated (three-character *ICD*-10 codes) and [ratios].[2] Disease categories newly included in the League of Nations/WHO surveillance records in the decade.
CNS = central nervous system. NEC = not elsewhere classified.

tick-borne diseases and chronic viral hepatitis) and the Eastern Mediterranean (congenital syphilis and other acute viral hepatitis).

(2) Consistent with the evidence in Figure 3.5 and Table 3.3, the 1980s are singled out in Table 3.4 by the rapid and widespread institution of regional surveillance for a number of new disease categories in tropical and sub-tropical zones. Especially noteworthy are a broad range of viral diseases (atypical and unspecified virus infections of the central nervous system (CNS), arenaviral and unspecified haemorrhagic fevers, and mosquito- and other arthropod-borne viral encephalitis) in Africa, South-East Asia, and the Western Pacific. To these can be added a range of fungal infections in Africa (histoplasmosis), Eastern Mediterranean (blastomycosis), South-East Asia (other mycoses, not elsewhere classified), and the Western Pacific (candidiasis), along with unspecified protozoal diseases and intestinal helminthiases.

3.2.4 Summary

In this section, we have drawn on the published records of the League of Nations/WHO to analyse the pattern of globally documented surveillance activities for a large sample of infectious and parasitic disease categories, 1923–83. A prominent finding of our analysis has been the rapid expansion in the number of disease categories for which surveillance was undertaken in the latter years of the observation period. So, while 'new' disease categories were added to the League of Nations/WHO surveillance records at various stages during the six-decade interval, 30 per cent of the sample categories were recorded for the first time in the 1970s and 1980s (Figure 3.5). This development reflected the extension of *ICD* recording classes to include a broad range of bacterial, fungal, helminthic, protozoal, and viral diseases (Table 3.3). When examined at the level of world region, the results in Table 3.4 highlight the regionally specific nature of globally documented disease surveillance activities, and the way in which these activities have evolved as both surveillance capacity and the number of recognized disease categories has expanded over time. Beginning with the Americas, Europe, and the Western Pacific in the early decades of the observation period, the geographical focus of monitoring activities for newly defined disease categories evolved to include Africa, the Eastern Mediterranean, and South-East Asia from the 1960s. Especially prominent in this latter development were a range of unspecified and atypical arthropod-borne viral fevers and infections of the CNS, viral haemorrhagic fevers, and bacterial, fungal, helminthic, and protozoal infections that were first included in the League of Nations/WHO surveillance records in the 1980s.

3.3 'Headline Trends' in Communicable Diseases: *MMWR Weekly*, 1952–2005

In this section, we examine the contents of one of the most familiar journals in the epidemiological world: *Morbidity and Mortality Weekly Report*. Universally abbreviated as *MMWR*, it has landed on thousands of desks each week since 1952—first in paper format and now electronically via the Internet. Published since 1961 by the CDC in Atlanta, *MMWR* contains a mix of current information on the distribution of outbreaks and epidemics around the world, reports on vaccines, protective devices, disease definitions, and other developments of epidemiological importance, as well as statistical tables of notifiable diseases in the states and territories of the United States.

The *MMWR* is valued for its timeliness and immediacy. Somewhat akin to the headlines of a newspaper, the mixture of reports, notices, and summaries contained within *MMWR* provides a means of tracking 'headline trends' in the contemporary occurrence of communicable diseases of national and international importance. It is the insights provided by an analysis of these headline trends that form the basis of the present section.

3.3.1 The MMWR Weekly *Data Set*

Volume 1, Number 1, of the weekly series of *MMWR* (now known as *MMWR Weekly*) appeared on Friday 11 January 1952 (Plate 3.2). In the 54 years since that first edition, 1952–2005 (volumes 1–54), a total of 2,798 issues of *MMWR Weekly* were published, including 2,785 regular issues, 11 double issues, and two special issues and supplements.[3] Aside from the core tables of notifiable diseases in the United States, the 2,798 issues included a total of 16,297 separate reports, articles, notices, updates, and related items that appeared under a variety of section headings, including 'Current Trends', 'Brief Reports', 'Epidemiologic Notes and Reports', 'International Notes', 'Special Reports', 'Surveillance Summaries', and 'Updates'. The topics covered in this class of item, which we refer to for convenience as 'entries' in the remainder of the present section, range from ciguatera fish poisoning to diabetic retinopathy, from iron deficiency to foetal alcohol syndrome, and from dental health to childhood pedestrian deaths during Hallowe'en. And scattered among these entries are the early notices and ground-breaking reports of a half-century-long series of newly emerging

[3] The count relates exclusively to *MMWR Weekly* and excludes additional publications in the *Recommendations and Reports*, *Surveillance Summaries*, *Supplements* and *Notifiable Diseases* series.

Morbidity and Mortality Weekly Report

FEDERAL SECURITY AGENCY Public Health Service

NATIONAL OFFICE OF VITAL STATISTICS

Vol. 1, No. 1 Washington 25, D.C. January 11, 1952

Provisional Statistics for Specified Notifiable Diseases in the United States for Week Ended January 5, 1952

For the current week there was a total of 9,284 cases of measles reported which was 14 percent higher than for the previous week and nearly 70 percent greater than the number reported for the same week of 1951. The disease is being reported in increasingly large numbers in several of the South Atlantic States. Incidence still remains high in the northeastern part of the country.

The revised list of diseases recommended for weekly reporting by States to the Public Health Service formed the basis for the current week. The diseases being reported for the first time are brucellosis, dengue, infectious hepatitis, trichiniasis, endemic typhus fever, and rabies in man. Cases of dengue and rabies in man will be shown only in footnotes when they occur.

Of the diseases reported for the first time on a regular weekly basis, there were few cases of brucellosis. A considerable number of cases of infectious hepatitis (157) were reported. States reporting the largest numbers were: Georgia with 48, Tennessee with 20, and Kentucky with 16. Only 2 cases of trichiniasis, and 3 of endemic typhus were reported.

In addition to the above changes all cases of scarlet fever and streptococcal sore throat will be combined in one figure. Paratyphoid fever has been ommitted, but typhoid fever cases will be reported. Influenza and pneumonia will no longer be included in morbidity tabulations.

EPIDEMIOLOGICAL REPORTS

Infectious Hepatitis

Dr. J. P. Ward, Arizona Director of Public Health, has reported an extensive outbreak (approximately 275 to 300 cases) of infectious hepatitis in a boarding school for Indians in Tuba City. Preliminary reports indicate that scattered cases occurred in October, but since that time increasing numbers have occurred. Staff members are also reported to be ill. A second nearby community consisting of 600 Indians has had frequent contact with the school, and it appears that some members of this group may be involved in the outbreak. Drs. L. A. Byers, and C. M. Clark, Jr., of the Indian Medical Service, and State health department officials in cooperation with other Federal officials are conducting an intensive investigation. Gamma globulin is being used in an attempt to prevent infection in those not yet ill.

Rabies in Man

Dr. C. R. Freeble, Ohio Department of Health, has reported a case of rabies in a man who died less than 24 hours after seeking medical advice. He had not been feeling well for several days, however. Profuse salivation and violence were noted a few hours before death. Microscopic examination of the brain demonstrated the presence of Negri bodies, which was confirmed by another laboratory. No animal inoculations were done. Three weeks prior to the patient's illness he shot a fox while hunting in an area where rabies was known to have occurred in these animals. However, no history of a bite was established. The family's hunting dogs had been well and had had antirabies vaccine.

Gastro-enteritis

Dr. Dean Fisher, Maine Director of Health, has reported an outbreak of food poisoning among 8 adults following a meal at which cooked chicken was eaten. Two chickens were cooked, and all 8 cases resulted from eating one of them. Persons eating the other were not ill.

Influenza

Dr. Morris Schaeffer, Public Health Service Communicable Disease Center, has reported through the Influenza Information Center, National Institutes of Health, that a set of paired serum specimens taken from a patient in Indiana showed a significant rise in titer to type A influenza virus. The pair of specimens was received from the Indiana State Board of Health on December 27, 1951. No date of onset was given nor was clinical information furnished.

Botulism

Dr. M. H. Merrill, California Department of Health, has reported 2 fatal cases of botulism which occurred in Fresno County. The onset of these cases was December 29 and both died on December 31. No other persons were present at the meal when infection took place. Laboratory examinations of food collected from the home have not been completed.

Primary Atypical Pneumonia

Dr. G. D. Carlyle Thompson, Executive Officer, Montana Board of Health, has supplied preliminary information on several cases of primary atypical pneumonia which occurred during the latter half of December at the Montana State Training School at Boulder, Montana. Considerable concern developed over this situation as the first 2 cases were severe, and the institution houses 550 individuals. Onset of the disease was sudden with slight sore throat, slight cough, chest pain, and temperatures ranging from 101° to 104°. Penicillin had little or no effect, but aureomycin promptly relieved all symptoms. However, as evidenced by X-ray, the pulmonary infiltration process continued after the administration of aureomycin. A total of 25 cases was hospitalized during a 3-week period. Cold-hemagglutinin tests were performed on these 25 cases. Ten of these gave findings significant of such an infection. Pharyngeal and nasal washings have been submitted to the Public Health Service Rocky Mountain Laboratory in order to isolate a specific virus, if possible.

Pl. 3.2. The inaugural issue of *Morbidity and Mortality Weekly Report* (*MMWR*) Vol. 1, no. 1, published by the US Public Health Service on Friday 11 Jan. 1952. Responsibility for the publication of *MMWR* passed to CDC in 1961.

infectious diseases (Plate 3.3). In this section, we undertake a content analysis of the 16,297 entries contained in *MMWR Weekly* to explore international and domestic (US) trends in the recognition and monitoring of infectious diseases, 1952–2005.

A

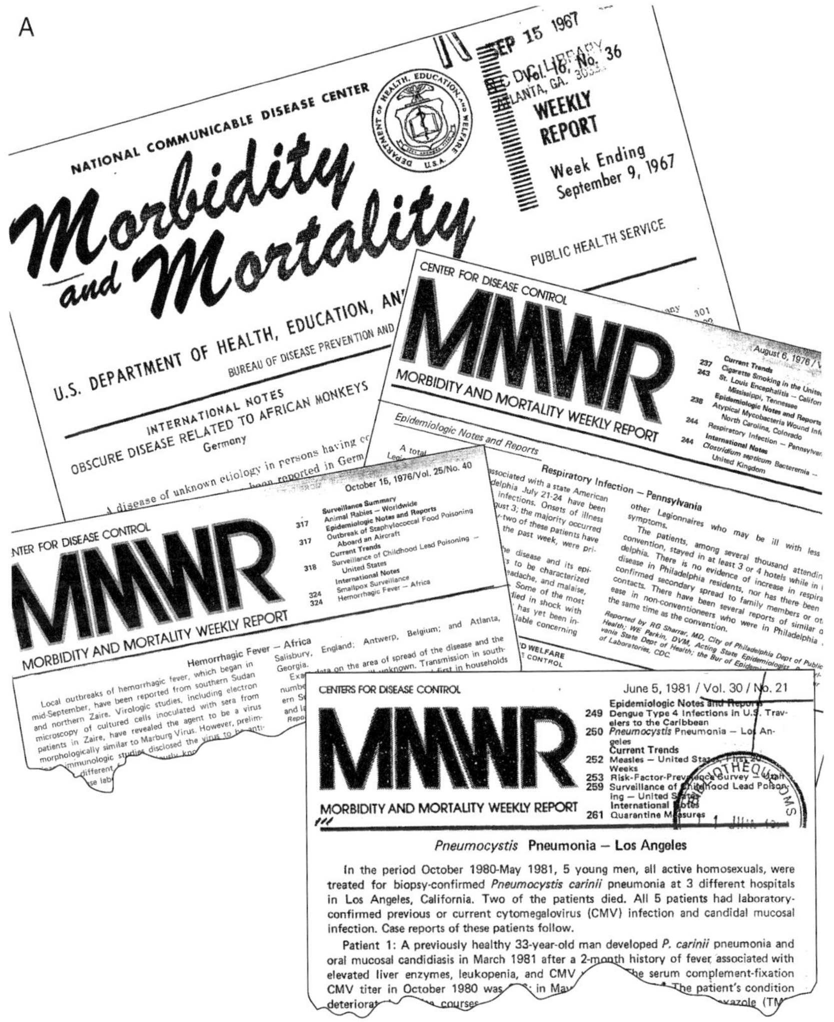
NATIONAL COMMUNICABLE DISEASE CENTER
Morbidity and Mortality
WEEKLY REPORT
Week Ending September 9, 1967
PUBLIC HEALTH SERVICE
U.S. DEPARTMENT OF HEALTH, EDUCATION, AND
INTERNATIONAL NOTES
OBSCURE DISEASE RELATED TO AFRICAN MONKEYS
Germany
CENTER FOR DISEASE CONTROL
MMWR
MORBIDITY AND MORTALITY WEEKLY REPORT
Epidemiologic Notes and Reports
Respiratory Infection – Pennsylvania
October 15, 1976/Vol. 25/No. 40
Hemorrhagic Fever – Africa
CENTERS FOR DISEASE CONTROL
June 5, 1981 / Vol. 30 / No. 21
Pneumocystis Pneumonia – Los Angeles
In the period October 1980-May 1981, 5 young men, all active homosexuals, were treated for biopsy-confirmed Pneumocystis carinii pneumonia at 3 different hospitals in Los Angeles, California. Two of the patients died. All 5 patients had laboratory-confirmed previous or current cytomegalovirus (CMV) infection and candidal mucosal infection. Case reports of these patients follow.
Patient 1: A previously healthy 33-year-old man developed P. carinii pneumonia and oral mucosal candidiasis in March 1981 after a 2-month history of fever associated with elevated liver enzymes, leukopenia, and CMV

Pl. 3.3. Reports of newly recognized diseases in *MMWR Weekly*, 1965–2005
(A) From top: Marburg viral disease, Germany (16/36, 9 Sept. 1967); Legionnaires' disease, US (25/30, 6 Aug. 1976); Ebola viral disease, Sudan and Zaire (25/40, 15 Oct. 1976); HIV-related disease (*Pneumocystis* pneumonia), US (30/21, 5 June 1981).
(B) From top: Hantavirus pulmonary syndrome, US (42/22, 11 June 1993); Nipah virus encephalitis, Malaysia and Singapore (48/13, 9 Apr. 1999); West Nile fever, US (48/38, 1 Oct. 1999); human infection with avian influenza A (H5N1) virus, Asia (53/5, 13 Feb. 2004).

B

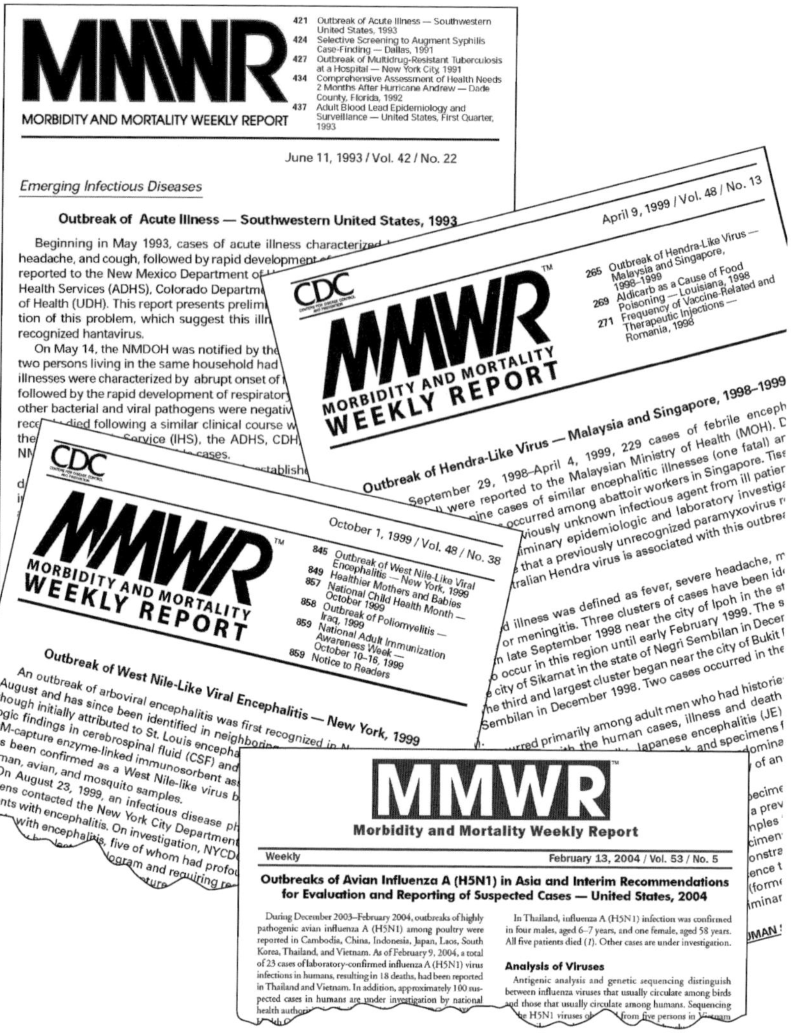

Pl. 3.3 (Continued)

DATABASE FORMATION

A database of the 16,297 entries in *MMWR Weekly*, 1952–2005, was formed to include the following fields: year, volume, number, and publication date; entry title; primary health issue; and, where applicable, primary geographical reference. On the basis of this information, entries were further classified by: (i) domestic (US) or international (non-US) status; (ii) WHO world region (Africa, Americas, Eastern Mediterranean, Europe, South-East Asia, and

Western Pacific; see Figure 3.1); (iii) *ICD* code, limited for the purposes of the present analysis to a sample set of 126 communicable disease categories drawn primarily from Chapter I ('Certain Infectious and Parasitic Diseases, A00–B99') of *ICD*-10;[4] and (iv) for the communicable disease entries in (iii), the category of disease agent (bacterium, helminth, protozoan, rickettsia, virus, and other). Summary details of the 16,297 entries are given by classifications (i)–(iv) in Table 3.5. Geographically, the majority of entries were related to domestic US issues (85 per cent) and the Americas region (87 per cent) more generally. Epidemiologically, just under two-thirds of all contributions were associated with the 126 sample communicable disease categories (64 per cent), with viral and bacterial agents and their associated diseases accounting for almost 60 per cent of the entries.

3.3.2 Global Trends

Our analysis of trends in *MMWR Weekly* begins at the global level. We then look at trends in domestic (US) (Section 3.3.3) and international (non-US) (Section 3.3.4) entries.

GENERAL TRENDS

Figure 3.8A plots the annual count of entries in *MMWR Weekly* for all topics (upper line trace) and sample categories of infectious and parasitic disease encompassed by *ICD*-10 codes A00–B99 (lower line trace). Underlying trends are depicted by the polynomial regression lines fitted by ordinary least squares. During the first three decades of the observation period, the annual count of entries for all topics waned gradually, from a peak of >400 per annum in the initial years to a low of <150 per annum in the early 1980s. From the late 1980s, the number of entries started to rise again, to reach >300 per annum from the late 1990s. The curve for infectious and parasitic diseases tracks the overall pattern—albeit at a reduced level—until the early 1980s. Thereafter, the divergence of the two curves reflects both (i) the establishment of new publications (*Recommendations and Reports* and *Surveillance Summaries*) as outlets for communicable-disease-related information in the *MMWR* series and (ii) the widening scope of *MMWR Weekly* as CDC's

[4] The 126 sample *ICD-10* disease categories include 110 in Chapter I ('Certain Infectious and Parasitic Diseases'), with additional categories from Chapters VI ('Diseases of the Nervous System'), VII ('Diseases of the Eye and Adnexa'), IX ('Diseases of the Circulatory System'), X ('Diseases of the Respiratory System'), XII ('Diseases of the Skin and Subcutaneous Tissue'), XIII ('Diseases of the Musculoskeletal System and Connective Tissue'), XVI ('Certain Conditions Originating in the Perinatal Period'), XIX ('Injury, Poisoning and Certain other Consequences of External Causes') and XXII ('Codes for Special Purposes').

Table 3.5. Summary details of entries in *MMWR Weekly*, 1952–2005

Category[1]	Number of entries
All entries	16,297
Domestic/international	
Domestic (US) only	13,838
International (non-US) only	1,650
Combined (domestic & international)/no geographical reference	809
WHO world region	
Africa	291
Americas	14,211
Eastern Mediterranean	184
Europe	514
South-East Asia	80
Western Pacific	208
Multiple region/other[1]	809
Sample infectious disease groups (*ICD*-10 code)	
Intestinal infectious diseases (A00–A09)	2,014
Tuberculosis (A15–A19)	244
Certain zoonotic bacterial diseases (A20–A28)	551
Other bacterial diseases (A30–A49)	889
Infections with a predominantly sexual mode of transmission (A50–A64)	394
Other spirochaetal diseases (A65–A69)	44
Other diseases caused by chlamydiae (A70–A74)	262
Rickettsioses (A75–A79)	112
Viral diseases of the central nervous system (A80–A89)	1,282
Arthropod-borne viral fevers and viral haemorrhagic fevers (A90–A99)	505
Viral infections characterized by skin and mucous membrane lesions (B00–B09)	1,284
Viral hepatitis (B15–B19)	495
HIV disease (B20–B24)	397
Other viral diseases (B25–B34)	76
Mycoses (B35–B49)	89
Protozoal diseases (B50–B64)	302
Helminthiases (B65–B83)	188
Influenza and pneumonia (J09–J18)	1,334
Severe acute respiratory syndrome (U04)	28
Infectious disease agents	
Bacteria	4,000
Helminths	188
Protozoa	345
Rickettsiae	111
Viruses	5,392
Multiple/other	156

Note: [1] Includes entries with no primary geographical reference.

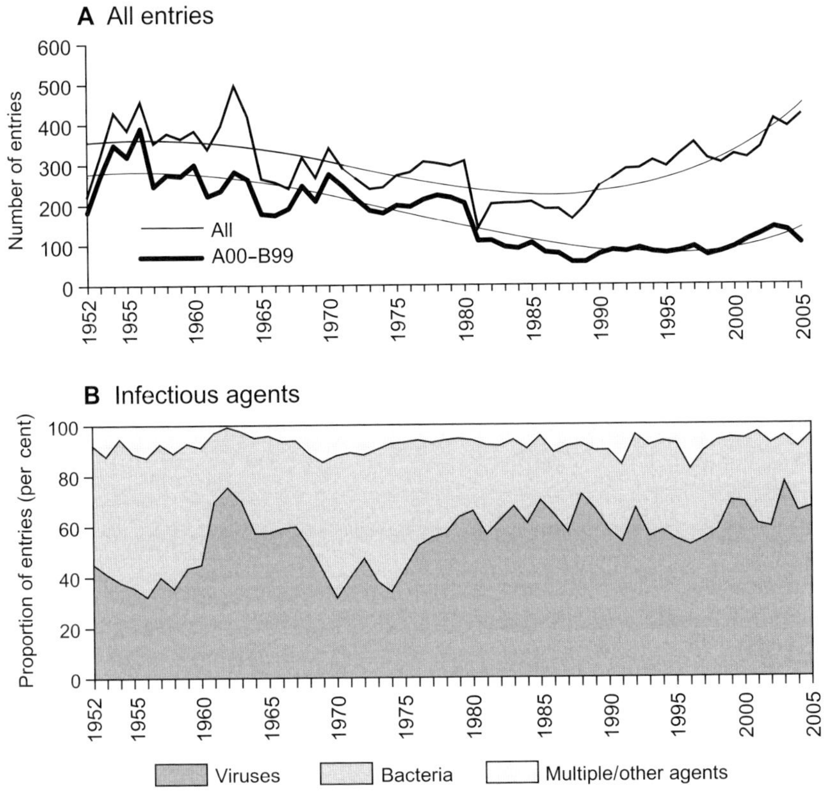

Fig. 3.8. Publishing trends in *MMWR Weekly*, 1952–2005
Graph A plots the annual count of entries on all topics (upper line trace) and sample infectious diseases encompassed by *ICD*-10 codes A00–B99 (lower line trace). Trends are depicted by polynomial regression lines fitted to the data by ordinary least squares. For the subset of entries relating to infectious agents, graph B plots the percentage proportion of entries associated with viruses, bacteria, and multiple/other infectious agents in each year. Note that graph B supplements sample diseases categorized in *ICD*-10 A00–B99 with infectious diseases included in other *ICD*-10 chapters.

activities expanded beyond communicable diseases (see Etheridge 1992; Centers for Disease Control and Prevention 1996*a*).

Trends in Infectious Disease Agents

Figure 3.8B plots, by annual period, the proportional distribution of a subset of 10,192 communicable disease entries in *MMWR Weekly* by type of agent (bacteria, viruses, and multiple/other agents). Although viruses and bacteria account for >90 per cent of entries in most years, noteworthy changes in the relative contribution of the two categories of disease agent are evident.

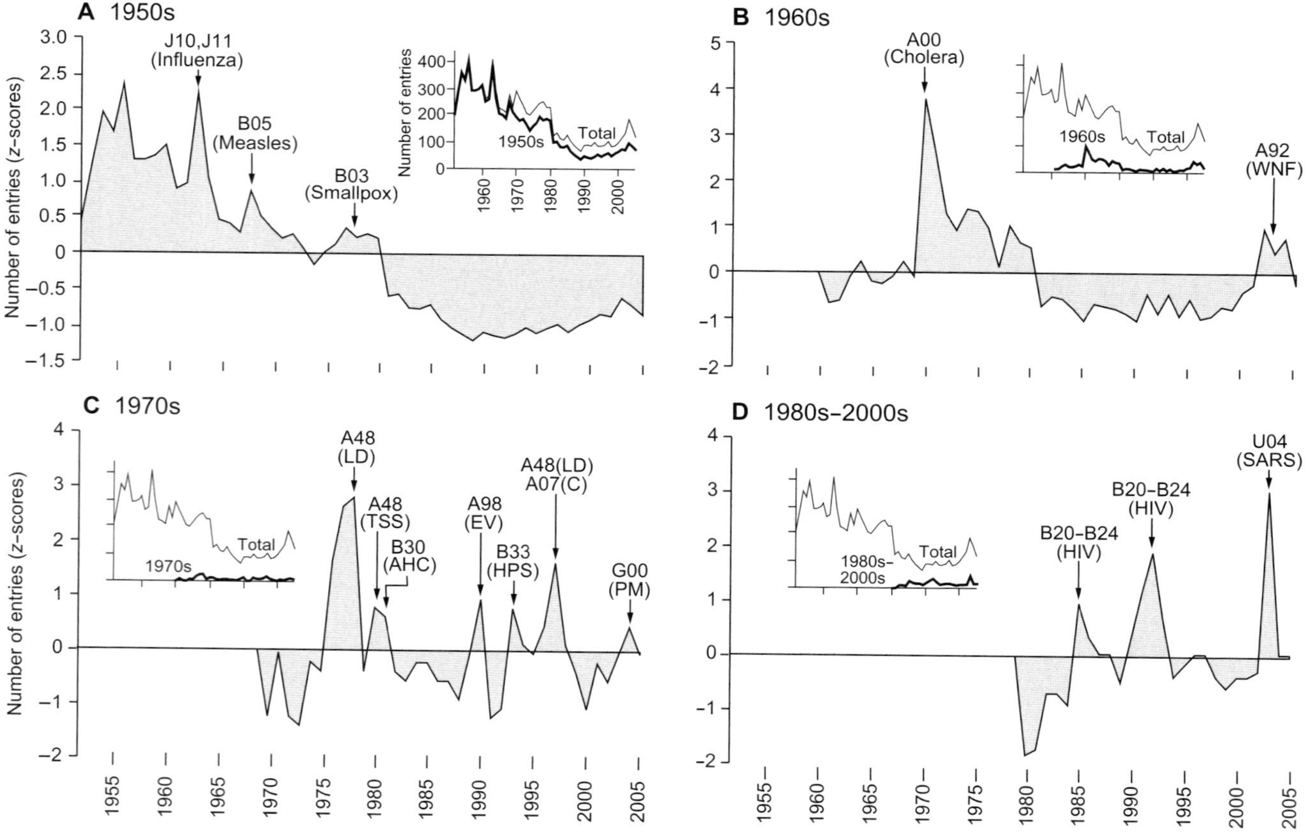
A 1950s
J10,J11
(Influenza)
B05
(Measles)
B03
(Smallpox)
Number of entries
1950s
Total
Number of entries (z-scores)
B 1960s
A00
(Cholera)
1960s
Total
A92
(WNF)
C 1970s
A48
(LD)
A48
(TSS)
B30
(AHC)
A98
(EV)
B33
(HPS)
A48(LD)
A07(C)
G00
(PM)
1970s
Total
Number of entries (z-scores)
D 1980s-2000s
1980s-
2000s
Total
B20-B24
(HIV)
B20-B24
(HIV)
U04
(SARS)

During the 1950s, viruses and bacteria each accounted for some 40–50 per cent of all entries. Thereafter, following a rise and fall in the 1960s and 1970s, viruses emerged as the most common type of disease agent—consistently accounting for 50–75 per cent of communicable disease entries in a given year—from the early 1980s.

NEW COMMUNICABLE DISEASE CATEGORIES

Figure 3.9 is based on the sample set of 126 communicable disease categories and plots, by year, the number of entries associated with diseases that were first included in *MMWR Weekly* in the 1950s (A), 1960s (B), 1970s (C), and 1980s–2000s (D). The main graphs plot the annual counts as standard Normal scores (*z*-scores); absolute counts are plotted in the inset graphs. Specific diseases associated with periods of increased coverage in *MMWR Weekly* are indicated for reference.

The main graphs in Figure 3.9 show a progressive shift in the pattern of publishing activity, with disease categories first included in the 1950s (graph A) and 1960s (graph B) displaying a pronounced reduction in levels of coverage in the pages of *MMWR Weekly* from the late 1970s. With the retreat of these longer-established diseases, the episodic spikes of activity associated with the graphs for the 1970s (graph C) and 1980s–2000s (graph D) flag the early reports of a range of apparently new diseases and disease agents. These include Legionnaires' (1976–8), toxic shock syndrome (1980), human immunodeficiency virus (HIV) (1985), Ebola virus infection in Asian primates (1990), hantavirus pulmonary syndrome (HPS) (1993), and severe acute respiratory syndrome (SARS) (2003). To these developments can be added the transatlantic extension of West Nile fever, evidenced by the early twenty-first-century resurgence of the curve in Figure 3.9B.

Fig. 3.9. Publishing trends for sample communicable diseases by decade of first inclusion in *MMWR Weekly*, 1952–2005.
The graphs are based on the sample set of 126 categories of communicable disease and plot the annual count of entries associated with the subset of categories first included in *MMWR Weekly* in the (A) 1950s, (B) 1960s, (C) 1970s, and (D) 1980s–2000s. Annual counts are plotted as standard Normal scores (*z*-scores) (main graphs) and as absolute counts (inset graphs, heavy line traces), with the latter also giving the annual count of entries for all 126 disease categories. Specific diseases (with their three-character *ICD*-10 codes) associated with periods of increased coverage in *MMWR Weekly* are indicated. AHC = acute haemorrhagic conjunctivitis. C = cyclosporiasis. EV = Ebola virus. HIV = human immunodeficiency virus. HPS = hantavirus pulmonary syndrome. LD = Legionnaires' disease. PM = pneumococcal meningitis. SARS = severe acute respiratory syndrome. TSS = toxic shock syndrome. WNF = West Nile fever.

Table 3.6. *MMWR Weekly*: leading disease categories by number of entries, 1952–2005

Rank	Disease	Number of entries
1	Influenza	1,180
2	Acute poliomyelitis	670
3	Smallpox	590
4	Viral hepatitis	495
5	Measles	491
6	Other salmonella infections[1]	428
7	Viral and other specified intestinal infections[2]	425
8	Rabies	415
9	HIV disease	397
10	Cholera	374
11	Other bacterial foodborne intoxications[3]	280
12	Syphilis	267
13	*Chlamydia psittaci* infection	259
14	Malaria	258
15	Tuberculosis	244
16	Diphtheria	240
17	Typhoid and paratyphoid fevers	221
18	Other septicaemia[4]	190
19	Shigellosis	185
20	Yellow fever	182

Notes: [1]*ICD*-10 A02 (including *Salmonella* enteritis, *Salmonella* septicaemia, and *Salmonella* infection, unspecified).[2]*ICD*-10 A08 (including rotaviral enteritis, acute gastroenteropathy due to Norwalk agent and adenoviral enteritis).[3]*ICD*-10 A05 (including botulism).[4]*ICD*-10 A41 (including septicaemia due to *Staphylococcus aureus*, septicaemia due to other specified *Staphylococcus*, septicaemia due to unspecified *Staphylococcus*, and septicaemia due to *Haemophilus influenzae*).

THE CHANGING IMPORTANCE OF COMMUNICABLE DISEASES

Based on the sample set of 126 of communicable disease categories, Table 3.6 compiles the top 20 disease categories as defined by the total number of entries in *MMWR Weekly*, 1952–2005. Influenza ranks as the disease with the highest number of entries (1,180 entries) (rank 1), with only two other diseases—acute poliomyelitis (rank 2) and smallpox (rank 3)—registering >500 entries. Classical infectious diseases (for example, cholera, diphtheria, malaria, measles, tuberculosis, typhoid and paratyphoid fevers, and yellow fever) dominate the remainder of the list, with HIV disease (rank 9) being the only disease category first included in *MMWR Weekly* in the period after the 1960s.

To check for temporal changes in the principal diseases covered in *MMWR Weekly*, Table 3.7 gives the top 20 disease categories for each of six successive time periods, 1952–2005. All told, 41 different disease categories were ranked in the top 20 at one point or another. On the basis of their sequence of appearance in Table 3.7, these categories can be classified into five broad groups:

(1) *Persistent disease categories*. Six disease categories ranked in the top 20 throughout the observation period (influenza, acute poliomyelitis, malaria, other salmonella infections, rabies, and viral hepatitis), with

Table 3.7. *MMWR Weekly*: leading disease categories by number of entries and time period, 1952–2005

	1952–9		1960–9		1970–9	
Rank	Disease	Number of entries	Disease	Number of entries	Disease	Number of entries
1	Gastroenteritis of assumed infectious origin	307	Influenza	440	Smallpox	276
2	Acute poliomyelitis	225	Acute poliomyelitis	247	Cholera	258
3	*Chlamydia psittaci* infection	224	Viral hepatitis	196	Influenza	214
4	Influenza	187	Smallpox	189	Syphilis	129
5	Rabies	140	Measles	156	Measles	104
6	Other salmonella infections[1]	134	Other salmonella infections[1]	121	Other salmonella infections[1]	103
7	Viral hepatitis	130	Other bacterial foodborne intoxications[3]	102	Yellow fever	96
8	Diphtheria	107	Rabies	96	Other bacterial foodborne intoxications[3]	84
9	Typhoid and paratyphoid fevers	105	Syphilis	96	Malaria	75
10	Anthrax	98	Pneumonia	95	Rabies	72
11	Shigellosis	72	Diphtheria	80	Viral hepatitis	65
12	Other septicaemia[2]	64	Malaria	75	Plague	53
13	Other bacterial foodborne intoxications[3]	62	Other septicaemia[2]	69	Shigellosis	52
14	Trichinellosis	55	Typhoid and paratyphoid fevers	69	Tuberculosis	50

(Continued)

Table 3.7. (Continued)

Rank	1952–9 Disease	1952–9 Number of entries	1960–9 Disease	1960–9 Number of entries	1970–9 Disease	1970–9 Number of entries
15	Malaria	44	Meningococcal infection	60	Typhoid and paratyphoid fevers	43
16	Smallpox	42	Gastroenteritis of assumed infectious origin	59	Acute poliomyelitis	42
17	Plague	39	Plague	53	Other bacterial diseases, NEC[4]	40
18	Meningococcal infection	37	Cholera	52	Pneumonia	40
19	Brucellosis	33	Dengue and dengue haemorrhagic fevers	43	Rubella	38
20	Leptospirosis	32	Yellow fever	43	Mosquito-borne viral encephalitis[5]	37

Rank	1980–9 Disease	1980–9 Number of entries	1990–9 Disease	1990–9 Number of entries	2000–5 Disease	2000–5 Number of entries
1	Influenza	183	HIV disease	189	Other mosquito-borne viral fevers[9]	125
2	Measles	125	Influenza	75	HIV disease	89
3	HIV disease	119	Acute poliomyelitis	68	Influenza	81
4	Tuberculosis	62	Tuberculosis	60	Acute poliomyelitis	68
5	Rabies	59	Measles	38	Tuberculosis	43
6	Smallpox	54	Viral hepatitis	35	Measles	37
7	Cholera	36	Rabies	33	Viral hepatitis	33
8	Viral hepatitis	36	Cholera	25	Severe acute respiratory syndrome (SARS)	28

9	Other salmonella infections[1]	33	Other bacterial intestinal infections[6]	23	Smallpox	27
10	Yellow fever	31	Malaria	22	Anthrax	24
11	Malaria	29	Other salmonella infections[1]	22	Bacterial meningitis, NEC	16
12	Rubella	29	Bacterial meningitis, NEC	21	Other salmonella infections[1]	15
13	Gonococcal infection	27	Bacterial infection of unspecified site	19	Rabies	15
14	Dengue and dengue haemorrhagic fevers	24	Other viral diseases, NEC[7]	18	Syphilis	15
15	Acute poliomyelitis	20	Other protozoal intestinal diseases[8]	16	Bacterial infection of unspecified site	14
16	Bacterial meningitis, NEC	18	Syphilis	15	Malaria	13
17	Other bacterial diseases, NEC[4]	18	Dengue and dengue haemorrhagic fevers	14	Viral and other specified intestinal infections[10]	13
18	Other bacterial foodborne intoxications[3]	17	Diphtheria	12	Whooping cough	11
19	Shigellosis	15	Viral and other specified intestinal infections[10]	12	Other bacterial intestinal infections[6]	9
20	Syphilis	12	Gonococcal infection	11	Varicella and zoster	9

Notes: [1]*ICD*-10 A02 (including *Salmonella* enteritis, *Salmonella* septicaemia, and *Salmonella* infection, unspecified).[2]*ICD*-10 A41 (including septicaemia due to *Staphylococcus aureus*, septicaemia due to other specified *Staphylococcus*, septicaemia due to unspecified *Staphylococcus* and septicaemia due to *Haemophilus influenzae*).[3]*ICD*-10 A05 (including botulism).[4]*ICD*-10 A48 (including gas gangrene, Legionnaires' disease, Pontiac fever, and toxic shock syndrome).[5]*ICD*-10 A83 (including Japanese encephalitis, Western equine encephalitis, Eastern equine encephalitis, St Louis encephalitis, Australian encephalitis, and California encephalitis).[6]*ICD*-10 A04 (including *Escherichia coli* infection).[7]*ICD*-10 B33 (including epidemic myalgia, Ross River disease, and viral carditis).[8]*ICD*-10 A07 (including cryptosporidiosis).[9]*ICD*-10 A92 (including West Nile fever).[10]*ICD*-10 A08 (including rotaviral enteritis, acute gastroenteropathy due to Norwalk agent, and adenoviral enteritis). NEC = not elsewhere classified.

influenza distinguished by a top 4 ranking in every period. An additional disease category (measles) continually ranked in the top 20 from the 1960s onwards.

(2) *Retreating disease categories.* Several disease categories featured prominently in the early time periods, but retreated from the top 20 ranking after the 1970s. Examples include plague and typhoid and paratyphoid fevers.

(3) *Emerging and retreating disease categories.* Certain disease categories waxed and waned over time in the rankings. Examples include cholera (1960s–1990s), dengue and dengue haemorrhagic fever (1980s–1990s), yellow fever (1960s–1980s), rubella (1970s–1980s), and shigellosis (1970s–1980s).

(4) *Recently emerging disease categories.* Consistent with the evidence in Figures 3.9C and D, some disease categories enter high into the rankings for the first time in the latter time periods of Table 3.7. Examples include HIV disease (1980s–2000s), other bacterial intestinal infections (including *Escherichia coli* infection) (1990s–2000s), viral and other specified intestinal infections (including norovirus gastroenteritis) (1990s–2000s), severe acute respiratory syndrome (SARS) (2000s), and other mosquito-borne viral fevers (including West Nile fever) (2000s).

(5) *Recently re-emerging disease categories.* Some established disease categories featured early in the rankings, disappeared, and then re-entered in the latter time periods of Table 3.7. Examples include smallpox and anthrax, whose coverage in *MMWR Weekly* in the 2000s was prompted by concerns over their use in bioterrorist attacks (see Section 8.5).

Fig. 3.10. Domestic (US) publishing trends for sample categories of communicable disease in *MMWR Weekly*, 1952–2005

Graphs plot, as the heavy line traces, the annual count of articles by *ICD*-10 code. (A) Intestinal infectious diseases (A00–A09). (B) Tuberculosis (A15–A19). (C) Certain zoonotic bacterial diseases (A20–A28). (D) Other bacterial diseases (A30–A49). (E) Infections with a predominantly sexual mode of transmission (A50–A64). (F) Viral infections of the central nervous system (A80–A89). (G) Arthropod-borne viral fevers and viral haemorrhagic fevers (A90–A99). (H) Viral infections characterized by skin and mucous membrane lesions (B00–B09). (I) HIV disease (B20–B24). (J) Protozoal diseases (B50–B64). (K) Helminthiases (B65–B83). (L) Influenza and pneumonia (J09–J18). Trends are depicted by polynomial regression lines fitted to the data by ordinary least squares. The principal diseases associated with sample periods of increased coverage are indicated on each graph. For reference, the bar chart on each graph plots, by year, the total number of entries associated with the entire sample set of 126 communicable diseases.

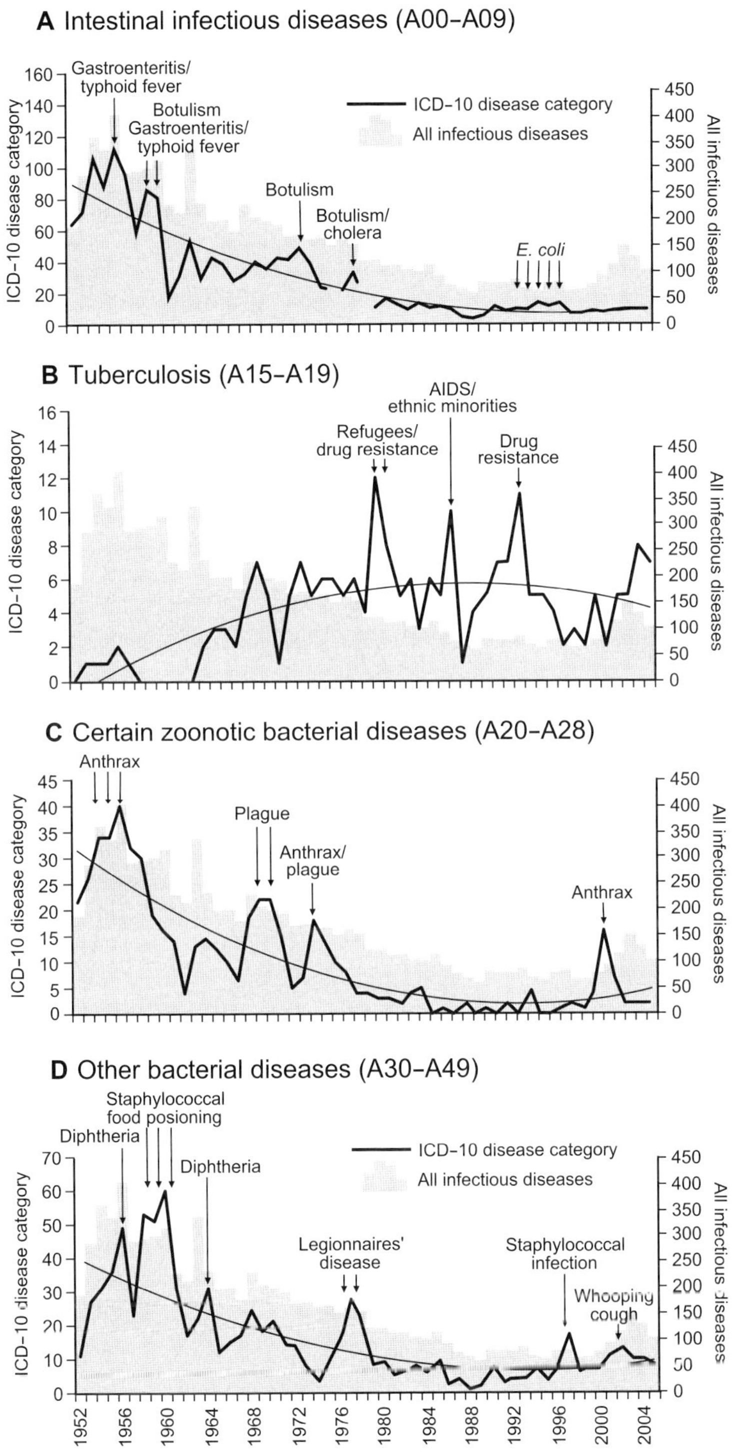

Fig 3.10. (Continued)

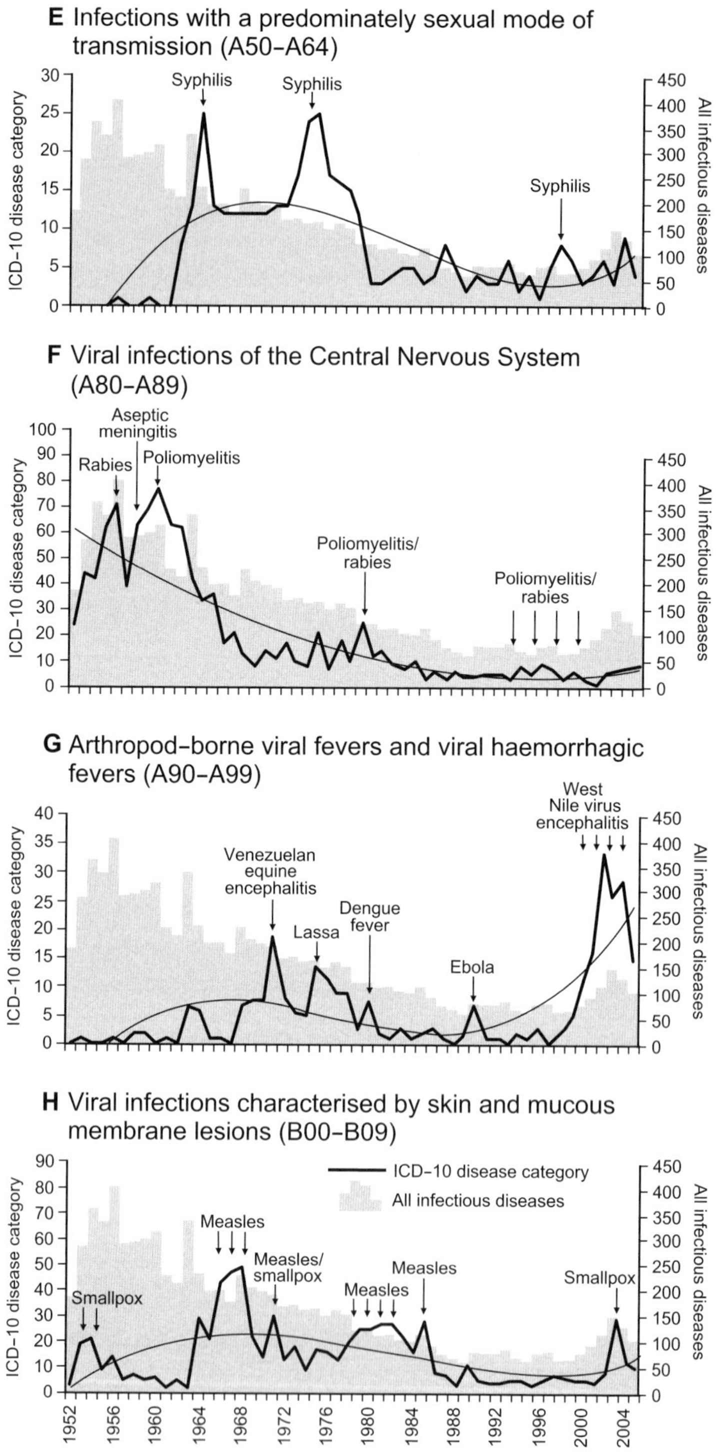

E Infections with a predominately sexual mode of transmission (A50–A64)
ICD-10 disease category
All infectious diseases
Syphilis
Syphilis
Syphilis
F Viral infections of the Central Nervous System (A80–A89)
ICD-10 disease category
All infectious diseases
Aseptic meningitis
Rabies
Poliomyelitis
Poliomyelitis/ rabies
Poliomyelitis/ rabies
G Arthropod-borne viral fevers and viral haemorrhagic fevers (A90–A99)
ICD-10 disease category
All infectious diseases
Venezuelan equine encephalitis
Lassa
Dengue fever
Ebola
West Nile virus encephalitis
H Viral infections characterised by skin and mucous membrane lesions (B00–B09)
ICD-10 disease category
All infectious diseases
Smallpox
Measles
Measles/ smallpox
Measles
Measles
Smallpox
1952
1956
1960
1964
1968
1972
1976
1980
1984
1988
1992
1996
2000
2004

Fig 3.10. (Continued)

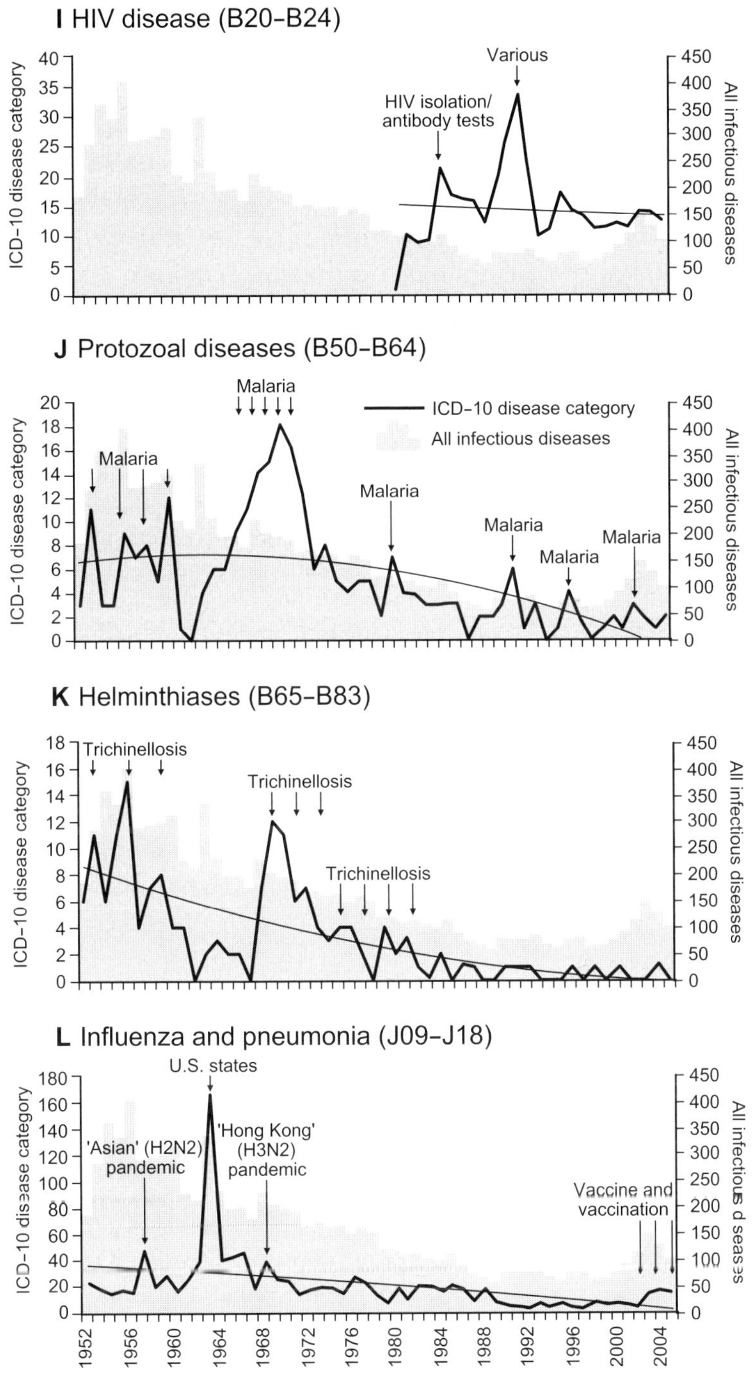

Fig 3.10. (Continued)

3.3.3 Domestic (US) Trends

In this subsection, we turn to an examination of the pattern of domestic (US) entries for communicable diseases in *MMWR Weekly*. We define domestic entries as the $n = 13{,}838$ entries (Table 3.5) relating exclusively to US locations; entries with combined US and non-US geographical references, or with no immediate geographical reference, have been omitted from the analysis.

GENERAL TRENDS IN COMMUNICABLE DISEASE CATEGORIES

Figure 3.10 plots as line traces in graphs A–K the annual count of domestic entries for each of 11 major divisions of Chapter I ('Certain Infectious and Parasitic Diseases, A00–B99') of *ICD*-10, 1952–2005; the equivalent information for an additional division ('Influenza and Pneumonia, J09–J18') in Chapter X ('Diseases of the Respiratory System, J00–J99') is plotted in graph L. Underpinning trends are shown by polynomial regression lines fitted by ordinary least squares. The principal diseases associated with sample periods of increased coverage in *MMWR Weekly* are indicated.

While most graphs display a secular reduction in coverage, approximately stable (HIV disease; graph I) or rising (tuberculosis, graph B; arthropod-borne viral fevers and viral haemorrhagic fevers, graph G) trends also occur. Superimposed on these trends, all graphs display occasional increases as developments in particular diseases or disease agents gained prominence in the epidemiological record. Especially noteworthy are the periodic increases in the coverage of botulism and *Escherichia coli* infection (graph A), tuberculosis (B), anthrax and plague (C), staphylococcal food poisoning and Legionnaires' disease (D), syphilis (E), poliomyelitis and rabies (F), Venezuelan equine encephalitis, Lassa fever, and, more especially, West Nile fever (G), measles and smallpox (H), malaria (J), trichinellosis (K), and influenza (L).

DISEASE RANKINGS

Paralleling the global analysis of Table 3.7, each of the 126 sample disease categories was ranked in terms of the number of domestic entries in *MMWR Weekly* (rank 1 = highest) for each of six time periods (1952–9, 1960–69, 1970–9, 1980–9, 1990–9, 2000–5). Changes in rank order, broadly categorized as rising (graph A), falling (graph B), and stable (graph C) trends, are illustrated for sample diseases in Figure 3.11. Consistent with the evidence in Figure 3.10, graph 3.11A highlights *Escherichia coli* infections, HIV disease, syphilis, tuberculosis, and West Nile fever, along with Lyme disease, as diseases that increased in rank importance over the course of the observation period. Other diseases (including leprosy, plague, and typhoid fever) reduced in rank importance (graph 3.11B), while yet others (including influenza, malaria, and rabies) changed little in their relative positions (graph 3.11C).

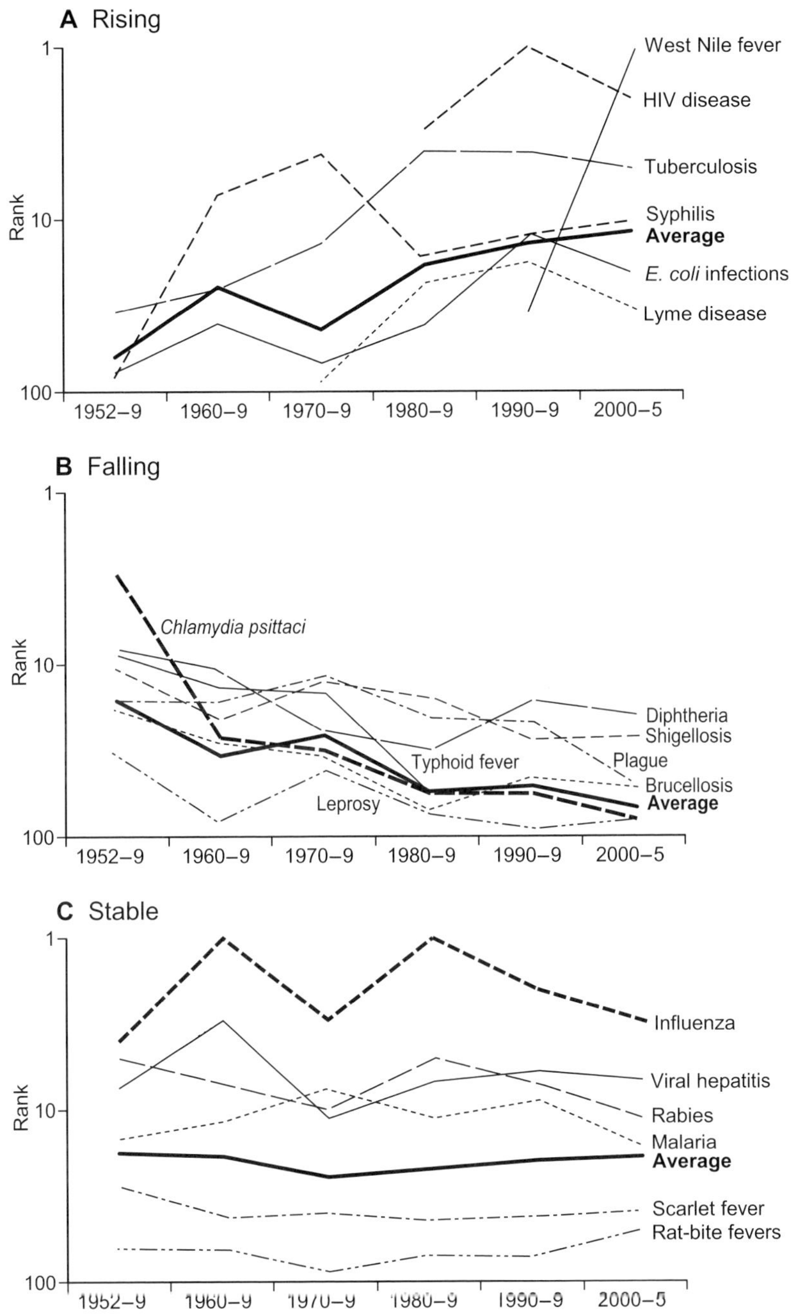

Fig. 3.11. Temporal changes in the rank importance of sample categories of communicable disease by number of domestic (US) entries in *MMWR Weekly*, 1952–2005 To form the graphs, diseases were ranked according to the number of entries (rank 1 = highest) in each of six time periods. Changes in rank order, broadly categorized as rising (A), falling (B), and stable (C), are illustrated for sample diseases. Heavy line traces show the average rank of the sample diseases on a given graph.

Table 3.8. Summary details of international (non-US) entries in *MMWR Weekly*, 1952–2005

World region[1]	Total	Number of entries			
		Communicable diseases[2]	Infectious agents[2]		
			Viruses	Bacteria	Multiple/other
Africa	291	239	148	66	25
Americas[3]	373	293	215	62	16
Eastern Mediterranean	184	163	88	65	10
Europe	514	444	295	129	20
South-East Asia	80	62	37	18	7
Western Pacific	208	182	119	55	8
TOTAL	1,650	1,383	902	395	86

Notes: [1] The six WHO world regions are mapped in Fig. 3.1.[2] Based on a sample set of 126 communicable disease categories.[3] Excludes the US.

3.3.4 International (Non-US) Trends

Approximately 10 per cent ($n = 1{,}650$) of all reports in *MMWR Weekly* were spatially referenced to non-US locations and are classified here as *international* entries (Table 3.5).[5] Summary details of these international entries, which form the basis of all analysis in the present subsection, are given by WHO region in Table 3.8.

TIME SERIES OF ENTRIES

Figure 3.12 plots as a histogram the annual count of international entries; counts of entries associated with viral, bacterial, and multiple/other disease agents are superimposed as line traces. The histogram is front-loaded, with the 1960s and 1970s marked out as decades of heightened international coverage in the journal. From an average of almost 60 entries per year (range 21–103) in these early years, international coverage fell away to just 17 entries per year (range 8–30) in the 1980s and beyond. As noted in Section 3.3.2, these developments coincided with the reorganization of CDC and a concomitant refocusing of the content of *MMWR Weekly*.

For the period of heightened international coverage, three major peaks of activity are evident in Figure 3.12: (i) 1961–5, associated with a pronounced increase in the coverage of two viral diseases (dengue and smallpox);

[5] For the purposes of the present analysis, international entries exclude the $n = 432$ entries which (i) encompass both US and non-US geographical locations, (ii) encompass geographical locations in more than one of the six standard WHO world regions or (iii) have a global / worldwide reference.

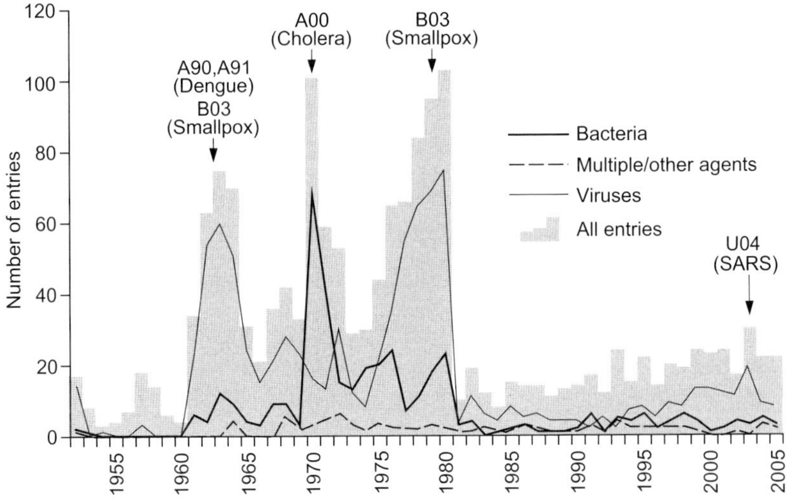

Fig. 3.12. Time series of disease agents associated with international entries in *MMWR Weekly*, 1952–2005
The histogram plots the annual count of all international (non-US) entries. The annual counts of entries associated with viral, bacterial, and multiple/other disease agents are superimposed as line traces. Diseases associated with raised numbers of entries are indicated, along with their three-character *ICD*-10 codes.

(ii) 1970–2, largely associated with an upsurge in entries relating to one bacterial disease (cholera); and (iii) 1976–80, related to the closing stages and immediate aftermath of the WHO Global Smallpox Eradication Programme. Finally, events associated with the 2003 epidemic of severe acute respiratory syndrome (SARS) are highlighted towards the end of the observation period.

World Regional Series

The geographical dimensions of the international coverage are shown in Figure 3.13 by the dark-shaded histograms which plot the annual count of entries geo-referenced to the WHO regions of: (A) Africa; (B) Americas, excluding the US; (C) Europe; and (D) the combined regions of Eastern Mediterranean, South-East Asia, and Western Pacific. Periodic upswings in regional coverage are evident, with smallpox in Europe (1962), dengue in the Americas (1963), cholera in Africa and Europe (1970), and smallpox in all regions (1976–80) underpinning the aggregate pattern. Thereafter, entries for each region continued at a low and approximately steady level. Inasmuch as there was a development in the regional focus of international coverage in the latter years of the observation period, a modest rise in entries for the combined regions of the Eastern Mediterranean, South-East Asia, and the Western Pacific from the early 1990s is apparent in Figure 3.13D. This was

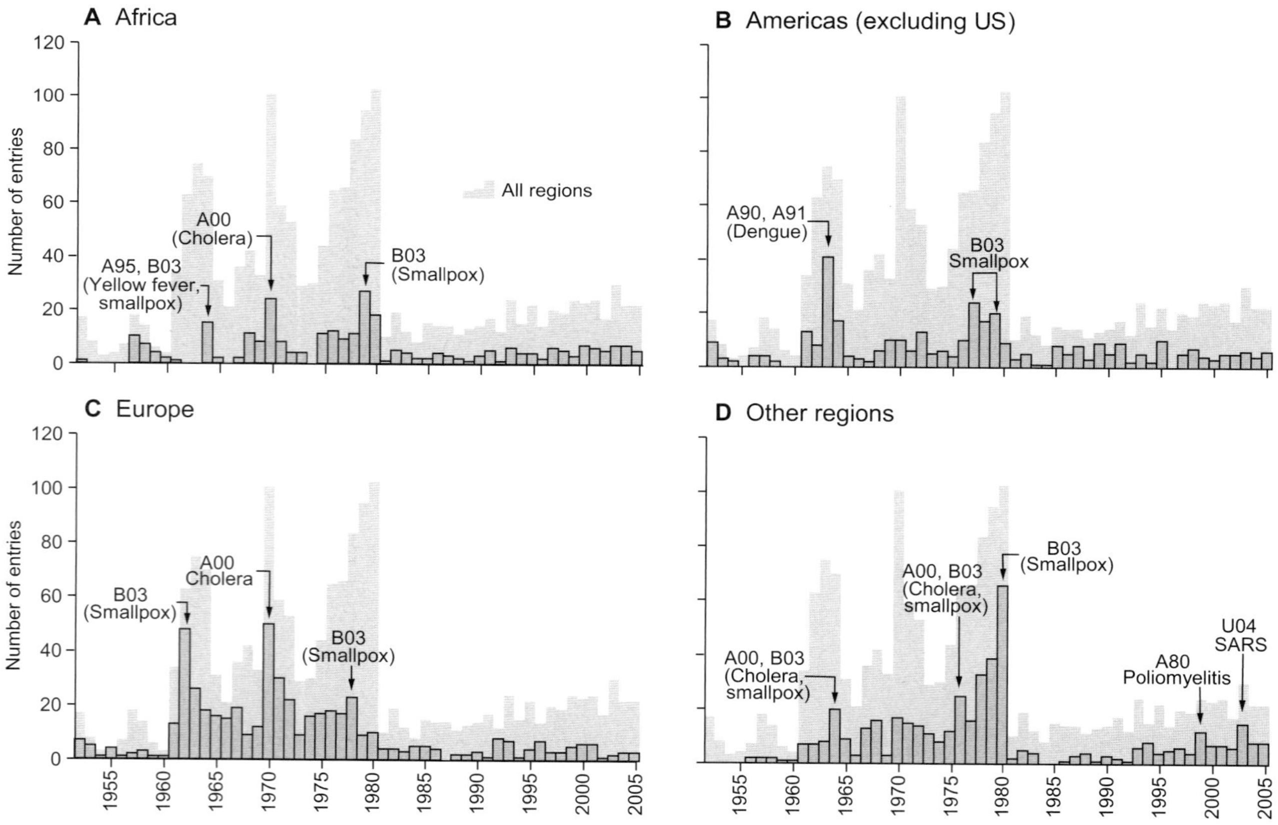

Fig. 3.13. International publishing trends in *MMWR Weekly*, 1952–2005
Dark-shaded histograms plot the annual count of international (non-US) entries by WHO region. (A) Africa. (B) Americas (excluding the US). (C) Europe. (D) Other world regions (Eastern Mediterranean, South-East Asia, and Western Pacific). The aggregate annual count of international entries, replotted from Fig. 3.12, is shown on each graph as the light-shaded histograms. Diseases associated with raised numbers of entries in a given region are indicated, along with their three-character *ICD*-10 codes. WHO world regions are mapped in Fig. 3.1.

associated, in part, with events related to (i) the progress of the WHO Global Polio Eradication Initiative in poliovirus-endemic countries of the Eastern Mediterranean and South-East Asia regions and (ii) the appearance and spread of SARS in countries of the Western Pacific region.

CENTROID ANALYSIS

Further insights into the geographical pattern of international entries in *MMWR Weekly* can be gained by examining the mean geographical centre of the entries over the observation period. The approach adopted is analogous to that outlined by Cliff, Haggett, Ord, and Versey (1981: 96–9) for the computation of epidemic centroids. For the six standard WHO world regions, let the location of the geographical centre of the *j*th world region be given a horizontal map coordinate (longitude) λ_j and a vertical map coordinate (latitude) ϕ_j.[6] For year t, let the number of entries in *MMWR Weekly* for j be denoted I_{jt}. The mean geographical centre at time t is then located at $\bar{\lambda}_t$, $\bar{\phi}_t$ where

$$\bar{\lambda}_t = \sum_{j=1}^{6} I_{jt}\lambda_j / \sum_{j=1}^{6} I_{jt}, \tag{3.2}$$

and

$$\bar{\phi}_t = \sum_{j=1}^{6} I_{jt}\phi_j / \sum_{j=1}^{6} I_{jt}. \tag{3.3}$$

For each year of the observation period, the geographical centre of international entries was computed for (i) the sample set of 126 communicable disease categories, and for entries associated with (ii) viral agents, (iii) bacterial agents, and (iv) multiple/other agents.

Results I: Map Patterns

Figure 3.14 summarizes the results of the centroid analysis for the sample set of communicable diseases (A) and for the sub-categories of entries associated with viral (B), bacterial (C), and multiple/other agents (D) disease categories. Broken lines link the latitude and longitude coordinates of centres in successive years, while, to capture the general pattern of movement, the heavy line traces link the average latitude and longitude coordinates of centres in sequential five-year periods (1955–9, ..., 2000–4). The locations of WHO regions, plotted as the average longitudes and latitudes of the constituent member states, are indicated for reference.

[6] The geographical centre of each of the six WHO world regions was computed as the average longitude and the average latitude of the capital city of the constituent member states.

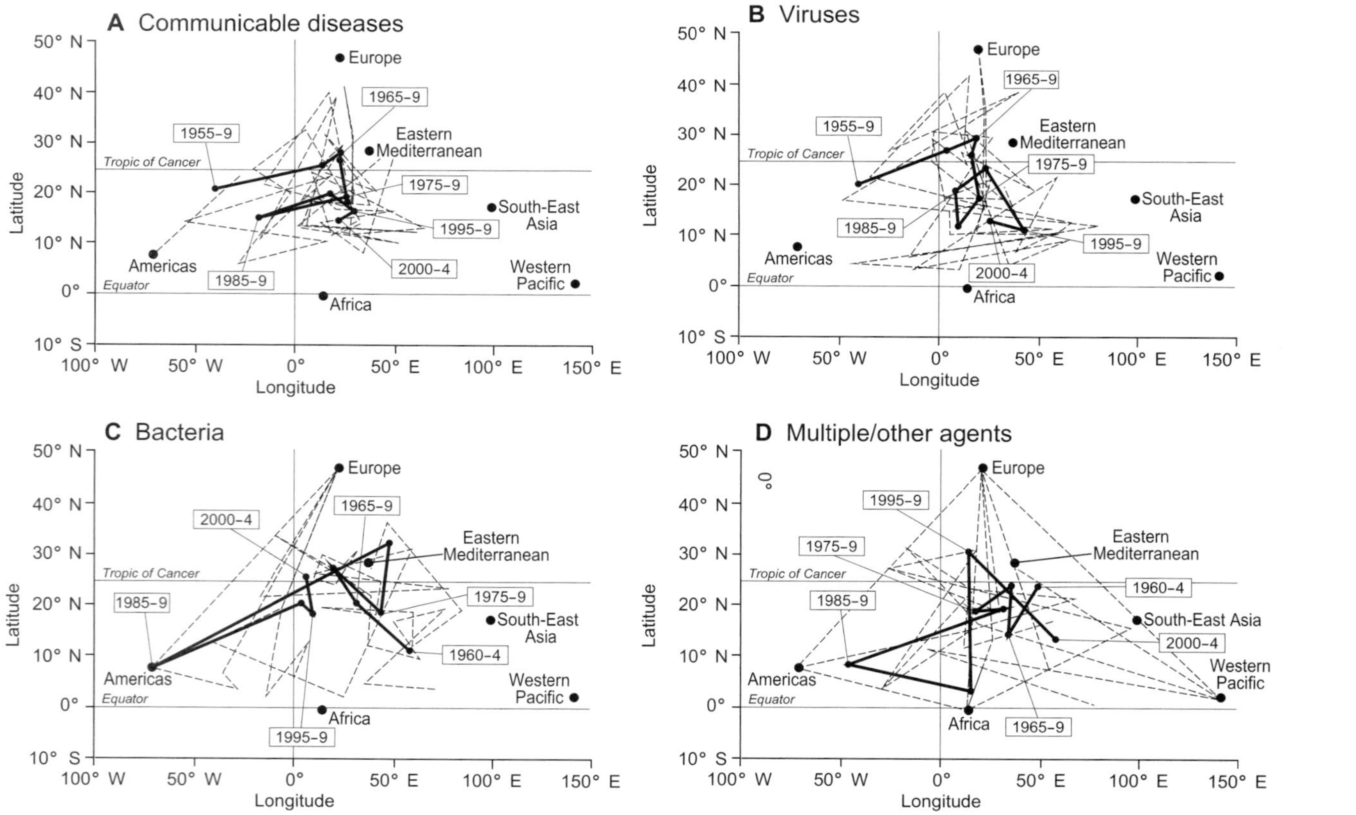

Fig. 3.14. Geographical centroids for international entries in *MMWR Weekly*, 1952–2005

Broken lines link successive positions of the annual coordinates of the centroids. Heavy lines link the average annual positions of the centroids by five-year period (1955–9, . . . , 2000–4). (A) Communicable diseases. (B) Viruses. (C) Bacteria. (D) Multiple/other agents. The locations of WHO world regions, plotted as the average longitudes and latitudes of the constituent member states, are indicated for reference.

For all communicable diseases, the broken line trace in Figure 3.14A shows that the annual centre of international coverage extended across a broad geographical area, bounded by the 5° N and 40° N parallels of latitude and the 65° E and 75° W meridians of longitude. When viewed in terms of five-year averages, the heavy line trace confirms that the centre was rooted in the tropical and subtropical northern latitudes that span the Africa and Eastern Mediterranean regions, but with periods of westerly extension towards the Americas. The same basic pattern is repeated on the remaining maps of Figure 3.14, but with a progressive increase in the longitudinal extent of the web of annual centres for entries associated with viruses (map B), through bacteria (map C), to multiple/other agents (map D).

Results II: Long-Term Trends

Figure 3.15 replots, as time series, the longitude (graph A) and latitude (graph B) coordinates of the sets of annual centres in Figure 3.14. For all communicable diseases (heavy line traces), two features of Figure 3.15 are evident:

(i) an underlying southwards trend in the latitude of entries in Figure 3.15B, with a progressive shift from a position north of the Tropic of Cancer (23.3° N) in the early 1960s towards the Equator by the early 1990s. Consistent with the evidence in Figure 3.13, this development marks a relative reduction in the contribution of temperate European latitudes to the overall pattern of international entries in the latter decades of the observation period;

(ii) from a centroid position fluctuating around 25° E in the period to the early 1980s, Figure 3.15A depicts a temporary westwards movement towards the Americas in the interval 1985–90. This feature cannot be attributed to a specific disease or condition, but appears to reflect the general tendency for international entries to focus on the Americas in the mid- to late 1980s (see Figure 3.13).

Figure 3.15 also confirms that features (i) and (ii) are broadly reflected in the centroid positions of entries associated with viruses, bacteria, and multiple/other disease agents.

3.3.5 *Summary*

In this section, we have sifted the contents of a half-century run of CDC's *MMWR Weekly* to determine 'headline trends' in the epidemiological monitoring of communicable diseases of national and international importance, 1952–2005. Although the general direction in the coverage of communicable diseases was downwards for much of the observation period, certain key features of the analysis emerge. First, viral and bacterial diseases and their agents have consistently dominated the coverage of communicable diseases

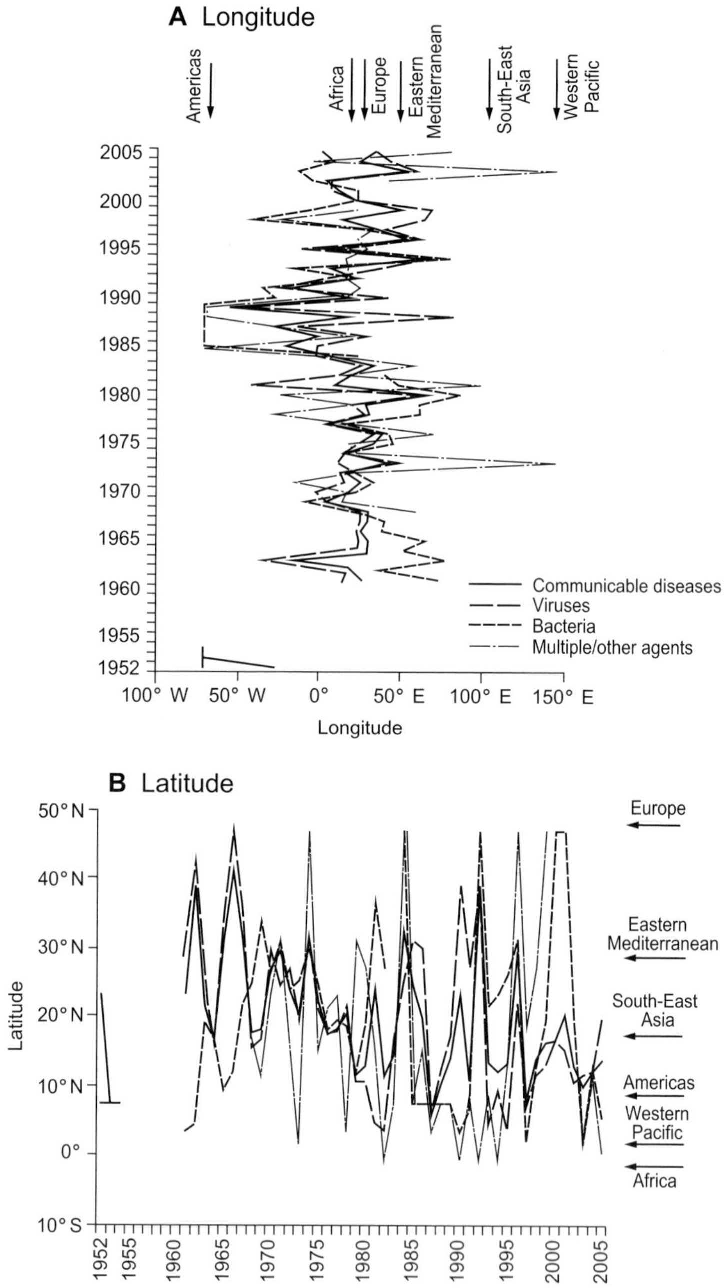

Fig. 3.15. Time series of geographical centroids for international entries in *MMWR Weekly*, 1952–2005

Graphs replot, as time series, the longitude (graph A) and latitude (graph B) coordinates of the sets of annual centroids in Fig. 3.14. The locations of WHO world regions, plotted as the average longitudes (upper graph) and latitudes of the constituent member states, are indicated for reference.

in *MMWR Weekly*, with viruses accounting for an increasing share of reports in the latter decades of the observation period (Figure 3.8). This is consistent with the findings in Section 1.5.3. Second, while some of the longer-established categories of communicable disease retreated from headline coverage, the global analysis in Section 3.3.2 highlights the sequence of emergence of a range of diseases in the epidemiological record: Legionnaires' disease in the 1970s, toxic shock syndrome, acute haemorrhagic conjunctivitis, and HIV disease in the 1980s, hantavirus pulmonary syndrome in the 1990s, and West Nile fever and severe acute respiratory syndrome (SARS) at the start of the new millennium (Figure 3.9 and Table 3.7). To these developments, the domestic (US) analysis in Section 3.3.3 adds Lyme disease (1970s), drug-resistant tuberculosis (1980s), *Escherichia coli* infection and norovirus gastroenteritis (1990s), while the looming threat of bioterrorism has served to resurrect fears over anthrax and smallpox (2000s) (Figures 3.10 and 3.11). Finally, the international (non-US) analysis in Section 3.3.4 highlights both the periodic upswings in the coverage of some long-established diseases (for example, cholera, dengue fever, poliomyelitis, and smallpox) and the relative shift in geographical areas of concern, away from Europe to other world regions (Figures 3.12–3.15).

3.4 Field Investigations: The US Epidemic Intelligence Service, 1946–2005

Since inception in 1951, the Epidemic Intelligence Service (EIS) of the CDC has been called on by state, federal, national, and international health authorities to assist in the field investigation of thousands of disease outbreaks and other events of public health importance. In this section, we undertake an examination of the inventory of EIS field investigations (1951–2005) and related investigations in earlier years (1946–51) to see what additional light they can cast on emerging patterns of communicable disease activity.

3.4.1 Background and Data

The history and operations of the EIS are reviewed by Langmuir (1980), Goodman *et al.* (1990), Koplan and Thacker (2001), and Thacker, Dannenberg, *et al.* (2001). The EIS Program was established by the Communicable Disease Center (forerunner of CDC) in July 1951 to provide capacity to respond to threats of bioterrorism. Underpinning the initiative, however, was a broader vision to provide a trained cohort of field epidemiologists that would be available at all times for the surveillance and control of diseases in outbreak situations. Since then, some 3,000 EIS officers have—among many other

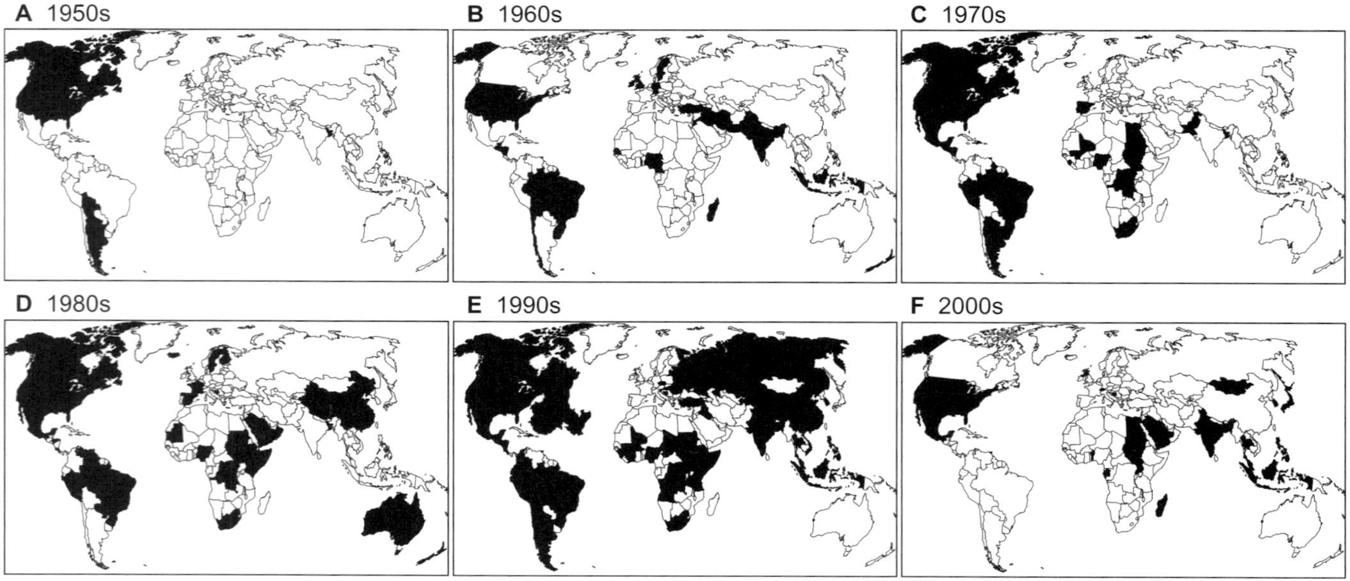

Fig. 3.16. Sites of EIS epidemic assistance investigations (Epi-Aids)
Countries in which investigations were undertaken in a given time period are shaded. (A) 1950s. (B) 1960s. (C) 1970s. (D) 1980s. (E) 1990s. (F) 2000s.

Source: Centers for Disease Control and Prevention (2005e).

Table 3.9. Selected investigations in which EIS officers participated, 1951–2007

1951–60
Contamination of killed poliovirus vaccine with live virus
Asian influenza epidemics
Nosocomial staphylococcal epidemics
Childhood lead poisoning from peeling paint
1961–70
Cases of poliomyelitis associated with oral vaccine
Smallpox epidemics (–1977)
Hong Kong influenza epidemics
Hurricane Camille after-effects
Salmonellosis in commercial chicken
1971–80
Salmonella in pet turtles
Oyster-associated hepatitis
Bacteraemia from contaminated intravenous fluids
Childhood lead poisoning from environmental exposure
Norwalk virus epidemic
Vinyl-chloride-associated liver cancer
Legionnaires' disease
Ebola virus in Zaire and Sudan
Guillain-Barré syndrome associated with swine influenza vaccine
Toxic shock syndrome
Heat-wave-associated morbidity and mortality in Missouri
Aspirin-associated Reye's syndrome
National Study of the Efficacy of Nosocomial Infection Control (SENIC)
National Cancer and Steroid Hormone Study (CASH)
Investigation of the health effects of the Three Mile Island nuclear incident (Pennsylvania)
1981–90
Health effects of the Mount St Helens volcano eruption (Washington State)
Acquired immunodeficiency syndrome (AIDS)
Accutane-associated birth defects
Escherichia coli O157:H7 associated with haemorrhagic diarrhoea and haemolytic uraemic syndrome
Role of parvovirus in erythema infectiosum (fifth disease)
Toxic oil syndrome in Spain
Eosinophilia-myalgia syndrome
Clusters of suicides by teenagers
Vietnam veterans studies
Mercury poisoning from commercial paint
1991–2000
Multistate outbreak of *Escherichia coli* O157:H7-associated diarrhoea and haemolytic uraemic syndrome from hamburgers
Hantavirus pulmonary syndrome
Health effects of Hurricane Andrew
Cryptosporidiosis from contaminated public drinking water in Milwaukee (Wisconsin)
Acute renal failure in Haiti from acetaminophen contaminated with diethylene glycol
Impact of physician-assisted suicide in Oregon
Multistate outbreak of salmonella associated with commercial ice cream
Suicide after natural disasters
Rotavirus vaccine recall
West Nile virus epidemic

(Continued)

Table 3.9. (Continued)

	Cardiac valvulopathy associated with fenfluramine (fen-phen)
	Violence against mothers of newborns of unintended pregnancies
	Definition of excess weight gain in pregnancy
2001–7	
	Aftermath of World Trade Center and Pentagon terrorist attacks and anthrax mailings
	Severe acute respiratory syndrome (SARS)
	Multistate outbreaks of *Escherichia coli* and salmonella associated with eating raw vegetables, puffed vegetable snack, frozen pizza, frozen pot pies, and dry dog food
	Zika virus in Micronesia
	Multiple investigations of methicillin-resistant *Staphylococcus aureus* (MRSA) in the hospital and the community
	Characteristics of perpetrators in homicide-followed-by-suicide in 17 states

Source: Based on Thacker, Dannenberg, *et al.* (2001, table 2, p. 987).

duties—participated in more than 4,000 epidemic assistance investigations in the United States and worldwide (Figure 3.16). In line with the original remit of CDC, the early investigations were largely concerned with outbreaks of communicable diseases. As the responsibilities of CDC have broadened, however, Table 3.9 shows that the public health problems addressed by EIS officers have expanded to include chronic diseases, injuries, drug/vaccine reactions, and reproductive, environmental, and occupational health issues (Goodman *et al.* 1990; Thacker, Dannenberg, *et al.* 2001).

Epidemic Assistance Investigations (Epi-Aids)

Within the framework of EIS operations, an epidemic assistance investigation (Epi-Aid) is a specific form of investigation that is undertaken by CDC in response to external requests for assistance by states, federal agencies, international organizations, and other countries. A request for assistance follows a prescribed administrative mechanism, which, if granted, results in the preparation of an initial memorandum ('Epi-1') and, following the investigation, a full report on the work undertaken ('Epi-2') (Plate 3.4). Although the Epi-1 and Epi-2 documents are for administrative use and have limited circulation, descriptions of investigations of special interest are frequently published in *MMWR Weekly* (see Section 3.3) and elsewhere in the scientific literature.

The Data Set

To analyse the pattern of EIS outbreak investigations, we draw on the systematic review of more than 2,700 Epi-Aid reports undertaken by Stroup and Thacker and published for each of four decadal periods, 1946–85, in the *EIS Bulletin* (Stroup and Thacker 2007; Thacker and Stroup 2007*a*,*b*, 2008). We supplement the statistical data included there with geo-referenced information for domestic (US) outbreak investigations abstracted for the period 1946–2005 from an expanded inventory of over 4,400 Epi-Aid report titles.

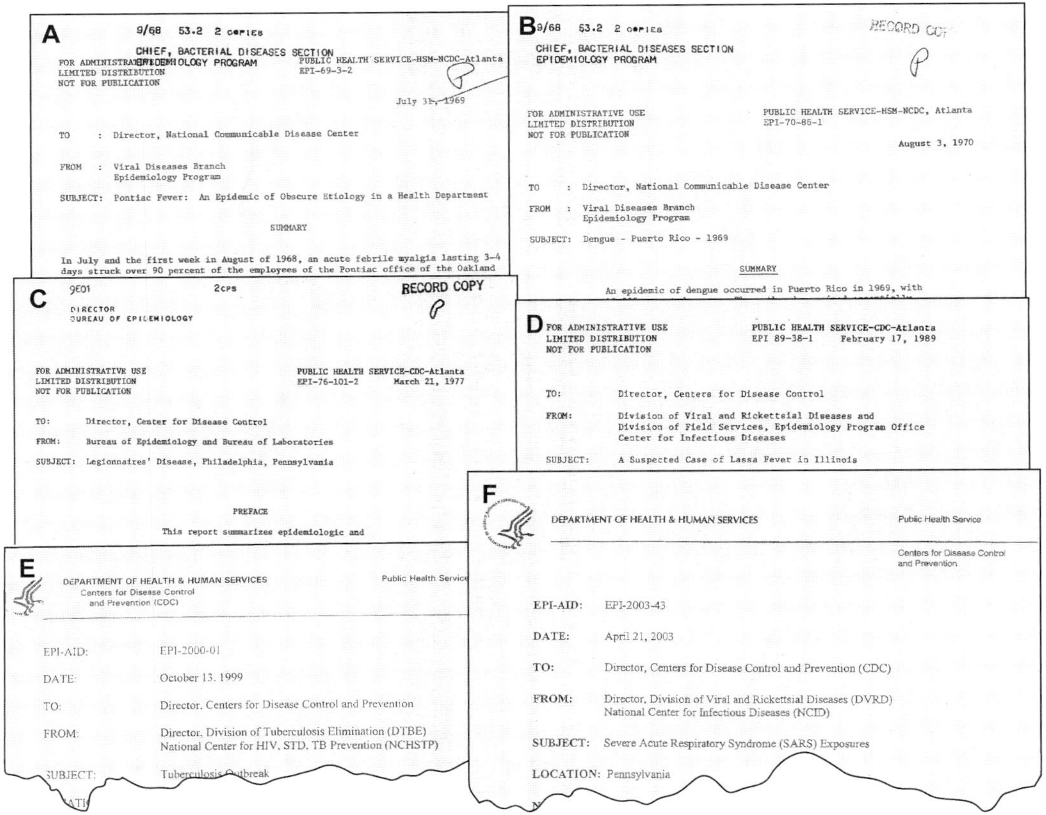

A 9/68 53.2 2 copies

CHIEF, BACTERIAL DISEASES SECTION
EPIDEMIOLOGY PROGRAM

FOR ADMINISTRATIVE USE
LIMITED DISTRIBUTION
NOT FOR PUBLICATION

PUBLIC HEALTH SERVICE-HSM-NCDC-Atlanta
EPI-69-3-2

July 31, 1969

TO : Director, National Communicable Disease Center

FROM : Viral Diseases Branch
Epidemiology Program

SUBJECT: Pontiac Fever: An Epidemic of Obscure Etiology in a Health Department

SUMMARY

In July and the first week in August of 1968, an acute febrile myalgia lasting 3-4 days struck over 90 percent of the employees of the Pontiac office of the Oakland

B 9/68 53.2 2 copies

RECORD COPY

CHIEF, BACTERIAL DISEASES SECTION
EPIDEMIOLOGY PROGRAM

FOR ADMINISTRATIVE USE
LIMITED DISTRIBUTION
NOT FOR PUBLICATION

PUBLIC HEALTH SERVICE-HSM-NCDC, Atlanta
EPI-70-86-1

August 3, 1970

TO : Director, National Communicable Disease Center

FROM : Viral Diseases Branch
Epidemiology Program

SUBJECT: Dengue - Puerto Rico - 1969

SUMMARY

An epidemic of dengue occurred in Puerto Rico in 1969, with

C 9E01 2cps

RECORD COPY

DIRECTOR
BUREAU OF EPIDEMIOLOGY

FOR ADMINISTRATIVE USE
LIMITED DISTRIBUTION
NOT FOR PUBLICATION

PUBLIC HEALTH SERVICE-CDC-Atlanta
EPI-76-101-2 March 21, 1977

TO: Director, Center for Disease Control

FROM: Bureau of Epidemiology and Bureau of Laboratories

SUBJECT: Legionnaires' Disease, Philadelphia, Pennsylvania

PREFACE

This report summarizes epidemiologic and

D FOR ADMINISTRATIVE USE
LIMITED DISTRIBUTION
NOT FOR PUBLICATION

PUBLIC HEALTH SERVICE-CDC-Atlanta
EPI 89-38-1 February 17, 1989

TO: Director, Centers for Disease Control

FROM: Division of Viral and Rickettsial Diseases and
Division of Field Services, Epidemiology Program Office
Center for Infectious Diseases

SUBJECT: A Suspected Case of Lassa Fever in Illinois

E DEPARTMENT OF HEALTH & HUMAN SERVICES
Centers for Disease Control
and Prevention (CDC)

Public Health Service

EPI-AID: EPI-2000-01

DATE: October 13, 1999

TO: Director, Centers for Disease Control and Prevention

FROM: Director, Division of Tuberculosis Elimination (DTBE)
National Center for HIV, STD, TB Prevention (NCHSTP)

SUBJECT: Tuberculosis Outbreak

F DEPARTMENT OF HEALTH & HUMAN SERVICES

Public Health Service

Centers for Disease Control
and Prevention

EPI-AID: EPI-2003-43

DATE: April 21, 2003

TO: Director, Centers for Disease Control and Prevention (CDC)

FROM: Director, Division of Viral and Rickettsial Diseases (DVRD)
National Center for Infectious Diseases (NCID)

SUBJECT: Severe Acute Respiratory Syndrome (SARS) Exposures

LOCATION: Pennsylvania

Pl. 3.4. US Epidemic Intelligence Service: sample field investigation memorandums (Epi-1) and reports (Epi-2) for selected outbreaks of infectious diseases

(A) Outbreak of Pontiac fever, Oakland County, Michigan, 1968. (B) Outbreak of dengue fever, Puerto Rico, 1969. (C) Outbreak of Legionnaire's disease, Philadelphia, 1976. (D) Suspected case of Lassa fever, Illinois, 1989. (E) Outbreak of tuberculosis, Columbia, South Carolina, 1999. (F) Hospital-based exposure to a probable SARS case in Pennsylvania, 2003.

3.4.2 Global Overview of Investigations, 1946–1985

A total of 2,720 Epi-Aid reports were filed in the 40 years to 1985 (Table 3.10), with the geographical reach of the investigations expanding from a primary concentration in North and South America in the 1950s (Figure 3.16A) to include representatives of each of the six WHO world regions in the 1960s–1980s (Figures 3.16B–D). As Table 3.10 shows, some 75 per cent of all investigations were associated with infectious diseases, but with non-infectious/unknown health problems accounting for an increasing share of all requests for assistance over the interval. For further details of the range of investigations undertaken in this period, see Goodman *et al.* (1990), Stroup and Thacker (2007), and Thacker and Stroup (2007*a*,*b*, 2008).

Infectious Diseases

Trends in infectious disease investigations are summarized in Figure 3.17. Figure 3.17A shows that the number of Epi-Aids for this category of health problem grew rapidly in the 1950s and 1960s. At a peak, in the period from the mid-1960s to the early 1970s, some 70–100 infectious disease investigations were undertaken annually. Thereafter, there was a modest fall in the annual count to 50–70 investigations in the latter years of the observation period. While Figure 3.17B indicates that bacteria and viruses accounted for the overwhelming majority (>80 per cent) of the annual count of infectious disease investigations, the pattern was underpinned by a perceptible shift in emphasis from viruses to bacteria over the 40-year interval.

Table 3.10. Number of EIS epidemic assistance investigations (Epi-Aids) by category of health problem, 1946–1985

	Interval				
Health problem	1946–55	1956–65	1966–75	1976–85	Total
Infectious	123	441	806	673	2,043
Bacteria	31	175	361	337	904
Mycobacteria	1	0	5	7	13
Virus	73	243	313	247	876
Parasite	8	10	92	50	160
Fungus	2	5	10	14	31
Rickettsia	0	1	7	8	16
Other/mixed	8	7	18	10	43
Non-infectious/unknown[1]	11	59	271	336	677
TOTAL	134	500	1,077	1,009	2,720

Note: [1] Including chronic diseases, environmental exposures and disasters, birth defects, genetic conditions, reproductive health, injuries, syndromes, and hysteria.

Sources: Stroup and Thacker (2007, table 1, p. 15) and Thacker and Stroup (2007*a*, table 1, pp. 40–1; 2007*b*, table 1, unpaginated; 2008, table 1, pp. 43–4).

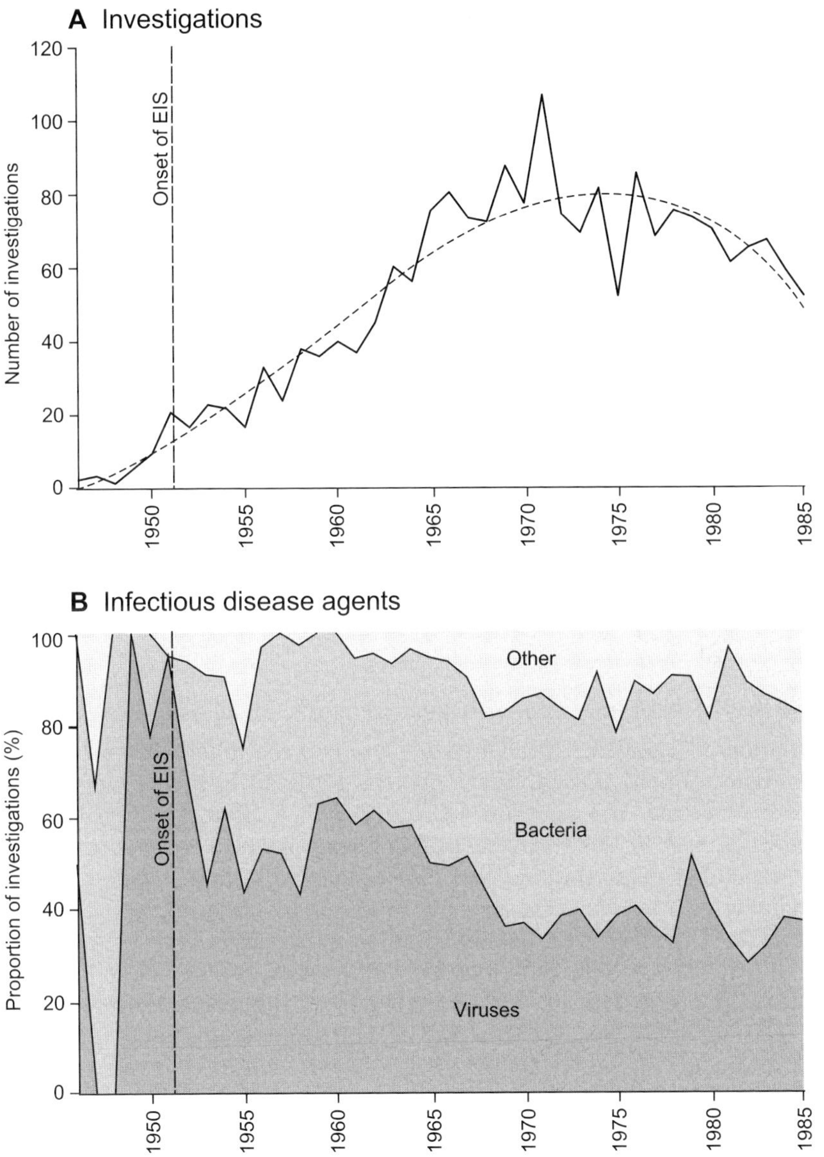

Fig. 3.17. EIS epidemic assistance investigations (Epi-Aids), infectious diseases, 1946–1985

(A) Annual count of investigations related to infectious diseases. The underlying trend is depicted by a polynomial regression line fitted to the data by ordinary least squares. (B) Percentage proportion of infectious disease investigations associated with viruses, bacteria, and other/mixed infectious agents in each year.

Sources: Drawn from Stroup and Thacker (2007, table 1, p. 15) and Thacker and Stroup (2007*a*, table 1, pp. 40–1; 2007*b*, table 1, unpaginated; 2008, table 1, pp. 43–4).

3.4.3 The Pattern of Domestic (US) Investigations, 1946–2005

In this subsection, we extend the examination in Section 3.4.2 to include a geographical analysis of approximately 4,000 Epi-Aid investigations in the conterminous United States, 1946–2005.

MAP PATTERNS

Figure 3.18 plots, for each of the nine standard census divisions of the conterminous United States (map A), the total number of Epi-Aid investigations in 1950–69 (map B), 1970–89 (map C), and 1990–2005 (map D). Investigations have been allocated to divisions on the basis of the states in which they were undertaken; to avoid multiple counting, multistate investigations that extended to include more than one division have been excluded from the analysis. While Figure 3.18B shows that all divisions registered ≥50 investigations in the period 1950–69, the largest number of investigations (100–99) were recorded in the Mountain, West North Central, and South Atlantic divisions. The South Atlantic states emerged as a primary focus of investigations in 1970–89 and 1990–2005 (Figures 3.18C,D), while the relative paucity of EIS investigations in the West Central and East South Central Divisions in 1990–2005 is noteworthy (Figure 3.18D).

GEOGRAPHICAL CENTROIDS OF INVESTIGATIONS

Equations 3.2 and 3.3 were used to compute the longitude and latitude coordinates of the geographical centroids of (i) all Epi-Aid investigations and (ii) Epi-Aid investigations associated with viral and bacterial agents. Centroids were formed on the basis of investigations in each of the 48 conterminous states and the District of Columbia; λ_j and ϕ_j were set as the longitude and latitude, respectively, of the mean geographical centres of the states. Centroids were computed on an annual basis for: (1) raw counts of investigations; and, to allow for variations in state population size, (2) investigation rates per 100,000 population. All rates (2) were formed using annual mid-point estimates of state populations included in the *Statistical Abstract of the United States* (Department of Commerce, Bureau of the Census, 1952–2007).

Results I: All Investigations

Figure 3.19 maps, for the period 1950–2005, the annual longitude and latitude coordinates of investigation centroids as computed for raw counts (grey triangles) and rates per 100,000 (black squares); lines link the centroid positions in successive years, while, for reference, state geographical centres are represented by the black circles. To assist in the interpretation of Figure 3.19, the graphs in Figure 3.20 replot the longitude (graph A) and latitude (graph B) coordinates of the investigation centroids as annual series. For reference, the

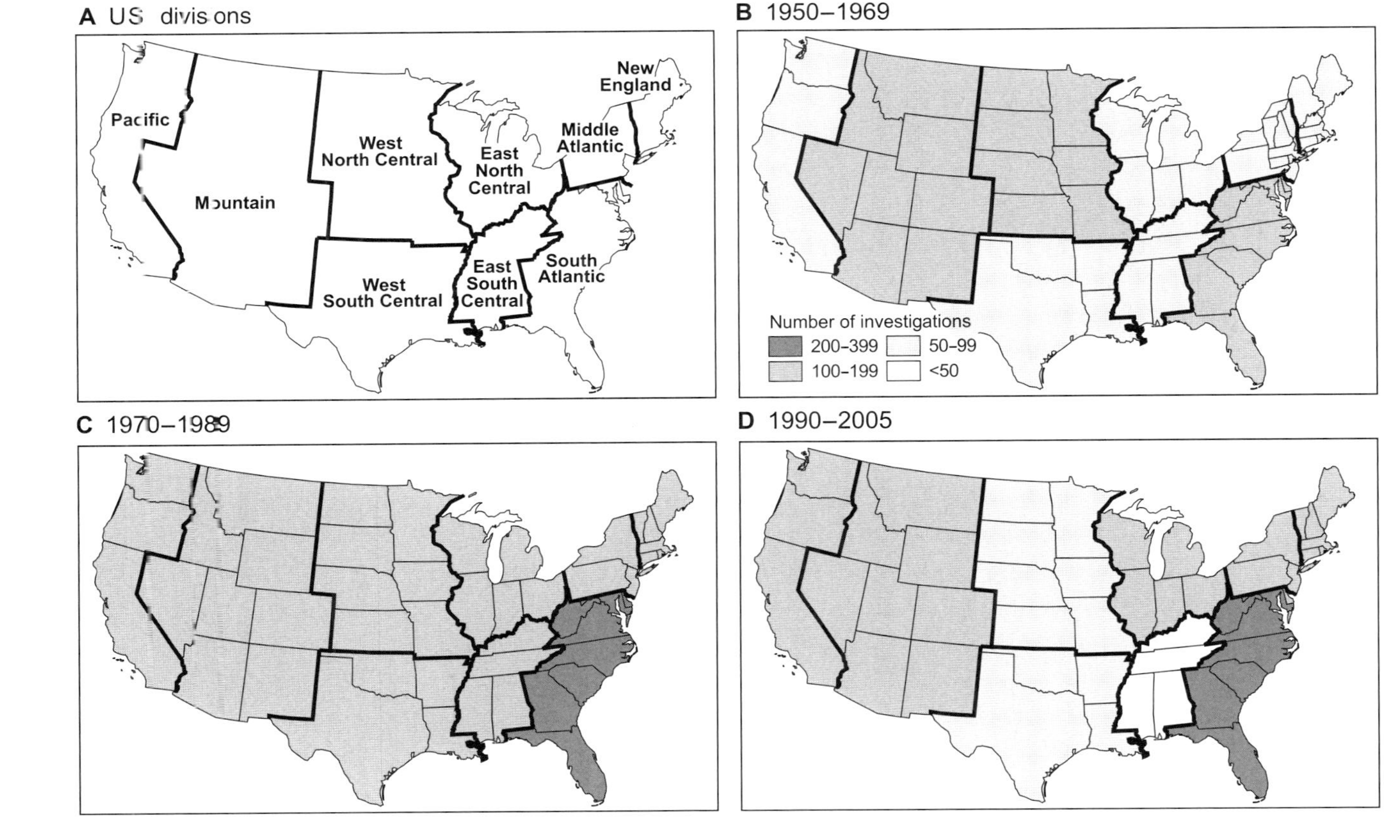

Fig. 3.18. EIS epidemic assistance investigations (Epi-Aids) in the conterminous United States: all investigations
Maps plot the total number of investigations undertaken in each of the nine standard divisions of the Unites States in 1950–69 (map B), 1970–89 (map C), and 1990–2005 (map D). Divisions are named in map A. Investigations that spanned more than one division have been excluded from the analysis.

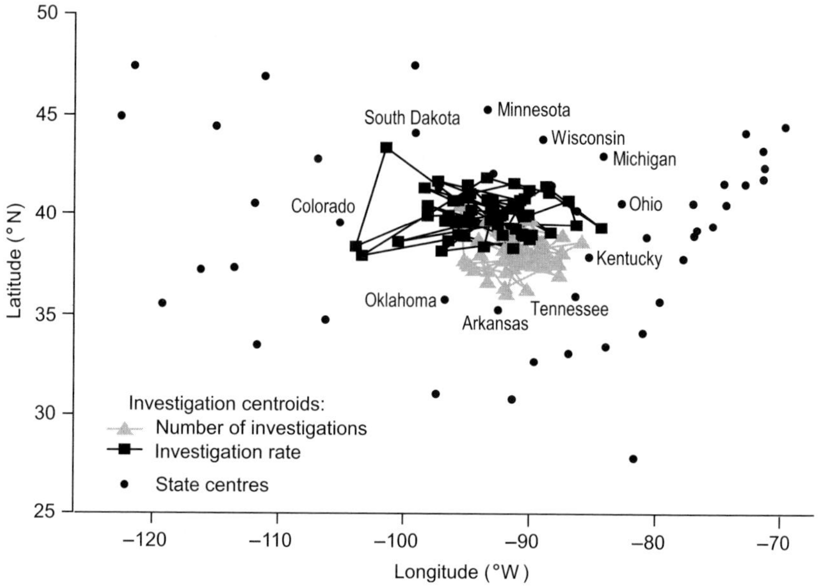

Fig. 3.19. Annual positions of the geographical centroids of EIS epidemic assistance investigations (Epi-Aids) in the conterminous United States, 1950–2005
Positions of centroids are shown for the raw count of investigations (grey triangles) and the investigation rate per 100,000 population (black squares). Lines link the centroid positions in successive years. State geographical centres are represented by circles.

corresponding coordinates of the mean population centre of the United States have been plotted as the broken line traces. Periods when the investigation centroids lay to the west (graph 3.20A) and north (graph 3.20B) of the mean population centre have been shaded.

Inspection of Figures 3.19 and 3.20 reveals that the investigation centroids ranged over a 1.6 million km^2 area of the central United States, from Ohio

Fig. 3.20. Geographical centroids of EIS epidemic assistance investigations (Epi-Aids) in the states of the conterminous United States, 1950–2005
Graphs plot the annual coordinates for longitude (A) and latitude (B) as computed from equations 3.2 and 3.3 using raw counts of investigations (fine line traces) and investigation rates per 100,000 population (heavy line traces). The annual position of the mean population centre of the United States, interpolated from decadal estimates of coordinates included in successive editions of the *Statistical Abstract of the United States* (Department of Commerce, Bureau of the Census, 1952–2007), is plotted on each graph as the broken line trace. Periods when investigation centroids were positioned to the west (graph A) and north (graph B) of the mean population centre have been shaded. The longitudes and latitudes of representative states are indicated for reference. Note that the centroid coordinates for 2005 are based on a sample of 41 investigations.

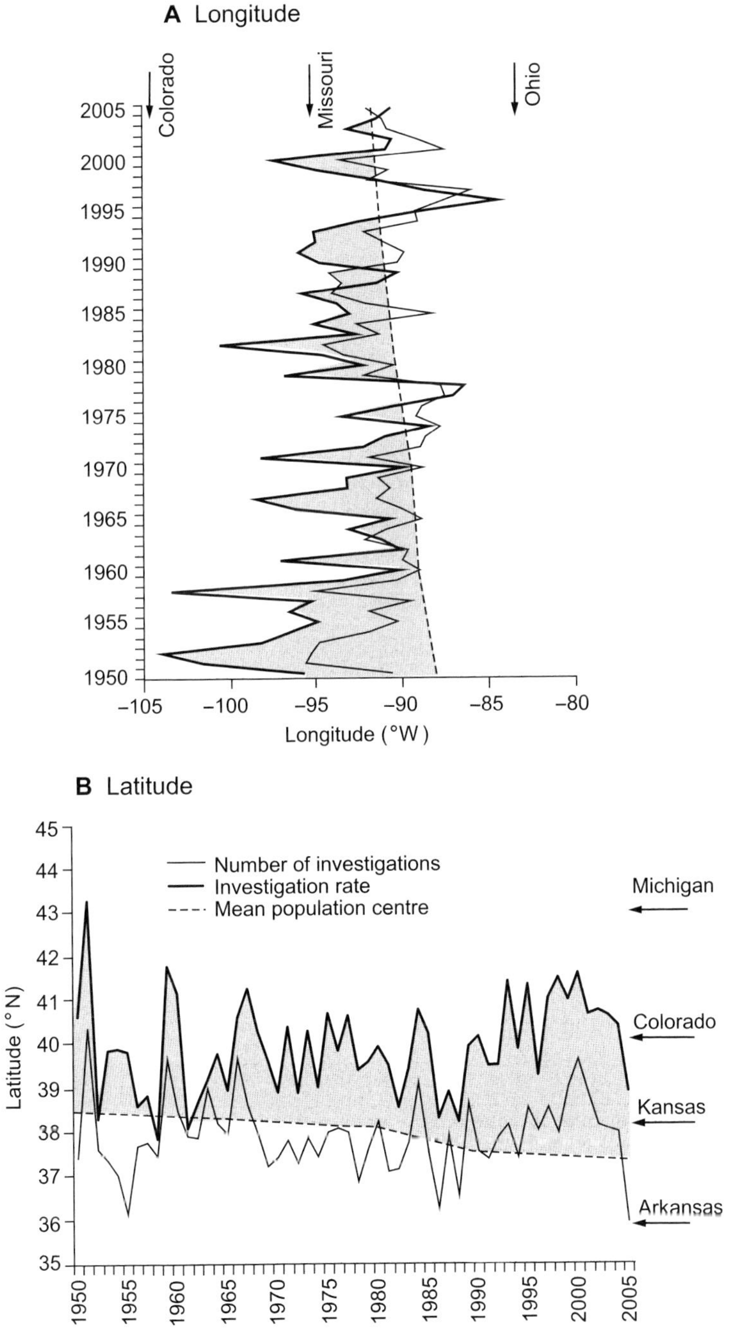
A Longitude
Colorado
Missouri
Ohio
2005
2000
1995
1990
1985
1980
1975
1970
1965
1960
1955
1950
−105
−100
−95
−90
−85
−80
Longitude (°W)
B Latitude
45
44
43
42
41
40
39
38
37
36
35
Latitude (°N)
Number of investigations
Investigation rate
Mean population centre
Michigan
Colorado
Kansas
Arkansas
1950
1955
1960
1965
1970
1975
1980
1985
1990
1995
2000
2005

(east) to Colorado (west) and South Dakota (north) to Arkansas (south). When viewed in terms of the raw count of investigations, the fine line traces in Figure 3.20 indicate that the centroids approximated the longitude and latitude positions of the mean population centre of the country. When scaled to state populations, however, the heavy line traces show a propensity for the investigation centroids: (i) to lie several degrees to the west (graph A) and north (graph B) of the mean population centre; and (ii) to migrate towards the westwards-drifting (graph A) and away from the southwards-drifting (graph B) mean population centre over time.

Results II: Infectious Diseases

Maps B in Figures 3.21 and 3.22 echo Figure 3.19 and plot, for Epi-Aid investigations of viral and bacterial diseases respectively, the annual longitude and latitude coordinates of investigation centroids, 1950–2005. For reference, the corresponding maps A give the associated number of investigations by standard census division. The web of centroid positions for both categories of disease agent, focused in an area between Kentucky (east) and Colorado (west) and Minnesota (north) to Arkansas (south), approximates the aggregate pattern in Figure 3.19. Thus, the analysis suggests that the broad pattern of investigations associated with the two major sub-categories of infectious disease agent did not deviate substantially from the overall pattern of domestic investigations undertaken by the EIS.

3.4.4 Summary

In this section, we have examined the pattern of EIS epidemic assistance investigations over a 60-year interval, 1946–2005. Although infectious diseases accounted for a declining share of all investigations, the work undertaken by the EIS extended across the United States and worldwide to include landmark investigations of many emerging infectious diseases, including Legionnaires' disease, Ebola viral disease, *Escherichia coli* O157:H7 infection, hantavirus pulmonary syndrome, and West Nile fever (Figure 3.16 and Table 3.9). Of the infectious disease agents, viruses and bacteria consistently accounted for the majority (>80 per cent) of investigations, but with a perceptible shift in the weight of investigations from the former to the latter in the period to the mid-1980s (Figure 3.17). Finally, the geographical analysis of domestic investigations in Figures 3.19–3.22 has demonstrated a propensity for the overall centre of investigative work to lie to the west and north of the mean population centre of the United States. In interpreting these patterns, we note that the investigations analysed here represent a biased sample of health events for which the assistance of CDC was requested. As Goodman *et al.* (1990) observe, many—if not most—investigations of health events in the United States are managed entirely by state and local health agencies.

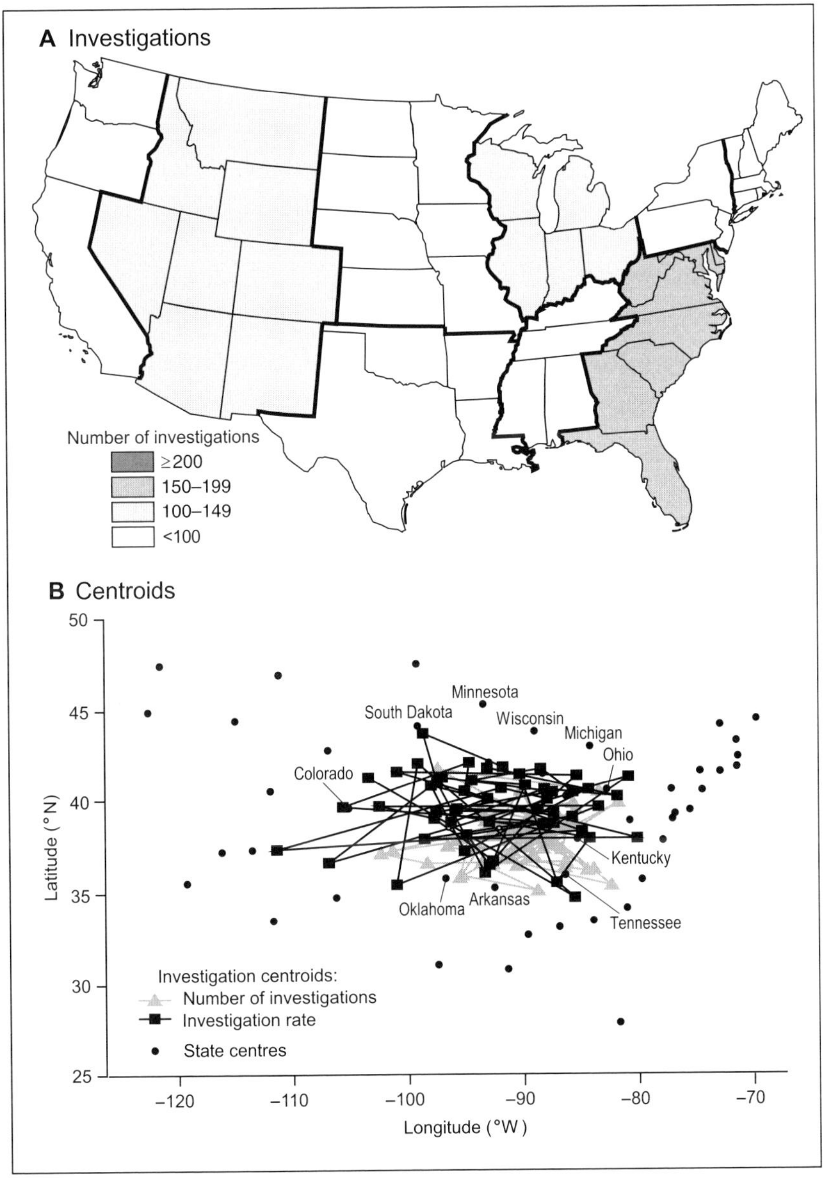

Fig. 3.21. EIS epidemic assistance investigations (Epi-Aids) associated with viral diseases in the conterminous United States, 1950–2005
(A) Count of investigations in each of the nine standard census divisions of the United States. Divisions are named in Fig. 3.18A. (B) Annual positions of centroids associated with the raw count of investigations (grey lines) and the investigation rate per 100,000 population (black lines). State geographical centres are represented by circles.

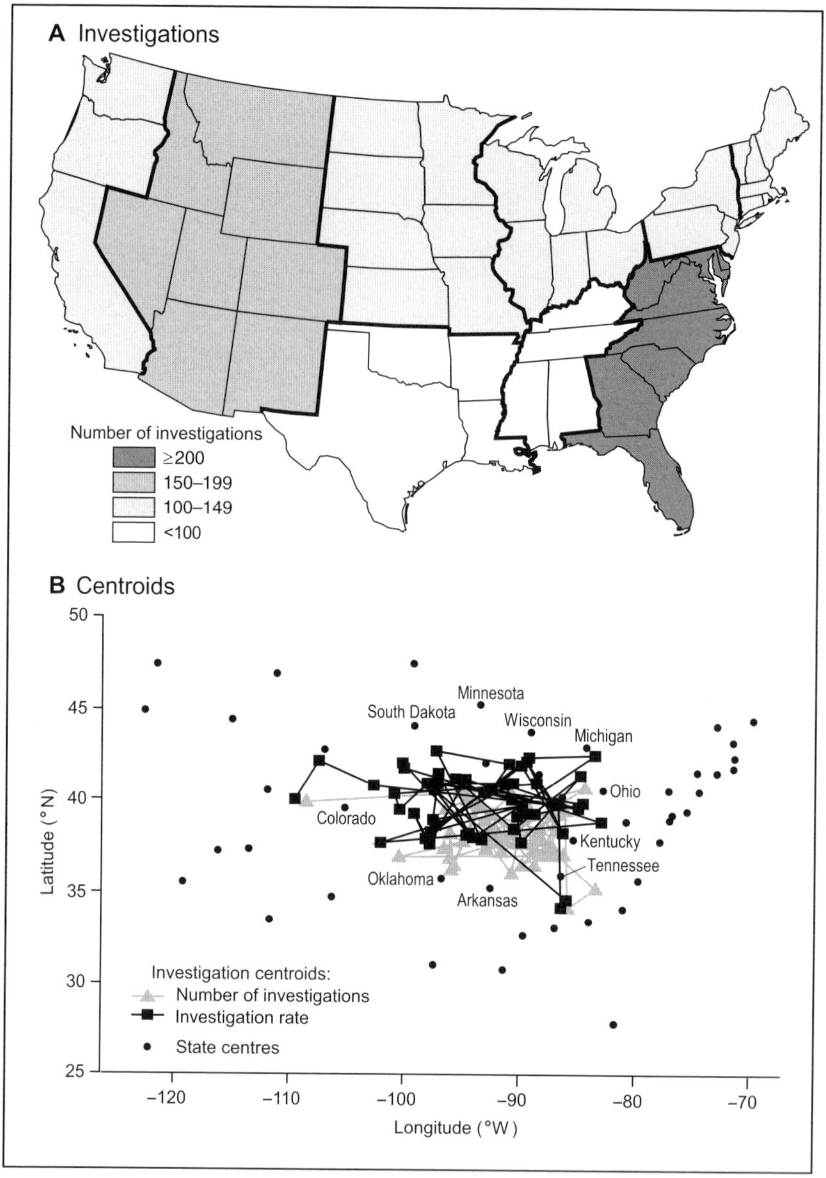

Fig. 3.22. EIS epidemic assistance investigations (Epi-Aids) associated with bacterial diseases in the conterminous United States, 1950–2005
(A) Count of investigations in each of the nine standard census divisions of the United States. Divisions are named in Fig. 3.18A. (B) Annual positions of centroids associated with the raw count of investigations (grey lines) and the investigation rate per 100,000 population (black lines). State geographical centres are represented by circles.

3.5 Conclusion

In this chapter, we have undertaken a content analysis of three major sources of epidemiological information—the global records of the League of Nations/WHO (1923–83), the regional and national coverage of *MMWR Weekly* (1952–2005), and the inventory of local EIS epidemic assistance investigations (1946–2005)—to identify patterns in the recognition and recording of communicable diseases of public health importance. Subject to biases in the sources used, certain broad patterns emerge from our analysis. First, throughout the observation period, both 'old' and 'new' communicable diseases have periodically emerged to prominence in the epidemiological record (Tables 3.2–3.4, 3.7, and Figures 3.4–3.6, 3.9–3.13). Second, the period from the 1970s is singled out by a rapid expansion in the number of newly recognized communicable diseases due to a variety of bacterial, fungal, helminthic, protozoal, and viral agents (Table 3.3 and Figure 3.5). Third, notwithstanding the widening range of diseases and disease agents in the latter decades of the observation period, viral and bacterial diseases continued to dominate the record of communicable diseases throughout the study interval (Figures 3.8 and 3.17).

SELECTION OF DISEASES FOR STUDY IN CHAPTERS 4–9

The combined analysis in Sections 3.2 and 3.3 yields evidence of well over 80 communicable diseases and disease categories that—at one time or another—gained prominence in the sources studied, either through an expansion of documented surveillance activities in the League of Nations/WHO records (Tables 3.2–3.4) or through increased headline coverage in *MMWR Weekly* (Figures 3.9–3.13). Informed by this 'long shortlist', a core set of 36 diseases was selected for consideration in Chapters 4–9. These diseases are listed in Table 3.11. Three principal criteria were applied in the selection process:

(i) *Criterion 1: Type examples*. This criterion required the selection of diseases that best illustrate the five themes in Figure II.1. On the basis of the scientific literature, these type examples were chosen to include, among others, influenza and tuberculosis ('Disease Changes', Chapter 4), *Escherichia coli* O157:H7 infection and Legionnaires' disease ('Technical Changes', Chapter 5), severe acute respiratory syndrome ('Population Changes', Chapter 6), hantavirus pulmonary syndrome ('Environmental Changes', Chapter 7), and Japanese encephalitis and Korean haemorrhagic fever ('Disease Amplifiers', Chapter 8).

(ii) *Criterion 2: Disease mix*. This criterion called for a broad mix of diseases in terms of both (*a*) the category of aetiological agent and (*b*) the status of the agent as 'emergent' or 're-emergent'. Consistent with the balance of evidence from *MMWR Weekly* (Section 3.3) and the EIS field investigations

Table 3.11. Diseases selected for analysis in Chapters 4–9

ICD-10 three-character classification	Disease	Agent	Category of agent	Status[1]
Cholera (A00)	Cholera	*Vibrio cholerae*	Bacterium	Re-emerging
Other bacterial intestinal infections (A04)	*Escherichia coli* O157:H7 disease	*Escherichia coli* O157:H7	Bacterium	Emerging
Tuberculosis (A15–A19)	Tuberculosis	*Mycobacterium tuberculosis*	Mycobacterium	Re-emerging
Plague (A20)	Plague	*Yersinia pestis*	Bacterium	Re-emerging
Anthrax (A22)	Anthrax	*Bacillus anthracis*	Bacterium	Re-emerging
Leprosy (A30)	Leprosy	*Mycobacterium leprae*	Mycobacterium	Re-emerging
Diphtheria (A36)	Diphtheria	*Corynebacterium diphtheriae*	Bacterium	Re-emerging
Whooping cough (A37)	Whooping cough	*Bordetella pertussis*	Bacterium	Re-emerging
Scarlet fever (A38)	Scarlet fever	Group A streptococci	Bacterium	Re-emerging
Meningococcal infection (A39)	Meningococcal disease	*Neisseria meningitidis*	Bacterium	Emerging
Other bacterial diseases, NEC (A48)	Legionnaires' disease	*Legionella pneumophila*	Bacterium	Emerging
Syphilis (A50–A53)	Syphilis	*Treponema pallidum*	Bacterium	Re-emerging
Other spirochaetal infections (A69)	Lyme disease	*Borrelia burgdorferi*	Bacterium	Emerging
Typhus fever (A75)	Typhus fever	*Rickettsia prowazekii*	Rickettsia	Re-emerging
Atypical virus infection of the CNS (A81)	Variant Creutzfeldt–Jakob disease	Prion protein	Prion	Emerging
Rabies (A82)	Australian bat lyssavirus disease	Australian bat lyssavirus	Virus	Emerging
Mosquito-borne viral encephalitis (A83)	Japanese encephalitis	Japanese encephalitis virus	Virus	Emerging
Dengue fever (A90)	Dengue fever	Dengue virus	Virus	Re-emerging
Other mosquito-borne viral fevers (A92)	Rift Valley fever	Rift Valley virus	Virus	Emerging
	West Nile fever	West Nile virus	Virus	Emerging
Arenaviral haemorrhagic fever (A96)	Argentine haemorrhagic fever	Junín virus	Virus	Emerging
Other viral haemorrhagic fevers, NEC (A98)	Ebola viral disease	Ebola virus	Virus	Emerging
	Korean haemorrhagic fever	Hantaan virus	Virus	Emerging
	Marburg viral disease	Marburg virus	Virus	Emerging
Smallpox (B03)	Smallpox	Variola virus	Virus	Re-emerging
Measles (B05)	Measles	Measles virus	Virus	Re-emerging
Viral hepatitis (B15–B19)	Hepatitis E	Hepatitis E virus	Virus	Emerging
HIV disease (B20–B24)	HIV/AIDS	HIV	Virus	Emerging
Other viral diseases, NEC (B33)	Hantavirus pulmonary syndrome	Sin Nombre virus	Virus	Emerging
	Hendra viral disease	Hendra virus	Virus	Emerging
	Menangle viral disease	Menangle virus	Virus	Emerging
	Nipah viral disease	Nipah virus	Virus	Emerging
Malaria (B50–B54)	Malaria	*Plasmodium* spp.	Protozoan	Re-emerging
Leishmaniasis (B55)	Visceral leishmaniasis	*Leishmania* spp.	Protozoan	Re-emerging
Influenza (J10, J11)	Influenza	Influenza virus	Virus	Re-emerging
Severe acute respiratory syndrome (U04)	Severe acute respiratory syndrome	SARS-coronavirus	Virus	Emerging

Notes: [1] Relative to known status as of mid-19th century; see Table 2.2. NEC = not elsewhere classified.

(Section 3.4), Table 3.11 shows that the majority of our sample diseases are of bacterial (11 diseases) and viral (19 diseases) aetiologies, although the selection also includes mycobacterial (leprosy and tuberculosis), rickettsial (typhus fever), prion (variant Creutzfeldt–Jakob disease), and protozoal (leishmaniasis and malaria) diseases. Judged relative to their known status in the mid-nineteenth century, the final column in Table 3.11 shows that the sample is approximately evenly split between diseases that may be classified as having 'emerged' (20) or 're-emerged' (16) at some point in the post-1850 period, with a skewed distribution towards viral diseases ('emerging' category) and bacterial diseases ('re-emerging' category).

(iii) *Criterion 3: Geographical coverage*. This criterion urged for a global coverage of examples in terms of countries, world regions, and latitudes. As the regional–thematic matrix in Table 3.12 shows, our sample diseases have been selected to illustrate aspects of disease emergence and re-emergence in representative countries of each of the six standard WHO world regions and at the inter-regional and global levels.

Although the 36 diseases in Tables 3.11 and 3.12 form the core of our analysis in Chapters 4–9, we include additional diseases where appropriate to the discussion. While we note that regional–thematic selections other than those in Table 3.12 could have been made, on grounds of length alone we have not tried to be exhaustive. Rather, we have attempted to gain a representative cross-section of disease examples that illustrate the principal themes. Readers will be able to add to the matrix of examples treated here.

DATA QUALITY: A CAUTIONARY NOTE

The mapping and analysis of infectious disease data is confronted by an insidious problem in epidemiological studies: the uneven quality of the data available for examination. Overviews of the limitations of public health surveillance data are provided by Thacker and colleagues (see, for example, Thacker, Choi, *et al.* 1983; Thacker and Berkelman 1988; and Thacker and Stroup 1994), while the geographical dimensions of the problem are reviewed by Cliff and Haggett (1988: 65–92). As described there, a plethora of issues relating to lack of surveillance capacity, delays in case reporting, limitations in the coordination of surveillance practice, and lack of funding for disease monitoring all conspire to limit the completeness, representativeness, and timeliness of communicable disease reporting. In the context of the present study, additional issues relating to the nature and structure of existing public health surveillance systems, the appropriateness of disease monitoring vis-à-vis population monitoring for the first-time detection of newly recognized diseases, and the effective linkage of different data sources also gain

Table 3.12. Matrix of core diseases for analysis in Chapters 4–9

	WHO region						
Chapter/theme	Africa	Americas	Eastern Mediterranean	Europe	South-East Asia	Western Pacific	Global/ inter-regional
4. Disease changes				Tuberculosis	Influenza, malaria		Influenza, malaria, tuberculosis
5. Technical changes		*Escherichia coli* O157:H7 disease, Legionnaires' disease		*Escherichia coli* O157:H7 disease, vCJD			
6. Population changes		Cholera, West Nile fever		Influenza, Marburg viral disease, meningococcal disease	Cholera, plague	Measles	Influenza, SARS
7. Environmental changes		AHF, HPS	Rift Valley fever			Nipah viral disease	Dengue fever, Lyme disease
8. Disease amplifiers	Typhus fever	Anthrax	Hepatitis E, visceral leishmaniasis			Japanese encephalitis, KHF, malaria, plague	
9. Temporal trends	Ebola viral disease, Marburg viral disease, meningococcal disease			Cholera, diphtheria, influenza, leprosy, measles, meningococcal disease, plague, scarlet fever, smallpox, syphilis, tuberculosis, whooping cough		Australian bat lyssavirus disease, Hendra viral disease, Menangle viral disease	Cholera, HIV/ AIDS, plague

Notes: AHF = Argentine haemorrhagic fever; HIV/AIDS = human immunodeficiency virus/acquired immunodeficiency syndrome; HPS = hantavirus pulmonary syndrome; KHF: Korean haemorrhagic fever; SARS = severe acute respiratory syndrome; vCJD = variant Creutzfeldt–Jakob disease.

prominence (Thacker and Stroup 1994). Recognizing the inherently variable nature and reliability of even the best available data sources, all analysis undertaken in this book is subject to the caveat of data quality.

With these points in mind, we move on in the next chapter to examine the first of our themes in disease emergence and re-emergence ('Disease Changes: Microbial and Vector Adaptation'; Figure II.1).

4

Disease Changes: Microbial and Vector Adaptation

4.1 Introduction

In this and the next four chapters, we examine five change agents which have facilitated the emergence and re-emergence of infectious human diseases. Each agent—*microbial and genetic adaptation*, *technology and industry*, *changes in host populations*, *environmental and ecological change*, and *war as a disease amplifier*—has underpinned over the centuries both the appearance of new diseases and the waxing and waning of familiar infections. As shown in Figure II.1, the agents are not independent and commonly interact in complex ways to facilitate microbe emergence and re-emergence at different times and in different geographical locations. Accordingly, we also explore

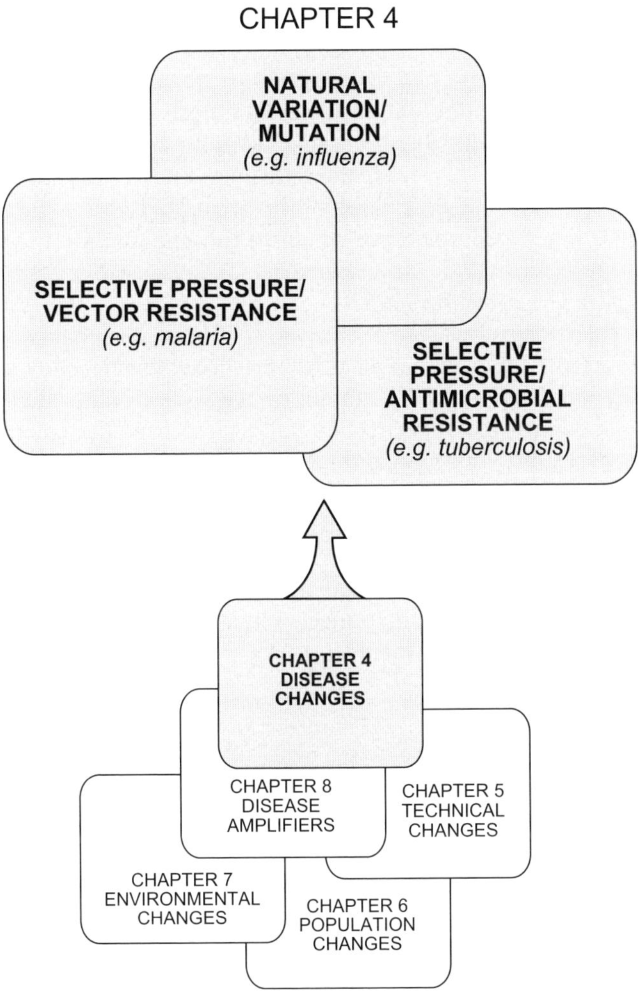

Fig. 4.1. (Upper) Venn diagram showing the facilitating factors for disease emergence and re-emergence associated with microbial and vector adaptation
The lower diagram is redrawn from Fig. II.1 and shows the position of microbial and vector adaptation (shaded box) within the suite of macro-factors associated with the processes of disease and emergence and re-emergence.

these interactions in our account. We begin here with *microbial and vector adaptation*.

THE PROBLEM

Disease microbes are in a continuous state of evolution, responding and adapting to the challenges and opportunities afforded by their hosts and their environments (Morse 1995). New pathogens are evolving, old pathogens are developing enhanced virulence and new clinical expressions, and susceptible pathogens are acquiring resistance to antimicrobial agents. In parallel, the environmental tolerance bands of both old and new pathogens are also changing (Cohen 1998). Not only are disease microbes in a continuous state of evolution. So, too, are the arthropod vectors that transmit many human pathogens. In the second half of the twentieth century, many of these vectors have developed tolerance to an expanding range of insecticides, larvicides, pupicides, and other chemical agents used in their control (World Health Organization 1992*c*).

Against this background, our examination of microbial change and vector adaptation is structured around the three interlinked themes shown in Figure 4.1. We begin in Section 4.2 by examining the issue of natural variation in pathogens and illustrate this with special reference to the emergence and spread of novel subtypes of influenza A virus. We then examine the topic of selective pressure and genetic change in the context of the man-made problems of pathogen resistance to antimicrobials (Section 4.3) and vector resistance to insecticides (Section 4.4).

The processes of microbial change and vector adaptation are not intrinsically geographical but they take place within, and are inextricably linked to, specific geographical environments. This gives a strong geographical emphasis to our discussion.

4.2 Genetic Change and Microbial Emergence

4.2.1 Nature of the Problem

Occasionally, complex evolutionary events can result in the emergence of entirely new genetic subtypes of known pathogens in the human population. Thus, many viruses display a predilection for rapid mutation and the evolution of novel variants. The genetically mutable influenza A virus is a prime example (Morse 1995; Fauci 2006). Likewise, among bacterial agents, the emergence of the virulent *Escherichia coli* O157:H7 has been attributed to the acquisition of *Shigella* genes by an enteropathogenic *E. coli* (Cohen 1998; Whittam *et al.* 1998). More rarely, novel subtypes of known pathogens can result in a new clinical expression of disease; the emergence of Brazilian purpuric fever due to invasive clones of *Haemophilus influenzae* biogroup *aegyptius* in the mid-1980s illustrates the point (Morens *et al.* 2004). Similarly, some recently recognized clinical manifestations of infection with group A *Streptococcus*, including streptococcal toxic shock syndrome and necrotizing fasciitis, might be the result of major changes in the virulence properties of the bacterium (Stevens 1995; Morens *et al.* 2004).

To illustrate the disease consequences of genetic change in a pathogen in more detail we consider the cyclical re-emergence of pandemic influenza.

4.2.2 Antigenic Shifts and the Cyclical Re-Emergence of Pandemic Influenza

The emergence of novel subtypes of influenza A virus, to which the human population has little or no existing immunity, underpins the great pandemics of influenza that have periodically rolled around the world (see Section 2.3.3). Historically, these events have been associated with large—sometimes massive—population losses. At an extreme, the Spanish influenza pandemic of 1918–19 is estimated to have killed 20–50 million or more worldwide (Jordan 1927; Oxford 2000; Johnson and Mueller 2002).[1] Other influenza pandemics have resulted in more modest death tolls, with the combined global excess mortality due to the so-called Asian (1957–8) and Hong Kong (1968–9) pandemics estimated at 3–4 million (World Health Organization 2005*d*). Whatever the associated mortality, however, the broader social and economic impacts of pandemic influenza are always substantial. The overloading of health services, high levels of worker absenteeism, the disruption of essential services, and the interruption of trade and commerce underline the status of influenza pandemics as global public health emergencies (Gust *et al.* 2001).

PANDEMIC EVENTS

An overview of the nature and history of influenza to AD 1850 appears in Section 2.3.3. As described there, pandemics and probable pandemics of influenza have occurred at irregular intervals over the last several centuries, although evidence for the period since 1850 yields an average interval of approximately 25 years (range 2–38 years) between major events (Table 4.1). While South-East Asia has been implicated as the likely source of many of these (Shortridge and Stuart-Harris 1982; Patterson 1986), considerable uncertainty surrounds the mechanisms by which the associated strains of the influenza A virus have emerged in the human population.

Antigenic Variation: Pandemic Shifts

Influenza A viruses are defined by the expression of their surface proteins, haemagglutinin (H) (governing the ability of the virus to bind to, and enter,

[1] Estimates of the global mortality associated with the 1918–19 pandemic vary widely. E. O. Jordan places the death toll at 21.6 million (Jordan 1927: 229–30). A revised estimate by Patterson and Pyle (1991: 19) places the mortality at 30 million, while, more recently, Oxford *et al.* (1999) and Oxford (2000) place the mortality at 40 million. Other, more extreme, estimates have ranged up to 100 million (see e.g. Burnet 1979: 203).

Table 4.1. Pandemics and probable pandemics of influenza, 1850–2005

Year(s)	Source of information: Hirsch (1883–6)[1,2]	Source of information: Patterson (1986)[3]	Interval since previous pandemic (years)	Influenza A subtype	Notes
1850–1	[4]		2	?	'Generally diffused over the Western and Eastern Hemispheres' (Hirsch 1883–6: i. 16)
1855	[4]		4	?	'General prevalence in Europe' (Hirsch 1883–6: i. 16)
1857–8	[4]		2	?	'Wide diffusion over the Western and Eastern Hemispheres' (Hirsch 1883–6: i. 17)
1874–5	[4]		16	?	'Widely spread over the Western and Eastern Hemispheres' (Hirsch 1883–6: i. 17)
1889–90	No information	[4]	14	H2?[5]	Global diffusion (Patterson 1986: 49)
1899–1900	No information	[4]	9	H3?[5]	
1918–19	No information	[4]	18	H1N1	Global diffusion in three pandemic waves (Patterson and Pyle 1991)
1957–8	No information	[4]	38	H2N2	Global diffusion
1968–9	No information	[4]	11	H3N2	Global diffusion

Notes: Table 2.5 provides a summary of pandemics and probable pandemics in the period 1500–1849.[1] Years 1850–75.[2] Excludes the 1873 'pandemic', listed by Hirsch (1883–6: i. 19) as exclusive to the Western Hemisphere.[3] Years 1850–1977.[4] Pandemics and probable pandemics.[5] See Dowdle (1999) for a further consideration of the subtypes associated with the events of 1889–90 and 1899–1900.

Sources: Abstracted from Smallman-Raynor and Cliff (2008, table 1, p. 555), originally based on information in Hirsch (1883–6: i. 7–54) and Patterson (1986, table 5.1, p. 83).

host cells), and neuraminidase (N) (governing the release of new virus particles from host cells). Antigenic changes in these proteins permit influenza A viruses to bypass existing immunity in the human host so that repeat infection and associated illness can occur. Antigenic changes are of two types: (i) frequent but minor *drifts* that result from the accumulation of mutations in the surface proteins and which yield influenza epidemics; and (ii) infrequent but major *shifts* that result in the emergence of novel surface proteins and which yield influenza pandemics (Glezen and Couch 1997). Known twentieth-century shifts in the H and N proteins of influenza A virus are summarized in Figure 4.2, while the associated pandemics are listed with

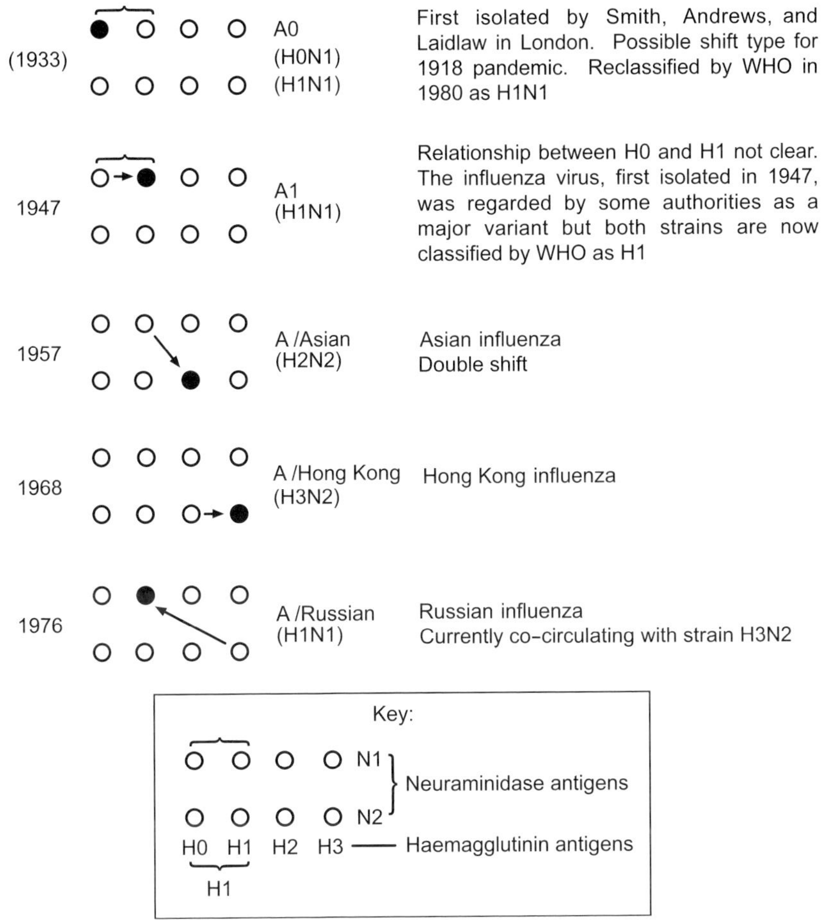

Fig. 4.2. Classification of human influenza A viruses by surface antigen characteristics The circles show in matrix form the various possible combinations of H and N antigens and should be referred to the key in lower part of the diagram. Solid circles represent the combinations that have occurred and the arrows indicate whether the shift involved a change in only one of the surface antigens (horizontal or vertical arrow) or both (diagonal arrow). Note the changed notation of the A0 virus.

Source: Redrawn from Cliff, Haggett, and Ord (1986, fig. 2.2, p. 14).

their designated virus subtypes (H1N1, H2N2, and H3N2) in Table 4.1.[2] One of the dramatic features of these documented virus shifts is the rapidity with which the new subtype becomes dominant and replaces the old as the main virus in circulation (Cliff, Haggett, and Ord 1986).

[2] Note that the Russian influenza (H1N1) of 1977, which is occasionally classified as a pandemic event (see e.g. Oxford 2000; Horimoto and Kawaoka 2001), has been excluded from Table 4.1 due to the similarities of the causative agent with previously circulating A/H1N1 viruses.

The cause of antigenic shifts in influenza A virus is not fully understood. Among the competing hypotheses (Oxford 2000), current evidence suggests that avian influenza viruses (influenza viruses for which birds are the natural reservoir) might play a pivotal role in the evolutionary process. In short, a new pandemic strain might emerge when an influenza A virus, possessing novel viral genes from an avian source, appears in the human population (Horimoto and Kawaoka 2001; Capua and Alexander 2004; de Jong and Hien 2006). Two principal mechanisms by which this might occur are generally recognized:

(1) *Reassortment events*, in which genetic material is exchanged between avian and human influenza A viruses during co-infection in 'reassortment vessels' (for example, pigs or humans). This process is believed to have underpinned the emergence of the virus subtypes associated with the Asian (H2N2) and the Hong Kong (H3N2) pandemics.
(2) *Adaptive mutation*, whereby an avian influenza A virus develops, through a process of genetic adaptation, an enhanced ability to bind to human cells. This process is believed to have underpinned the emergence of the virus subtype associated with the 'Spanish' (H1N1) pandemic of 1918–19. A recent study by Tumpey *et al.* (2007) indicates that minor adaptations in the H protein of the H1N1 virus, resulting in a predilection for virus receptors in human airways rather than in bird intestines, might have served to trigger the transmissibility of the virus between humans.

Pandemic Origins: The 'Influenza Epicentre' Hypothesis

The hypothesis that Asia in general—and southern China in particular—might be a source of new pandemic strains of influenza A virus is outlined by Shortridge and Stuart-Harris (1982) and Shortridge (1992). Informed by the apparent emergence of the Asian and Hong Kong pandemics in South-East Asia, the 'influenza epicentre' hypothesis is founded on (i) the high diversity of avian influenza viruses that circulate in aquatic and terrestrial birds in the region and (ii) the existence of intensive rice/duck/pig farming systems and live animal markets. Together these factors are viewed as providing ideal opportunities for the cross-species transfer and reassortment of influenza viruses and their genes—in a part of the world with massive, densely packed human populations in which any new strain might take hold. As discussed below, the influenza epicentre hypothesis has gained particular prominence with the recent emergence and spread of highly pathogenic avian influenza A (H5N1) in China and other countries of East Asia.

PANDEMIC AND POST-PANDEMIC INFLUENZA WAVES: THE KILBOURNE MODEL

Figure 4.3 shows Kilbourne's (1973) schematic model of the relationship between the number of cases produced by a pandemic of influenza A virus

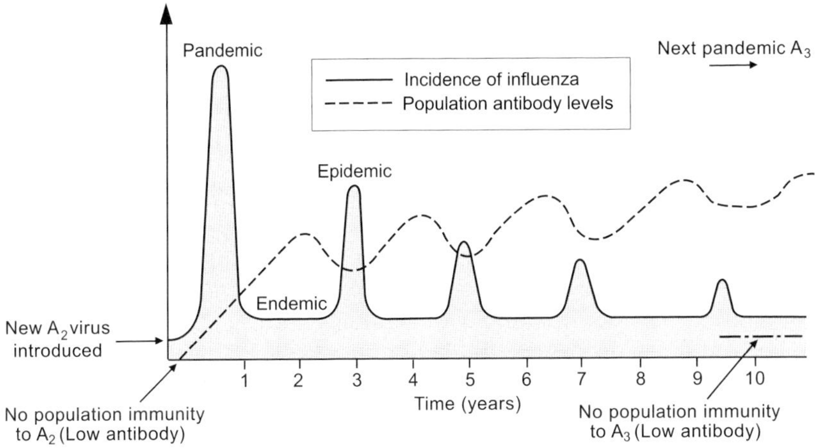

Fig. 4.3. Kilbourne's model of the decline in severity of influenza epidemics in a post-pandemic period
The broken line shows the rise in specific A_2 antibody levels in the exposed population.
Sources: Redrawn from Cliff, Haggett, and Ord (1986, fig. 2.8, p. 25), originally from Kilbourne (1973, fig. 3, p. 480).

and later epidemics due to the same virus subtype. Once the new virus subtype, denoted A_2 in Figure 4.3, is introduced into the population and individuals become infected, so antibody levels to the virus build up over time (pecked line). This process leads to a diminishing stock of susceptibles and so to successively smaller epidemics with a greater time interval between them (solid line). As a result of the natural selection pressure forced upon the virus, antigenic drift will occur. In time, an antigenic shift will result in the appearance of a new subtype of influenza A virus (A_3 in Figure 4.3) to which antibody levels in the population are low. This new virus causes the next pandemic and the process is repeated. Statistical methods for the monitoring of pandemic shifts in influenza time series are examined in Sections 10.3 and 10.5.1.

4.2.3 Avian Influenza A (H5N1) I: Epizootic emergence and Panzootic Transmission

While the pandemic transmission of human influenza has attracted a substantial geographical literature,[3] little is known of the antecedent spread of the avian influenza viruses from which many human pandemic strains are believed to have evolved (Horimoto and Kawaoka 2001; de Jong and Hien 2006). In this

[3] See e.g. Hunter and Young (1971); Patterson and Pyle (1983, 1991); Cliff, Haggett, and Ord (1986); Patterson (1986); Pyle (1986); and Smallman-Raynor, Johnson, and Cliff (2002).

subsection, we examine the emergence and spread of the highly pathogenic avian influenza A (H5N1) virus—a virus that, according to the weight of international scientific opinion, has the potential to trigger the first human influenza pandemic of the twenty-first century (World Health Organization 2005*d*,*g*). Our examination draws on the study of Smallman-Raynor and Cliff (2008).

BACKGROUND: THE CURRENT PANDEMIC ALERT

On Thursday 15 May 1997, a 3-year-old boy was admitted to a Hong Kong hospital with fever, sore throat, and cough of six days' duration. The child's condition deteriorated rapidly, with acute respiratory distress, multi-organ failure, and death on the twelfth day of illness. An atypical influenza virus, recovered from the child's upper respiratory tract, was typed as avian influenza A (H5N1)—a novel and highly pathogenic virus of poultry that had been identified first in China the previous year (Centers for Disease Control and Prevention 1997*b*, 1998*c*). Further 'dead-end' jumps of H5N1 from birds to humans were recorded in Hong Kong in late 1997 and again in early 2003 (Claas *et al.* 1998; Peiris *et al.* 2004) (Table 4.2). But it was the unprecedented events of the winter of 2003–4 that raised international concerns over H5N1 to a new level. Beginning in the latter part of 2003, poultry-based outbreaks of avian influenza, caused by genetic variants of the H5N1 virus, erupted in geographically disseminated form in East Asia. From this early epicentre, the

Table 4.2. Documented human infections with avian influenza A viruses, 1959–2005

Year	Geographical location	Strain	Cases	Deaths	Symptoms	Source
1959	US	H7N7	1	0	Respiratory	Overseas travel
1995	UK	H7N7	1	0	Conjunctivitis	Pet ducks
1997	Hong Kong SAR	H5N1	18	6	Respiratory/ pneumonia	Poultry
1998	China (Guangdong)	H9N2	5	0	Unknown	Unknown
1999	Hong Kong SAR	H9N2	2	0	Respiratory	Poultry; unknown
2003 (Feb.)	Hong Kong SAR	H5N1	2	1	Respiratory	Unknown
(Mar.)	Netherlands	H7N7	89	1	Conjunctivitis[1]	Poultry
(Dec.)	Hong Kong SAR	H9N2	1	0	Respiratory	Unknown
2003–5	Vietnam	H5N1	93	42	Respiratory	Poultry
2004	Canada	H7N3	2	0	Conjunctivitis	Poultry
2004–5	Thailand	H5N1	22	14	Respiratory	Poultry
2005	Cambodia	H5N1	4	4	Respiratory	Poultry
	China	H5N1	8	5	Respiratory	Poultry
	Indonesia	H5N1	17	11	Respiratory	Poultry

Note: [1] Pneumonia and respiratory insufficiency in solitary fatal case.

Sources: Smallman-Raynor and Cliff (2008, table 2, p. 556), originally based on World Health Organization (2005*d*, table 3, p. 40).

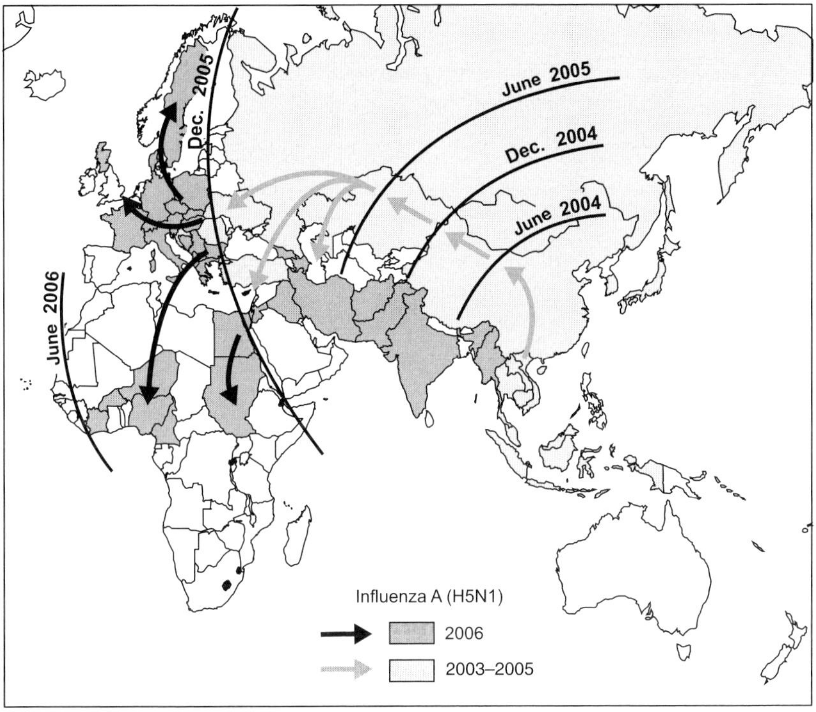

Fig. 4.4. Countries in which avian influenza A (H5N1) was reported in wild birds and poultry, December 2003–May 2006
Shading categories identify OIE member states in which outbreaks were first confirmed in the period 1 Jan.–18 May 2006 (dark shading) and in prior time periods (light shading). Isochrones are modified from evidence presented by the Emergency Preparedness and Response Branch, UN World Food Programme, and show the approximate position of the panzootic wave-front at six-monthly intervals. Vectors indicate the inferred corridors of panzootic diffusion.

Sources: Redrawn from Smallman-Raynor and Cliff (2008, fig. 1, p. 556), based on information in *Disease Information* (Paris: OIE).

virus has spread westwards to Siberia, Europe, the Middle East, and Africa (Figure 4.4). As of 18 February 2008, poultry-based outbreaks of avian influenza (H5N1) had been confirmed in a total of 48 countries, with a number of additional countries having documented the virus in wild bird species (Organisation Mondiale de la Santé Animale 2008).

Although still primarily an infection of avian species, the H5N1 virus has demonstrated a disturbing propensity to extend its host range to include several mammalian species;[4] the World Health Organization (WHO)

[4] Outbreaks of H5N1 among big cats in zoos and rescue centres have been documented in Cambodia (2003) and Thailand (2003, 2004) (see e.g. Food and Agriculture Organization 2004; Keawcharoen *et al.* 2004). The largest outbreak was recorded at a zoo in Si Racha district, Chon Buri province,

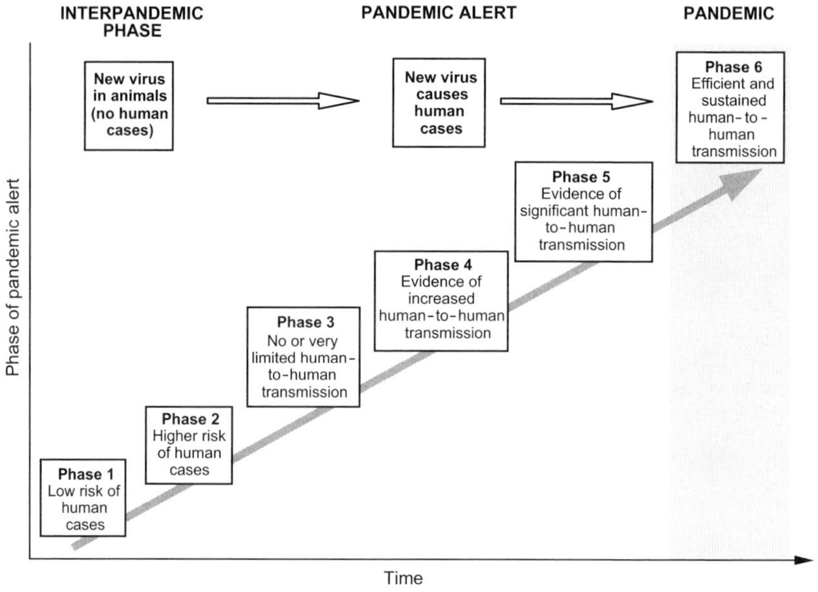

Fig. 4.5. Phases of global pandemic alert for influenza
The WHO *Global Influenza Preparedness Plan* identifies six phases of pandemic alert. Each phase of alert is associated with a series of recommended responses and activities to be implemented by the WHO, the international community, governments, and industry. The epidemiological behaviour of the disease and the characteristics of circulating viruses, among other factors, determine changes from one phase to another.
Sources: Redrawn from Smallman-Raynor and Cliff (2008, fig. 2, p. 557), based on information in World Health Organization (2005*g*).

confirmed cases of human infection exceeded 360 by February 2008 (World Health Organization 2008*a*). This capacity to cross the species barrier, and to cause severe disease and death in humans, has raised grave concerns over the pandemic potential of the virus. In the words of the late Dr Lee Jong-wook, former Director-General of the WHO, the advent of the H5N1 virus has moved the world 'closer to a further [influenza] pandemic than... at any time since 1968' (World Health Organization 2005*d*: 3). In recognition of the heightened concern, the WHO currently classifies the world at Phase 3 of the operative six-phase system of global pandemic alert for influenza (Figure 4.5):

Thailand, in October 2004 and resulted in the death (through disease and slaughter) of 147 tigers (*Panthera tigris*). Feed, consisting of chicken carcasses, was identified as the most likely source of infection (Organisation Mondiale de la Santé Animale 2004*e*). Naturally occurring infections with H5N1 have also been reported in domestic cats, dogs, and stone martens among other mammalian species (Butler 2006*b*; Songserm *et al.* 2006).

Phase 3. Human infection(s) with a new [influenza virus] subtype, but no human-to-human spread, or at most rare instances of spread to a close contact. (World Health Organization 2005g: 2)

The level of global alert is under constant review as epidemiological, laboratory, and other relevant data are made available to the WHO.

THE NATURE OF AVIAN INFLUENZA A

Avian influenza is a disease of birds and, occasionally, certain terrestrial and marine mammals (including horses, humans, pigs, seals, and whales) caused by infection with type A strains of avian influenza virus. Although the majority of wild and domestic bird species are known to be susceptible to infection with influenza A viruses, and the viruses are widespread in nature, particular interest attaches to wild aquatic birds as natural reservoirs of infection and to domestic poultry as birds of economic significance.

Wild aquatic birds. Wild aquatic birds (ducks, gulls, and shore birds) are the principal reservoir of influenza A viruses in nature. Infection in these species is usually asymptomatic and is indicative of the optimal adaptation of the viruses to their reservoir hosts. Studies of wild ducks have revealed that influenza A viruses replicate in both the respiratory systems and intestines of infected birds; virus is shed in large quantities in faeces, with the faecal contamination of surrounding waters serving as an efficient route for the onwards transmission of virus. Virus is also shed in the respiratory secretions of infected birds and this might serve as an additional source of environmental contamination (Tollis and Di Trani 2002; World Health Organization 2005*c*,*d*).

Domestic poultry. Domestic poultry (including chickens, turkeys, ducks, and geese) can become infected with influenza A viruses through direct contact with infected wild waterfowl or other wild birds, other infected poultry, or through contact with surfaces and materials (including water) that have been contaminated with virus. Two principal forms of clinical disease, distinguished on the basis of severity, are recognized:

(1) *Low pathogenic avian influenza (LPAI)*, a mild disease associated with influenza viruses of low virulence and characterized by minor respiratory disorders, depression, ruffled feathers and a drop in egg production in laying birds. This mild form of the disease might go undetected in affected birds.
(2) *Highly pathogenic avian influenza (HPAI)*, a severe disease associated with influenza viruses of high virulence and characterized by depression, loss of appetite, cessation of egg laying, disturbances of the nervous system, swelling and discolouration of combs and wattles, coughing, sneezing, and diarrhoea. The disease can affect many

internal organs and has a mortality rate which, for infected flocks, can approach 100 per cent within 48 hours.

Highly pathogenic avian influenza viruses have no natural reservoir, and the evolution of virulent viruses in poultry from avirulent viruses in wild birds is not completely understood. Experimental evidence suggests the operation of a two-stage process: (i) wild waterfowl introduce influenza viruses of low pathogenicity into poultry populations; (ii) when allowed to circulate in poultry, rapid genetic drift results in the mutation of low pathogenic viruses into highly pathogenic viruses (Capua and Alexander 2004).

Subtypes of Avian Influenza Viruses

As described for human influenza A viruses in Section 4.2.2, subtypes of avian influenza virus are defined by the expression of their H and N surface proteins. Wild birds demonstrate infection with the largest variety of subtypes of influenza A virus; indeed, the majority of possible combinations of the currently recognized 16 H subtypes (H1–H16) and nine N subtypes (N1–N9) have been identified in avian species. However, on the basis of current evidence, viruses that cause HPAI are restricted to the H5 and H7 subtypes, although not all H5 and H7 subtypes are highly pathogenic (Tollis and Di Trani 2002; Capua and Alexander 2004).

Geographical Spread

Avian influenza A viruses (of low and high pathogenicity) are readily transmitted from farm to farm by the movement of live poultry, and by people and equipment contaminated with virus. Until recently, the detection of HPAI viruses in wild birds was a rare event, with cases usually limited to small numbers of birds found dead or moribund within the flight range of a poultry outbreak. This observation has been interpreted as evidence that wild waterfowl are not agents for the onward transmission of influenza viruses in their highly pathogenic form. However, recent events have indicated that some migratory birds do have the capacity to spread the highly pathogenic H5N1 virus over extended distances (World Health Organization 2005*c*).

AVIAN INFLUENZA A (H5N1)

Although descriptions of poultry-based outbreaks of HPAI can be traced to the latter part of the nineteenth century,[5] the first confirmed report of the disease dates to 1959 and an outbreak of a highly pathogenic H5N1 virus (designated A/chicken/Scotland/59) in two flocks of chickens in Aberdeen, Scotland (Pereira *et al.* 1965). During the next 30 years, reports of HPAI were relatively uncommon and were limited to Europe, North America, and

[5] The initial recognition of HPAI is attributed to Edoardo Perroncito and his description of a poultry-based outbreak of a contagious disease on farms near Turin, Italy, in 1878 (Perroncito 1878).

Oceania (Capua and Alexander 2004). Many of these early outbreaks were geographically localized (occasionally restricted to a single farm or flock), with no evidence of transmission across international borders. But, beginning in the 1990s, there was an upsurge in the global record of HPAI activity, with outbreaks noted for the first time in Africa, Asia, and Latin America.[6]

Origins: The Emergence of the Influenza A (H5N1) Virus in Asia

A prominent feature of the recent upsurge of HPAI is the occurrence of outbreaks due to the H5N1 virus in East Asia. The known evolution of highly pathogenic H5N1 influenza viruses in the region can be traced to an outbreak of HPAI on a goose farm in Guangdong province, southern China, in the summer and early autumn of 1996 (Xu *et al.* 1999). Since then, multiple genotypes of the H5N1 virus have been detected in ducks and geese in southern China (Sims *et al.* 2005; de Jong and Hien 2006), with the so-called 'Z' genotype of H5N1 having emerged as the dominant genotype of the virus in East Asia by 2003 (Sims *et al.* 2005; Webster, Guan, *et al.* 2005).[7] In summarizing the evidence regarding the geographical source of H5N1, Chen, Smith, *et al.* (2006) infer that the virus originated in southern China—an inference that is consistent with the 'influenza epicentre' hypothesis outlined in Section 4.2.2.

GEOGRAPHICAL CORRIDORS OF H5N1 PANZOOTIC TRANSMISSION

Global surveillance for influenza A (H5N1) in avian and other animal species is undertaken by the World Organization for Animal Health (Organisation Mondiale de la Santé Animale, OIE), Paris. The disease is subject to urgent notification (within 24 hours of outbreak identification), with summary details of reported outbreaks in OIE member states included in the weekly editions of *Disease Information* (Paris: OIE). Details of the data source are provided in Smallman-Raynor and Cliff (2008), where a review of data-associated

[6] The Food and Agriculture Organization (2005: 5–11) attributes the global increase in HPAI activity since the 1990s to a combination of factors, including: (i) enhanced disease surveillance; (ii) changes in the nature of circulating influenza viruses; and (iii) increases in poultry populations in the absence of appropriate developments in biosecurity. Prominent among these factors, the global trend towards the intensification of poultry production, with the rapid growth of industrial-scale farming and a concomitant increase in the concentration of susceptible birds, has provided ideal conditions for the spread of LPAI viruses—a precondition for the emergence of HPAI viruses. Outbreaks of HPAI in Pennsylvania in 1983 (H5N2), Australia in 1992 (H7N3), and Canada in 2004 (H7N3), among others, are known or suspected to have been attributable to these developments in farming methods. At the same time, an associated increase in the international movement of poultry and poultry products has raised the spectre of the long-distance transfer of avian influenza viruses, as illustrated by the suspected role of imported turkey meat in the introduction of the H5N1 virus to a poultry plant in Suffolk, England, in 2007 (see Section 11.2.4).

[7] Subsequent studies have traced the evolution of the Z genotype of H5N1 back to the viruses responsible for the outbreaks in China and Hong Kong in the mid-1990s (Li, Guan, *et al.* 2004; de Jong and Hien 2006). It is assumed that these viruses, in turn, emerged from low pathogenic viruses of aquatic birds, although no such precursor viruses have yet been identified (Sims *et al.* 2005).

problems is also provided. In this section, we use the outbreak reports included in *Disease Information* to trace the international spread of highly pathogenic H5N1 in wild birds and poultry during the first 30 months of the recognized panzootic, December 2003–May 2006. To assist our discussion, Figure 4.4 shades the 53 OIE member states in which avian outbreaks of H5N1 had been confirmed in the 30-month observation period; the isochrones give the approximate position of the panzootic wave-front at six-monthly intervals, while the vectors depict the inferred spatial corridors of H5N1 transmission.[8]

Global and World Regional Time Series

As Figure 4.4 shows, the H5N1 panzootic diffused as a spatially contagious wave of infection, pushing outwards from an apparent source in East Asia and moving progressively westwards across the Eurasian landmass to Europe and Africa. This diffusion process was underpinned by three distinct phases of outbreak activity. By way of illustration, the bar chart in Figure 4.6 is based on information included in the OIE's *Disease Information* and plots, by month of report, the global count of H5N1 outbreaks in wild birds and poultry, January 2004–April 2006. A polynomial regression line, fitted to the monthly series of reported outbreaks by ordinary least squares, is shown for reference. Inspection of the graph reveals a brief and intense primary wave of outbreak activity in January–February 2004 (denoted Wave I), followed by two extended and less intense secondary waves in July 2004–April 2005 (Wave II) and July 2005–April 2006 (Wave III). The world regional manifestations of each wave are indicated by the bar charts in Figure 4.7. We examine the spread of Waves I–III in turn.

(1) Wave I: Epizootic Onset in East Asia (January–February 2004). Although genotypes of H5N1 are known to have been circulating in waterfowl and terrestrial poultry in East Asia since the mid-1990s, occasional detections of the virus gave way to an epizootic upsurge in the latter part of 2003. The first indication of the upsurge can be traced to a commercial chicken farm in the central province of Chungcheong-buk, Republic of Korea, in mid-December 2003 (Organisation Mondiale de la Santé Animale 2003).[9] While measures to stamp out the disease were swiftly implemented by the Korean authorities (Wee *et al.* 2006), the New Year presented evidence that H5N1 was already widely distributed in other parts of the region. Figure 4.8 plots the monthly count of outbreaks of avian influenza A (H5N1) as reported to the OIE from countries of Asia, December

[8] Summary details of the timing and location of the first confirmed avian outbreaks of H5N1 in OIE member states, Dec. 2003–May 2006, are provided by Smallman-Raynor and Cliff (2008, app. 1, pp. 579–82).

[9] The source of the virus to spark the early farm-based outbreaks in the Republic of Korea is unknown, although some connection with the seasonal appearance of migratory birds in late Oct. and Nov. 2003 is suspected (Organisation Mondiale de la Santé Animale 2003; Wee *et al.* 2006).

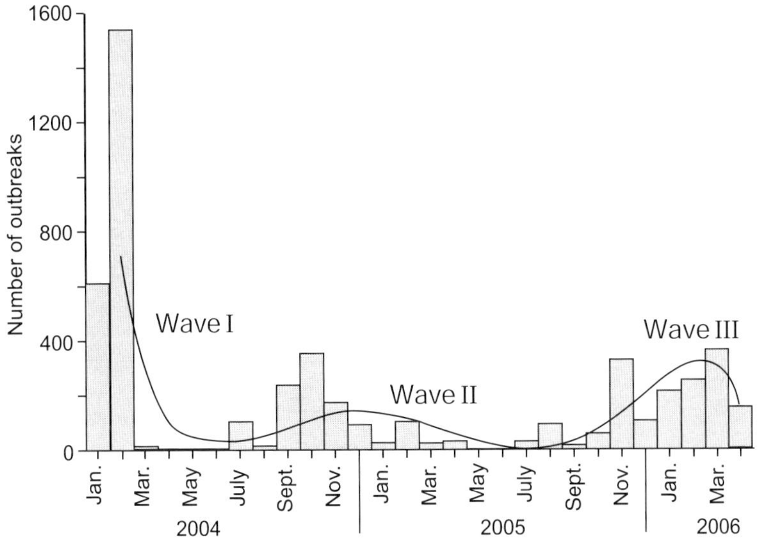

Fig. 4.6. Global time series of outbreaks of avian influenza A (H5N1) in wild birds and poultry, January 2004–April 2006
The bar chart plots the global count of outbreaks by month of report to OIE. A polynomial regression line, fitted to the monthly series of reported outbreaks by ordinary least squares, is shown for reference.
Sources: Redrawn from Smallman-Raynor and Cliff (2008, fig. 3, p. 562), based on information in *Disease Information* (Paris: OIE).

2003–February 2004. Emergency reports of poultry-based outbreaks were issued in rapid succession by Vietnam (8 January), Japan (12 January), Thailand (23 January), Cambodia (24 January), Lao PDR (27 January), Indonesia (2 February), and China (4 February),[10] with Thailand and Vietnam forming the epicentre of outbreak activity (Figure 4.8). The early and widespread dissemination of the virus in the region appears to have been fuelled by wild birds, silently infected domestic waterfowl, and the large-scale movement and trade of poultry (Food and Agriculture Organization 2005).[11]

Whatever the mechanisms involved in the seeding of the virus, H5N1 rapidly colonized the poultry populations of some countries. In the week to 30 January 2004, for example, Thailand recorded 156 outbreaks in 32 provinces, with reports of the disease extending to include chickens, ducks, geese,

[10] An additional report of H5N1 in a dead peregrine falcon was issued by Hong Kong SAR on 26 Jan. 2004 (Organisation Mondiale de la Santé Animale 2004*b*).

[11] Illegal trade, in particular, has been identified by the Food and Agriculture Organization (2005: 19) as having played a potentially important role in the international transmission process: 'Long land borders exist between many of the infected countries in the region and smuggling of poultry and poultry products across many of these is acknowledged. Movement of live poultry (including fighting cocks) across borders is considered to be the most likely source of infection in some places.'

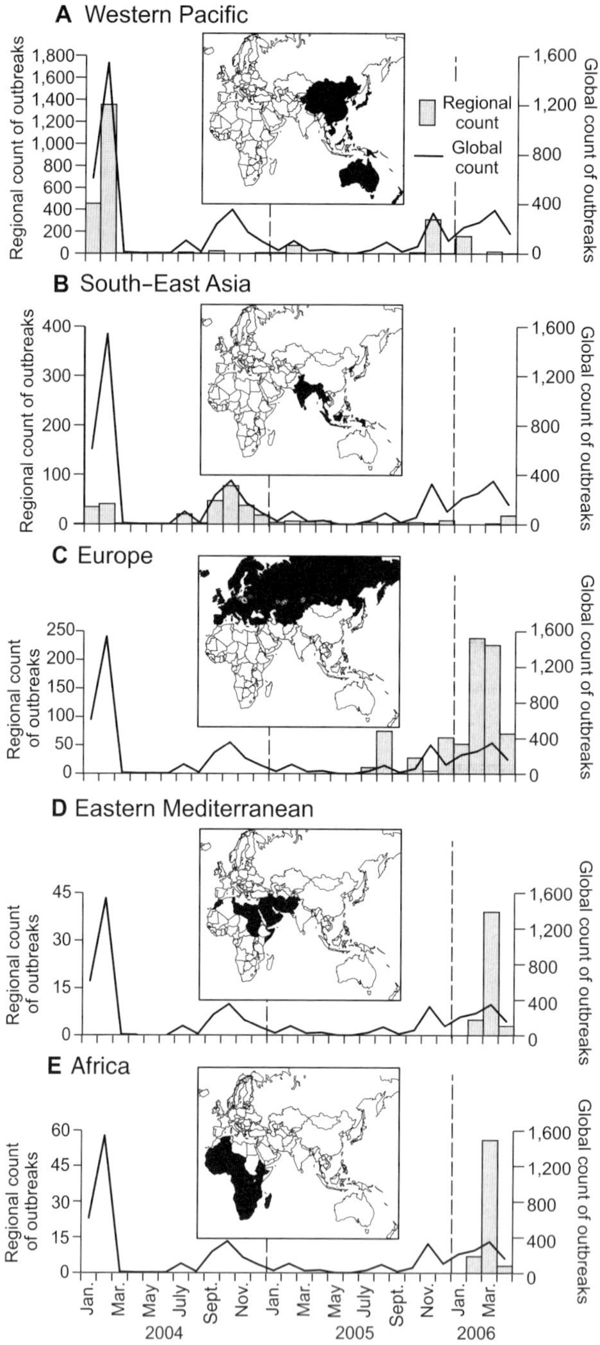

Fig. 4.7. World regional time series of outbreaks of avian influenza A (H5N1) virus in wild birds and poultry by world region, January 2004–April 2006
Bar charts plot the number of outbreaks by month of report to OIE. (A) Western Pacific. (B) South-East Asia. (C) Europe. (D) Eastern Mediterranean. (E) Africa. Geographical divisions A–E relate to the standard WHO world regions (shaded on inset maps), with regions time-ordered according to the estimated date of onset of the first recognized outbreak of the H5N1 virus. The global count of outbreaks is replotted from Fig. 4.6 as the line trace on each graph.

Source: Based on information in *Disease Information* (Paris: OIE).

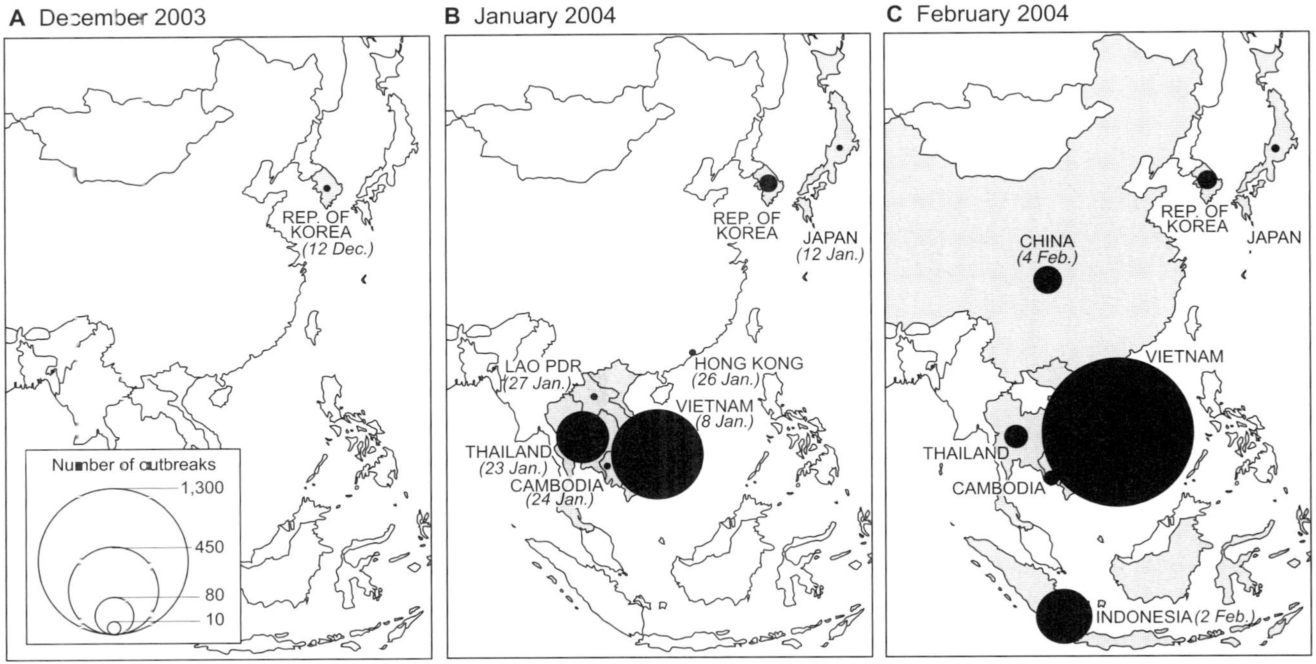

Fig. 4.8 Wave I of the panzootic transmission of avian influenza A (H5N1)

Proportional circles are based on information in *Disease Information* (OIE: Paris) and plot, by country, the count of reported outbreaks of H5N1 in wild birds and poultry in Jan. (map B) and Feb. (map C) 2004. The initial outbreaks in Dec. 2003 are shown for reference (map A). The date of report of the first outbreak of H5N1 in each affected country is given in parentheses.

Source: Redrawn from Smallman-Raynor and Cliff (2008, fig. 4, p. 563).

turkeys, ostriches, quail, and peacocks in commercial and backyard settings (Organisation Mondiale de la Santé Animale 2004*c*) (Figure 4.8B). An even more extreme situation emerged in Vietnam, where, between 24 January and 19 February, 1,282 poultry-based outbreaks—resulting in the death and destruction of some 6.62 million birds—were recorded across the country (Organisation Mondiale de la Santé Animale 2004*d*) (Figures 4.8B,C).

(2) Wave II: Epizootic consolidation (July 2004–April 2005). In some countries, such as Japan and the Republic of Korea, the early outbreaks of H5N1 were quickly contained in commercial poultry flocks and the virus eliminated. Elsewhere in the region, the summer of 2004 heralded fresh poultry-based outbreaks of H5N1 in Cambodia, China, Indonesia, Thailand, and Vietnam, while, in mid-August, Malaysia issued its first report of the disease. As Figure 4.9A shows, Thailand formed the epicentre of reported outbreaks in this second wave. Such were the developments that, by January 2005, the WHO could conclude that H5N1 was enzootic in some parts of the region, the virus having 'established a permanent ecological niche' in Asian poultry (World Health Organization 2005*d*: 16).

(3) Wave III: Panzootic expansion (July 2005–April 2006). A two-month lull in reported outbreak activity gave way, in July 2005, to the fastest and geographically most extensive spread of highly pathogenic avian influenza ever recorded. In a period of 10 months, the virus expanded beyond its initial focus in Asia, sweeping westwards across large tracts of Eurasia and Africa, affecting more than 50 countries and resulting in the loss from disease and culling activities of >200 million birds. The sequence of extension of the panzootic, first to include lands east of the Urals, and then the eastern Mediterranean, Europe, and West Africa, is tracked in Figures 4.4 and 4.9B.

The rapid spatial expansion of the panzootic was linked to a rarely observed phenomenon in the epizootiology of avian influenza: the apparent ability of migratory wildfowl to carry H5N1 in highly pathogenic form over extended distances, and to seed the virus along principal flyways. The first substantial evidence of the phenomenon came in late April 2005, when a mass die-off of some 6,000 migratory birds was recorded at the Qinghai Lake nature reserve (a major rendezvous and breeding site for birds on Asia–Siberia migratory routes) in central China. The source of H5N1 which sparked the die-off is unknown, although an importation with bar-headed geese (*Anser indicus*) arriving from areas of enzootic infection via one of the Asian flyways is suspected (Liu *et al.* 2005; Chen, Li, *et al.* 2006). From here, Qinghai-like viruses began to appear in northern and north-western China, Mongolia, and, to the west, Siberia and the Black Sea region. The latter location, in turn, served as a bridgehead for the carriage of H5N1 by migratory waterfowl to countries of southern, central, and northern Europe, eastern Mediterranean, and West Africa in the early months of 2006. At about the same time, outbreaks of H5N1 also began to be reported from parts of South Asia and the Middle

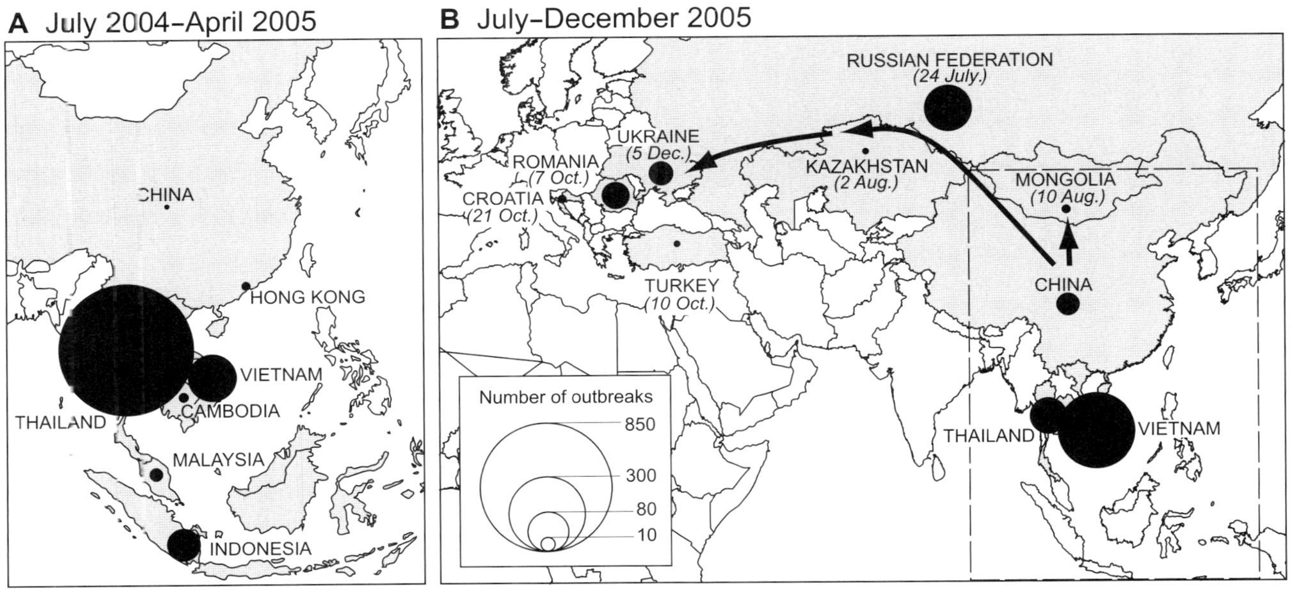

Fig. 4.9. Waves II and III (part) of the panzootic transmission of avian influenza A (H5N1), July 2004–December 2005 Proportional circles are based on information included in *Disease Information* (OIE: Paris) and plot, by country, the count of reported outbreaks of H5N1 in wild birds and poultry. (A) Wave II (July 2004–Apr. 2005). (B) Wave III (part) (July–Dec. 2005). Vectors in map B plot the postulated routes of transmission of H5N1 from a primary focus of infection in East Asia, with the date of report of the first documented outbreak in a given country indicated. Infected countries are shaded.

Source: Redrawn from Smallman-Raynor and Cliff (2008, fig. 5, p. 564).

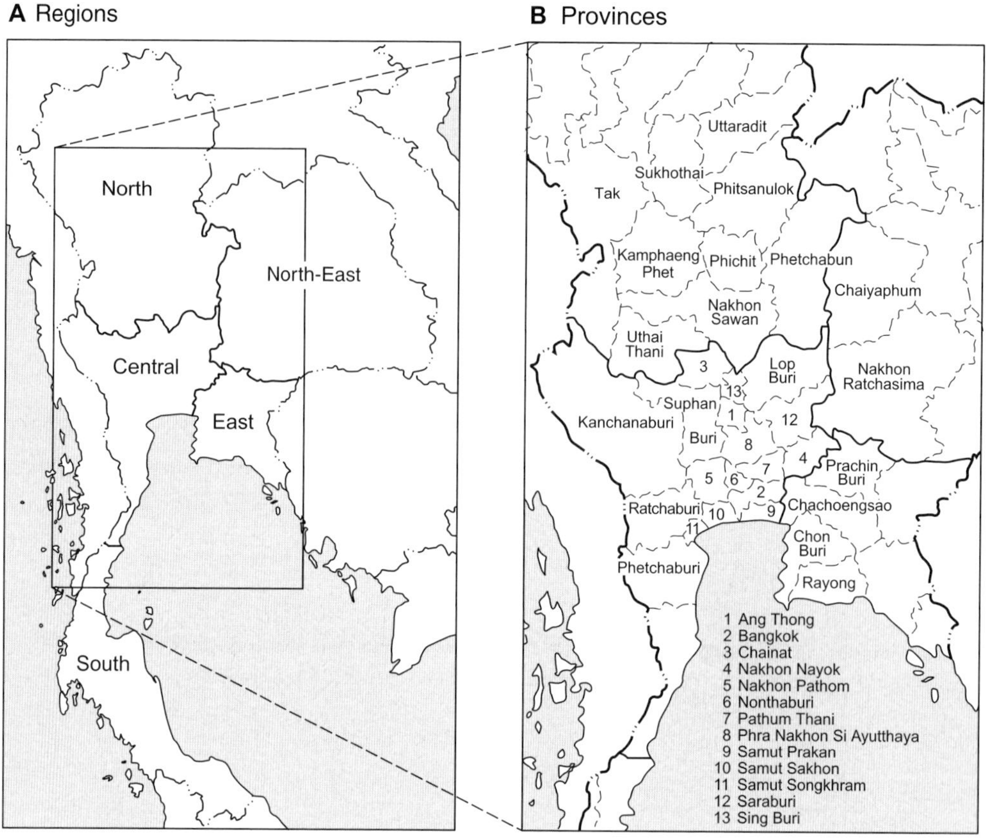

Fig. 4.10. Location map of Thailand (A) Regions. (B) Provinces.

East, including Afghanistan, India, Iran, Iraq, and Pakistan. Countries in which highly pathogenic H5N1 was recorded for the first time in the period January–May 2006 are identified by the dark shading in Figure 4.4.

NATIONAL EPIZOOTICS: THAILAND

To examine the epizootic spread of avian influenza A (H5N1) at the national level, we draw on evidence relating to one of the earliest and most severely affected countries of the East Asian epicentre—Thailand (Figure 4.10). Although large-scale die-offs of poultry were observed in the Central and North regions of Thailand in the latter part of 2003 (Tiensin *et al.* 2005), official confirmation of the presence of H5-related HPAI in the country came with the submission of an emergency report to OIE on 23 January 2004

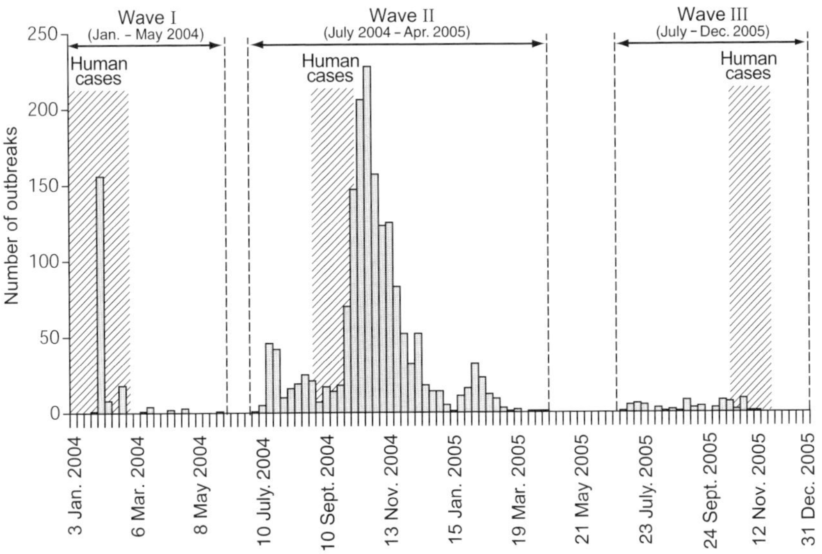

Fig. 4.11. Time series of confirmed outbreaks of HPAI caused by H5N1 in poultry, Thailand, January 2004–December 2005
Outbreaks are plotted by week of report, with summary details of the three main waves of outbreak activity (Waves I–III) given in Table 4.3. Intervals associated with WHO-confirmed human cases of avian influenza A (H5N1) are delimited by the diagonal shading.
Sources: Based on Department of Livestock Development (2008) and *Disease Information* (Paris: OIE).

(Organisation Mondiale de la Santé Animale 2004*a*). A nationwide surveillance programme for the detection of HPAI in avian species was established by the Department of Livestock Development, Ministry of Agriculture and Cooperatives, with the system bolstered by the implementation of intensive surveillance ('x-ray survey') from October 2004 (Tiensin *et al.* 2005). In the analysis to follow, we draw on poultry-based outbreak reports collated by the Department of Livestock Development during the main phase of recorded epizootic activity, July 2004–December 2005 (Department of Livestock Development 2008). We supplement these data with earlier outbreak reports submitted by the Thai authorities to OIE, January–June 2004, and included in *Disease Information*.

Epizootic Waves

Over 1,900 poultry-based outbreaks of HPAI due to the H5N1 virus were detected in Thailand during the 24-month period to December 2005. Consistent with the global pattern in Figure 4.6, Figure 4.11 shows that the outbreaks in Thailand occurred as three distinct waves of epizootic activity (again, denoted Waves I–III), with each wave associated with confirmed human cases of H5N1-related disease (diagonal shading). Summary details

Table 4.3. Waves of highly pathogenic avian influenza A (H5N1) outbreaks, Thailand, January 2004–December 2005

	Avian species					Human infections	
Wave	Onset[1]	End[1]	Peak	Duration (weeks)	Total number of outbreaks	Total	Deaths
I	24 Jan. 2004	29 May 2004	31 Jan. 2004	19	194[2]	12	8
II	3 July 2004	16 Apr. 2005	23 Oct. 2004	42	1,680	5	4
III	2 July 2005	12 Nov. 2005	29 Oct. 2005	20	70	5	2

Notes: [1] Last day of calendar week.[2] Estimate based on reports to the World Organization for Animal Health (OIE).

Sources: Based on Department of Livestock Development (2008) and *Disease Information* (Paris: OIE).

of the magnitude and timing of the three epizootic waves, along with the number of associated human infections and deaths, are given in Table 4.3. As the table shows, Wave II (July 2004–April 2005) was the largest and most sustained of the three epizootic waves. It is to an examination of the geographical spread of this second wave that we turn.

Map Sequences of Wave II Transmission

Wave II of the H5N1 epizootic in Thailand lasted for 284 days, beginning with the first outbreak report on Saturday 3 July 2004 and ending with the last outbreak report on Tuesday 12 April 2005. For this interval, information relating to each of 1,680 poultry-based HPAI outbreaks in Table 4.3 was abstracted from the records of the Thai Department of Livestock Development (2008) to form 76 (province) × 284 (day of report) matrices of H5N1 outbreak counts for (i) all poultry, (ii) chickens, and (iii) ducks. For each of the matrices, the daily counts were then combined by seven-day calendar period to yield 42-week time series of outbreak counts.[12]

The spatial evolution of Wave II is traced in Figure 4.12. For consecutive fortnightly periods over a 24-week interval, 27 June–10 July (map A) to 28 November–11 December (map L) 2004, the maps give the province-level count of newly reported H5N1 outbreaks in all poultry. The first confirmed outbreaks were recorded among domestic chickens in provinces of the Central (Pathum Thani and Phra Nakhon Si Ayutthaya) and North (Sukhothai and Uttaradit) regions in early July (Figure 4.12A). From this apparent onset, HPAI spread to adjacent provinces of the Central, East, North, and North-East regions in the period to mid-September (Figures 4.12B–F)—a spatial pattern that was reinforced as the wave escalated to a peak in late

[12] Weekly calendar periods (Sunday to Saturday) were formed by dividing the 284-day observation period into 42 seven-day units, beginning with the period Sunday 27 June–Saturday 3 July 2004 (week 1) and ending with the period Sunday 10–Saturday 16 Apr. 2005 (week 42).

October (Figures 4.11 and 4.12G–I). Thereafter, spatial decay of the epizootic wave set in from November (Figures 4.12 J–L).

Alternative Spatial Frameworks: Avian Spaces

Previous studies of the epizootic pattern of HPAI in Thailand have identified significant and positive spatial associations between (i) the recorded count of H5N1 outbreaks in poultry and (ii) size estimates of type-specific poultry populations (Gilbert, Chaitaweesub, *et al.* 2006). To examine the hierarchical pattern of outbreak activity implied by these associations, Thailand was converted into a series of 'avian spaces' that reflected the size-ordered distribution of poultry species. For each of the 76 provinces of Thailand, January 2003 estimates of the count (head) and density (head/km^2) of sample categories of poultry (general poultry,[13] native chickens, and ducks) were derived from information included in *Agricultural Statistics of Thailand 2003/04* (Office of Agricultural Economics 2004). Thailand was then treated as a series of graphs consisting of a set of nodes (76 provinces; Figure 4.10) and the links between them, with the graphs configured so that all provinces were joined to their next largest and next smallest provinces in terms of size (variously, head and head/km^2) for each of the three sample categories of poultry. We refer to the resulting avian spaces associated with each pair of size-ordered graphs as *general poultry spaces*, *native chicken spaces*, and *duck spaces* in the subsequent discussion.

Method. To examine the pattern of outbreak activity within each of the avian spaces, we draw on a measure of local spatial association known as the $G_i(d)$ statistic (Getis and Ord 1992; Ord and Getis 1995). The $G_i(d)$ statistic provides a measure of the spatial concentration of a given variable x (in the present analysis, the count of reported H5N1 outbreaks) within distance d of a specified reference point i. High values of $G_i(d)$ are generated when large values of x cluster within distance d of reference point i, while low values of $G_i(d)$ are generated when the converse is true. Following Getis and Ord (1992: 190), $G_i(d)$ is defined as

$$G_i(d) = \frac{\sum_{j=1}^{n} w_{ij}(d)x_j}{\sum_{j=1}^{n} x_j}, j \neq i, \qquad (4.1)$$

where n is the number of Thai provinces, d is the distance between the reference province i and province j, x_j is the reported number of H5N1 outbreaks in j, and $\{w_{ij}\}$ is a symmetric binary spatial weights matrix in which $w_{ij} = 1$ if province j is within distance d of province i and $w_{ij} = 0$

[13] For the purposes of the present analysis, the category 'general poultry' was formed by aggregating the estimated count of broilers, native chickens, and ducks as recorded in *Agricultural Statistics of Thailand 2003/04* (Office of Agricultural Economics 2004).

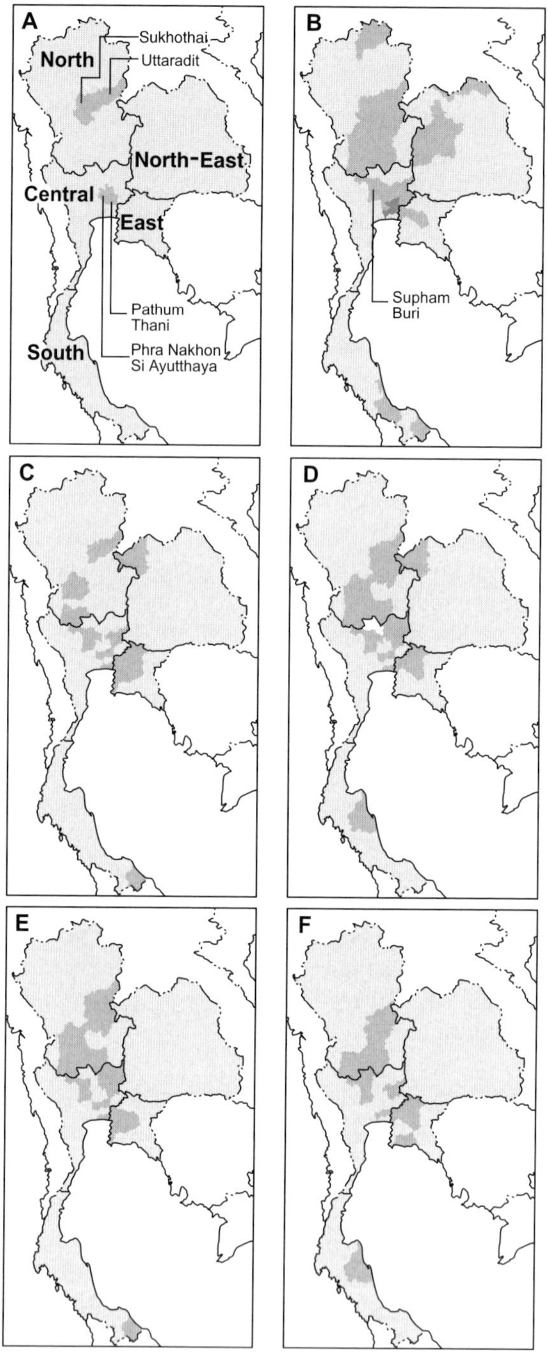

Fig. 4.12. Time-ordered sequence of development of Wave II of the HPAI epizootic due to H5N1 in poultry, Thailand, June–December 2005

The maps relate to the first 24 weeks of Wave II of the epizootic (27 June–11 Dec. 2004) and plot the fortnightly count of newly reported HPAI outbreaks by province. (A) Weeks 1–2 (27 June–10 July). (B) Weeks 3–4 (11–24 July). (C) Weeks 5–6 (25 July–7 Aug.). (D) Weeks

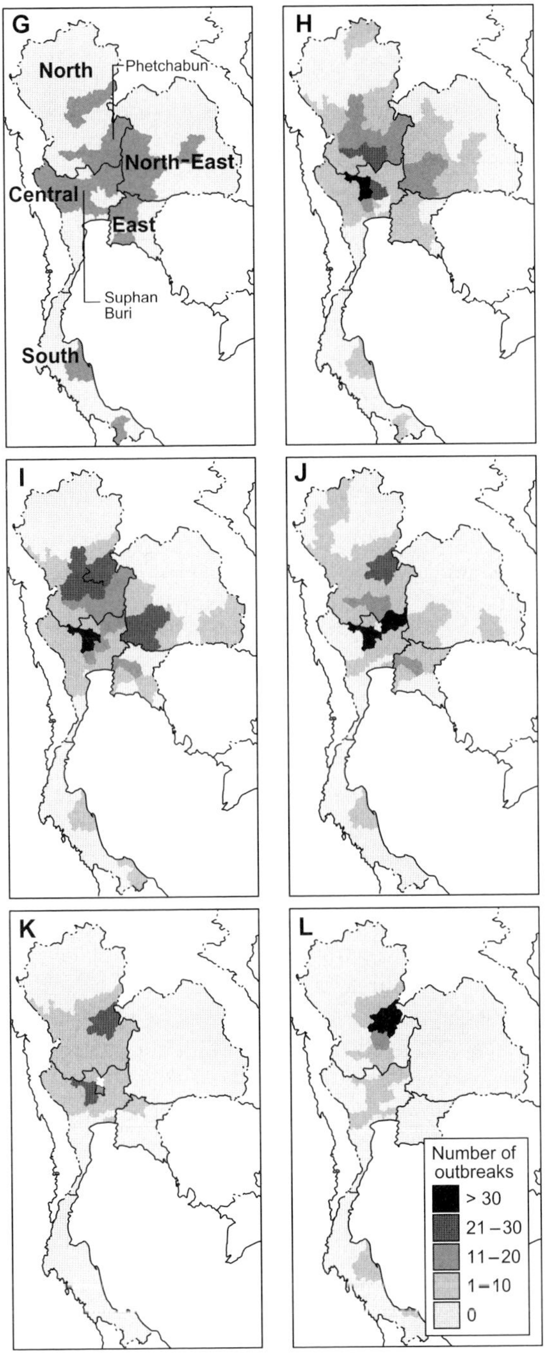

Fig. 4.12 (Continued)
7–8 (8–21 Aug.). (E) Weeks 9–10 (22 Aug.–4 Sept.). (F) Weeks 11–12 (5–18 Sept.). (G) Weeks 13–14 (19 Sept.–2 Oct.). (H) Weeks 15–16 (3–16 Oct.). (I) Weeks 17–18 (17–30 Oct.). (J) Weeks 19–20 (31 Oct.–13 Nov.). (K) Weeks 21–2 (14–27 Nov.). (L) Weeks 23–4 (28 Nov.–11 Dec.). Summary details of outbreak activity in Wave II are given in Table 4.3.

otherwise. For large values of n, $G_i(d)$ can be tested for significance as a standard Normal deviate, $Z[G_i(d)]$. Formulae for the computation of the expectation and variance under the null hypothesis of no spatial association are given in Getis and Ord (1992: 192).

For the purposes of the present analysis, local indicator i in equation 4.1 was fixed as the largest (rank 1) province in each of the (3 poultry categories $\times$ 2 size measures =) 6 size-ordered avian spaces, with $G_i(d)$ evaluated for each of the 75 increments of distance d associated with the provinces j. Analysis of H5N1 outbreak activity in each of the poultry spaces was undertaken for each week of the 42-week observation interval, July 2004–April 2005, for: (i) values of x_j associated with H5N1 outbreaks in all poultry; and (ii) values of x_j associated with H5N1 outbreaks in chickens and ducks.

Results I: All Poultry

Equation 4.1 was first evaluated for values of x_j associated with H5N1 outbreaks in all poultry. The contour plots in Figure 4.13 chart the values of $G_i(d)$, as a standard Normal deviate $Z[G_i(d)]$, for alternative avian spaces as defined by count (head) (upper plots) and density (head/km^2) (lower plots) of (A) general poultry, (B) native chickens, and (C) ducks. For each space, values of $Z[G_i(d)]$ are plotted by week (vertical axis) and rank of distance from the largest province (horizontal axis), with the peak week of outbreak activity (week ending 23 October 2004) identified on each plot by the horizontal pecked line. Periods of epizootic build-up (pre-peak) and fade-out (post-peak) are indicated for reference.

Figure 4.13 yields little (plots A) or no (plots B) evidence for the temporally sustained clustering of H5N1 outbreaks in the upper tiers ($d < 20$) of the general poultry spaces and native chicken spaces, suggesting that the province-level size hierarchies of these two poultry categories played only a limited role in the spatial mediation of the H5N1 epizootic. Rather, consistent with evidence for the role of domestic ducks as silent carriers of highly pathogenic H5N1 virus in Thailand (Gilbert *et al.* 2006; Songserm *et al.* 2006), strong and temporally sustained evidence of outbreak clustering is associated with the duck space in the upper map of plot 4.13C. The spatial correspondence between the province-level counts of H5N1 outbreaks and ducks waxed and waned with the progress of the epizootic wave, with the darker shading categories $\{Z[G_i(d)] > 2.0\}$ in the upper plot of Figure 4.13C consistent with a four-stage model of epizootic development.

(1) *Stage 1 (3 July–21 August 2004; weeks 1–8)*. An early phase of epizootic build-up, with the first evidence of the temporally sustained clustering of H5N1 outbreaks—manifesting in the middle tiers of the duck space—in mid-August (week 8).

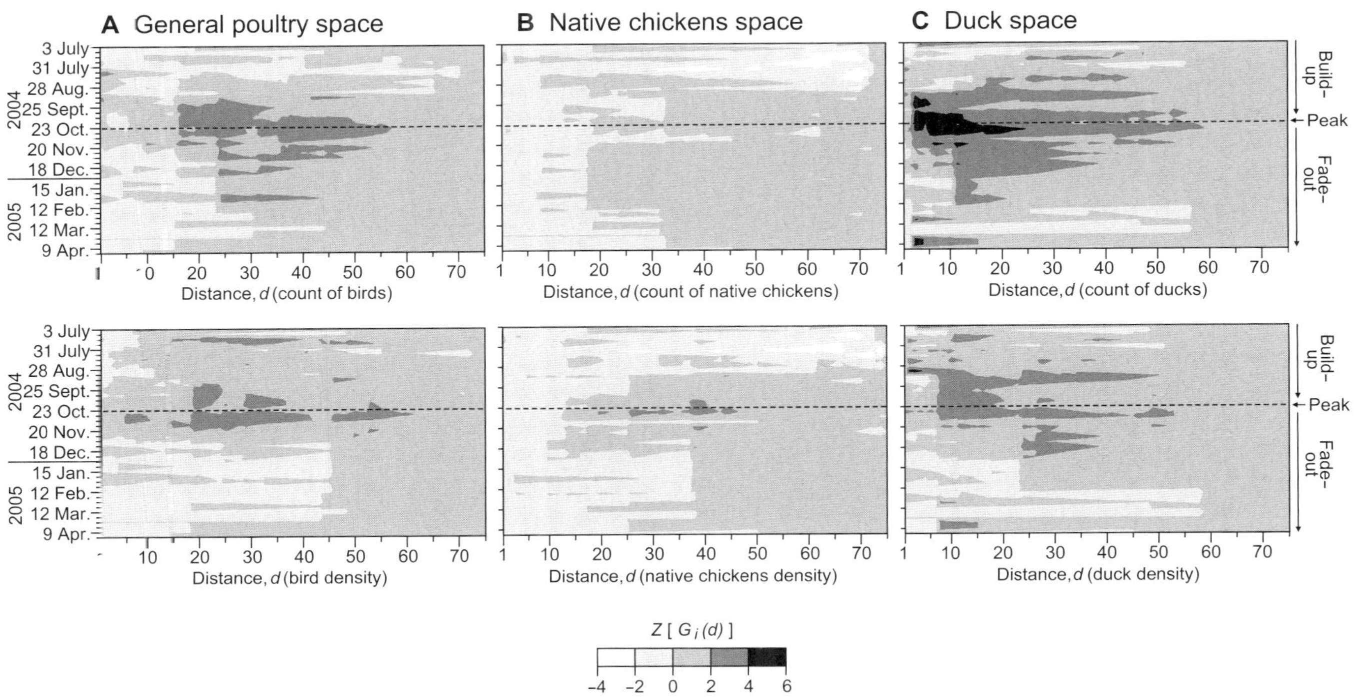

Fig. 4.13. Clustering of HPAI outbreaks due to H5N1 in alternative avian spaces of Thailand, July 2004–April 2005: all poultry outbreaks The contour plots show the value of the $G_i(d)$ statistic as a standard Normal deviate, $Z[G_i(d)]$, by week and rank of province (d) from the first-ranked province in each of six spaces formed to reflect the size distribution of poultry in Thailand. (A) General poultry space, formed by aggregating the count of broilers, native chickens, and ducks. (B) Native chickens space. (C) Duck space. Within A–C, contour plots of the $Z[G_i(d)]$ statistic are given for spaces as defined by the total count of birds (upper) and density of birds (lower). The peak week of reported outbreak activity at the national level (week ending 23 Oct. 2004; Fig. 4.11) is indicated on each plot by the broken line.

(2) *Stage 2 (22 August–18 September 2004; weeks 9–12)*. Continued intensification of H5N1 activity, with a rapid extension of the outbreak cluster to include the upper tiers of the duck space by early September (week 12).
(3) *Stage 3 (19 September–6 November 2004; weeks 13–19)*. The maximum limit of the cluster in the upper and middle tiers of the duck space was reached around the peak of the epidemic in mid-October (week 17), with the most intense levels of clustering $\{Z[G_i(d)] > 4.0\}$ identified in the uppermost tiers of the duck space at this time.
(4) *Stage 4 (7 November 2004–12 February 2005; weeks 20–33)*. The strength of the cluster began to wane in the post-peak period, with a noteworthy retreat of outbreak activity from the uppermost tiers of the hierarchy by early December 2004 (week 23) and with a collapse of spatial association from early February 2005 (week 33).

Results II: Chickens and Ducks

Figures 4.14 and 4.15 have been formed in the manner described for Figure 4.13 and plot, for each of the six poultry spaces, the weekly values of $Z[G_i(d)]$ associated with outbreaks in chickens and ducks. As for the epizootic in all poultry (Figure 4.13), two features of Figures 4.14 and 4.15 are especially noteworthy:

(1) the strongest and temporally most sustained clustering of outbreak activity in both chickens and ducks is associated with the duck space in the upper plots of 4.14C and 4.15C; and
(2) the pattern of outbreaks in both chickens and ducks was independent of the native chicken spaces in plots 4.14B and 4.15B.

Inasmuch as there are between-species differences in observation (1), these relate to the generally earlier onset and cessation of outbreak clustering in ducks as compared with chickens, and the greater maximum extent of the cluster in chickens as compared with ducks at the epidemic peak.

Interpretation. Consistent with the findings of Gilbert *et al.* (2006), evidence for the strong and temporally sustained clustering of H5N1 outbreaks in the upper plots of Figures 4.13C–4.15C suggests that the spatial evolution of the epizootic pattern in Figure 4.12—both overall, and for individual poultry species—was mediated through the size hierarchy of the duck population of Thailand. Although not shown, techniques of cross-correlation analysis and cross-correlogram analysis indicate that the space–time pattern of outbreak activity for chickens (upper plot, Figure 4.14C) lagged that for ducks (upper plot, Figure 4.15C) by 1–2 weeks. Taken together, these findings reflect the documented role of free-grazing ducks as a source of H5N1 infection in domestic chickens in Thailand, and serve to underscore the biosecurity risks associated with 'open' duck-raising systems in the country (Songserm *et al.* 2006).

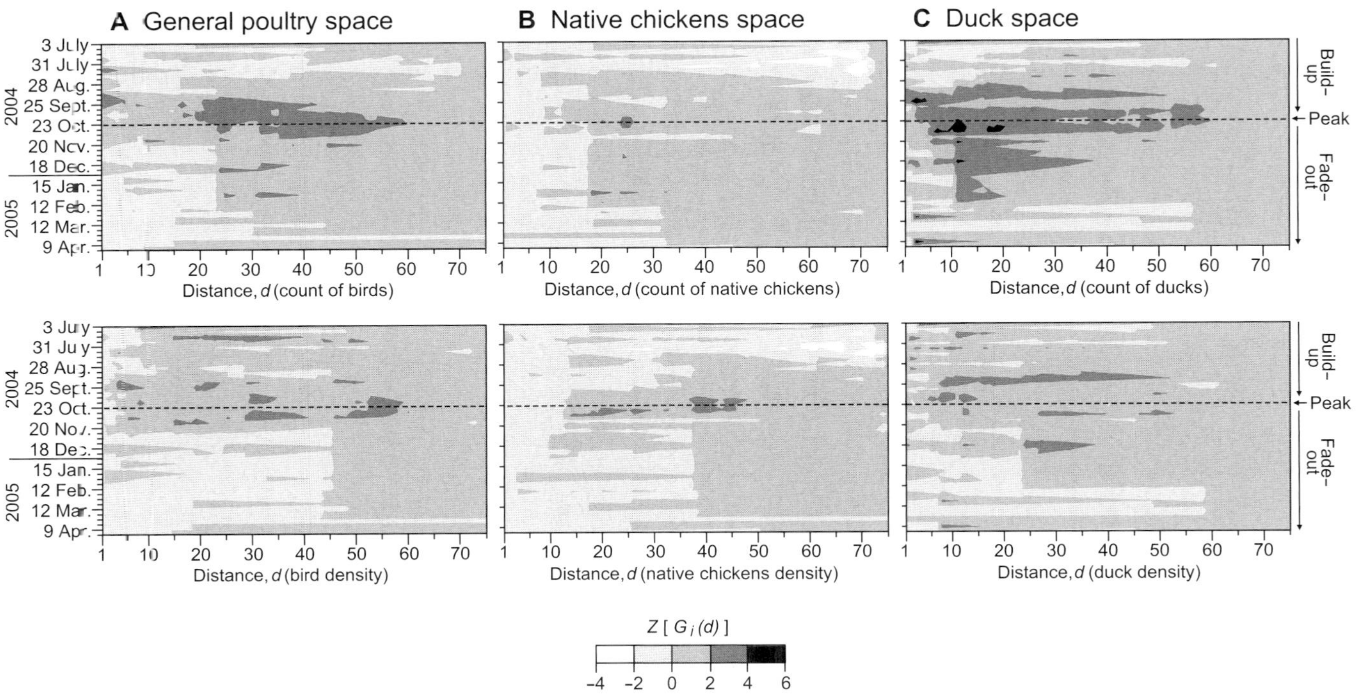

Fig. 4.14. Clustering of HPAI outbreaks due to H5N1 in alternative avian spaces of Thailand, July 2004–April 2005: outbreaks in chickens Contour plots A–C have been formed in the manner described in the caption to Fig. 4.13.

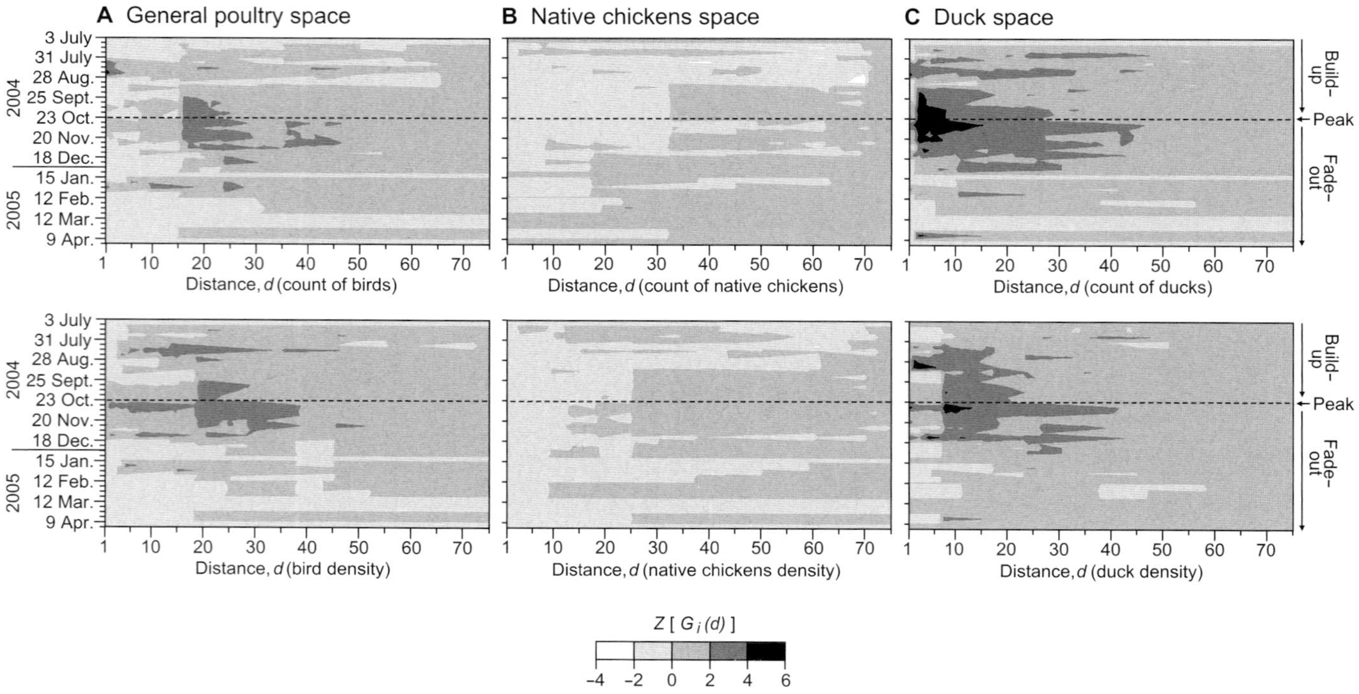

Fig. 4.15. Clustering of HPAI outbreaks due to H5N1 in alternative avian spaces of Thailand, July 2004–April 2005: outbreaks in ducks Contour plots A–C have been formed in the manner described in the caption to Fig. 4.13.

4.2.4 Avian Influenza A (H5N1) II: Human Infections and Pandemic Potential

In response to the public health risks of H5N1, a framework for the enhanced global surveillance of H5 viral infections in humans was established by the WHO in February 2004 (World Health Organization 2005*d*). All WHO member states are requested to submit notifications of probable and confirmed human cases of H5N1 to WHO headquarters, with details of confirmed cases summarized in WHO's *Situation Updates—Avian Influenza* (Geneva: WHO). To parallel the foregoing examination of the panzootic transmission of H5N1, the analysis to follow draws upon Smallman-Raynor and Cliff's (2008) examination of the WHO records of human cases of avian influenza A (H5N1), December 2003–May 2006.

NATURE OF HUMAN H5N1 INFECTION AND THE PANDEMIC RISK

Avian influenza viruses are highly species-specific. As Table 4.2 shows, reports of human infection with avian influenza viruses are few in number and have been limited to just four virus subtypes (H5N1, H7N3, H7N7, and H9N2). Clinically, these infections have usually manifested as mild respiratory illnesses and viral conjunctivitis, although infection with the H5N1 subtype has been associated with severe illness and a high case-fatality rate.

Clinical Course

Current knowledge of the clinical spectrum of human infection with avian influenza A (H5N1) virus is based on the surveillance of hospital patients with moderate and severe disease. The frequency of milder illness and subclinical infection has yet to be determined, although epidemiological studies suggest that both occur (Thorson *et al.* 2006). In confirmed cases, an incubation period of 2–8 days gives way to high fever (>38°C) and a typical influenza-like illness, sometimes accompanied by diarrhoea, vomiting, abdominal pain, and bleeding from the nose and gums. Breathing difficulties usually begin on the fifth or sixth day of illness, with the development of clinically apparent pneumonia in the majority of cases. Multi-organ failure with signs of renal dysfunction and, occasionally, cardiac compromise have been reported in some patients, with death (primarily due to progressive respiratory failure) typically occurring 9–10 days (range 2–31 days) after onset of the clinical illness. The observed case-fatality rate is >50 per cent (Writing Committee of the WHO Consultation on Human Influenza A/H5 2005; World Health Organization 2006*b*).

Transmission Routes

As judged by the exposure histories of confirmed human cases of avian influenza A (H5N1), present evidence is consistent with bird-to-human, environment-to-human, and limited, non-sustained, human-to-human

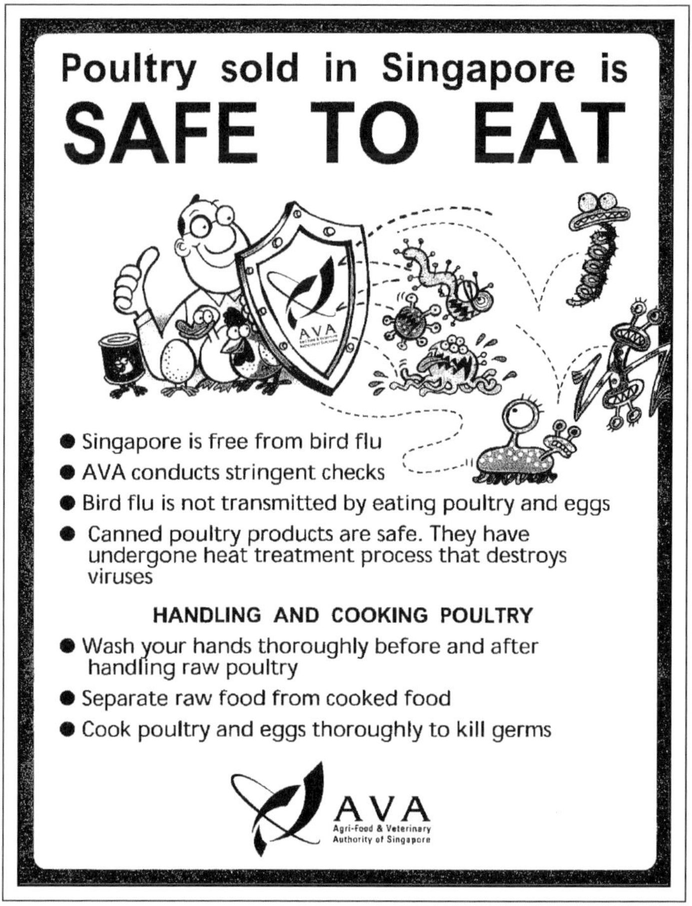
Poultry sold in Singapore is
SAFE TO EAT
AVA
• Singapore is free from bird flu
• AVA conducts stringent checks
• Bird flu is not transmitted by eating poultry and eggs
• Canned poultry products are safe. They have undergone heat treatment process that destroys viruses
HANDLING AND COOKING POULTRY
• Wash your hands thoroughly before and after handling raw poultry
• Separate raw food from cooked food
• Cook poultry and eggs thoroughly to kill germs
AVA
Agri-Food & Veterinary Authority of Singapore

Pl. 4.1. Avian influenza A (H5N1) information poster
English-language version of information poster issued by the Agri-Food and Veterinary Authority (AVA), Singapore, for supermarkets and hawkers. Chinese, Malay, and Tamil versions of the poster are also available.
Source: Agri-Food and Veterinary Authority (2008).

transmission. Direct contact with sick and dead birds, or with surfaces and objects contaminated by poultry faeces, is believed to represent the primary route of human exposure. The slaughter, plucking, and preparation of poultry for consumption has been identified by WHO as a particular risk factor (Plate 4.1), while environmental exposure to poultry-contaminated land and water bodies is another potential source of infection (World Health Organization 2006*a*). Limited human-to-human transmission has been implicated in some family clusters (see, for example, Ungchusak *et al.* 2005).

Pandemic Potential of the Influenza A (H5N1) Virus

As Alvarado de la Barrera and Reyes-Terán (2005) observe, the occurrence of a pandemic of human influenza is dependent on three conditions: (i) a new influenza virus emerges; (ii) the new virus has the ability to cause disease in humans; and (iii) the new virus can spread from human to human in an efficient and sustained manner. The H5N1 virus currently meets conditions (i) and (ii), but not the transmissibility condition (iii). Reassortment events and adaptive mutation (see Section 4.2.2) are generally recognized as the principal mechanisms by which increased transmissibility among humans might arise. As the World Health Organization (2005*c*) observes, the risk that the H5N1 virus might acquire the ability to spread efficiently from human to human via either mechanism will persist as long as the opportunities for human infection occur. As the highly pathogenic H5N1 virus is now considered to be enzootic in avian species in some parts of Asia, this risk is likely to continue for the foreseeable future.

GLOBAL TIME SERIES

Beginning in late October 2003—coincident with the inferred time of onset of the epizootic spread of H5N1 in domestic poultry in East Asia—sporadic human cases of severe respiratory illness began to present at hospitals in Hanoi and neighbouring provinces of northern Vietnam. Among the series of 14 suspicious cases, a 12-year-old girl from Ha Nam province, admitted to hospital in Hanoi on 27 December, was subsequently identified as the first WHO-confirmed human case of avian influenza A (H5N1) associated with the nascent panzootic (World Health Organization 2004*e*).[14] From this putative beginning, a global total of 216 confirmed human cases of avian influenza A (H5N1), including 122 deaths, was documented by the WHO in the 30 months to May 2006 (Table 4.4). These cases are plotted, by week of report in the WHO's *Situation Updates*, as the bar chart in Figure 4.16.[15] The corresponding global time series of outbreaks of H5N1 in wild birds and poultry is represented by the line trace in Figure 4.16. Consistent with an avian → human transmission route, the weekly time series of human case reports reveals pronounced periods of raised disease activity (January–March 2004, January–June 2005, and October 2005–May 2006), with each period coincident with upswings in outbreak activity associated with Waves I–III of the avian panzootic (Figure 4.6).

[14] An earlier WHO-confirmed human case of avian influenza A (H5N1), with symptom onset on 25 Nov. 2003, has been retrospectively identified by Chinese scientists. The patient (a 24-year-old male in military service) was hospitalized with a severe respiratory illness in Beijing, China, and died on 3 Dec. 2003. It was initially suspected that the patient was infected with the severe acute respiratory syndrome (SARS) virus. Stored specimens from the man tested positive for H5N1 (Zhu *et al.* 2006).

[15] Cases in Figure 4.16 are plotted by week of report, rather than week of symptom onset or week of hospital admission, on account of the large number of early cases for which onset and/or hospital admission data is unavailable in the published WHO statistics.

Table 4.4. Confirmed human cases of influenza A (H5N1), 2003–2006

	Cases (deaths)				
Country	2003	2004	2005	2006[1]	Total
Vietnam	3 (3)	29 (20)	61 (19)	0	22 (14)
China	0	0	8 (5)	10 (7)	18 (12)
Cambodia	0	0	4 (4)	2 (2)	6 (6)
Indonesia	0	0	17 (11)	23 (20)	40 (31)
Azerbaijan	0	0	0	8 (5)	8 (5)
Djibouti	0	0	0	1 (0)	1 (0)
Egypt	0	0	0	14 (6)	14 (6)
Iraq	0	0	0	2 (2)	2 (2)
Turkey	0	0	0	12 (4)	12 (4)
TOTAL	3 (3)	46 (32)	95 (41)	72 (46)	216 (122)

Note:[1] 1 Jan.–18 May.

Sources: Smallman-Raynor and Cliff (2008, table 3, p. 566), based on the World Health Organization's *Situation Updates–Avian Influenza* (Geneva: WHO).

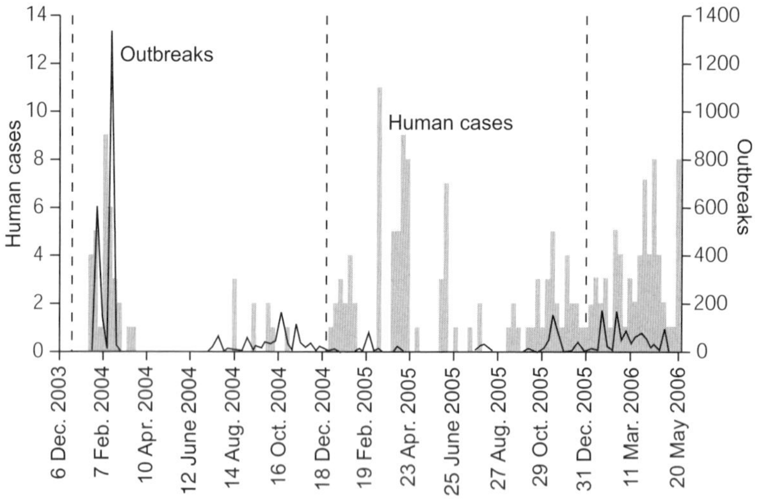

Fig. 4.16. Global time series of WHO-confirmed human cases of avian influenza A (H5N1), December 2003–May 2006

The bar chart plots the number of confirmed human cases by week of report in the WHO's *Situation Updates–Avian Influenza.* For reference, the line trace plots the number of confirmed outbreaks of avian influenza A (H5N1) in domestic and wild birds by week of report in OIE's *Disease Information.*

GEOGRAPHICAL PATTERNS

While the H5N1 panzootic wave had spread to over 50 countries by May 2006, WHO-confirmed human cases of the disease were limited to just 10 countries (Table 4.4). Figure 4.17 plots the geographical incidence of these human cases in the periods December 2003–December 2004 (map A), January–December 2005 (map B), and January–May 2006 (map C). Countries in which H5N1 had been confirmed in avian species by the end of each time period are shaded, while, for reference, the isochrones in maps 4.17B and C are replotted from Figure 4.4 and show the approximate position of the panzootic wave-front at six-monthly intervals. Finally, the bar charts in Figure 4.18 plot the weekly time series of human cases by reporting country; the corresponding national series of outbreaks in wild birds and poultry are represented on each graph as the line traces.

WHO-confirmed human cases of avian influenza A (H5N1) were confined to East Asia in the period to December 2004 (Figure 4.17A), with major clusters of disease activity in northern and southern Vietnam and central Thailand associated with strongly defined peaks of epizootic activity (Figures 4.18A,B). Notwithstanding the rapid westwards movement of the panzootic wave-front, reported human cases of the disease remained concentrated in East Asia in 2005 (Figure 4.17B), with Cambodia, Indonesia, and, by the end of year, China reporting their first cases (Figure 4.18C–E). Finally, trailing the panzootic wave-front, human cases of the disease were reported for the first time in countries of Europe (Azerbaijan and Turkey) and the eastern Mediterranean (Djibouti, Egypt, and Iraq) in the period January–May 2006 (Figure 4.17C).

In deciphering the evolution of cases in Figure 4.17, Smallman-Raynor and Cliff (2008) note that the spatial pattern of human cases has tracked—albeit imperfectly—the spatial pattern of poultry-based H5N1 outbreaks. Evidence of human infection due to contact with migratory waterfowl and other wild birds has been reported on only rare occasions,[16] and no human cases of avian influenza A (H5N1) have been documented in countries for which outbreaks have been limited to wild bird species. Thus, the pattern highlights the pivotal role of poultry in the pan-continental extension of human infection with H5N1.

EPIDEMIOLOGICAL FACETS

To date, confirmed human cases of avian influenza A (H5N1) have been relatively few in number, and many epidemiological aspects of the disease in

[16] The first recorded outbreak worldwide for which wild birds are the most likely source of human infection is described by Gilsdorf *et al.* (2006). The outbreak manifested in Feb.–Mar. 2006 as a cluster of seven laboratory-confirmed human cases of avian influenza A (H5N1), including six members of a single family, in the village of Daikyand, Salyan district, south-eastern Azerbaijan. The outbreak was coincident with a die-off of swans, with the human cases having been involved in the de-feathering of the dead birds.

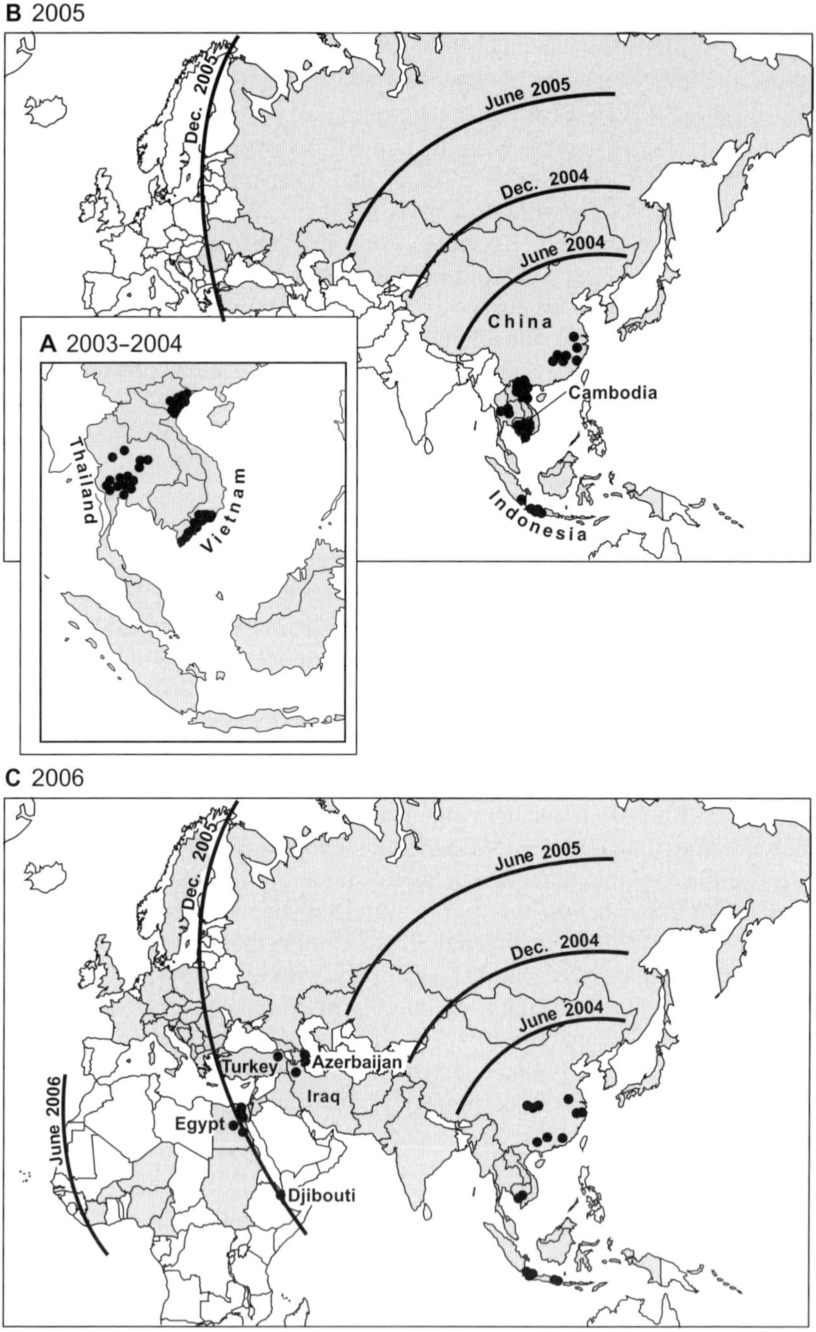

Fig. 4.17. Geographical distribution of WHO-confirmed human cases of avian influenza A (H5N1), December 2003–May 2006
Circles show the distribution of the 216 human cases reported to 18 May 2006. (A) Dec. 2003–Dec. 2004. (B) Jan.–Dec. 2005. (C) Jan.–May 2006. Countries in which avian influenza A (H5N1) had been confirmed in wild birds and/or poultry by the end of each time period are shaded. Isochrones are replotted from Fig. 4.4 and show the approximate position of the panzootic wave-front at six-monthly intervals.
Source: Redrawn from Smallman-Raynor and Cliff (2008, fig. 7, p. 568).

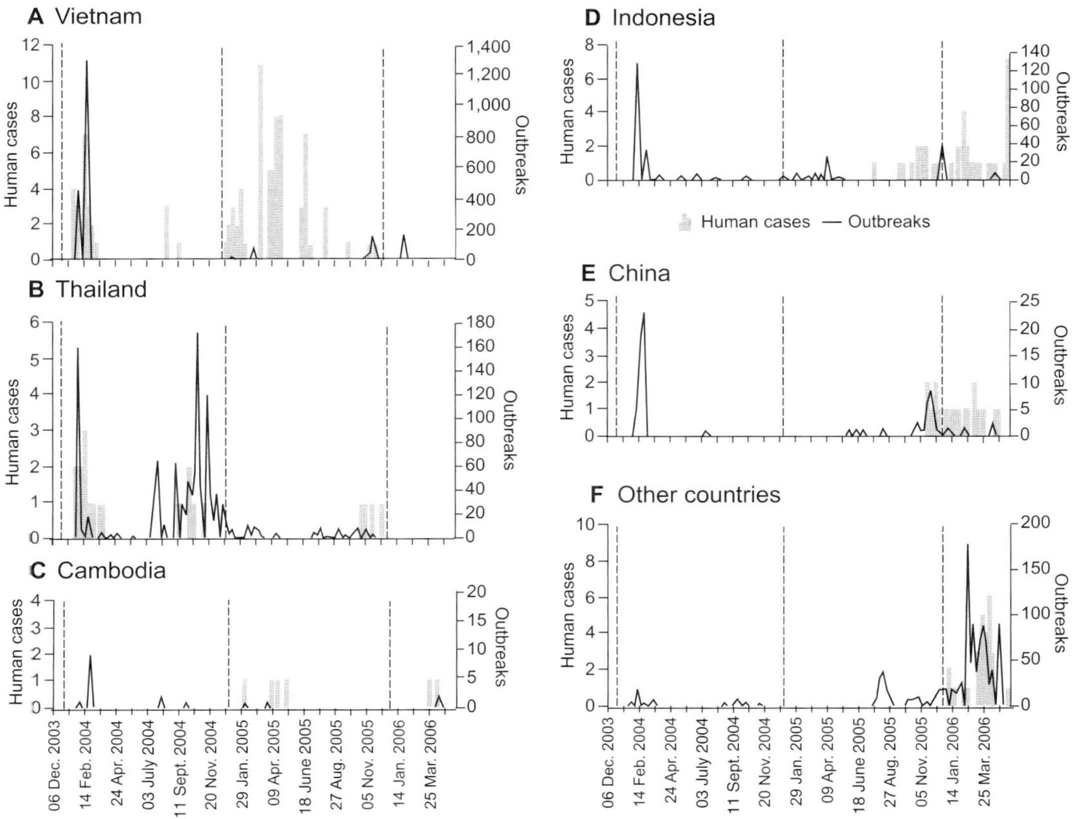

Fig. 4.18. National time series of WHO-confirmed human cases of avian influenza A (H5N1), December 2003–May 2006 The bar charts plot the number of confirmed human cases by week of report in the WHO's *Situation Updates–Avian Influenza*. Countries are ordered according to the date of first report of human cases. (A) Vietnam. (B) Thailand. (C) Cambodia. (D) Indonesia. (E) China. (F) Other countries. Counts of human cases are given by country in Table 4.4. For reference, the line traces plot the national count of confirmed outbreaks of H5N1 in wild birds and poultry by week of report in *Disease Information* (Paris: OIE).

Source: Redrawn from Smallman-Raynor and Cliff (2008, fig. 8, p. 569).

humans are still poorly understood (World Health Organization 2006*b*). In this section, we examine three prominent epidemiological facets of the disease so far identified: (i) the age bias of cases towards children and young adults; (ii) the seasonal bias of cases towards the winter and spring months; and (iii) the occurrence of cases in family clusters.

(i) Age Distribution

One noteworthy epidemiological feature of WHO-confirmed human cases of avian influenza A (H5N1) is the skewed distribution towards children and young adults, with relatively few cases in older age categories (World Health Organization 2006*b*). To illustrate the phenomenon, the box-and-whisker plots in Figure 4.19 are based on a sample of 169 cases (77 males and 92 females) in Table 4.4 and show the age distribution of patients by gender (A), year of report (B), patient outcome (C), and country (D).[17] The mean age of the 169 sample cases was 19.8 years (median 18.0; range 0.3–75.0), with estimated age-specific case rates per million population of 0.15 (0–9 years), 0.15 (10–19 years), 0.13 (20–9 years), 0.08 (30–9 years), and 0.02 ($\geq$40 years).[18] The skewed age distribution is reflected in each field of Figure 4.19, with the third quartiles of the plots (Q_3, defined by the box tops) demarcating an age band (30–5 years) above which proportionally very few cases ($<$10 per cent overall) occurred.

Behavioural factors that increase the risk of H5N1 exposure in younger persons, including the engagement of children and young adults in the slaughter, de-feathering, and cooking of poultry, have been proposed by the WHO as one determinant of the skewed age distribution in Figure 4.19 (World Health Organization 2006*b*). Biological mechanisms, too, might account for the apparent selective demographic targeting of H5N1. A recent experimental study by Kash *et al.* (2006) suggests that the 1918 (H1N1) pandemic influenza virus provoked a greatly enhanced immune response, resulting in massive damage to lung tissue. The immune response was most potent in young people with healthy immune systems, giving rise to an excess mortality among those in early adulthood (Patterson 2005). A similar hyperactive immune response has been reported from studies of the pathogenesis of H5N1 in Vietnamese patients (de Jong *et al.* 2006), and again might account for the apparently higher levels of severe disease in younger subjects. Finally, we note that a biological model of geographically widespread immunity in persons born prior to 1969 (that is, $\sim$35 years prior to the onset of the currently recognized panzootic in domestic poultry) might also account for some of the demographic pattern in Figure 4.19 (Smallman-Raynor and Cliff 2007).

[17] Age-related information for an additional 47 cases in Table 4.4 could not be ascertained from published WHO sources and have been omitted from the analysis in Fig. 4.19.

[18] Case rates were derived from age-specific national population estimates for 2005 included in Population Division of the Department of Economic and Social Affairs of the United Nations Secretariat (2006).

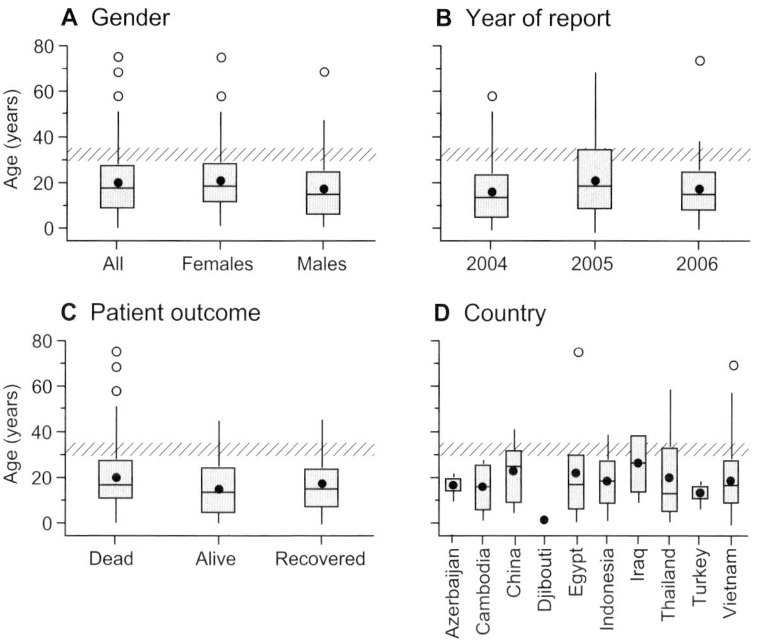

Fig. 4.19. Age distribution of confirmed human cases of avian influenza A (H5N1), December 2003–May 2006

Box-and-whisker plots show the age distribution of cases by (A) gender, (B) year of report, (C) patient outcome, and (D) country. The horizontal line and bullet mark in each box give, respectively, the median and mean age of cases. The variability in age is shown by plotting, as the outer limits of the shaded box, the first and third quartiles, Q_1 and Q_3, of the ages. Whiskers encompass all ages that satisfy the criteria $Q_1 - 1.5(Q_3 - Q_1)$ (lower limit) and $Q_3 + 1.5(Q_3 - Q_1)$ (upper limit). Points beyond the whiskers denote outliers. Information in graph C is based on the recorded status of patients according to WHO sources, with the category 'alive' formed to include patients who were last reported as hospitalized (alive) or discharged (recovered). The age category 30–5 years (shaded band) is marked on each graph for reference.

Source: Redrawn from Smallman-Raynor and Cliff (2007, unnumbered fig., p. 511).

(ii) Seasonality

A long-recognized epidemiological feature of human influenza is the marked seasonality of the disease, usually manifesting as a sharply defined peak of activity in the winter hemisphere (Glezen and Couch 1997). While the cause of this phenomenon is not fully understood, a combination of both human host- and environment-related factors is generally suspected (Cliff, Haggett, and Ord 1986). To check for a seasonal dimension to the human disease pattern, the average count of WHO-confirmed human cases of avian influenza A (H5N1) for a given calendar month (January, February, ...,

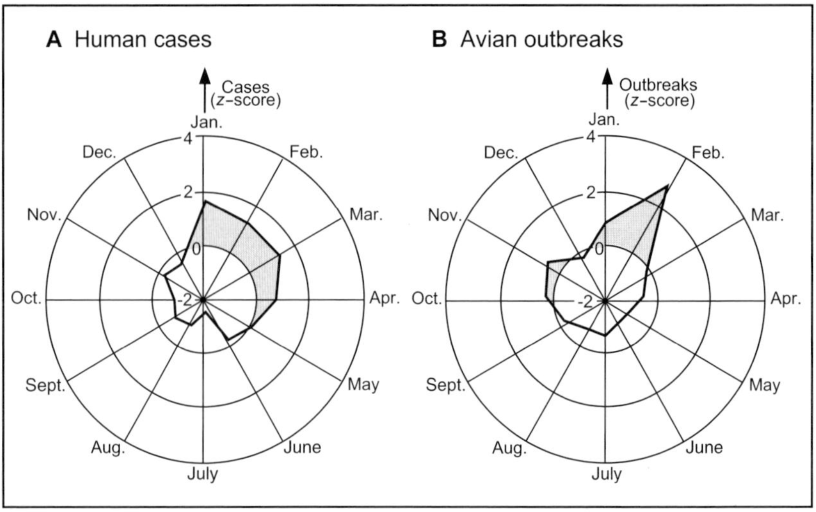

Fig. 4.20. Seasonal distribution of avian influenza A (H5N1)
Cobweb charts plot, as an average for each calendar month, the reported global occurrence of avian influenza A (H5N1), Jan. 2004–May 2006. Monthly averages are expressed in standard Normal (z-) score form. Periods with above-average levels of disease activity ($z > 0$) are shaded. (A) WHO-confirmed human cases. (B) Avian outbreaks.

Source: Redrawn from Smallman-Raynor and Cliff (2008, fig. 10, p. 571).

December) was computed over corresponding months in the period December 2003–May 2006. The average monthly count is plotted as the cobweb chart in Figure 4.20A. For reference, the corresponding average monthly count of avian outbreaks of H5N1 is plotted in Figure 4.20B. To facilitate interpretation of the cobweb charts, all monthly values are expressed in standard Normal (z-) score form, with months of above average levels of disease activity ($z > 0$) identified by the shaded sectors.

Recognizing that WHO-confirmed human cases of avian influenza A (H5N1) were restricted to the Northern Hemisphere in the period to May 2006 (Figure 4.17), Figure 4.20A shows that H5N1 follows a typical seasonal pattern for influenza, with peak levels of human activity in the winter–early spring months (January–April). The summer–autumn months (July–October), by contrast, are associated with a marked reduction in reported disease activity. As judged by Figure 4.20B, the winter–spring increase in human cases is coincident with (or presaged by) a seasonal upswing in the epizootic activity of H5N1 in autumn–winter (October–February). As most confirmed human infections have arisen through contact with infected poultry, Figure 4.20 implies the existence of some as yet undetermined seasonal environmental control (possibility related to the enhanced survival and viability of influenza A virus at lower temperatures) on H5N1 activity in birds (Li, Guan, *et al.* 2004).

(iii) Family Clusters: Local Transmission Chains

As Figure 4.5 shows, the pandemic potential of H5N1 is contingent on the development of the capacity to spread between humans in an efficient and sustained manner. In monitoring for this development, particular interest attaches to family clusters of H5N1 illness as these might provide the first indication of the viral or epidemiological change associated with enhanced person-to-person transmission. In a review of the evidence to July 2005, Olsen, Ungchusak, *et al.* (2005) identified a total of 15 family clusters of avian influenza A (H5N1) in four East Asian countries: Vietnam (11 clusters), Thailand (two clusters), Cambodia (one cluster), and Indonesia (one cluster). Clusters varied in size from two to five persons, and involved 41 (37.6 per cent) of the first 109 WHO-confirmed human cases of H5N1 infection. With the exception of one family cluster in Thailand, where limited person-to-person transmission was suspected on epidemiological grounds (Ungchusak *et al.* 2005), insufficient evidence was available to determine whether the clusters had resulted from person-to-person transmission or a common source of exposure (Olsen, Ungchusak, *et al.* 2005).

More recently, additional family clusters of H5N1 illness have been documented in Iraq (January–February 2006), Azerbaijan (March–April 2006), Egypt (April 2006), and Indonesia (April–May 2006).[19] The epidemiological associations involved in the latter cluster, formed to include members of an extended family in the north Sumatran villages of Kubu Simbelang and Kabanjahe, are shown in Figure 4.21. The cluster consisted of an initial (suspected) case and seven confirmed cases, including adult siblings and their children in four separate households. As Figure 4.21 indicates, the case cluster can be divided into three generations, with each generation representing a particular time–space association in the infection pattern.

(1) *Generation 1* (one case). The initial case in the cluster was a 37-year-old female who developed symptoms of respiratory disease on 24 April and died 10 days later on 4 May 2006. Although the patient died before H5N1 infection could be confirmed, epidemiological evidence indicates that she was exposed to sick and dying household poultry in the days preceding the onset of her illness.
(2) *Generation 2* (six cases). Between 3 and 5 May, six members of the initial case's extended family (one sister, one brother, and four children) developed symptoms of an illness that was subsequently confirmed as avian influenza A (H5N1). Epidemiological investigations revealed that, on 29 April—at a time when the initial case was severely ill and coughing heavily—a number of family members had spent the night in the same

[19] See the WHO's *Situation Updates–Avian Influenza* (Geneva: WHO) for further information.

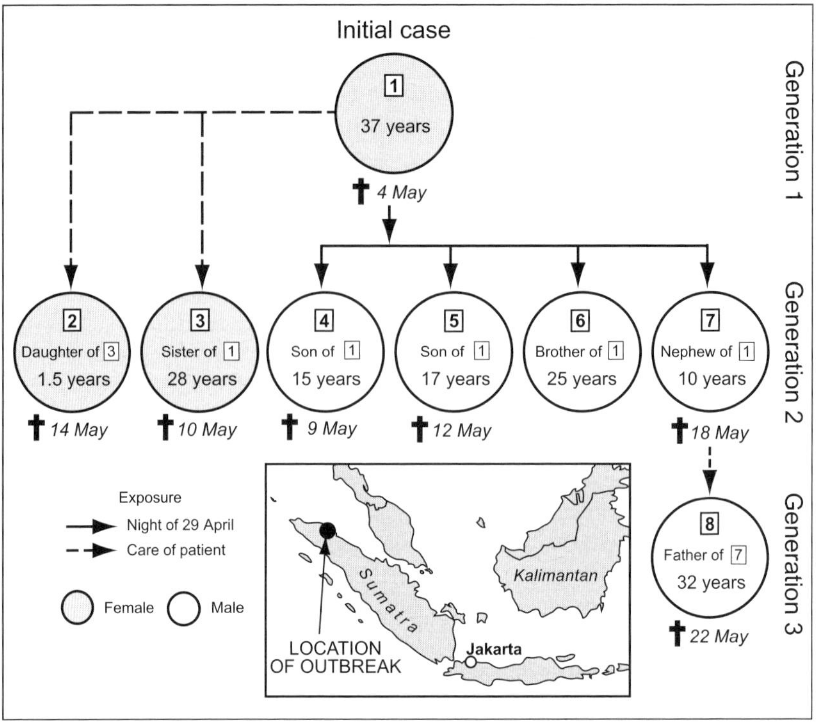

Fig. 4.21. Extended family cluster of avian influenza A (H5N1) in the villages of Kubu Simbelang and Kabanjahe, north Sumatra, Indonesia, April–May 2006 Confirmed ($n = 7$) and probable ($n = 1$) cases are represented by circles (coded 1–8). The vectors indicate inferred routes of virus exposure. The age, date of death, and relationship of cases are indicated. The inset map gives the location of the cluster.
Sources: Redrawn from Smallman-Raynor and Cliff (2008, fig. 11, p. 572), after Butler (2006*a*).

room as the index patient, while her sister had provided ongoing care. Five of the six cases in Generation 2 had died by mid-May.

(3) *Generation 3* (one case). The final case in the cluster was the 32-year-old father of a 10-year-old boy in Generation 2. The father had provided care for his son while in hospital; father and son died within four days of each other.

Virological investigations of viruses isolated from the patients in Generations 2 and 3 revealed a number of minor genetic mutations, with evidence suggestive of the person-to-person transmission chain implied by the vectors in Figure 4.21 (Butler 2006*a*). As far as the epidemiological evidence allows, the inferred chain of human transmission stopped with the death of the final case on 22 May.

CONCLUSION: PANDEMIC PREPAREDNESS AND RESPONSE

Preparations for a human pandemic of influenza, with the H5N1 virus as a likely trigger, have been identified as a global health priority by the WHO. Working in cooperation with national governments, the operations of the WHO's strategic Global Influenza Preparedness Plan are structured according to the six-phase system of pandemic alert in Figure 4.5 (World Health Organization 2005*g*). Each phase of alert is associated with a series of actions (including: sensitive surveillance for human-to-human H5N1 transmission events; the development and manufacture of vaccines; and the production and stockpiling of antiviral drugs) which seek to contain, delay, and, ultimately, to minimize the impact of a pandemic virus. As described by Ferguson *et al.* (2006), mathematical simulations of alternative pandemic mitigation strategies in economically more developed countries have highlighted the potential effectiveness of combined control measures (notably, household-based antiviral prophylaxis, along with school closure) in reducing the influenza attack rate. The same models suggest that border and/or internal travel restrictions are unlikely to prove effective in halting or substantially delaying the geographical spread of a pandemic virus (Ferguson *et al.* 2006).

4.3 Antimicrobial Resistance

4.3.1 Nature of the Problem

Antimicrobial agents (antibiotics, antivirals, and related drugs) have formed a cornerstone of the therapeutic response to infectious diseases for almost 70 years. The achievements have been dramatic, with antimicrobials—combined with wider societal improvements in sanitation and hygiene, nutrition, and immunization programmes—driving the stark decline in infectious disease morbidity and mortality in the post-1945 period. Recent developments have, however, raised questions over the continued effectiveness of antimicrobial agents. The emergence of drug-resistant strains of many micro-organisms, including those responsible for common conditions such as acute respiratory infections, diarrhoeal diseases, malaria, and tuberculosis, has rendered some 'first-line' (first-choice) drugs ineffective. Pathogen resistance to more expensive (and, sometimes, more toxic) 'second-line' and 'third-line' drugs has also been reported in some instances, while, to add to the problems, the development of new and effective antimicrobials has begun to falter in recent years. As Cohen (1992: 1055) warns, 'the post-antimicrobial era may be rapidly approaching in which infectious disease wards housing untreatable conditions will again be seen'.

MECHANISMS AND AMPLIFYING FACTORS

The biological phenomenon of antimicrobial resistance has been recognized for many decades (Figure 4.22). Although the processes involved are complex, the basic Darwinian principles are straightforward. Antimicrobial drugs exert a selective pressure that allows microbes with resistance traits to survive and flourish at the expense of their susceptible counterparts. While some microbes display an inherent resistance to antimicrobial agents, others can acquire resistance through genetic mutation or by gene transfer from one microbial subpopulation to another. Resistance genes encode a range of

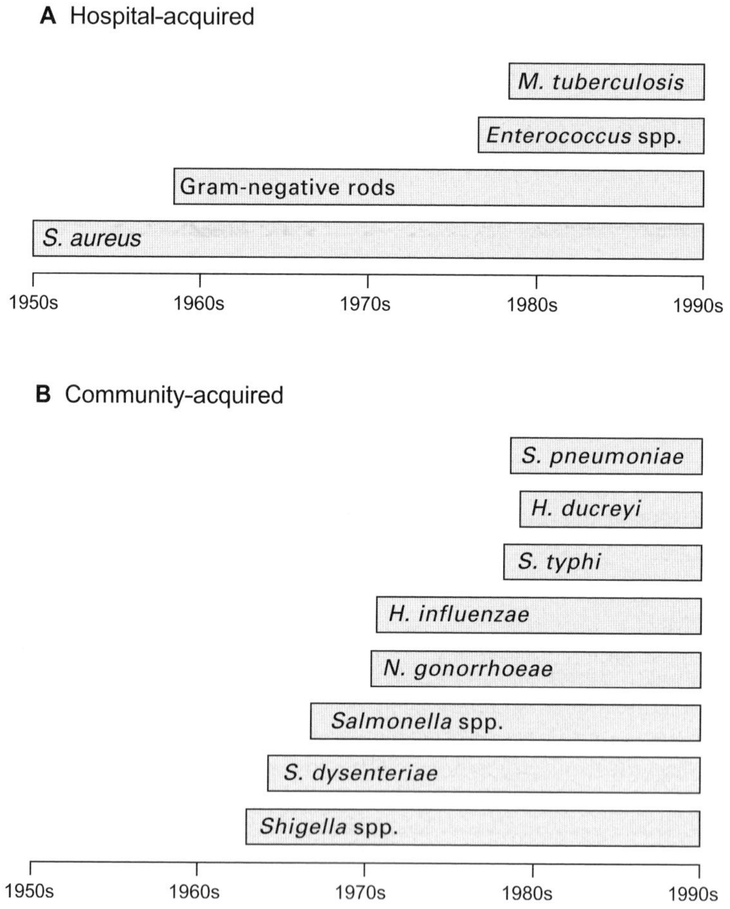

Fig. 4.22. Emergence of clinically important antimicrobial resistance in selected human pathogens, 1950s–1990s
(A) Hospital-acquired infections. (B) Community-acquired infections.
Source: Redrawn from Cohen (1992, fig. 1, p. 1051).

mechanisms that inhibit the growth-suppressing or microbicidal action of specific antimicrobial agents and, potentially, additional agents of the same and other classes (Neu 1992; World Health Organization 2001b; Amábile-Cuevas 2007).

Amplifying Factors

Factors that amplify the emergence of antimicrobial resistance in various ecosystems are reviewed by Cohen (1992), Levy (1997), O'Brien (2002), and Stokes (2002). Epidemiological studies have highlighted the use and misuse of antimicrobials as a critical factor in the selection of drug-resistant micro-organisms, with over-prescription, inappropriate prescription, and non-adherence to treatment regimens all contributing to the phenomenon. Unrestricted (over-the-counter) access and self-medication, sometimes with low-potency or counterfeit drugs, have further compounded the problem, as has the widespread use of antimicrobials in animal husbandry and agriculture. Demographic and societal changes have resulted in increased numbers of elderly, immunocompromised, and other 'at-risk' people, with a concomitant increase in the demand for antimicrobial drugs (Section 1.4.2). Hospitals and other niche environments provide reservoirs for the maintenance, development, and transmission of drug-resistant organisms, while global travel and trade networks have promoted their rapid international dissemination. As O'Brien (2002: S81) observes: 'The history of antimicrobial resistance, in examples where it can be delineated, has often been that of a successful resistance construct evolving under selection somewhere, emerging under further selection, and then spreading everywhere.'

ECOSYSTEMS: HOSPITAL- AND COMMUNITY-ACQUIRED INFECTIONS

The hospital and the community form two linked ecosystems in the emergence of antimicrobial resistance (Cohen 1992). Examples of resistance emergence in each ecosystem are given in Figure 4.22, while Table 4.5 summarizes the importance of the hospital- and community-based use and misuse of antimicrobials for resistance development in sample pathogens. We consider hospital-acquired and community-acquired infections in turn.

Hospital-Acquired (Nosocomial) Infections

The intensive use of antimicrobials, combined with the attendant risk of cross-infections, makes hospitals a fertile environment for the emergence, maintenance, and spread of drug-resistant pathogens. Specific factors involved in the development of antimicrobial resistance in healthcare settings are reviewed by Shlaes *et al.* (1997); see Table 4.6. Among the hospital-acquired infections in Figure 4.22 and Table 4.5, penicillin-resistant staphylococci were first recognized in healthcare settings in the 1950s, with the identification of resistant Gram-negative organisms (including *Escherichia* spp. and *Enterobacter* spp.), vanomycin-resistant enterococci, and

Table 4.5. Contribution of hospital and community misuse of antimicrobials in the emergence and spread of drug resistance in sample bacterial pathogens

Pathogen	Antimicrobial misuse in hospitals[1]	Antimicrobial misuse in the community[1]
Hospital-acquired infections		
Staphylococcus aureus	+++	+
Streptococci	+	–
Enterococci	+++	–
Escherchia coli	++	+
Enterobacter spp.	+++	+
Klebsiella spp.	+++	+
Pseudomonas aeruginosa	++	–
Diarrhoeal diseases		
Campylobacter spp.	–	+/–
Shigella spp.	–	++
Salmonella Typhi & *Salmonella* Paratyphi	–	++
Non-typhoidal salmonellae	–	–/+
Vibrio cholerae	–	+
Respiratory tract infections and meningitis		
Streptococcus pneumoniae	+	+++
Haemophilus influenzae	–	++
Neisseria meningitidis	–	+
Sexually transmitted infections		
Neisseria gonorrhoeae	–	+++
Haemophilus ducreyi	–	+++
Treponema pallidum	–	–
Chlamydia trachomatis	–	–
Other		
Mycobacterium tuberculosis	–	++

Note: [1] Scale ranges from low (–) to high (+++).
Source: From World Health Organization (2001*b*, tables 2–7, pp. 72–4).

Table 4.6. Factors that may increase antimicrobial resistance in hospitals

Greater severity of illness of hospital patients
More severely immunocompromised patients
Newer devices and procedures in use
Increased introduction of resistant organisms from the community
Ineffective infection control and isolation practices and compliance
Increased use of antimicrobial prophylaxis
Increased empiric polymicrobial therapy
High antimicrobial usage per geographic area per unit time

Source: Shlaes *et al.* (1997, table 4, p. 281).

multidrug-resistant (MDR) *Mycobacterium tuberculosis* in subsequent decades (Cohen 1992). To these developments can be added the establishment of epidemic methicillin-resistant *Staphylococcus aureus* (MRSA) infections (Richards and Jarvis 1999; Beović 2006) and, more recently, fluoroquinolone-resistant *Clostridium difficile* infections (Kazakova *et al.* 2006; Drudy *et al.* 2007) in a range of European and North American healthcare settings.

Community-Acquired Infections

Drug resistance in community-acquired infections arises from (i) the selective pressure of antimicrobial use in the community and (ii) the geographical transmission of drug-resistant microbes from hospitals, farms, and other ecosystems. A number of community-acquired drug-resistant pathogens, transmitted by a variety of routes, have been recognized as significant public health problems in recent decades. As Figure 4.22 and Table 4.5 show, these pathogens include *Shigella* spp. (faecal–oral), *Salmonella* spp. (foodborne), *Haemophilus ducreyi* and *Neisseria gonorrhoeae* (sexual contact), and *H. influenzae* and *Streptococcus pneumoniae* (respiratory). In addition, some infections that have commonly been associated with healthcare settings, including MRSA, have emerged as the cause of community-based outbreaks since the 1980s (Beović 2006).

HUMAN AND ECONOMIC IMPACTS

Excess morbidity and mortality are the immediate and direct human consequences of antimicrobial resistance. To these human costs must be added the increased healthcare expenditure that arises from the treatment of prolonged illness, the substitution of ineffective therapies with newer and potentially more costly treatment regimens, and the containment and control of hospital- and community-based outbreaks (Howard *et al.* 2001; McGowan 2001). In the United States, the annual costs of treating resistant infections have been placed at \$7 billion (Smith and Coast 2002) with the costs of MRSA, alone, estimated at upwards of \$830 million in 2005 (Klein *et al.* 2007). But concerns over antimicrobial resistance extend well beyond the immediate human and economic consequences of the phenomenon to include issues of national security and the political stability of countries and regions (World Health Organization 2001*b*).

4.3.2 Global Patterns of Anti-Tuberculosis Drug Resistance

Antimicrobial resistance is a problem of global proportions. The genetic changes that effect antimicrobial resistance can occur anywhere in the world and in a wide variety of settings (Smith and Coast 2002; Stokes 2002; O'Brien 2002). However, as we illustrate for one bacterial disease (tuberculosis) in this subsection, antimicrobial resistance is not evenly distributed and pronounced international variations in the prevalence of resistance in individual pathogens are evident.

BACKGROUND

Tuberculosis (*ICD*-10 A15–A19) is a potentially severe disease caused by *Mycobacterium tuberculosis*. The principal route of human-to-human transmission is via exposure to bacilli in the airborne exhalations of infected individuals. The initial infection usually goes unnoticed. Lesions at the site of lodgement of the organism commonly heal, leaving no residual changes except occasional pulmonary or tracheobronchial lymph node calcifications. Approximately 95 per cent of those initially infected enter this latent phase, from which there is a lifelong risk of reactivation. In approximately 5 per cent of cases, the initial infection progresses directly to *pulmonary tuberculosis* or, by lymphohaematogenous dissemination of bacilli, to pulmonary, miliary, meningeal, or other extra-pulmonary involvement. Serious outcome of the initial infection is more frequent in infants, adolescents, and young adults. *Extrapulmonary* tuberculosis is much less common than the pulmonary form. It can affect any organ or tissue and includes tuberculous meningitis, acute haematogenous (miliary) tuberculosis, and involvement of lymph nodes, pleura, pericardium, kidneys, bones and joints, larynx, skin, intestines, peritoneum, and eyes. *Progressive* pulmonary tuberculosis arises from exogenous reinfection or endogenous reactivation of a latent focus remaining from the initial infection. If untreated, over half the patients will die within a five-year period (Heymann 2004: 560–72).

Global Disease Patterns

Historical trends in tuberculosis activity are summarized by Cliff, Haggett, and Smallman-Raynor (2004: 56–61). We note here that, since the nineteenth century, improvements in living standards have been associated with a secular decline in tuberculosis morbidity and mortality in Europe and North America. The decline gained further momentum when effective chemotherapy was ushered in with the development of streptomycin in 1946. During the 1980s and 1990s, however, there was a resurgence of tuberculosis activity in some developed countries in which the disease was believed to be under control. This, coupled with the continued high prevalence of the disease in many developing countries, prompted the WHO to declare tuberculosis a 'global emergency' in April 1993 (World Health Organization 1994). To illustrate the international dimensions of the problem, Figure 4.23 shows the global pattern of tuberculosis notification rates per 100,000 population for 2005. The map marks out much of sub-Saharan Africa and parts of Central and South-East Asia and South America as areas with very high notification rates (≥100 cases per 100,000 population). The HIV/AIDS pandemic (Section 9.2.3) is recognized as an important factor in this distribution, with HIV prevalences of >50

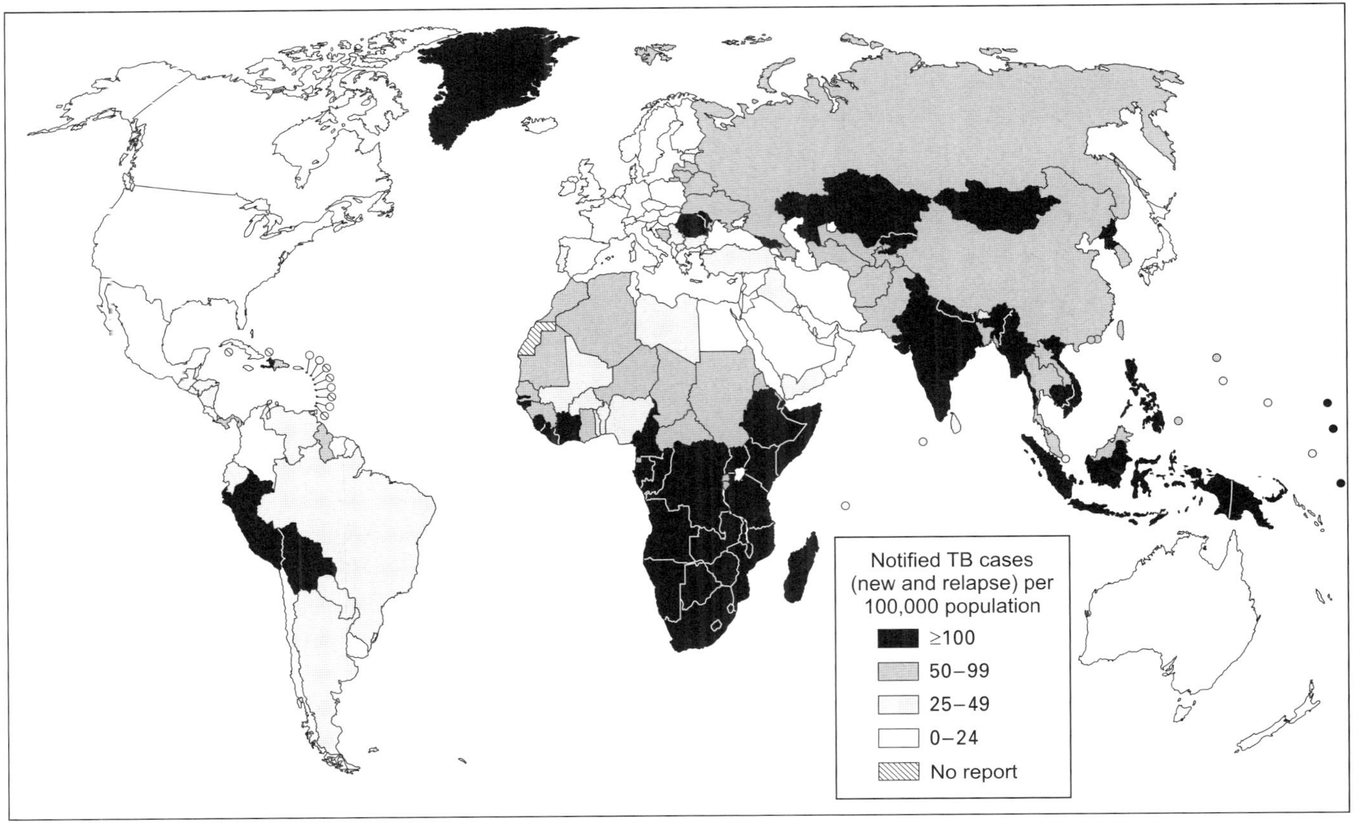

Fig. 4.23. Global pattern of tuberculosis notification rates per 100,000 population, 2005

Source: Redrawn from World Health Organization (2007*h*, fig. 1, p. 23).

per cent among new tuberculosis cases in the countries of southern Africa (World Health Organization 2007*h*).

ANTI-TUBERCULOSIS DRUG RESISTANCE

Espinal (2003) provides a historical overview of the problem of anti-tuberculosis drug resistance, while Fox *et al.* (1999) describe the ground-breaking research on the subject by the British Medical Research Council (MRC). The first recognition of drug resistance in *M. tuberculosis* was documented in MRC multi-centre trials of streptomycin in 1946–7. Subsequent MRC studies laid the foundations for a modern understanding of anti-tuberculosis drug resistance and its treatment, including the development of methods for the measurement of drug resistance, the establishment of the principle of drug combination therapy, and the initiation of fully supervised antibiotic treatment (Fox *et al.* 1999). Informed by the work of the MRC, evidence for the international extent of anti-tuberculosis drug resistance began to accrue in the 1960s. At this time, reports of the prevalence of primary resistance to at least one drug ranged between 3.0–13.0 per cent (sample developed countries) and 14.7–22.0 per cent (sample developing countries) (Espinal 2003). Such observations, however, were insufficient to halt the dismantling of national and international tuberculosis control programmes. Surveys of anti-tuberculosis drug resistance in the United States were suspended in 1985; the MRC's tuberculosis units were finally closed in 1986; while, at the global level, the number of professional staff dedicated to tuberculosis at WHO Headquarters had shrunk to two in 1989 (Raviglione and Pio 2002; Espinal 2003).

Types and Causes of Anti-Tuberculosis Drug Resistance

Two types of anti-tuberculosis drug resistance are usually recognized. *Acquired resistance* arises due to the multiplication of drug-resistant bacilli in a patient undergoing anti-tuberculosis therapy, whereas *primary resistance* arises from primary infection with drug-resistant bacilli. The nexus of factors associated with the development of anti-tuberculosis drug resistance is shown in Figure 4.24. As the World Health Organization (2004*d*: 23–4) explains, patient- and health system-related issues are especially prominent in discussions of the phenomenon:

> The emergence of drug-resistant *M. tuberculosis* has been associated with a variety of factors related to management, health providers and patients. In some countries, management factors may include the lack of a standardized therapeutic regimen, poor programme implementation, compounded by frequent or prolonged shortages of drugs, inadequate resources, political instability, or lack of political commitment. Use of anti-TB drugs of unproven quality is an additional concern, as is the sale of these medications over the counter and on the black market. Moreover, incorrect management of individual cases, difficulties in selecting the appropriate chemotherapeutic

regimen with the right dosage, and patient non-adherence to prescribed treatment also contribute to the development of drug resistance.

Among the additional factors identified in Figure 4.24, particular attention has been paid to the possible contribution of HIV infection to the development of anti-tuberculosis drug resistance. Although HIV infection is not generally recognized as an independent factor for the development of resistance (note, however, that intermittent rifamycin use in HIV-infected tuberculosis patients has been associated with the development of rifamycin resistance), high tuberculosis caseloads in areas of raised HIV prevalence might result in the increased transmission of resistant bacilli (World Health Organization 2004*d*).

Multidrug-Resistant (MDR) Tuberculosis

The term multidrug-resistant (MDR) tuberculosis refers to clinical disease arising from infection with strains of *M. tuberculosis* that are resistant to at least two first-line anti-tuberculosis drugs: isoniazid and rifampicin. Treatment of MDR tuberculosis requires the use of other drugs, including second-line drugs that may be less effective and more toxic. The phenomenon of MDR tuberculosis was first observed in the United States in the early 1990s and, as we describe below, has subsequently been recognized as a problem of global proportions (Sharma and Mohan 2006).

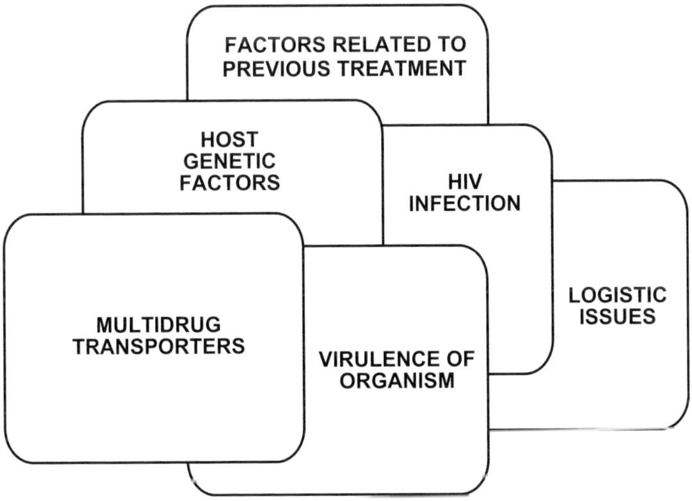

Fig. 4.24. Venn diagram showing factors that have contributed to the emergence of drug-resistant tuberculosis

Source: Based on Sharma and Mohan (2006: 262–5).

GLOBAL PATTERNS OF ANTI-TUBERCULOSIS DRUG RESISTANCE

Data Sources: The WHO/IUATLD Global Project

In early 1994, the WHO Global Programme on Tuberculosis, in association with the International Union Against TB and Lung Disease (IUATLD), established the Global Project on Anti-Tuberculosis Drug Resistance to collect and analyse standardized data on the magnitude and extent of anti-tuberculosis drug resistance worldwide (World Health Organization 1996; Espinal 2003; Zager and McNerney 2008). Since inception, the Global Project has expanded to include survey data for a global sample of 35 (*First Global Report*, 1997), 58 (*Second Global Report*, 2001), and 77 (*Third Global Report*, 2004) geographical settings.[20] In this subsection, we draw on the materials included in the *Third Global Report* (World Health Organization 2004*d*) to examine patterns of drug resistance in the four-year survey period 1999–2002. The 77 geographical settings included in the 1999–2002 survey, spanning 62 countries and including representatives from each of the six standard WHO world regions, are mapped in Figure 4.25.

Definition of resistance categories. In analysing the WHO/IUATLD data, an important distinction is drawn between:

(i) *drug resistance among new tuberculosis cases*, serving as a proxy for the measurement of levels of primary resistance. Estimates for this category are based on a total of 55,779 surveyed patients in 75 of the geographical settings in Figure 4.25;
(ii) *drug resistance among previously treated tuberculosis cases*, serving as a proxy for the measurement of levels of acquired resistance. Estimates for this category are based on a total of 8,405 surveyed patients in 66 of the geographical settings in Figure 4.25.

Two additional categories of drug resistance are defined. The term *any resistance* refers to isolates of *M. tuberculosis* that display resistance to at least one anti-tuberculosis drug, while, as defined above, the term *multidrug resistance* refers to isolates of *M. tuberculosis* that display resistance to at least isoniazid and rifampicin. Limitations of the WHO/IUATLD data are summarized in World Health Organization (2004*d*: 35–6).

Global Patterns

The box-and-whisker plots in Figure 4.26 provide a global overview of the WHO/IUATLD survey results for 1999–2002. Based on the sample evidence in Figure 4.26, the median global prevalence of anti-tuberculosis drug resistance is estimated at 10.2–18.4 per cent (any resistance; left-hand plots) and 1.1–7.0 per cent (multidrug resistance; right-hand plots). The substantially higher estimates

[20] Since this section was written, the *Fourth Global Report* of the Global Project has been published. See World Health Organization (2008*c*).

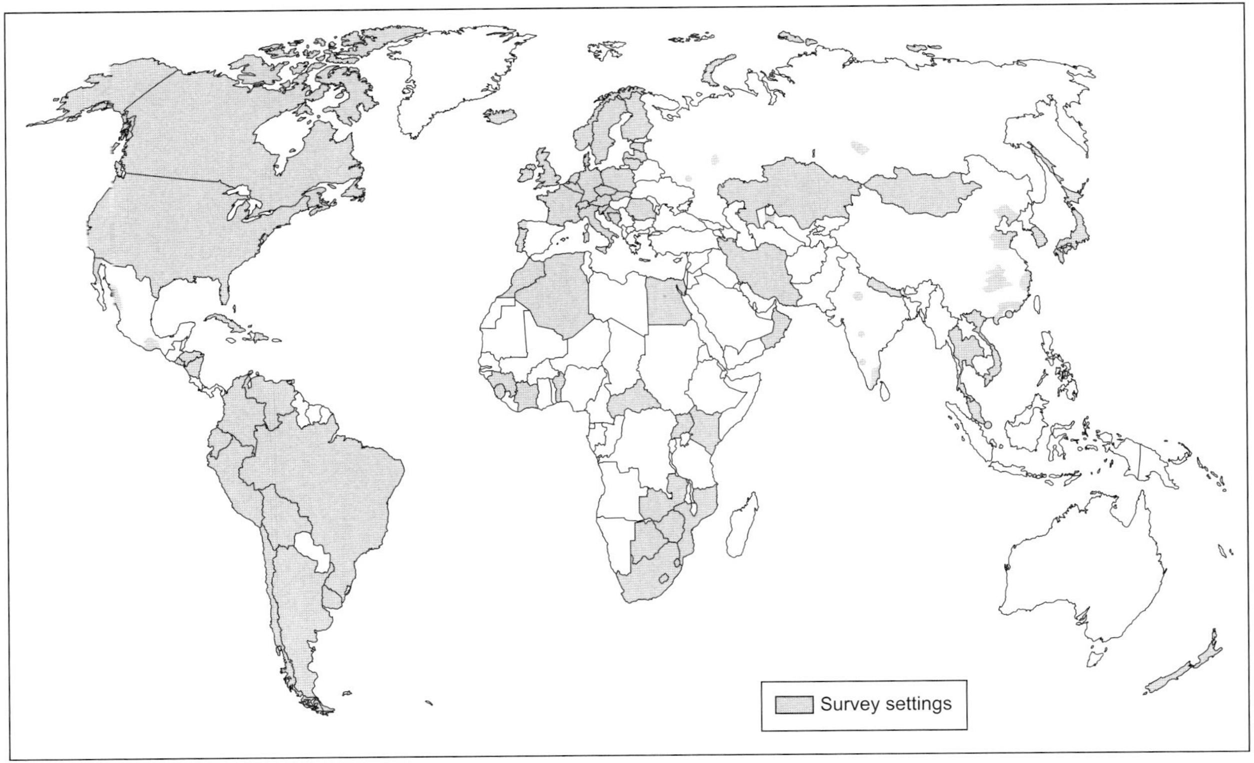

Fig. 4.25. Geographical settings surveyed by the WHO/IUATLD Global Project on Anti-Tuberculosis Drug Resistance, 1999–2002

Source: Based on Sharma and Mohan (2006: 262–5).

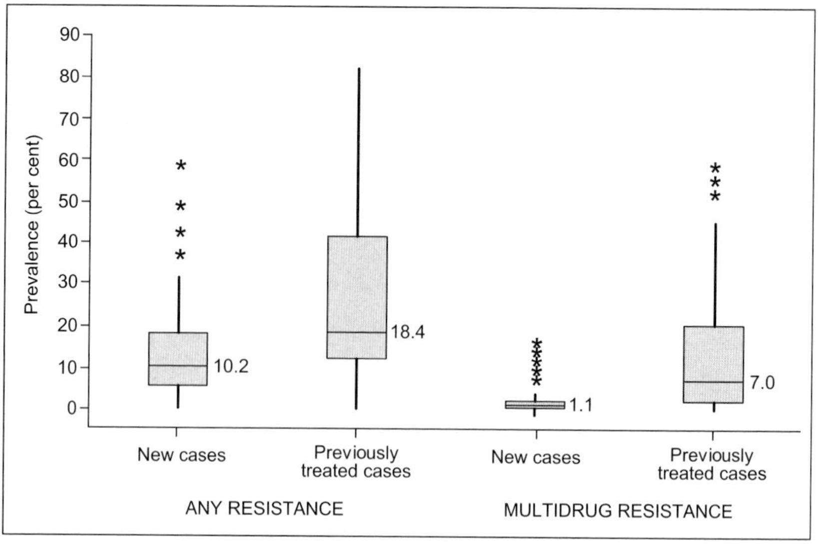

Fig. 4.26. Box-and-whisker plots of the global prevalence of drug resistance among tuberculosis cases, 1999–2002

Plots are based on information gathered by the WHO/IUATLD Global Project on Anti-Tuberculosis Drug Resistance from 77 sample locations in 62 countries worldwide (Fig. 4.25). The horizontal line in each box gives the median prevalence of any resistance (left-hand plots) and multidrug resistance (right-hand plots) among new and previously treated cases of tuberculosis; exact values of the median prevalence are given in numerical form. The variability in prevalence is shown by plotting, as the outer limits of the shaded boxes, the first and third quartiles, Q_1 and Q_3, of the prevalence scores. Whiskers encompass all prevalences that satisfy the criteria $Q_1 - 1.5(Q_3 - Q_1)$ (lower limit) and $Q_3 + 1.5(Q_3 - Q_1)$ (upper limit). Points beyond the whiskers denote outliers.

Source: Drawn from World Health Organization (2004*d*, annexes 1 and 3, pp. 96–8, 102–4).

of prevalence for previously treated cases of tuberculosis as compared with new cases implies that acquired, rather than primary, resistance was the principal driver of the global pattern of anti-tuberculosis drug resistance at the millennium.

World Regions

The box-and-whisker plots in Figure 4.27 echo Figure 4.26 and show, for each of the six standard WHO world regions, the prevalence of resistance in new (left-hand plots, A and C) and previously treated (right-hand plots, B and D) cases of tuberculosis cases. The horizontal dashed line on each plot marks the corresponding global median prevalence as depicted in Figure 4.26, while the six WHO regions are mapped in Figure 3.1. We consider the evidence for new (primary resistance) and previously treated (acquired resistance) cases in turn.

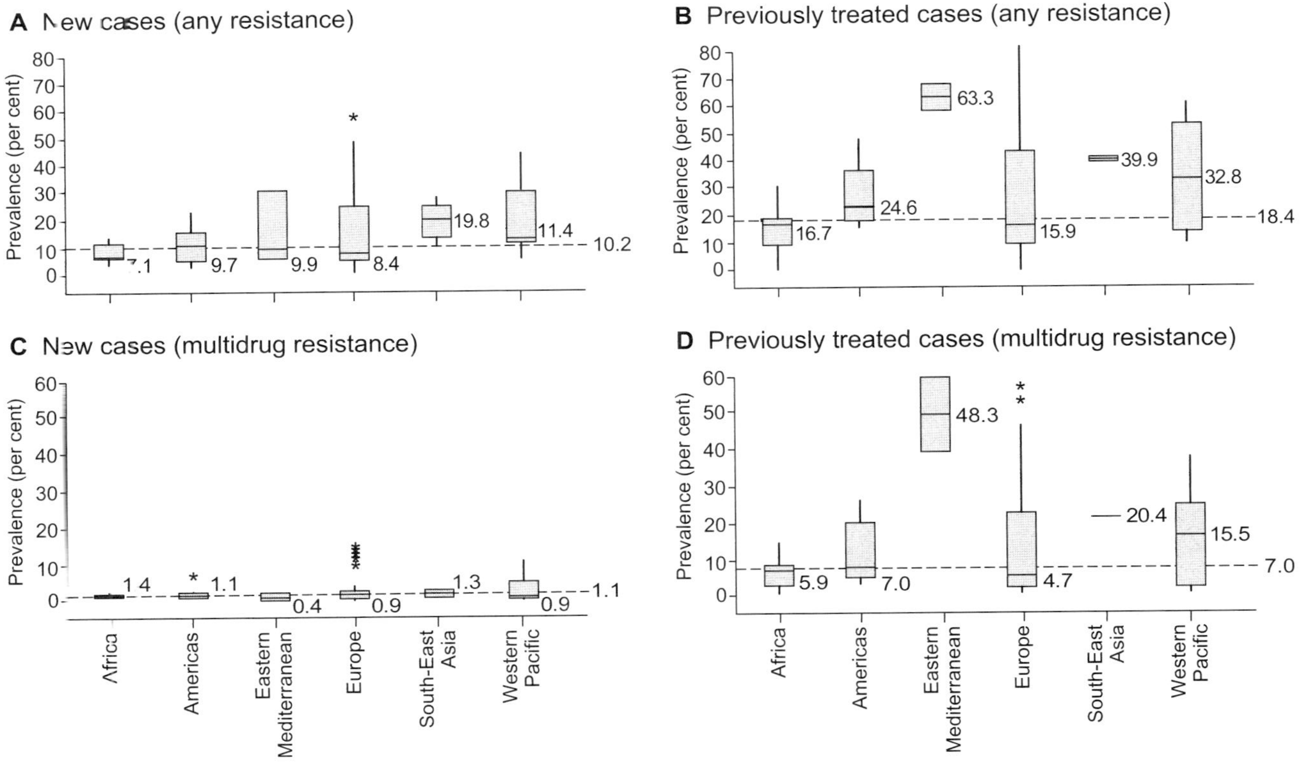

Fig. 4.27. Box-and-whisker plots of the world regional prevalence of drug resistance among tuberculosis cases, 1999–2002
Plots are based on information gathered by the WHO/IUATLD Global Project on Anti-Tuberculosis Drug Resistance for sample locations in each of the six standard WHO world regions. Upper graphs show the prevalence of any resistance among new (A) and previously treated (B) tuberculosis cases. Lower graphs show the prevalence of multidrug resistance among new (C) and previously treated (D) tuberculosis cases. The broken horizontal lines on each graph indicate the global median prevalence for each of the four categories of patient/resistance. Plotting conventions of the box-and-whisker plots are given in the caption to Fig. 4.26.

Source: Drawn from World Health Organization (2004*d*, annexes 1 and 3, pp. 96–8, 102–4).

New Cases—proxy for primary resistance (Figures 4.27A,C). As judged by the median prevalences (horizontal bars), a marked feature of Figures 4.27A and C is the geographical homogeneity of the prevalence of primary resistance as inferred from new cases of tuberculosis. In the majority of instances, the regional medians for any resistance (plot A) and multidrug resistance (plot C) are positioned close to the global medians of 10.2 per cent and 1.1 per cent respectively. One important difference between Figures 4.27A and C, however, is the substantially larger ranges (boxes) associated with any resistance (A) than multidrug resistance (C). This observation reflects a much higher degree of intra-regional variability in the any resistance category.

Previously treated cases—proxy for acquired resistance (Figures 4.27B,D). In contrast to the evidence for new cases, a striking feature of Figures 4.27B and D is the high degree of regional variation in the prevalence of acquired resistance as inferred from previously treated cases of the disease. Although the sample sizes for some regions are small and must be treated with caution, median prevalences (horizontal bars) of >30.0 per cent (any resistance; Figure 4.27B) and >15.0 per cent (multidrug resistance; Figure 4.27D) are recorded for the WHO Eastern Mediterranean, South-East Asia, and Western Pacific regions.

Inspection of Figure 4.27 reveals considerable ranges in the prevalence of resistance (boxes) in many world regions. To illustrate the phenomenon, the box-and-whisker plots in Figure 4.28 show variations in the prevalence of drug resistance in three sub-regions (denoted Central, Eastern, and Western) of the WHO Europe region. Geographical locations included in the three regions are indicated in the inset map. When examined for any resistance (Figure 4.28A) and multidrug resistance (Figure 4.28B), a striking feature of the plots is the substantially higher prevalences of resistance in the Eastern sub-region as compared with the Central and Western sub-regions. Anti-tuberculosis drug resistance in the Eastern sub-region, which includes a number of states of the former Soviet Union (Estonia, Kazakhstan, Lithuania, Latvia, Russian Federation, Turkmenistan, and Uzbekistan), is now recognized as a public health problem of potentially catastrophic proportions and remedial responses are urgently required (World Health Organization 2004*d*).

MDR Tuberculosis 'Hot Spots'

While MDR tuberculosis has been identified in every region of the world (Figure 4.27), considerable variation in prevalence rates is recognized at all geographical scales. To capture areas of high MDR activity, we follow the World Health Organization (2004*d*) in defining 'hot spots' for MDR tuberculosis as locations with prevalences of ≥3.0 per cent for multidrug resistance among new cases of tuberculosis. Hot spots identified by the WHO/IUATLD survey data in the period 1999–2002 are represented by the black circles in Figure 4.29 and include a number of Baltic (Estonia, Latvia, and Lithuania)

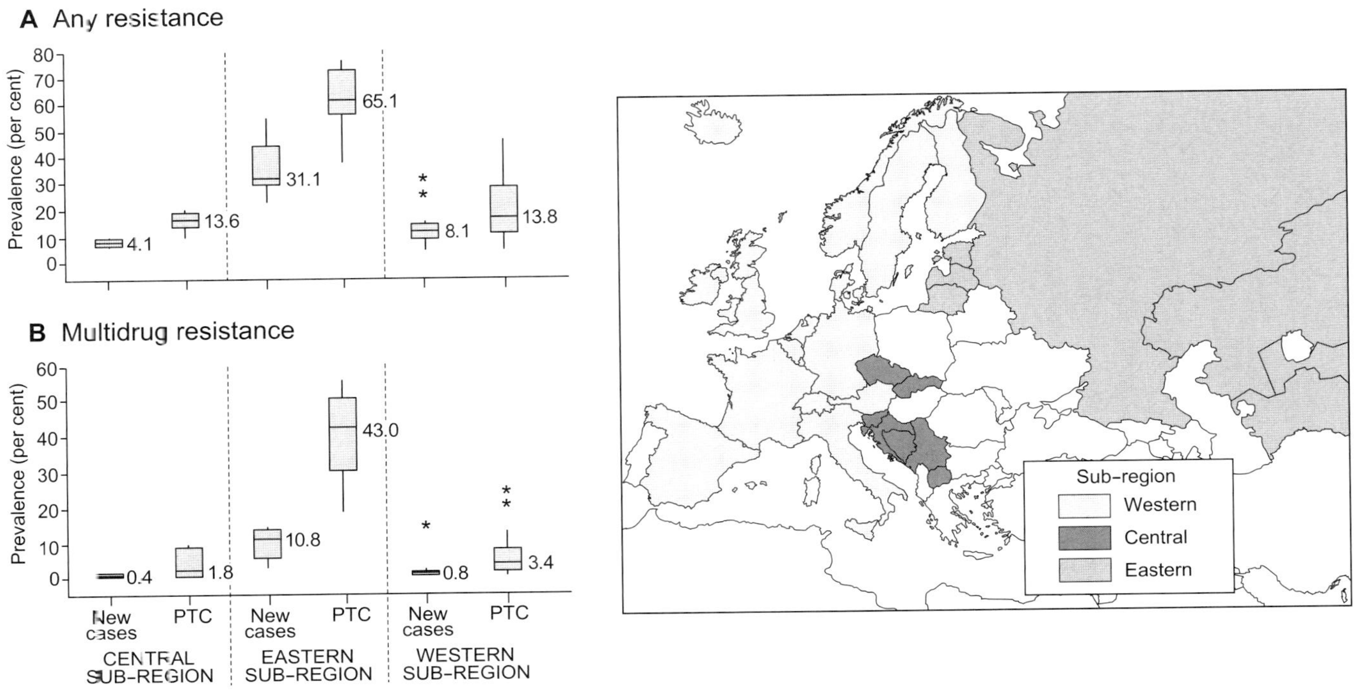

Fig. 4.28. Box-and-whisker plots of the prevalence of drug resistance among tuberculosis cases in Europe, 1999–2002
Plots are based on information gathered by the WHO/IUATLD Global Project on Anti-Tuberculosis Drug Resistance for sample locations in each of three sub-regions of the WHO European region. (A) Prevalence of any resistance among new cases and previously treated cases of tuberculosis. (B) Prevalence of multidrug resistance among new cases and previously treated cases of tuberculosis. The map identifies locations included in each of the three sub-regions. PTC = previously treated cases. Plotting conventions of the box-and-whisker plots are given in the caption to Fig. 4.26.

Source: Drawn from World Health Organization (2004*d*, annexes 1 and 3, pp. 96–8, 102–4).

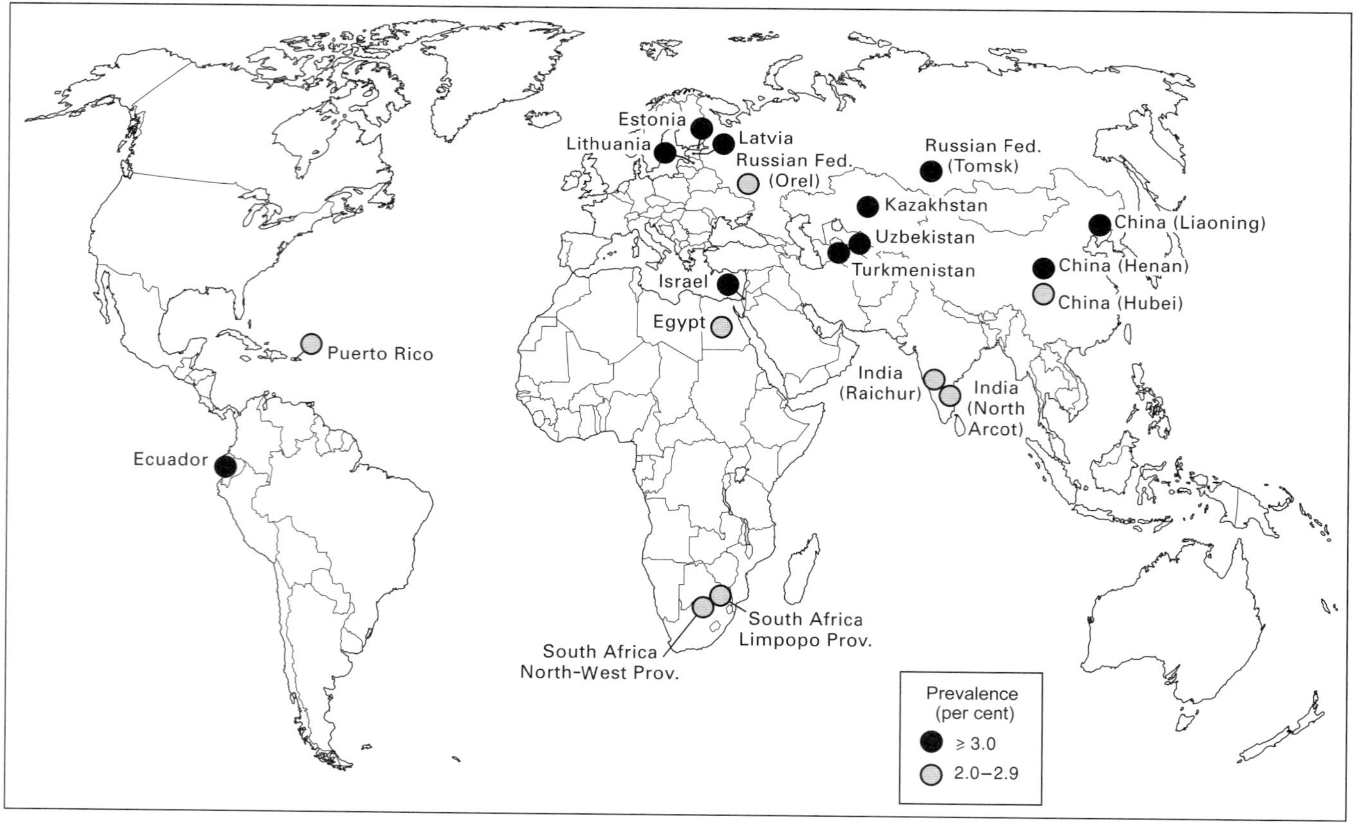

Fig. 4.29. Global hot spots of MDR tuberculosis, 1999–2002

The map is based on survey data gathered by the WHO/IUATLD Global Project on Anti-Tuberculosis Drug Resistance and plots, as the black circles, locations with ≥3.0 per cent prevalence of multidrug resistance among new cases of tuberculosis. Locations with 2.0–2.9 per cent prevalences of multidrug resistance among new cases are identified by the grey circles.

Source: Drawn from World Health Organization (2004*d*, annex 1, pp. 96–8).

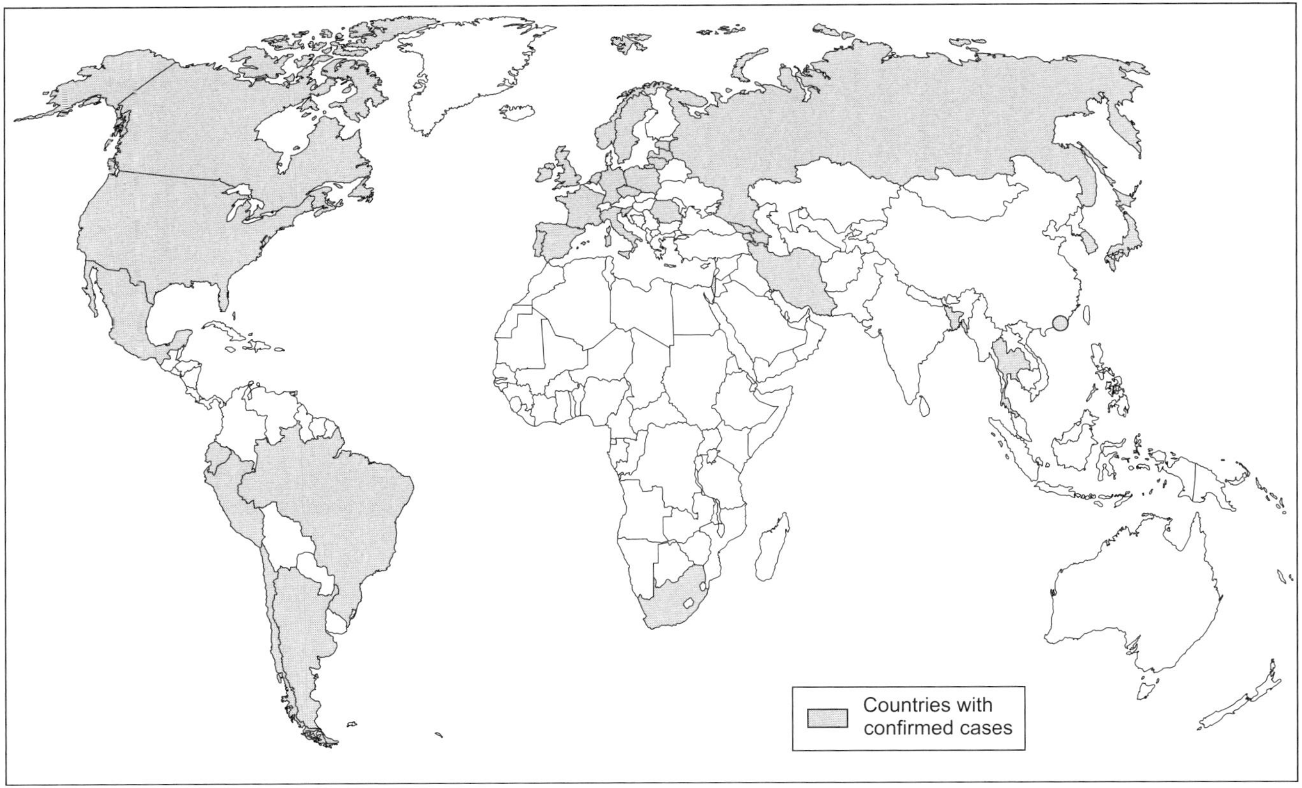

Fig. 4.30. Countries with confirmed cases of XDR tuberculosis as of 1 May 2007
Source: Redrawn from World Health Organization (2007*d*, unnumbered fig.).

and Central Asian (Kazahkstan, Turkmenistan, and Uzbekistan) states, the Russian Federation (Tomsk Oblast), China (Henan and Liaoning), Israel, and, in the Americas, Ecuador. For reference, the grey circles in Figure 4.29 identify those locations that fall just below the hot spot criterion (2.0–2.9 per cent prevalence) and identify further potential problem areas in the WHO Africa (South Africa), Eastern Mediterranean (Egypt), and South-East Asia (India) regions.

THE EMERGENCE OF XDR TUBERCULOSIS

Beginning in 2000, reports began to emerge of cases of tuberculosis that were resistant to two or more second-line anti-tuberculosis drugs—a phenomenon known as extensively drug-resistant (XDR) tuberculosis. XDR tuberculosis is formally defined as MDR tuberculosis with additional resistance to (i) any *fluoroquinolone* and (ii) at least one of three other second-line injectable drugs (amikacin, kanamycin, or capreomycin). Cases of XDR tuberculosis have been identified in multiple settings in all world regions (Figure 4.30). The further spread of untreatable disease due to XDR bacilli threatens to undermine global tuberculosis control efforts and is recognized as an urgent public health priority (Centers for Disease Control and Prevention 2006*e*).

4.4 Vector Adaptation and Insecticide Resistance

4.4.1 Nature of the Problem

In Section 1.5.1, we observed how vector-borne pathogens are over-represented among emerging species of human disease agents. While the factors involved in the emergence and re-emergence of vector-borne pathogens are complex (Gubler 1998), one technical consideration—the development of resistance to insecticides used in vector control—has underpinned the resurgence of some major insect-borne diseases, and is anticipated to have a profound impact on the future control of others (Brogdon and McAllister 1998).

NATURE OF INSECTICIDE RESISTANCE

The public health importance of vector resistance to insecticides was first recognized in the early post-war period when resistance to DDT was noted among *Musca domestica* (houseflies) and *Culex molestus* (mosquitoes) in 1946, *Pediculus humanus capitis* (head lice) and *Anopheles sacharovi* (mosquitoes) in 1951, and, soon thereafter, other species of anopheline mosquito (Shidrawi 1990). Since then, resistance to one or more classes of insecticide have been identified in all insect groups that serve as vectors of human infections.

However, vector control only becomes compromised when the prevalence of resistance becomes sufficiently high that the interruption of disease transmission is compromised. Thus, the presence of insecticide resistance is not necessarily a barrier to vector control, and insecticide resistance and vector control can coexist in a given geographical area (Brogdon and McAllister 1998).

Resistance Mechanisms

The mechanisms of insecticide resistance have a biochemical basis. Two major types of resistance are usually recognized: (1) *target-site resistance*, arising when the insecticide is no longer able to bind to its target; and (2) *detoxification enzyme-based resistance*, arising when the insecticide is prevented from reaching its site of action. As Brogdon and McAllister (1998: 608) observe, 'Innumerable genetic, biologic, and operational factors influence the development of insecticide resistance' and each manifestation of resistance is potentially unique. Geographically, resistance in a particular vector species tends to be focal rather than widespread, with empirical studies demonstrating higher resistances in areas of intensive vector control—whether arising from the agricultural or public health use of insecticides (Brogdon and McAllister 1998).

Rates of Resistance Evolution

The evolution of insecticide resistance in a given vector population is dependent on a combination of factors, including the volume and frequency of insecticide application and the inherent characteristics of the species involved (Hemingway and Ranson 2000). Table 4.7 shows the results of mathematical modelling to determine the characteristic time for 'significant' (or observable) resistance to develop to two insecticides (DDT and dieldrin) in sample species of anopheline mosquito that are recognized as important or poten-

Table 4.7. Characteristic time (in years) for the development of significant resistance to DDT and dieldrin in sample species of anopheline mosquito

	Insecticide	
Mosquito	DDT	Dieldrin
Anopheles sacharovi	4–6	8
A. stephensi	7	5
A. culicifacies	8–12	—
A. annularis	3–4	—
A. sundaicus	3	1–3
A. quadrimaculatus	2–7	2–7
A. pseudopunctipennis	>20	<1

Source: Anderson and May (1991, table 22.1, p. 612).

tially important vectors of malaria parasites. Assuming the application of insecticides at a specified and constant rate, Table 4.7 yields estimates of between 2 and 7 years (*Anopheles quadrimaculatus*) and >20 years (*A. pseudopunctipennis*) for significant resistance to DDT, and between <1 year (*A. pseudopunctipennis*) and 8 years (*A. sacharovi*) for significant resistance to dieldrin. The same mathematical models indicate that resistance problems might emerge relatively suddenly, possibly after many years of insecticide application, in a vector population (Anderson and May 1991).

4.4.2 Temporal and Spatial Patterns of Vector Resistance

HISTORICAL SERIES OF VECTOR RESISTANCE, 1947–1985

Vectors of important human diseases include:

(i) mosquitoes, notably those of the *Aedes* (dengue, dengue haemorrhagic fever, and yellow fever), *Anopheles* (malaria), and *Culex* (filariasis and Japanese encephalitis) genera;
(ii) flies, including those of the *Simulium* (onchocerciasis) and *Phlebotomus* (leishmaniasis) genera; and
(iii) other arthropods, including ticks (e.g. tick-borne relapsing fever), fleas (e.g. plague), and lice (e.g. epidemic typhus fever).

For each of the three vector groups (i)–(iii), the graphs in Figure 4.31 are based on the historical records of the WHO and plot the cumulative number of arthropod species of medical and veterinary importance that were documented to have developed resistance to one or more insecticides in successive time periods, 1947–85. Taken together, graphs A–C depict a progressive rise in the cumulative number of insecticide-resistant arthropods, from 12 (1947–50) to 186 (1981–5). Mosquitoes constituted almost two-thirds of all resistant species, possibly reflecting a bias towards the screening of this insect. As for the specific insecticides to which the arthropod species in Figure 4.31 were resistant, Shidrawi (1990: 407) observes that the proportion of tests indicating resistance was highest for dieldrin (56.9 per cent), DDT (48.4 per cent), chlorphoxim (38.1 per cent), and deltamethrin (30.7 per cent).

LATE TWENTIETH-CENTURY PATTERNS: IMPACTS ON DISEASE CONTROL PROGRAMMES

Figure 4.32 is based on information assembled by the WHO Expert Committee on Vector Biology and Control (World Health Organization 1992*c*) and summarizes the known status of vector resistance to insecticides in the late twentieth century. The graphs plot, for the world and for each of the six WHO world regions, the percentage proportion of countries for which resistance had been documented in one or more species of anopheline

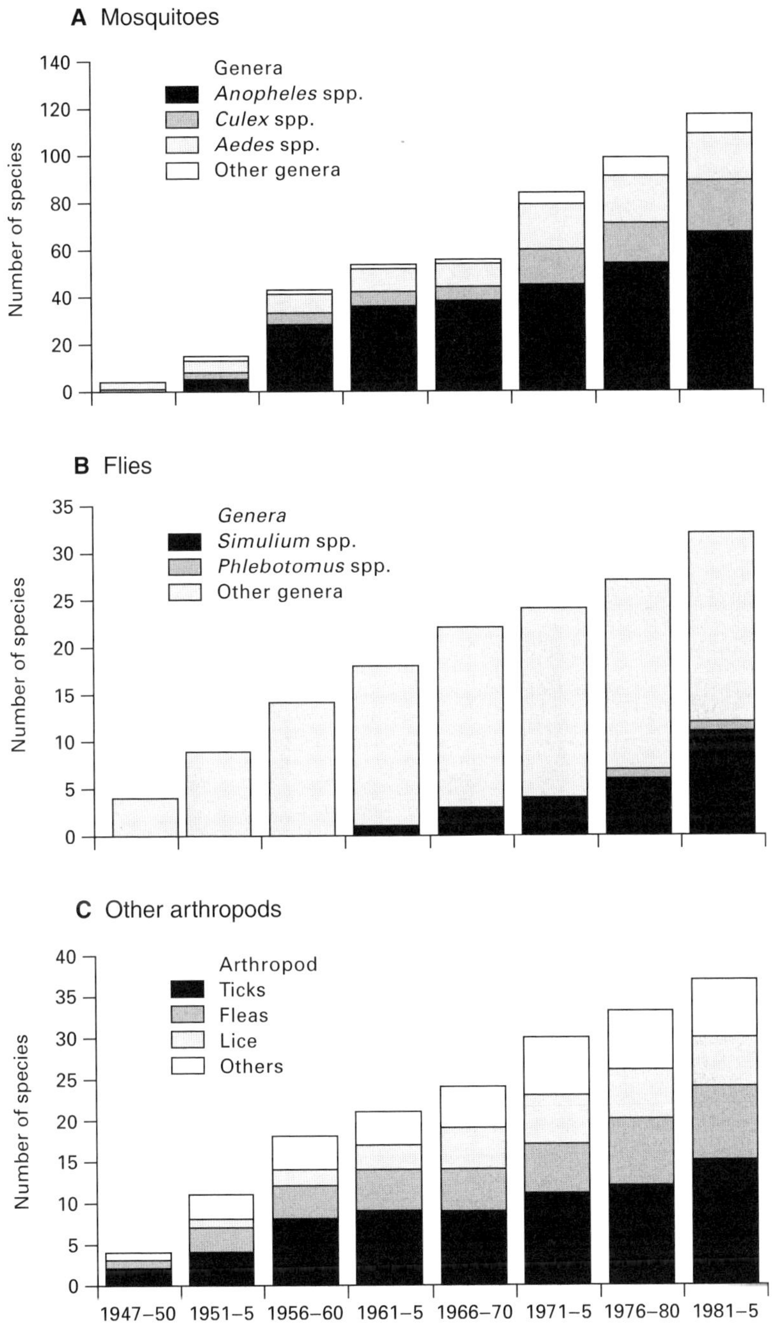

Fig. 4.31 Arthropod resistance to pesticides
Graphs plot the cumulative number of arthropod species of medical and veterinary importance identified by the WHO as resistant to one or more pesticides, 1947–85. (A) Mosquitoes. (B) Flies. (C) Other arthropods (including flea, lice, bedbug, reduviid bug, tick, and cockroach species).

Source: Drawn from Shidrawi (1990, table 2, p. 406).

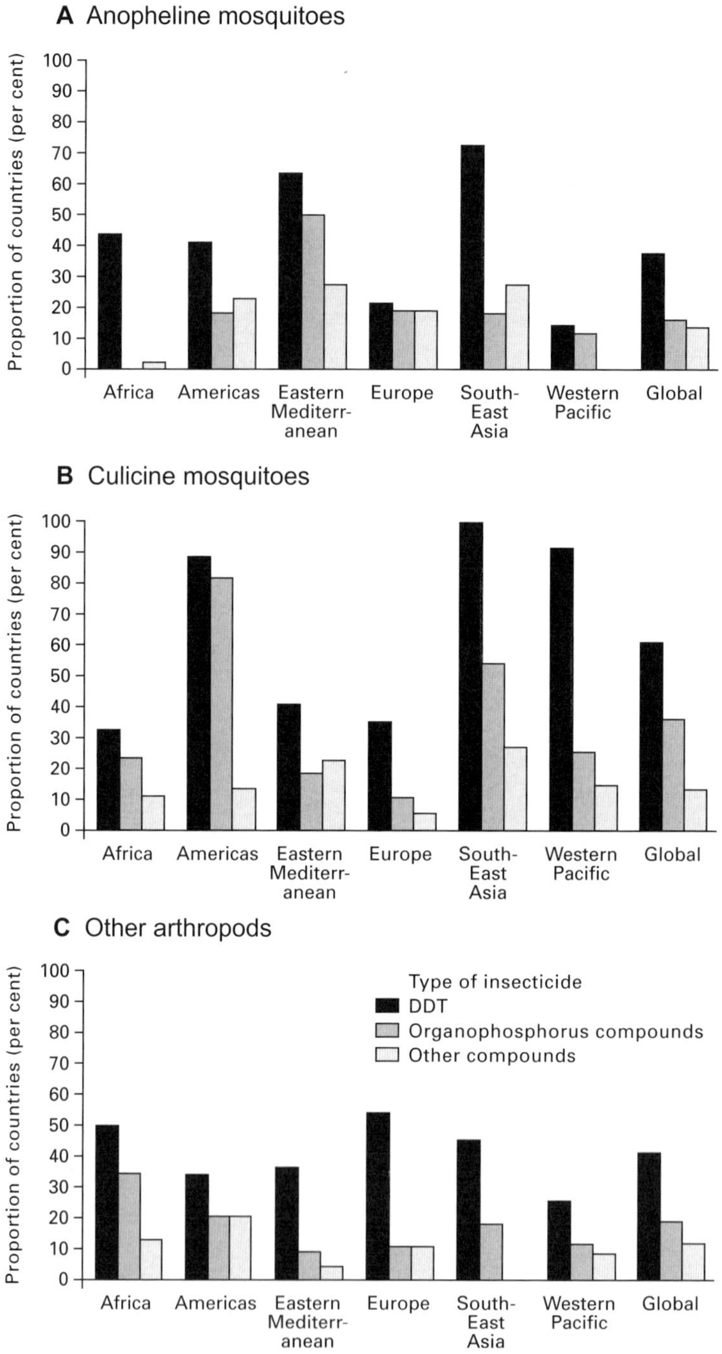
A Anopheline mosquitoes
Proportion of countries (per cent)
100
90
80
70
60
50
40
30
20
10
0
Africa
Americas
Eastern Mediterr-anean
Europe
South-East Asia
Western Pacific
Global
B Culicine mosquitoes
C Other arthropods
Type of insecticide
DDT
Organophosphorus compounds
Other compounds

mosquito (A), culicine mosquito (B), and other arthropods (C) of public health or veterinary importance. Information is shown for resistance to DDT, organophosphorus compounds, and other compounds.

While Figure 4.32 highlights the global nature of the problem of vector resistance to insecticides, pronounced variations in resistance to a given insecticide are evident between (i) regions and (ii) vectors. As Table 4.8 indicates, the impact of these resistance patterns on disease control programmes have ranged from minor (for example, trypanosomiasis in the WHO Africa region) to substantial (for example, malaria in the WHO South-East Asia region).

4.4.3 Mosquitoes, Insecticide Resistance, and the Global Malaria Eradication Campaign

The introduction of DDT revolutionized the post-war control of mosquitoes and the diseases that they carry. With the combined virtues of low cost, ready availability, and high and long-lasting potency for insects, early reports of the residual application of DDT in parts of southern Europe and the Americas demonstrated the potential for the insecticide to interrupt malaria transmission in endemic areas. Thus prompted, the Eighth World Health Assembly in Mexico City in May 1955 resolved that the WHO should spearhead a programme for the global eradication of malaria. The resolution was facilitated by mounting evidence that anopheline mosquitoes were developing resistance to DDT in parts of the world where malaria control programmes had already been implemented, and a desire to achieve worldwide eradication before insecticide resistance became general or widespread (Wright *et al.* 1972).

THE GLOBAL MALARIA ERADICATION CAMPAIGN

At the time of its launch, the Global Malaria Eradication Campaign was the largest and most ambitious public health programme ever undertaken. For a given malarious country or region, the eradication campaign consisted of four phases: (*a*) *preparatory phase*, characterized primarily by geographical reconnaissance and staff training; (*b*) *attack phase*, with

---

Fig. 4.32. Geographical distribution of resistance to insecticides in the late twentieth century Graphs plot, for the world and each of the six WHO world regions, the percentage proportion of countries for which resistance had been documented in one or more species of anopheline mosquito (A), culicine mosquito (B), and other arthropods (C) of public health or veterinary importance. Information is shown for resistance to DDT, organophosphorus compounds, and other compounds. The WHO world regions are delimited in Fig. 3.1.

Source: Drawn from World Health Organization (1992*c*, tables 1–3, pp. 3–15).

Table 4.8. Impact of insecticide resistance on the control of sample vectored diseases by WHO world region

WHO region	Disease	Vector	Comments on vector resistance
Africa	Malaria	*Anopheles* spp.	Main vectors (*A. arabiensis*, *A. gambiae* and *A. funestus*) have developed widespread resistance to some insecticides, although impact on malaria control is limited due to preferred use of drugs to limit morbidity and mortality.
	Filariasis	*Culex* spp.	Resistance to many types of insecticides reported, although no information available on impact on filariasis transmission.
	Onchocerciasis	*Simulium* spp.	Resistance to temephos has developed over much of the savannah area of the Onchocerciasis Control Programme in West Africa; temephos can no longer be used alone in the control of onchocerciasis in this region.
	Trypanosomiasis	*Glossina* spp.	No substantial resistance reported.
	Yellow fever	*Aedes aegypti*	Resistance to DDT has developed in many West African countries; organochlorine compounds are no longer used in control operations.
Americas	Malaria	*Anopheles* spp.	Main vectors (*A. albimanus*, *A. pseudopunctipennis*, *A. darlingi*, and *A. vestidipennis*) have demonstrated resistance to one or more insecticides.
	Dengue	*Aedes* spp.	Resistance to one or more insecticides documented in North, Central, and South America and the Caribbean (*A. aegypti*) and North America (*A. albopictus*), although no reported operational failures in vector control programmes.
	Chagas' disease	*Reduviidae* spp.	*Rhodnius prolixus* displays high levels of resistance to several insecticides focally in Venezuela, resulting in a switch in insecticide use.
Eastern Mediterranean	Malaria	*Anopheles* spp.	Fifteen of the 18 vector species have developed resistance to one or more groups of insecticides, including six major vectors (*A. culicifacies*, *A. stephensi*, *A. arabiensis*, *A. sacharovi*, *A. sergenti*, and *A. pharoensis*) that are resistant to organochlorines and organophosphorus compounds.

	Leishmaniasis	*Phlebotomus* spp.	Most widely distributed vector (*P. papatasi*) still susceptible to all insecticides.
	Filariasis	*Culex* spp.	The two most important vectors (*C. pipiens* and *C. quinquefasciatus*) have developed resistance to several insecticides, although impact on transmission cannot be assessed.
Europe	Malaria	*Anopheles* spp.	Broad-spectrum resistance to organophosphorus compounds and carbamates recorded in *A. sacharovi* in Turkey, prompting a switch in insecticide use.
South-East Asia	Malaria	*Anopheles* spp.	Resistance of *A. culicifacies* and *A. stephensi* to DDT and other insecticides has developed in India. High levels of resistance of *A. aconitus* to DDT have developed in Yogyakarta, Indonesia. Emergence of DDT resistance in *A. culicifacies* in the late 1960s was a major factor in the failure to control malaria in Sri Lanka.
	Dengue and dengue haemorrhagic fever	*Aedes* spp.	*A. aegypti* has developed resistance to DDT and other insecticides in most countries of the region.
	Japanese encephalitis	*Culex* spp.	Several vectors of Japanese encephalitis (*C. tritaeniorhynchus*, *C. fuscocephalus*, and *C. vishnui*) have developed resistance to DDT and other pesticides.
Western Pacific	Malaria	*Anopheles* spp.	DDT cannot be used to control *A. sinensis* by indoor residual spraying.
	Japanese encephalitis	*Culex* spp.	Resistance of *C. pipiens* and *C. tritaeniorhynchus* includes several organophosphorous compounds and some other insecticides.

Source: Based on World Health Organization (1992*c*: 17–24).

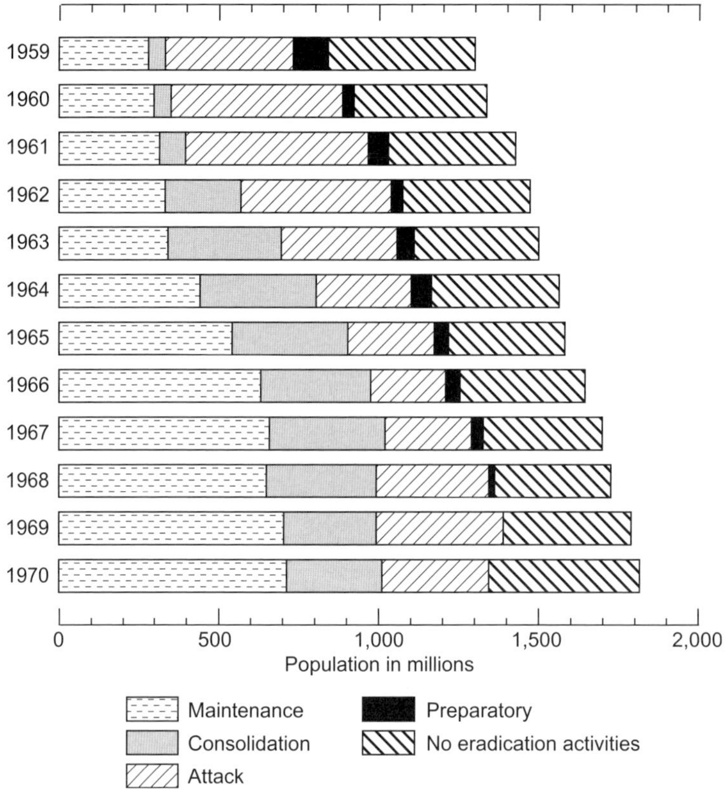

Fig. 4.33. Annual distribution of population in areas originally classified as malarious, by phase of the WHO Global Malaria Eradication Programme, 1959–1970
The category 'no eradication activities' includes countries with anti-malaria activities that were not classified as eradication operations.
Source: Redrawn from Wright *et al.* (1972, fig. 1, p. 77).

total coverage spraying of insecticides; (*c*) *consolidation phase*, during which total coverage spraying ceased and surveillance was carried out; and (*d*) *maintenance phase* from the time malaria was eradicated. The attack phase (*b*) in each country was dominated by the use of residual insecticides (DDT and, later, other insecticides) against the adult *Anopheles* mosquito. In addition, anti-larval measures such as marsh draining were used to restrict breeding grounds, while improved therapeutic and prophylactic drugs were also administered.

Progress of the Campaign

By 1959, eradication programmes had been launched in 60 of the 148 countries and territories that were classified as malarious, with a further 24 undertaking necessary preparatory work for the launch of eradication initiatives. Some indication of the subsequent progress of the eradication campaign can be gained from Figure 4.33. Between 1959 and 1970, the total population of areas classified in the maintenance phase (malaria eradicated) of the programme grew from ~280 million to ~710 million, while, in any given year, a further 500–700 million were resident in areas classified within the consolidation and attack phases (Wright *et al.* 1972). Although issues of the feasibility of eradication resulted in the exclusion of most countries of sub-Saharan Africa from the global campaign, large tracts of subtropical Asia and Latin America were all but free of infection by 1965 (Learmonth 1988; Trigg and Kondrachine 1998).

By the late 1960s, a number of technical and other obstacles to the global eradication of malaria had become apparent. These obstacles included the emergence of substantial vector resistance to DDT and other chlorinated hydrocarbons (Figure 4.31A), the development of drug-resistant strains of the malaria parasite, logistical difficulties relating to both manpower and the accessibility of areas for insecticide spraying, along with a broad array of other technical, administrative, financial, and political issues. In 1969, the Twenty-Second World Health Assembly re-examined the eradication strategy, with the conclusion that the aims of the programme should be switched from eradication to control. The effective ending of the malaria eradication initiative resulted in a considerable reduction in financial support for anti-malaria programmes, with the problems compounded by the rise in price of insecticides and anti-malaria drugs with the world economic crisis of the early 1970s (Bruce-Chwatt 1987; Trigg and Kondrachine 1998). The dramatic resurgence of malaria that accompanied these developments is illustrated for one country (India) in Figure 4.34.

Insecticide Resistance and the Failure of the Global Eradication Initiative

The overall contribution of insecticide resistance to the ultimate failure of the malaria eradication initiative cannot be readily quantified, although available evidence indicates that the resistance problem was present—to a greater or lesser extent—in all malarious regions of the world. As part of a more general attempt to assess the impact of insecticide resistance on vector control activities in the late 1960s, a WHO questionnaire survey of 114 public health authorities worldwide yielded the following insights on malaria:

> Resistance has occurred in the principal malaria vectors in many places during malaria eradication programmes. The effects have ranged from being an inconvenience to an apparently insuperable obstacle. Thus, in temperate regions, such as Europe, where malaria does not reach hyper-endemic levels, resistance has not prevented the achievement of eradication ...
>
> In warmer climates, where malaria is more fully established, there are ... areas where resistance challenges the outcome of the campaigns (e.g., the areas around the Persian Gulf, Mexico, and several countries in Central America) ...

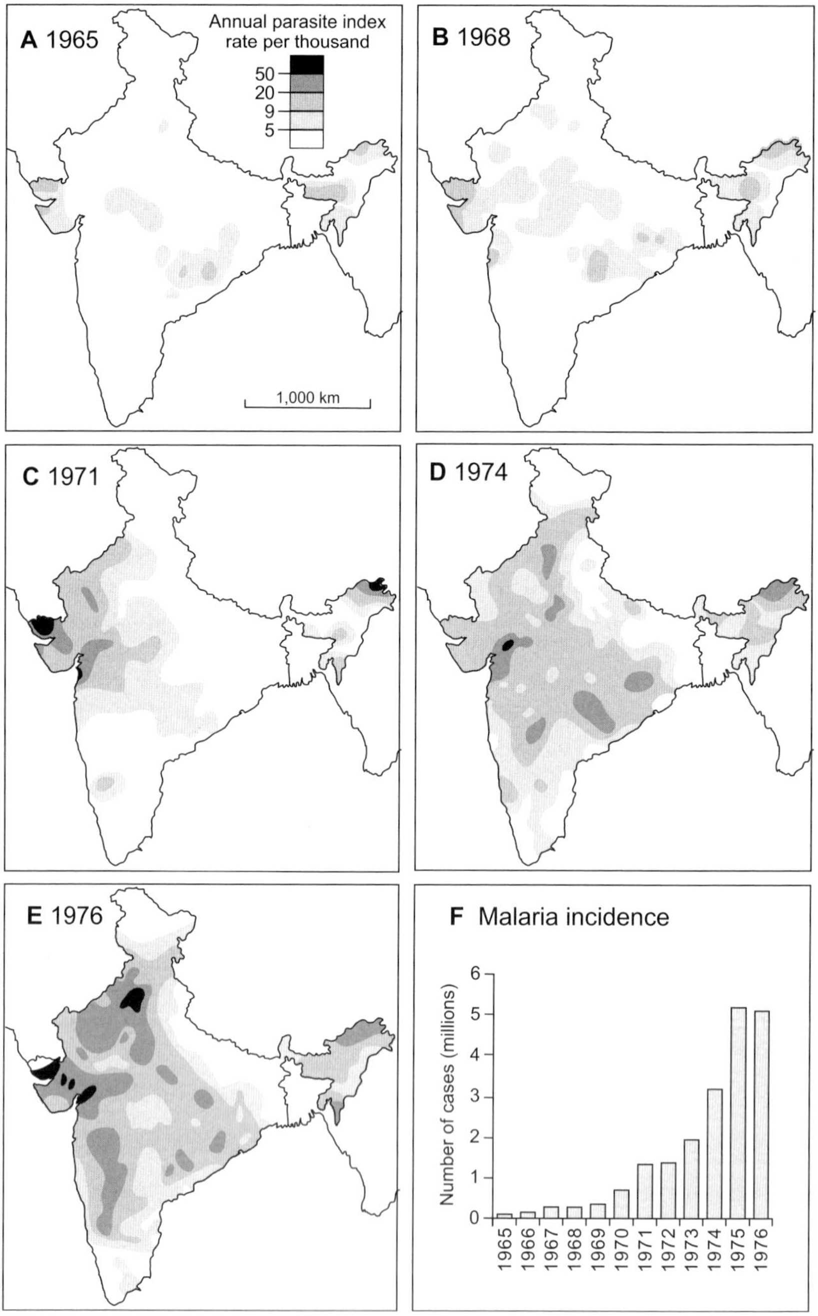
A 1965
Annual parasite index rate per thousand
50
20
9
5
1,000 km
B 1968
C 1971
D 1974
E 1976
F Malaria incidence
Number of cases (millions)
0
1
2
3
4
5
6
1965
1966
1967
1968
1969
1970
1971
1972
1973
1974
1975
1976

In the African continent, the difficulties of control and eradication are very considerable and could be attacked only by a highly effective insecticide. DDT is not completely satisfactory and the widespread dieldrin resistance in West Africa renders both this compound and HCH useless. (World Health Organization 1970*b*: 20–1)

At the time of the WHO survey, a total of 19 species of malaria vector had been found to display resistance to DDT, 28 to dieldrin and benzene hexachloride, and two to malathion and other organophosphorus insecticides. Within a restricted area of central America, one vector (*Anopheles albimanus*) was found to display resistance to all four of the insecticides, while resistance to the two main groups of chlorinated hydrocarbons (DDT group and HCH-dieldrin group) was recognized in a number of vectors in all six WHO regions (World Health Organization 1970*b*; Wright *et al.* 1972) (Figure 4.35)

4.5 Conclusion

Disease microbes are continually adapting to the challenges and opportunities afforded by their hosts and their environments, rendering them not only remarkable survivors but also genetically moving targets for the purposes of disease management and control. Few pathogens illustrate the principles of natural mutability as vividly and dramatically as influenza A virus (Fauci 2006), with periodic shifts in the antigenic structure of the virus allowing it to evade any existing immunity in the human population. As we have seen in this chapter, the WHO believes that the advent of highly pathogenic avian influenza A (H5N1) has moved the world closer to a global pandemic of human influenza than at any time since the Hong Kong pandemic of 1968–9. The immediacy of the perceived threat is underscored by the current classification of the world at Phase 3 of the WHO's operative six-phase system of pandemic alert, with H5N1 having met all the prerequisites for the onset of a human pandemic but one: the efficient and sustained person-to-person transmission

---

Fig. 4.34. The resurgence of malaria in India, 1965–1976
Maps A–E plot the annual parasite index (number of malaria cases per 1,000 population per year) by malaria control area for sample years. The annual incidence of malaria in India is plotted in graph F. From residual foci of disease activity in central, north-eastern, and western parts of India in 1965, the map sequence displays a spatial resurgence of malaria activity that, in the words of Chapin and Wasserstrom (1983: 273), constituted a 'major ecological disaster'. Widespread tolerance to organochlorines in some important malaria vectors has been identified as one of the factors that contributed to the resurgence (Chapin and Wasserstrom 1983; Learmonth 1988; Sharma 1996).

Sources: Maps A–E drawn from Learmonth (1988, fig. 10.9, pp. 212–13); graph F drawn from data in Learmonth (1988, table 10.1, p. 210).

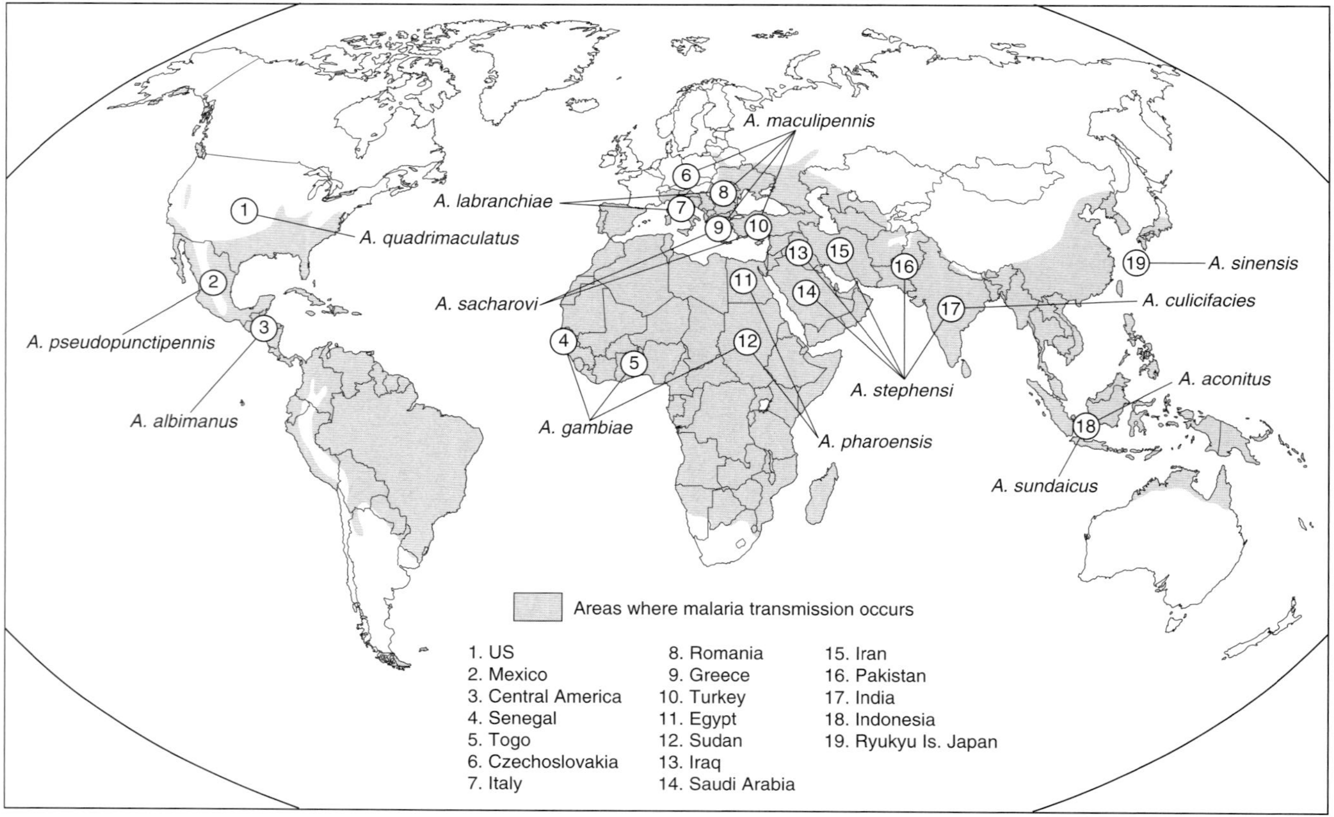

Fig. 4.35. Countries in which resistance to chlorinated hydrocarbon insecticides (DDT group and HCH-dieldrin group) had been detected in malaria vectors, *c.*1970

Countries in which vector resistance had been detected (circles) are shown against the global distribution of malaria transmission at the onset of the eradication initiative (shading). Resistant *Anopheles* spp. in a given country are named.

Source: Drawn from Wright *et al.* (1972).

of the virus. Should H5N1 acquire the ability to spread from human to human in an efficient and sustained manner, interrelated and interdependent systems of travel, trade, and commerce have the capacity to accelerate the pace, and magnify the amplitude, of any ensuing pandemic (World Health Organization 2005*c*).

The human-induced phenomenon of antimicrobial resistance has been recognized since the early clinical applications of antibiotics in the 1940s. Over the ensuing decades, the use and misuse of antimicrobial agents has resulted in the emergence of a number of pathogens that are resistant to first-line drugs and, in the high-profile instance of tuberculosis, several of the more costly and potentially more toxic second-line drugs. Within the framework of the WHO Global Strategy for Containment of Antimicrobial Resistance, current efforts to contain the global problem of drug resistance hinge on limiting both the emergence and transmission of resistance. Cornerstones of the WHO strategy include: improving access to, and the use of, appropriate antimicrobials; strengthening surveillance capacity; and promoting the development of effective new drugs and vaccines (World Health Organization 2001*b*; Smith and Coast 2002).

Insect vectors, like the microbes they transmit, are in a continuous state of evolution, responding and adapting to the human-induced pressures applied by chemicals used in their control. Vector resistance to insecticides is now widespread. It has contributed to the resurgence of some major insect-borne diseases—illustrated here by malaria. And it has the potential to have a profound impact upon the future control of others. As Brogdon and McAllister (1998) observe, surveillance lies at the heart of the effective management of insecticide resistance, with emphasis placed on (i) the collection of baseline data for programme planning and effective implementation and (ii) continuous monitoring for the timely detection of the emergence of resistance in vector species.

5

Technical Changes: Technology and Industry

5.1 Introduction

In this chapter, we examine the second of the five overlapping drivers of disease emergence and re-emergence shown in Figure II.1—*technology and industry*.

THE PROBLEM

Technological developments have yielded immeasurable benefits to society. In the field of medicine, for example, improvements in sanitation and hygiene, along with the widespread use of vaccines and antimicrobial drugs, have served to control and prevent the spread of infectious diseases. Likewise, improvements in intensive care, surgical techniques, cancer therapy, and therapies for other conditions have led to prolonged survival and an enhanced quality of life for many millions of people. But negative effects, too, have sometimes resulted from technological developments. Not least, such developments can provide, occasionally unwittingly, supportive environments for the proliferation and spread of pathogenic micro-organisms. Following Breiman (1996), Figure 5.1 identifies several key areas to these developments.

(i) Food Safety

The impact of technology on food production, distribution, and processing has had a substantial effect on the spread of infectious diseases, with potential contamination occurring at all stages of production and processing. The centralization of production and the increased international sourcing of foodstuffs has also had an impact on foodborne disease activity. In addition, current methods of storing foods have resulted in the emergence of foodborne pathogens; an example is provided by outbreaks of *Listeria monocytogenes*. This bacterium has been found in a variety of raw foods, such as uncooked meats and vegetables, as well as in processed foods that become contaminated after processing, such as soft cheeses and cold cuts from delicatessens, in unpasteurized (raw) milk, and in foods made from unpasteurized milk. *Listeria* thrives in refrigerated environments and, in its presence, widespread contamination of stored refrigerated food products can occur.

(ii) Plumbing and Cooling Systems

Legionnaires' disease is the paradigmatic disease associated with technological innovation, with cooling towers, evaporative condensers, whirlpools, spas, and showers providing temperatures which promote the survival and proliferation of the causative bacterium, *Legionella pneumophila*.

(iii) Municipal Water Systems

Municipal water systems are efficient conduits for the dissemination of pathogenic micro-organisms. While most water supplies in developed countries are effectively treated in municipal water treatment facilities, the treatment may occasionally be ineffective owing to faulty procedures or the development of resistance of an organism to routine procedures. In 1993, for example, an estimated 400,000 residents of Milwaukee, Wisconsin, experienced severe diarrhoea and other gastrointestinal symptoms attributed to the dissemination of *Cryptosporidium* in the water supply (MacKenzie, Hoxie, *et al.* 1994). Prior to this event, *Cryptosporidium* as a cause of human disease was believed to be limited to the immunosuppressed, children attending day-care facilities, and animal workers. It is now believed that municipal water systems may be responsible for the emergence of what is now recognized as a common gastrointestinal infection in many cities. Other disease agents, too, may be transmitted through the domestic water supply, including *Vibrio cholerae* and *Mycobacterium avium* complex.

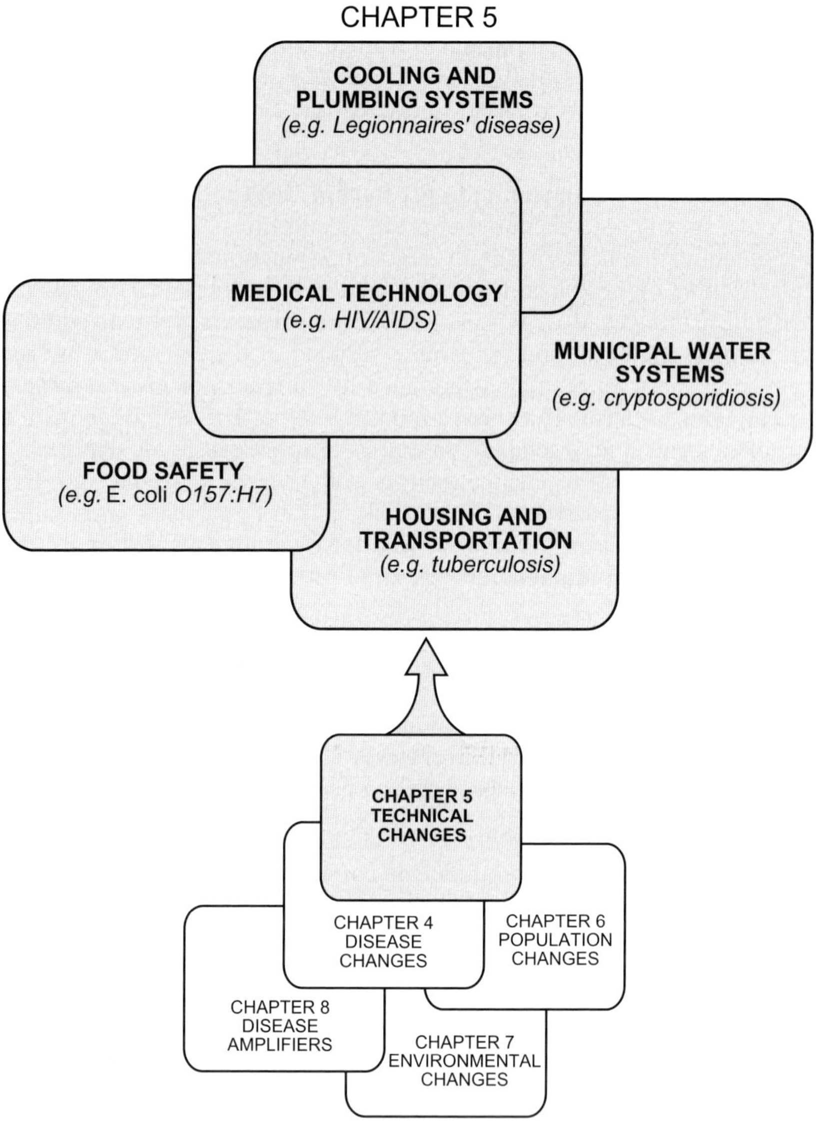

Fig. 5.1. (Upper) Venn diagram showing the facilitating factors for disease emergence and re-emergence associated with technology and industry
The lower diagram is redrawn from Fig. II.1 and shows the position of technology and industry (shaded box) within the suite of macro-factors associated with the processes of disease and emergence and re-emergence.

(iv) Housing and Transportation

Outbreaks of respiratory infections can be facilitated by overcrowding, especially where there is inadequate or faulty ventilation. Institutions such as prisons are especially prone. Such conditions provide appropriate settings for the spread of *Mycobacterium tuberculosis*, as well as many other disease agents. Both commercial aircraft and ships have come under scrutiny with regard to the on-board transmission of infectious diseases between and among crew and passengers, while aircraft particularly can transport disease vectors (e.g. mosquitoes) as well as passengers from one location to another; see Sections 6.3–6.5, later.

(v) Medical Technology

The emergence of some infectious diseases has been a side-effect of progress in medical technology. Surgical procedures, injections, and implantable devices have led to systemic or deep-tissue infections with a host of organisms (for example, *Staphylococcus epidermidis* and *Mycobacterium fortuitum/chelonae*) that historically would not have progressed beyond epidermal layers. Antimicrobial drugs have resulted in the development of drug-resistant strains of a number of infectious disease agents, while blood and blood products have been associated with the transmission of such disease agents as HIV and hepatitis B, among other pathogens.

LAYOUT OF THE CHAPTER

Given the countless ways in which technology and industry impinge on our daily lives, with corresponding windows of opportunity for infectious disease agents to emerge and spread in the human population, our approach in the present chapter is necessarily selective. We begin in Section 5.2 by examining the issue of food safety, with particular reference to the ways in which technological developments in food production, processing, and distribution have influenced the emergence and spread of a number of apparently ‘new’ foodborne illnesses such as *Escherichia coli* O157:H7 disease and variant Creutzfeldt–Jakob disease. We then turn in Section 5.3 to one of the type examples of technology-driven disease emergence: Legionnaires’ disease and its association with cooling and plumbing systems. The chapter is concluded in Section 5.4.

5.2 Food Safety and Disease Emergence

Foodborne diseases can be defined as illnesses that result from the ingestion of foodstuffs contaminated with microbial pathogens, chemical agents, or biotoxins (Snowdon *et al.* 2002). The contaminants may be inherent constituents of the food, or they may arise from inadvertent addition during the production, processing, and preparation of food products. While twentieth-century developments in sanitation and hygiene (e.g. sewage treatment, the availability of refrigeration, pasteurization, on-farm infection controls, and food industry regulations) have resulted in the retreat of familiar foodborne diseases such as typhoid fever, bovine tuberculosis, and trichinosis, as these diseases have retreated others have emerged to take their place. An example is provided by the growing incidence of non-typhoidal salmonella in the United States in the post-war period. Tauxe (1997) and Cliver (2002) discuss a number of foodborne pathogens—newly described or newly associated with food vehicles—which have emerged as major threats to public health.

5.2.1 Background to the Problem

As discussed by Motarjemi and Adams (2006), a large number of factors have contributed to the emergence of foodborne diseases in recent decades. We consider these factors under the headings of (1) changes in disease agents and disease surveillance, (2) changes in the food industry, and (3) changes in the population.

(1) CHANGES IN DISEASE AGENTS AND DISEASE SURVEILLANCE

New Foodborne Pathogens

The last half-century has witnessed a rapid expansion in the number of recognized foodborne pathogens. In the United States, for example, only a handful of disease agents (*Salmonella* Typhi and other *Salmonellae*, *Shigella* spp., and intoxications from *Clostridium botulinum* and *Staphylococcus aureus*) were implicated in the aetiology of foodborne disease in the 1950s (Cliver 2002). Several decades on, the number of microbial and chemical agents involved in reported outbreaks of foodborne disease as detected by the US Foodborne Disease Outbreak Surveillance System had increased to >15 (early 1990s) and >20 (early 2000s) (Centers for Disease Control and Prevention 1996*b*, 2006*g*). Cliver (2002) recognizes three broad categories of emerging foodborne pathogen:

(i) New agents, previously unknown to medical science. This category includes *E. coli* O157:H7, first identified in association with outbreaks of haemorrhagic colitis in 1982 and now recognized as a major cause of zoonotic foodborne illness worldwide. Other examples of recently recognized foodborne pathogens include norovirus, *Vibrio vulnificus*, and *Cyclospora cayetanensis*.

(ii) Known agents, not previously recognized as foodborne. This category includes *Campylobacter jejuni*, formerly believed to be a rare opportunistic bloodstream infection and now known to be a common cause of diarrhoeal disease.

(iii) Known agents in food, not previously recognized as pathogenic. This category includes *L. monocytogenes*, historically believed to be rarely

pathogenic for humans and now known as a potentially life-threatening bacterium. Likewise, as described in Section 5.2.5, bovine spongiform encephalopathy (BSE) was recognized in the national herd of the United Kingdom for a decade before the first cases of variant Creutzfeldt–Jakob disease (vCJD) in humans was described.

Foodborne Disease Surveillance

The increasing recognition of foodborne pathogens has been contingent on the enhanced capacity for foodborne disease surveillance in recent years (Tauxe 1997). In the United States, surveillance of foodborne pathogens via the Foodborne Disease Outbreak Surveillance System and the National Notifiable Diseases Surveillance System has been supplemented by such systems as PulseNet and FoodNet to monitor, analyse, and respond to foodborne disease events (see Section 5.2.3). As described in more detail below, enhanced surveillance and improved diagnostics have resulted in an upsurge in reported foodborne disease outbreaks since the 1980s.

(2) CHANGES IN THE FOOD INDUSTRY

Fresh Food Processing and Handling

The increased consumption of fresh produce in Western nations, with concomitant developments in produce processing and handling, has been associated with a rise in foodborne outbreaks in recent years (Beuchat and Ryu 1997; Swerdlow and Altekruse 1998). Contamination of fresh produce can occur at the pre-harvest, harvest, and post-harvest stages, as Swerdlow and Altekruse (1998: 280–1) explain:

> There are many points where produce can become contaminated during growth and harvesting, processing and washing, distribution (usually by truck), and final processing (slicing, shredding, and peeling)... The surface of plants and fruits may be contaminated by soil, manure, or feces of animals or agricultural workers... Use of unclean water supplies can lead to the contamination of produce because water is used to irrigate and wash produce and to make ice used to keep produce cool during trucking. The extra handling required to prepare salads and salad bars may increase the potential for produce to cause illness... Pathogens on the surface of produce such as melons can be transferred to the inner surface of produce during cutting and can then multiply if held at room temperature.

Centralization of Food Supply and Widening Distribution Networks

The increasing centralization of food production has played an important role in the recent emergence of foodborne diseases (Swerdlow and Altekruse 1998; Sobel *et al.* 2002). The tendency towards larger livestock holdings has been implicated in the efficient and rapid dissemination of such disease agents as *Salmonella* Enteritidis (chickens), while larger slaughter facilities and centralized processing plants have served to increase the risk of the cross-contamination of meat products with agents such as *E. coli* O157:H7 (cattle).

At the same time, widening food distribution networks have promoted the occurrence of foodborne disease outbreaks as geographically diffuse and widespread events, with 'multistate' and 'multicountry' outbreaks underscoring the transboundary nature of the public health problem (Käferstein *et al.* 1997; Tauxe 1997; Motarjemi and Adams 2006).

New Food Vehicles

A number of new food vehicles have been implicated in the transmission of foodborne disease agents in recent years, including raw and lightly cooked eggs (*Salm.* Enteritidis), beef and raw milk (*E. coli* O157:H7), shellfish (norovirus), fruit and vegetables (*Cyclospora* and *E. coli* O157:H7), and beverages such as apple cider (*E. coli* O157:H7). These newly recognized food vehicles are typically associated with contamination at a relatively early stage in the production process, they frequently lack salt, sugar, or preservatives that may limit microbial growth, and, for reasons outlined above, they include an increasing range of fresh produce (Tauxe 1997).

(3) CHANGES IN THE POPULATION

Changes in the human population that have contributed to the emergence of foodborne diseases in recent decades encompass a multiplicity of considerations relating to consumer lifestyle and behaviour, host susceptibility, and travel; see Swerdlow and Altekruse (1998) and Motarjemi and Adams (2006). The principal issues are succinctly summarized by Snowdon *et al.* (2002: 49):

> People are more mobile, which increases the probability of exposure to a pathogen [see Chapter 6] as well as the ability to carry (in the intestines) pathogens anywhere that the person goes. The population is changing: more people are living longer and their vulnerability to foodborne disease is increasing as a result of aging, AIDS, cancer, and organ transplants. Influential changes in society result in more food being consumed away from home; food service workers remain important in protecting the food supply. There are new dietary patterns, an interest in new foods, and new merging and mixing of cultures and their cuisines.

SUMMARY OBSERVATIONS

A number of common features of emerging foodborne pathogens can be identified. First, many are zoonoses and are frequently associated with asymptomatic infection in their animal hosts. Limited research suggests that the animals acquire the infections from contaminated fodder and water, indicating that issues of public health safety extend to what animals (as well as humans) eat. Second, a number of the pathogens have been associated with rapid global transmission. *Yersinia enterocolitica*, for example, spread globally among swine in the 1970s, while *Salm.* Enteritidis appeared almost simultaneously in many parts of the world in the 1980s. Third, a number of emerging foodborne pathogens, including *Salmonella* spp. in North America and *Campylobacter* in Europe, are increasingly acquiring resistance to antimicrobials. Fourth, pathogens are demonstrating an ability to survive traditional preparation techniques; *E. coli* O157:H7 can survive the gentle heating of hamburgers, *Salm.* Enteritidis can persist in omelettes, and noroviruses can survive the steaming of oysters. Fifth, contaminated food can look, smell, and taste normal, thereby eluding traditional visual inspection procedures (Tauxe 1997).

5.2.2 The Global Burden of Foodborne Disease

Estimating the global occurrence of foodborne diseases is complicated by the lack of adequate surveillance data for many countries, especially in the developing nations. In 2005 alone, 1.8 million people are reckoned to have died from diarrhoeal diseases—a large (but indeterminate) proportion arising from the consumption of contaminated food and drinking water. While some 30 per cent of the population of more economically developed countries is estimated to experience at least one foodborne illness each year, fragmentary evidence suggests that levels of foodborne disease activity may be even higher in less economically developed countries (World Health Organization 2007*e*).

WORLD REGIONAL ASSESSMENTS

Table 5.1 is taken from Motarjemi and Käferstein (1997) and presents a semi-quantitative assessment of the world regional occurrence of sample diseases that are known to be (or which may be) foodborne. Some bacterial (*Bacillus cereus* gastroenteritis, campylobacteriosis, *Clostridium perfringens* enteritis, salmonellosis, *Staph. aureus* intoxication), viral (hepatitis A and rotavirus gastroenteritis), and protozoal (cryptosporidiosis) diseases are geographically ubiquitous, occurring at estimated annual rates of $\geq$1 cases per 100,000 population in all world regions. Others, notably the helminthiases and certain bacterial and protozoal conditions, display more complex geographical patterns, with pronounced inter- and intra-regional variations in estimated levels of disease activity.

5.2.3 Foodborne Outbreak Patterns in the United States

MAGNITUDE OF THE PROBLEM

Foodborne diseases are estimated to account for 76 million cases of illness, 325,000 hospital admissions, and 5,000 deaths in the United States each year (Mead *et al.* 1999). While the organisms responsible for the majority of this disease burden are unknown or unidentified, Table 5.2 provides late twentieth-/early twenty-first-century estimates of the annual number of cases of illness (~13.8 million), hospital admissions (~61,000), and deaths (~1,800)

Table 5.1. Estimation of the occurrence of diseases that are or may be foodborne by WHO region[1]

Disease	WHO region[2]							
		Americas					Western Pacific	
	Africa	North	Central & South	Eastern Mediterranean	Europe	South-East Asia	Australia, New Zealand, & Japan	Other member states
Bacterial infections and toxications								
Bacillus cereus gastroenteritis	+++	++	+++	+++	++	+++	++	+++
Botulism	+	+	+	+	+	+	+	+
Brucellosis	+/++[3]	+	++	+/++[3]	– /+/++[3]	+/++[3]	+	+/++[3]
Campylobacteriosis	+++	++	+++	+++	++	+++	++	+++
Cholera	+/++[3]	– /+	+/++[3]	+	–	+	– /+	+
Clostridium perfringens enteritis	+++	++	+++	+++	++	+++	++	+++
Escherichia coli disease	+++	+	+++	+++	+/++[3]	+++	+	+++
Listeriosis	+	+	+	+	+	+	+	+
Typhoid and paratyphoid fevers	++	+	++	++	+	++	+	++
Salmonellosis	+++	++	+++	+++	++/+++[3]	+++	++	+++
Shigellosis	+++	++	+++	+++	+/++[3]	+++	++	+++
Staphylococcus aureus intoxication	+++	++	+++	+++	++	+++	++	+++
Vibrio parahaemolyticus enteritis		+			+	++	+/++[3]	++
Vibrio vulnificus septicaemia		+			+/++[3]		+/++[3]	++
Yersiniosis		+			+/++[3]		+	
Viral infections								
Hepatitis A	++	++	++	++	++	++	++	++
Norovirus gastroenteritis	+	+	+	+	+	+	+	+
Rotavirus gastroenteritis	+++	++	+++	+++	++	+++	++	+++
Protozoal infections								
Amoebiasis	+++	+	+++	++/+++	+	+++	+	+++

Cryptosporidiosis	+++	++	+++	+++	++	+++	++	+++
Giardiasis	+++	++	+++	++/+++	+/++[3]	+++	++	+++
Toxoplasmosis	++	+	++	+/++	+	+/++	++	++
Helminthiases								
Ascariasis	+++	+	+++	+++	+/++[3]	+++	+/++	+++
Clonochiasis	–	–	–	–	– /++[3]	–	– /+[3]	++/+++[3]
Fascioliasis	– /++[3]	–	++/+++[3]	++	– /+++[3]	–	–	– /++
Hydatidosis	+/++[3]			+/++	+		+	
Opisthorchiasis (*O. felineus*)					– /+++[3]			
Opisthorchiasis (*O. viverrini*)						– /+++[3]		+/+++[3]
Taeniasis/cysticercosis	+/+++[3]	+	++	+	+			
Trichinellosis	+/++	+	+/++	– /+[3]	+/++[3]	+/++[3]	+/++	++
Trichuriasis	+++	+	+++	+++	+/++[3]	+++	++	++

Notes: [1] WHO regions are mapped in Figure 3.1. [2] Occurrence of diseases measured on a four-point scale (– absent; + occasional or rare, reported annual incidence of <1 case per 100,000 population; ++ frequent, reported annual incidence of 1–100 cases per 100,000 population; +++ very frequent, reported annual incidence of >100 cases per 100,000 population). [3] Major regional variations.

Source: Motarjemi and Käferstein (1997, table 1, pp. 8–9).

Table 5.2. Estimated annual number of illnesses, hospital admissions, and deaths due to known foodborne pathogens, United States[1]

Disease agent	Illnesses[2]	Hospital admissions[2]	Deaths[2]
Bacterial			
Campylobacter spp.	1,963,141 (14.2)	10,539 (17.3)	99 (5.5)
Salmonella, non-typhoidal	1,341,873 (9.7)	15,608 (25.6)	553 (30.6)
Clostridium perfringens	248,520 (1.8)	41 (0.1)	7 (0.4)
Staphylococcus food poisoning	185,060 (1.3)	1,753 (2.9)	2 (0.1)
Shigella spp.	89,648 (0.6)	1,246 (2.0)	14 (0.8)
Yersinia enterocolitica	86,731 (0.6)	1,105 (1.8)	2 (0.1)
Escherichia coli O157:H7	62,458 (0.5)	1,843 (3.0)	52 (2.9)
E. coli, enterotoxigenic	55,594 (0.4)	15 (0.0)	0 (0.0)
Streptococcus, foodborne	50,920 (0.4)	358 (0.6)	0 (0.0)
Other	91,620 (0.7)	3,959 (6.5)	568 (31.4)
Subtotal	4,175,565 (30.2)	36,466 (59.9)	1,297 (71.7)
Parasitic			
Giardia lamblia	200,000 (1.4)	500 (0.8)	1 (0.1)
Toxoplasma gondii	112,500 (0.8)	2,500 (4.1)	375 (20.7)
Cryptosporidium parvum	30,000 (0.2)	199 (0.3)	7 (0.4)
Cyclospora cayetanensis	14,638 (0.1)	15 (0.0)	0 (0.0)
Trichinella spiralis	52 (0.0)	4 (0.0)	0 (0.0)
Subtotal	357,190 (2.6)	3,219 (5.3)	383 (21.2)
Viral			
Noroviruses	9,200,000 (66.6)	20,000 (32.9)	124 (6.9)
Rotavirus	39,000 (0.3)	500 (0.8)	0 (0.0)
Astrovirus	39,000 (0.3)	125 (0.2)	0 (0.0)
Hepatitis A	4,170 (0.0)	90 (0.1)	4 (0.2)
Subtotal	9,282,170 (67.2)	21,167 (34.8)	129 (7.1)
TOTAL	13,814,924 (100.0)	60,854 (100.0)	1,809 (100.0)

Notes: [1] All estimates relate to cases and deaths arising from transmission of pathogens via food vehicles. [2] Percentage proportion of respective grand totals in parentheses.
Source: Mead *et al.* (1999, table 3, p. 611).

due to known foodborne pathogens. All estimates relate to cases and deaths arising exclusively from transmission of the organisms via food vehicles. As the table shows, most cases of illness are due to viral (67 per cent) and bacterial (30 per cent) agents, with noroviruses identified as the single most common cause of morbidity. In terms of severity, bacterial agents account for the majority of hospital admissions (60 per cent) and deaths (72 per cent), with the bacterial non-typhoidal salmonella and the parasitic *Toxoplasma gondii* as the leading causes of mortality.

Economic Costs

The Economic Research Service of the US Department of Agriculture estimates the total direct and indirect economic costs of foodborne diseases in the US at $6.9 billion per year, with the highest costs associated with non-typhoidal salmonella ($2.4 billion), *L. monocytogenes* ($2.3 billion), *Campylobacter* spp. ($1.2 billion), and *E. coli* O157:H7 ($0.7 billion). The overall estimate of $6.9

billion per year, however, is based on a small number of known pathogens and excludes the costs of morbidity and premature mortality arising from the chronic sequelae of foodborne infections (Snowdon *et al.* 2002).

SURVEILLANCE FOR FOODBORNE DISEASES IN THE UNITED STATES

The methods used for the surveillance of foodborne pathogens in the United States are outlined by Braden and Tauxe (2006). The Foodborne Disease Outbreak Surveillance System was established by Centers for Disease Control and Prevention (CDC) in 1967, with this system forming a channel for the reporting of outbreak investigations by local, state, and national public health authorities. Surveillance was enhanced in the mid-1990s by the implementation of active sentinel (FoodNet)[1] and laboratory-based (PulseNet USA)[2] networks for the detection and investigation of foodborne diseases. In addition to these dedicated systems, information on selected foodborne diseases is routinely reported to CDC through the National Notifiable Diseases Surveillance System (NNDSS), the Public Health Laboratory Information System (PHLIS), and the National Antimicrobial Resistance Monitoring System for Enteric Bacteria (NARMS-EB). The limitations of the data gathered through these various systems, including problems of outbreak recognition, case ascertainment, laboratory diagnosis, and food vehicle attribution, are summarized by Braden and Tauxe (2006) and Centers for Disease Control and Prevention (2006*g*).

FOODBORNE OUTBREAK PATTERNS, 1988–2002

For surveillance purposes, CDC defines a foodborne disease outbreak as 'the occurrence of two or more cases of a similar illness resulting from ingestion of a food in common' (Centers for Disease Control and Prevention 2006*g*: 3). To examine the pattern of outbreaks in the US, we draw on a 15-year series of outbreak reports to the Foodborne Disease Outbreak Surveillance System, 1988–2002, published in CDC's *MMWR Surveillance Summaries* (Atlanta: CDC). For the period under review, the *Surveillance Summaries* include the annual count of reported foodborne disease outbreaks by aetiology and

[1] The Foodborne Diseases Active Surveillance Network (FoodNet) was established in 1996 as a collaborative programme of CDC, the US Department of Agriculture (USDA), the Food and Drug Administration (FDA), and selected state health departments. FoodNet operates under the aegis of CDC's Emerging Infections Program (EIP) as an active sentinel site surveillance system for the monitoring of selected foodborne infections (including *Campylobacter*, *Cyclospora*, *Cryptosporidium*, *E. coli* O157, *Listeria*, *Salmonella*, *Shigella*, *Vibrio*, and *Yersinia enterocolitica*). The FoodNet partner states currently include: California, Colorado, Connecticut, Georgia, Maryland, Minnesota, New Mexico, New York, Oregon, and Tennessee.

[2] As described in Section 10.6.3, PulseNet USA was established in 1996 as a national network of state health departments, local health departments, and federal agencies (CDC, USDA, FDA) to perform molecular subtyping of foodborne disease-causing bacteria by pulsed-field gel electrophoresis (PFGE). This technique is used to distinguish strains of *E. coli* O157:H7, *Salmonella*, *Shigella*, *Listeria*, and *Campylobacter* at the DNA level.

vehicle of transmission, along with the associated number of cases and deaths. Data limitations and categories of outbreak excluded from the surveillance system are summarized by Centers for Disease Control and Prevention (2006*g*). We emphasize here that reported outbreaks represent only a small proportion of the actual number of foodborne outbreaks in the United States, and that the available data are subject to surveillance biases.

Temporal Trends

In total, 11,820 outbreaks, 291,793 cases of illness, and 189 deaths were reported to CDC's Foodborne Disease Outbreak Surveillance System in the 15-year observation period, 1988–2002. Annual trends in the recorded number of outbreaks (bar chart) and cases of illness (line trace) are depicted in Figure 5.2A. As the graph shows, a step function increase in the number of outbreak reports occurred between 1988–97 and 1998–2002, probably reflecting the implementation of enhanced surveillance in the second time interval (Centers for Disease Control and Prevention 2006*g*). While some two-thirds of all outbreaks were of unknown aetiology, and these accounted for most of the increase in the period 1988–2002, specific features relating to events associated with bacterial and viral agents are evident.

Bacterial agents. For the events associated with known foodborne pathogens in Figure 5.2A, bacterial agents accounted for 65.1 per cent of all outbreaks, 73.3 per cent of all cases, and 90.5 per cent of all deaths. Figure 5.2B has been formed in the manner of Figure 5.2A and plots, by year, the number of outbreaks associated with specified bacterial agents. *Salmonella* was the single most common cause of bacterial outbreaks, but there was a marked increase in events due to *Staph. aureus*, *E. coli*, and *C. perfringens* over the observation period. As the line trace shows, the annual count of cases associated with bacterial agents peaked in 1996—a reflection of the relatively large number of cases of salmonella (12,450 cases) reported in that year.

Viral agents. A prominent feature of Figure 5.2A is the increase in the number of events due to viruses, rising from 7 per cent (1988) to 42 per cent (2002) of all reported outbreaks of known aetiology over the 15-year observation period. Contributory factors in this development include the recognition of noroviruses as the most common cause of infectious gastroenteritis in the United States (cf. Section 6.3.1)—a finding contingent on the introduction of reverse transcription–polymerase chain reaction (RT–PCR) and other diagnostic techniques since the early 1990s (Widdowson, Sulka, *et al.* 2005; Centers for Disease Control and Prevention 2006*g*).

Places of Consumption, Vehicles, and Contributing Factors, 1998–2002

Of the total of 6,647 foodborne outbreaks reported to the Foodborne Disease Outbreak Surveillance System in the five-year interval of enhanced surveillance, 1998–2002, the majority were associated with the consumption

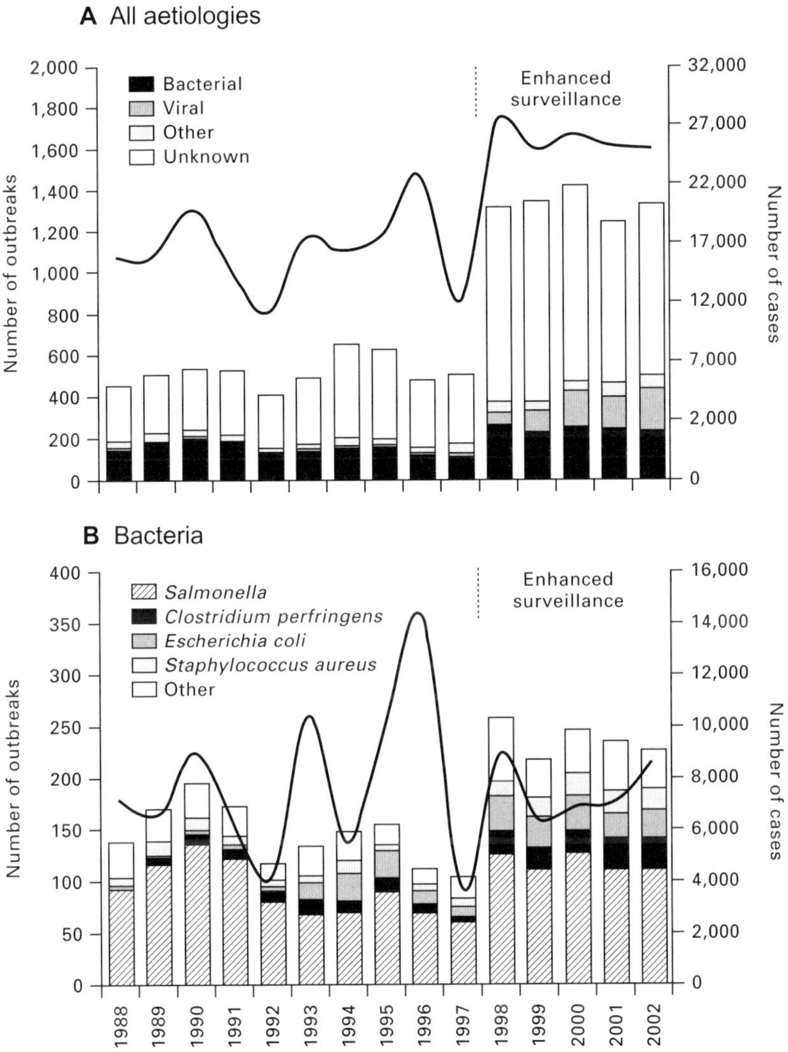

Fig. 5.2. Foodborne disease outbreaks in the United States, 1988–2002
Graphs are based on the number of foodborne disease outbreaks as recorded by CDC's Foodborne Disease Outbreak Surveillance System. Bar charts show the annual count of recorded outbreaks by aetiology. Line traces plot the associated number of documented cases of illness. (A) Outbreaks due to all aetiologies. (B) Outbreaks attributed to bacterial agents.

Sources: Drawn from Centers for Disease Control and Prevention (1996b, tables 1–5, pp. 16–20; 2000*b*, tables 2–6, pp. 12–16; 2006*g*, tables 2–6, pp. 10–14).

Table 5.3. Vehicle of transmission of sample foodborne disease outbreaks in the United States, 1998–2002[1]

Commodity category	Number of outbreaks (%)
Meats and poultry	701 (10.5)
Fish and shellfish	488 (7.3)
Vegetables	192 (2.9)
Dairy and eggs	175 (2.6)
Fruits and nuts	87 (1.3)
Grains	81 (1.2)
Oils and sugars	12 (0.2)
Unclassifiable vehicle[2]	232 (3.5)
Complex vehicle[3]	2,079 (31.3)
Unknown vehicle	2,600 (39.1)
TOTAL	6,647 (100.0)

Notes: [1] Outbreaks reported to the CDC's Foodborne Disease Outbreak Surveillance System. [2] Outbreaks associated with vehicles that cannot be categorized in a single commodity category. [3] More than one food implicated, or implicated food contains ingredients from multiple commodity categories.

Source: Centers for Disease Control and Prevention (2006*g*, tables 9–13, pp. 18–19).

of food in restaurants/delicatessens (3,334 outbreaks) and in private residences (1,297 outbreaks). Among the other places of consumption, schools (285 outbreaks), workplace cafeterias (201 outbreaks), and churches (115 outbreaks) each experienced >100 outbreaks (Centers for Disease Control and Prevention 2006*g*). The accompanying tables give summary details of the principal food vehicles (Table 5.3) and the contributory factors involved in food contamination, and pathogen proliferation and survival (Table 5.4), for outbreaks reported in the observation period.

MULTISTATE OUTBREAKS

One important feature of foodborne disease outbreaks in the United States is their increasing tendency to occur as geographically widespread (multistate) events. This development reflects a growing trend towards the centralization of food production, with many thousands of products sourced from domestic and international producers and supplied to consumers through an ever-widening distribution network (Sobel *et al.* 2002). To illustrate the phenomenon, Table 5.5 provides summary details of sample multistate outbreaks as reported in the epidemiological literature, 1988–2006. Among the largest and geographically most widespread of the events, a nationwide outbreak of *Salm.* Enteritidis associated with contaminated ice cream, resulted in an estimated 224,000 cases of illness in 1994. The outbreak is believed to have been due to the carriage of the ice cream base (premix) in tanker trailers that had previously carried non-pasteurized eggs (Hennessy *et al.* 1996). Other

Table 5.4. Factors contributing to sample foodborne disease outbreaks in the United States, 1998–2002[1]

Contributing factors	Number of outbreaks
1. Contamination factors	
Bare-handed contact by handler/worker/preparer	765
Inadequate cleaning of processing/preparation equipment/utensils	668
Handling by an infected person or carrier of pathogen	600
Cross-contamination from raw ingredient of animal origin	382
Raw product/ingredient contaminated by pathogens from animal or environment	345
Glove-handed contact by handler/worker/preparer	187
Storage in contaminated environment leads to contamination of vehicle	174
Other	635
2. Proliferation factors	
Allowing foods to remain at room or warm outdoor temperature for several hours	891
Inadequate cold-holding temperatures	568
Slow cooling	330
Insufficient time and/or temperature during hot holding	320
Preparing foods a half-day or more before serving	253
Other	181
3. Survival factors	
Insufficient time and/or temperature during initial cooking/heat processing	373
Insufficient time and/or temperature during reheating	250
Insufficient thawing, followed by insufficient cooking	33
Other	148

Note: [1] Outbreaks reported to CDC's Foodborne Disease Outbreak Surveillance System.
Source: Centers for Disease Control and Prevention (2006g, table 19, pp. 30–4).

multistate outbreaks have arisen through a variety of mechanisms including the distribution of shellfish harvested from unapproved waters (Desenclos *et al.* 1991), fresh produce exposed to faecally contaminated wash waters (Hilborn *et al.* 1999), and meat products contaminated at food processing plants (Olsen, Patrick, *et al.* 2005); see Table 5.5.

5.2.4 The Emergence of Enterohaemorrhagic E. coli *O157:H7*

The pathogenic nature of *Escherichia coli* O157:H7 was first recognized in the course of two outbreaks of a clinically distinctive gastrointestinal disease linked to the consumption of hamburgers from a fast food restaurant chain in the US states of Michigan and Oregon in 1982 (Riley *et al.* 1983). Since then, the organism has been identified as a cause of large-scale foodborne outbreaks in Canada (MacDonald *et al.* 2004), Japan (Sugiyama *et al.* 2005), the United Kingdom (Pennington Group 1997), and the United States (Rangel *et al.* 2005); sporadic cases of the illness have been documented in many other countries (Griffin and Tauxe 1991).

Table 5.5. Sample multistate outbreaks of foodborne disease in the United States, 1988–2006

Date	Disease agent	Vehicle	States involved	Cases	Deaths	Notes	Source
1988	Hepatitis A	Raw oysters	Alabama, Florida, Georgia, Hawaii, Tennessee	61	0	Contaminated oysters illegally harvested from unapproved waters	1
1992–3	*Escherichia coli* O157:H7	Hamburgers	California, Idaho, Nevada, Washington	583	3	Source unidentified	2
1994	*Salmonella* Enteritidis	Ice cream	Nationwide	224,000[1]	—	Contamination of premix in tanker that had previously transported non-pasteurized liquid eggs	3
1996	*Escherichia coli* O157:H7	Mesclun lettuce	Connecticut, Illinois	49	0	Faecally contaminated wash water	4
1997	*Escherichia coli* O157:H7	Alfalfa sprouts	Michigan, Virginia	82	0	Contaminated seeds	5
1998	*Salmonella* Agona	Toasted oats cereal	11 states	209	0	Contaminated manufacturing facility	6
1998–9	*Listeria monocytogenes*	Hot dogs	24 states	108	14[2]		7
	Salmonella Baildon	Tomatoes	Alabama, Arizona, California, Georgia, Illinois, Kansas, Tennessee, Virginia	86	0	Contamination on farm or during packing	8
1999–2000	*Salmonella* Newport	Imported mangoes	13 states	78	2	Hot-water treatment on farm	9

2000	*Shigella sonnei*	Commercially prepared dip	10 states	406	0	Contamination at dip-production facility	10
	Norovirus	Salad	13 states	333	0	Contamination of salad stuffs by handler during preparation	11
	Listeria monocytogenes	Turkey deli meat	11 states	30	4[2]	Contaminated food processing plant	12
2002	*Listeria monocytogenes*	Turkey deli meat	Connecticut, Delaware, Illinois, New Jersey, Maryland, Massachusetts, Michigan, Pennsylvania, New York	54	8[2]	Contaminated food processing plant	13
2002–3	*Salmonella* Typhimurium	Unpasteurized milk	Illinois, Indiana, Ohio, Tennessee	62	0	Local dairy/restaurant	14
2003–4	*Salmonella* Typhimurium	Ground beef	Connecticut, Maine, Massachusetts, New Hampshire, Vermont	30	0	Contaminated meat processing plant	15
2004	*Salmonella* Braenderup	Roma tomatoes	16 states	125	0	Contamination in a packing house	16
2006	*Escherichia coli* O157:H7	Fresh spinach	26 states	183	1	Faecally contaminated wash water	17
2006–7	*Salmonella* Tennessee	Peanut butter	47 states	628	0	Source of contamination unknown	18

Notes: [1] Estimated number of cases. [2] Excluding foetal deaths in pregnant patients.

Sources: (1) Desenclos *et al.* (1991); (2) Centers for Disease Control and Prevention (1993*a*); (3) Hennessy *et al.* (1996); (4) Hilborn *et al.* (1999); (5) Breuer *et al.* (2001); (6) Centers for Disease Control and Prevention (1998*b*); (7) Graves *et al.* (2005); (8) Cummings *et al.* (2001); (9) Sivapalasingam *et al.* (2003); (10) Kimura *et al.* (2004); (11) Anderson *et al.* (2001); (12) Olsen, Patrick, *et al.* (2005); (13) Gottlieb *et al.* (2006); (14) Centers for Disease Control and Prevention (2003*a*); (15) Dechet *et al.* (2006); (16) Centers for Disease Control and Prevention (2005*a*); (17) Centers for Disease Control and Prevention (2006*a*); (18) Centers for Disease Control and Prevention (2007*b*)

NATURE OF *E. COLI* O157:H7

E. coli O157:H7 is one of a large number of strains of the *E. coli* bacterium (family *Enterobacteriaceae*) that inhabit the gut of humans, warm-blooded animals, and birds. Although the O157:H7 serotype has been isolated from a wide range of wild, farmyard, and domestic animals, the main reservoirs are believed to be the rumens and intestines of cattle and other ruminants. Human infection may occur through direct contact with infected animals and their faeces, or indirectly through the consumption of contaminated meat, meat products, and other foods (including milk, cheese, and apple juice). *E. coli* O157:H7 can endure frozen storage and, although the bacterium is killed by heating, it can survive if food is not properly cooked. In addition, cross-contamination between uncooked and cooked meats can result from non-compliance with appropriate hygiene measures. Finally, human-to-human transmission via the faecal–oral route represents a potentially important source of infection, especially in day-care facilities, nursing homes, hospitals, prisons, and other institutional settings (Griffin and Boyce 1998; Slutsker *et al.* 1998; Fratamico *et al.* 2002).

The Disease in Man: Enterohaemorrhagic E. coli *(EHEC)*

E. coli O157:H7 is the principal agent of enterohaemorrhagic *E. coli* (EHEC) (*ICD*-10 A04.3), the most severe of several categories of human enteric disease caused by pathogenic strains of *E. coli*. In EHEC, a typical incubation period of 3–4 days (range 2–8 days) gives way to the onset of severe abdominal cramps and watery diarrhoea that may progress to highly haemorrhagic stools. Diarrhoea usually lasts for about four days, with vomiting seen in approximately 50 per cent of cases. Most patients make a complete recovery within 10 days of clinical onset, although a small proportion of patients (particularly young children and the elderly) may develop life-threatening complications such as haemolytic uraemic syndrome (HUS) and thrombotic thrombocytopaenic purpura (TTP). HUS is the most common cause of acute renal failure in young children, with an estimated case-fatality rate of 3–5 per cent and with chronic renal sequelae in about 50 per cent of survivors (Heymann 2004: 160–4).

The Emergence of E. coli *O157:H7*

Several lines of evidence point to the relatively recent emergence of pathogenic *E. coli* O157:H7 as a significant public health problem, as Griffin and Tauxe (1991: 60) explain:

> Infections caused by this organism are being recognized more frequently, which in part reflects increased interest in the organism and the availability of commercial reagents for detection, but also a real increase in its incidence and geographic scope. The distinctive colitis it causes appears to have been uncommon until recently; outbreaks of this disease would have attracted close scrutiny whenever they occurred, and the organism was first identified using classic microbiologic techniques. The

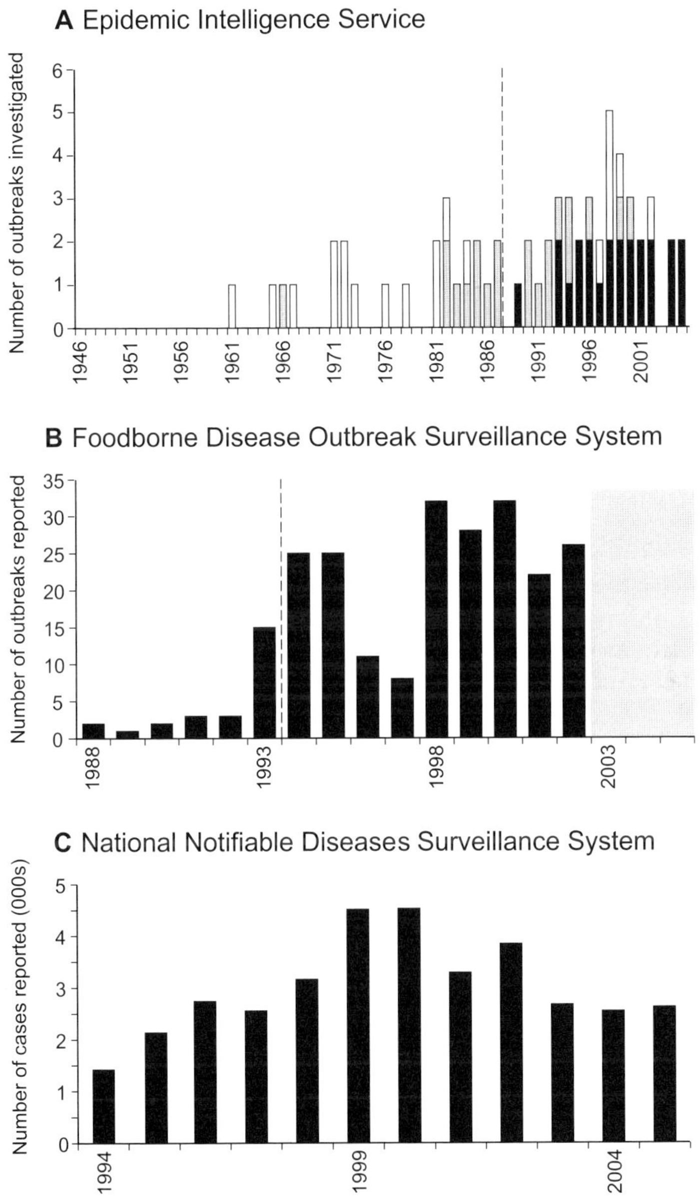

Fig. 5.3. *E. coli* surveillance in the United States

(A) Annual count of sample *E. coli* outbreak investigations by the US Epidemic Intelligence Service, 1946–2005. Investigations are coded according to whether the outbreaks were: (i) stated to be due to *E. coli* O157:H7 (black bars); (ii) of unstated aetiology but associated with clinical conditions (haemorrhagic colitis and haemolytic uraemic syndrome for which *E. coli* O157:H7 and other enterohaemorrhagic strains hemolytic uremic syndrome was first described in 1955. Thus, *E. coli* O157:H7 and the diseases it causes have only recently become common. The organism is a prototype both for the enterohemorrhagic *E. coli* group and for new and emerging bacterial pathogens in general.

As for the events involved in the evolution of the organism, evidence suggests that pathogenic *E. coli* O157:H7 may have arisen from the horizontal transfer of virulence genes between an *E. coli* O157:H7 ancestor and *Shigella dysenteriae* or a *S. dysenteriae*-like organism; see Whittam *et al.* (1998) and LeClerc *et al.* (1999).

E. COLI O157:H7 OUTBREAKS IN THE UNITED STATES

In the United States, foodborne infection with *E. coli* O157:H7 is estimated to cause upwards of 62,000 cases of illness, 1,800 hospital admissions, and 50 deaths each year (Table 5.2).[3] While most cases of infection are sporadic in nature, Rangel *et al.* (2005) document no less than 183 foodborne outbreaks of *E. coli* O157 in the two decades to 2002, including 24 multistate events of the type illustrated in Table 5.5.[4] Where ascertained, the majority of outbreaks have been linked to the consumption of ground beef (notably, hamburgers), although other products (including roast beef, lettuce, apple cider, apple juice, melons, raw milk, and other dairy products) have also been implicated (Griffin and Tauxe 1991; Rangel *et al.* 2005).

Time Series

Figure 5.3A is based on a content analysis of the report titles of US Epidemic Intelligence Service investigations (Section 3.4), and plots, for the period 1946–2005, the annual count of sample outbreaks that were (i) stated to be due to *E. coli* O157:H7 (black bars), (ii) of unstated aetiology but which were associated with clinical conditions (haemorrhagic colitis and HUS) for which

---

of *E. coli* are a recognized cause (grey bars); and (iii) stated to be due to non-O157:H7 or unspecified strains of *E. coli* (white bars). (B) Annual count of *E. coli* outbreaks as reported to CDC's Foodborne Disease Outbreak Surveillance System, 1988–2002. (C) Annual count of *E. coli* O157:H7 cases reported to the US National Notifiable Diseases Surveillance System, 1994–2005.

Sources: Graph A drawn from the records of the US Epidemic Intelligence Service; graph B drawn from Centers for Disease Control and Prevention (1996*b*, tables 1–5, pp. 16–20; 2000*b*, tables 2–6, pp. 12–16; 2006*g*, tables 2–6, pp. 10–14); graph C drawn from annual editions of the Centers for Disease Control and Prevention's *MMWR Summary of Notifiable Diseases* (Atlanta: CDC).

[3] An additional ~11,000 cases of illness, ~300 hospital admissions, and ~10 deaths are estimated to result from the non-foodborne transmission of *E. coli* O157:H7 each year. See Mead *et al.* (1999).

[4] Outbreaks of *E. coli* O157 are formed to include those due to *E. coli* O157:H7 and Shiga toxin-producing *E. coli* O157:NM. In addition to the 183 foodborne outbreaks, Rangel *et al.* (2005) document a further 167 outbreaks due to other (person-to-person, animal contact, water, and laboratory-related) and unknown transmission routes.

E. coli O157:H7 and other enterohaemorrhagic strains of *E. coli* are a recognized cause (grey bars), and (iii) stated to be due to non-O157:H7 or unspecified strains of *E. coli* (white bars). Consistent with the recognition of *E. coli* O157:H7 as a pathogen of public health significance in 1982, a prominent feature of Figure 5.3A is the upsurge in *E. coli*-related outbreak investigations from the early 1980s. This upsurge was initially led by investigations of HUS and haemorrhagic colitis (grey bars), with *E. coli* O157:H7 as the specified agent of outbreaks from the late 1980s (black bars). The upsurge in outbreak investigations was associated with a more general increase in the number of *E. coli* outbreaks reported to CDC's Foodborne Disease Outbreak Surveillance System from the mid-1990s (Figure 5.3B), with the national count of *E. coli* O157:H7 reports to the US National Notifiable Diseases Surveillance System peaking at approximately 4,500 cases per annum in 1999–2000 (Figure 5.3C). As noted above, however, the latter figure is likely to be a gross underestimate of the actual level of morbidity due to *E. coli* O157:H7 in the United States.

EIS Outbreak Investigations

To provide a flavour of the factors that have promoted the foodborne transmission of *E. coli* O157:H7 in the United States, we sample from the investigations of the Epidemic Intelligence Service (Figure 5.3A). Our account draws on published evidence in *Morbidity and Mortality Weekly Report* (Section 3.3) and other sources, and extends to include outbreaks associated with the consumption of meat, fresh vegetables, and dairy products.[5]

(1) Outbreak linked to hamburger patties, Western US, 1992–3. Between 15 November 1992 and 28 February 1993, a multistate outbreak comprising >500 laboratory-confirmed cases of *E. coli* O157:H7 infection (including four deaths) occurred in Washington (477 cases), Nevada (58 cases), California (34 cases), and Idaho (14 cases) (Table 5.5). The outbreak was epidemiologically linked to the consumption of undercooked hamburger patties from a single chain of restaurants. A meat traceback identified five slaughter plants in the US and one in Canada as the likely sources of carcasses used in the contaminated lots of meat. Meat contamination may have occurred during the slaughter of animals, with the grinding of beef resulting in the internal contamination of the product (Centers for Disease Control and Prevention 1993*a*).

(2) Outbreak linked to alfalfa sprouts, Michigan, 1997. As part of a multistate outbreak of *E. coli* O157:H7 in June and July 1997, 38 laboratory-confirmed cases of infection were documented in the state of Michigan (Table 5.5). The

[5] We note here that, for the purposes of surveillance, waterborne outbreaks of *E. coli* O157:H7 and other disease-causing organisms are usually distinguished from foodborne outbreaks and fall beyond the remit of CDC's Foodborne Disease Outbreak Surveillance System.

outbreak was epidemiologically linked to the consumption of produce (alfalfa sprouts) that could be traced back to seed lots from a single supplier. A contemporaneous outbreak, linked to the same seed supplier, was recorded in Virginia. The specific mechanism of seed contamination is unknown, although it is noted that exposure to animal faeces that harbour *E. coli* O157:H7 may occur at various points in the seed production and sprouting process (Centers for Disease Control and Prevention 1997*a*; Breuer *et al.* 2001).

(3) Outbreak linked to fresh cheese curds, Wisconsin, 1998. In June 1998, 55 laboratory-confirmed cases of *E. coli* O157:H7 infection were reported in association with an outbreak of bloody diarrhoea in Wisconsin. The outbreak was epidemiologically linked to the consumption of fresh cheese curds that were traced back to a dairy plant that made both pasteurized and unpasteurized products. Investigations revealed that the curds had inadvertently been contaminated with unpasteurized (raw) milk (Centers for Disease Control and Prevention 2000*a*).

E. COLI O157:H7 OUTBREAKS IN SCOTLAND

Since the mid-1990s, the annual incidence of laboratory-confirmed cases of *E. coli* O157 infection in Scotland has varied between 3.0 and 10.0 per 100,000 population—higher than the equivalent rate for any other country of the United Kingdom (Locking *et al.* 2006) or continental Europe (Webster,

Table 5.6. Documented foodborne outbreaks of *E. coli* O157 infection in Scotland, 1994–2003

Year	Location	Persons affected	Food vehicle
1994	Grampian	22	Unpasteurized farm cheese
	Lothian	71[1]	Contaminated pasteurized milk
	Fife	22[1]	Burgers linked to butcher's shop chain
1996	Forth Valley	2	Burger from café
	Central Scotland	496[2]	Meat products from butcher's shop
1997	Borders	6	Cold meat served at public house
	Borders	15	Cold meat and meat paste from butcher's shop
1998	Grampian	4	Unpasteurized farm cheese
1999	Greater Glasgow	3	Cold meat from butcher's shop
	Grampian	27	Inadequately pasteurized goat's cheese
	Lothian	4	Undercooked homemade beefburgers
	Forth Valley	3	Contact with raw milk and calves on dairy farm[3]
2000	Forth Valley	2	Unpasteurized milk on farm[3]
2001	Argyll and Clyde	2	Cold meat from butcher's shop
2002	Grampian	5	Home barbecue including burgers
2003	Ayrshire and Arran	3	Minced beef pie served at home

Notes: [1] Microbiologically confirmed symptomatic cases only. [2] Case count from Pennington Group (1997). [3] Outbreak includes cases associated with environmental exposure.

Source: Based primarily on Strachan *et al.* (2006, table 2, p. 132).

Cowden, *et al.* 2007). Although the majority of Scottish cases are sporadic, with exposure to the faeces of farm animals as the main risk factor (Locking *et al.* 2006), foodborne transmission of *E. coli* O157 has been implicated in a number of outbreaks (Strachan *et al.* 2006); see Table 5.6

The Central Scotland Outbreak, 1996

Among the events listed in Table 5.6, the notorious outbreak of *E. coli* O157: H7 that spread in Lanarkshire and contiguous areas of central Scotland in 1996 is the largest (496 cases) and most severe (18 deaths) outbreak of the organism yet recorded in the United Kingdom. The course of the outbreak, from onset in mid-November to termination in late December 1996, is summarized in Figure 5.4 and Table 5.7. Initial reports of the disease were centred on residents of the north Lanarkshire town of Wishaw (inset map, Figure 5.4) and occurred in association with (i) a lunch attended by *c.*100 people at Wishaw parish church (17 November) and (ii) a birthday party held at the Cascade public house (23 November). Preliminary investigations traced the source of these infections to meat products from the local retail outlet of John M. Barr & Son, Butchers, a wholesale producer and supplier of raw and cooked meats to outlets in the central belt of Scotland (Plate 5.1). Through this distribution network, the outbreak extended from Wishaw to elsewhere in Lanarkshire and the Forth Valley, with additional cases in Greater Glasgow and Lothian (Table 5.7). The majority of recorded deaths occurred among elderly people (>65 years) who attended the lunch at Wishaw parish church (eight deaths) and residents of a nursing home in the Forth Valley (six deaths). The official report on the outbreak concluded that inadequate hygiene practices in Barr's shop resulted in the cross-contamination of meats handled there (Pennington Group 1997).

5.2.5 Transmissible Spongiform Encephalopathies and Variant CJD (vCJD)

Transmissible spongiform encephalopathies (TSEs) form a group of sub-acute degenerative neurological diseases that affect humans and animals (Table 5.8). Although much remains unknown about the aetiology of TSEs, the infectious agents are believed to be filterable, self-replicating proteinaceous particles known as prions. Infection is characterized by a long incubation period, with no measurable immunological response and with central nervous system (CNS) symptoms in the advanced stages of disease. Routes of transmission vary between TSE strains and their host species, although indirect horizontal pathways via the environment (e.g. scrapie), animal feed (e.g. bovine spongiform encephalopathy), and the human food chain (e.g. variant Creutzfeldt–Jakob disease) appear to be of particular importance (Doherr 2007). To illustrate the role of food production systems in the recent emergence of a human TSE, we focus here on

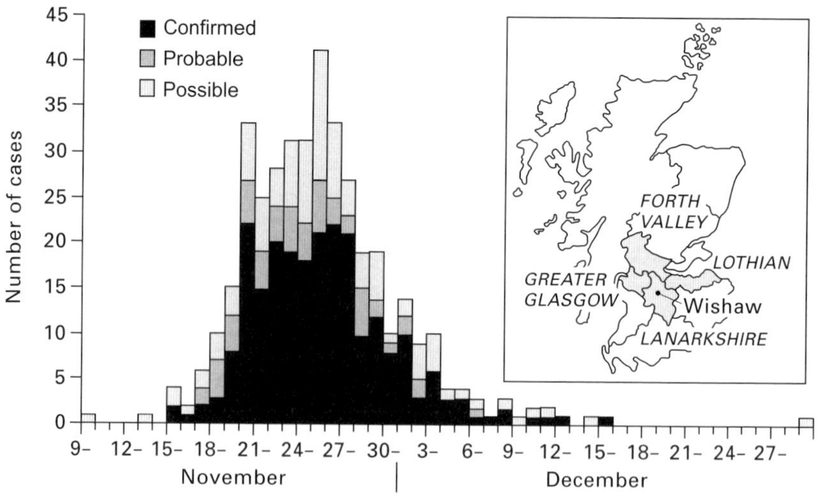

Fig. 5.4. Outbreak of *E. coli* O157:H7 in central Scotland, November–December 1996
Histogram plots the number of confirmed, probable, and possible cases by day of onset. Inset map shades NHS Scotland health boards in which cases associated with the outbreak were reported. The location of Wishaw, Lanarkshire, site of the butcher's shop implicated in the outbreak, is indicated.

Source: Adapted from Pennington Group (1997, sect. 2.15, p. 6).

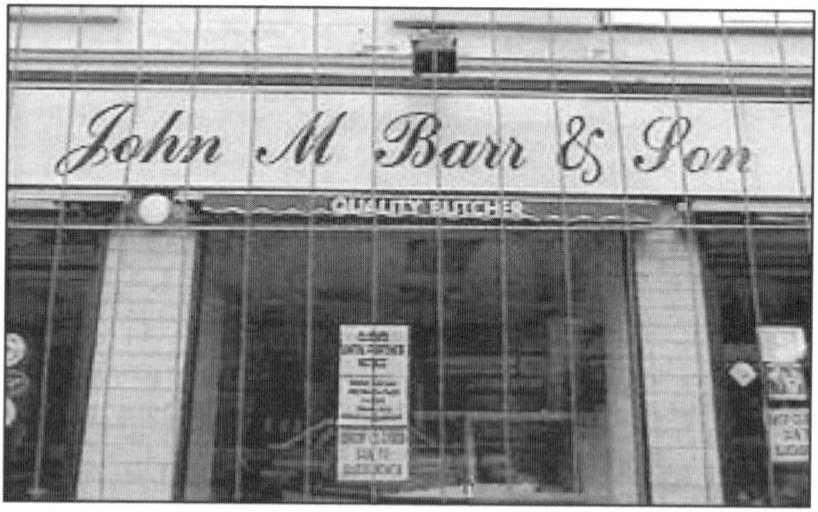

Pl. 5.1. John M. Barr & Son, Butchers, Wishaw
Butcher's shop implicated in the outbreak of *E. coli* O157:H7 in central Scotland, Nov.–Dec. 1996. The shop was closed for three months in the wake of the outbreak, but reopened in late Feb. 1997. The shop closed again in Apr. 1998 owing to mining subsidence. The business had been named Best Scottish Beef Butcher of the Year in the months prior to the outbreak.

Source: British Broadcasting Corporation (2002).

Table 5.7. Cases of infection with *E. coli* O157:H7 in the central Scotland outbreak, November–December 1996

	Number of cases by geographical area[1]				
Case classification	Lanarkshire	Forth Valley	Lothian	GGHB[2]	Total
Confirmed[3]	195	73	4	0	272
Probable[4]	50	10	0	0	60
Possible[5]	128	35	0	1	164
Total	373	118	4	1	496

Notes: [1] See inset map to Figure 5.4 for locations. [2] Greater Glasgow Health Board. [3] Person with *E. coli* O157 identified in their stool, irrespective of clinical history. [4] Person with bloody diarrhoea and positive serology. [5] Person who has non-bloody diarrhoea with positive serology *or* person who has no symptoms with positive serology *or* person who has bloody diarrhoea without positive serology.

Source: Pennington Group (1997, unnumbered table, p. 7).

variant Creutzfeldt–Jakob disease (vCJD) and its postulated link to bovine spongiform encephalopathy (BSE) in the United Kingdom.

THE NATURE OF CREUTZFELDT–JAKOB DISEASE

Creutzfeldt–Jakob disease (CJD) (*ICD*-10 A81.0) was first recognized by Creutzfeldt and Jakob in the 1920s (Table 5.8). It occurs throughout the world as an uncommon (1.0 case per million population per year) condition. As indicated in Table 5.8, there are four types of CJD (sporadic, sCJD; iatrogenic, iCJD; familial, fCJD; and variant, vCJD), with sCJD accounting for 80–90 per cent of recorded cases. Classically, the disease affected older adults (50–75 years). A highly variable (but typically long) incubation period of months or years gives way to the subacute onset of disease, with confusion, rapidly progressing dementia, and ataxia. The typical duration of CJD is 2–5 months, although patients may survive for up to two years. There is no specific therapeutic treatment, and the disease is invariably fatal. As for the mode of acquisition, spontaneous generation of the prion agent has been posited in sCJD. Iatrogenic cases may arise through the inadvertent transmission of the prion agent from cases of sCJD during medical treatment, while vCJD has been linked to the consumption of contaminated foodstuffs (Heymann 2004: 191–4).

Variant CJD

The first recorded cases of vCJD occurred in the United Kingdom in the mid-1990s. In 1996, R. G. Will and colleagues described a series of 10 atypical cases of CJD that had been reported to the National CJD Surveillance Unit, Edinburgh. The cases had onset between February 1994 and October 1995 and were distinguished from other forms of CJD by their distinctive neuropathological profile, their unusual concentration in adolescents and young adults (<45 years), and a clinical course that included the early onset of behavioural changes,

Table 5.8. Transmissible spongiform encephalopathies (TSEs) in animals and man

Disease	Disease name/ abbreviation	Known affected species	Year of first report in the scientific literature
Classical scrapie in small ruminants (sheep and goats)	Scrapie, SR TSE	Sheep and goats	1732
Sporadic Creutzfeldt–Jakob disease in humans	CJD, sCJD	Humans	1920/1
Gerstmann–Sträussler–Scheinker syndrome in humans	GSS	Humans	1936
Kuru in humans	Kuru	Humans	1957
Transmissible mink encephalopathy in captive mink	TME	Mink	1965
Iatrogenic Creutzfeldt–Jakob disease in humans	CJD, iCJD	Humans	1974
Chronic wasting disease in deer and elk	CWD	Deer and elk	1980
Fatal familial insomnia in humans	FFI	Humans	1986
Bovine spongiform encephalopathy in cattle	BSE	Cattle	1987
TSE in zoo ungulates and big cats	BSE	Big cats	1988
Familial Creutzfeldt–Jakob disease in humans	CJD, fCJD	Humans	1989
BSE (feline spongiform encephalopathy) in domestic cats	FSE	Domestic cats	1990
New-variant of Creutzfeldt–Jakob disease in humans	vCJD	Humans	1996
Sporadic fatal familial insomnia in humans	SFI	Humans	1999
Atypical form of TSE in small ruminants	SR TSE, atypical scrapie, Nor98	Small ruminants	2003
BSE in goats	SR TSE (BSE)	Goats	2005
Atypical form of BSE in cattle	BSE	Cattle	2005

Source: Adapted from Doherr (2007, table 1, p. 5620).

dysaesthesiae, and ataxia (Will *et al.* 1996). Since then, >200 cases of vCJD have been documented in 11 countries worldwide, with the United Kingdom accounting for the majority of reports (Table 5.9).

BSE AND THE ORIGINS OF vCJD

Since the first descriptions of vCJD appeared in the mid-1990s, considerable speculation has surrounded the possible origins of the disease with the

Table 5.9. Cumulative count of reported cases of vCJD by country (status: February 2008)

Country	Cases
United Kingdom	166
France	23
Republic of Ireland	4
US	3
Netherlands	2
Portugal	2
Spain	2
Canada	1
Italy	1
Japan	1
Saudi Arabia	1
TOTAL	206

Source: European and Allied Countries Collaborative Study Group of CJD (2008).

massive epizootic of bovine spongiform encephalopathy (BSE)—a prion disease that produces a progressive degeneration of the CNS in cattle—in the national herd of the United Kingdom.

The BSE Epizootic

The story of BSE in the United Kingdom is described in detail in *The BSE Inquiry: The Report*, the outcome of a two-year investigation that was established by Parliament on 12 January 1998 (Phillips 2000). The disease first came to the attention of British veterinarians in November 1986 when cases of a novel neurological disease, characterized by nervousness, heightened reactivity to external stimuli, and impaired movement, were observed in domestic cattle (Wells *et al.* 1987). The number of cases of the newly named BSE grew rapidly in subsequent years, reaching a peak in 1992 and declining sharply thereafter (Figure 5.5). By the late 1990s, the cumulative case total had exceeded 170,000, with approximately two-thirds of all dairy herds in the United Kingdom having had at least one confirmed case of BSE (Pattison 1998)—a clinical epizootic consistent with an estimated 1.0 million infections with the BSE agent in the national herd (Anderson, Donnelly, *et al.* 1996).

Although scientific opinion on the origins of BSE is divided (Colchester and Colchester 2005), the cross-species transmission of the agent of another TSE (sheep scrapie) via animal feed containing ruminant-derived protein has been postulated as one likely source of the disease in cattle (Figure 5.5); see Nathanson *et al.* (1997) and Brown, Will, *et al.* (2001). Further details of the hypothesized link between BSE and scrapie, including a possible connection with changes in the rendering practices of abattoir-derived ruminant wastes in the late 1970s, are provided by Nathanson *et al.* (1997). Irrespective of the exact source of BSE, however, the subsequent recycling of BSE-infected cattle waste

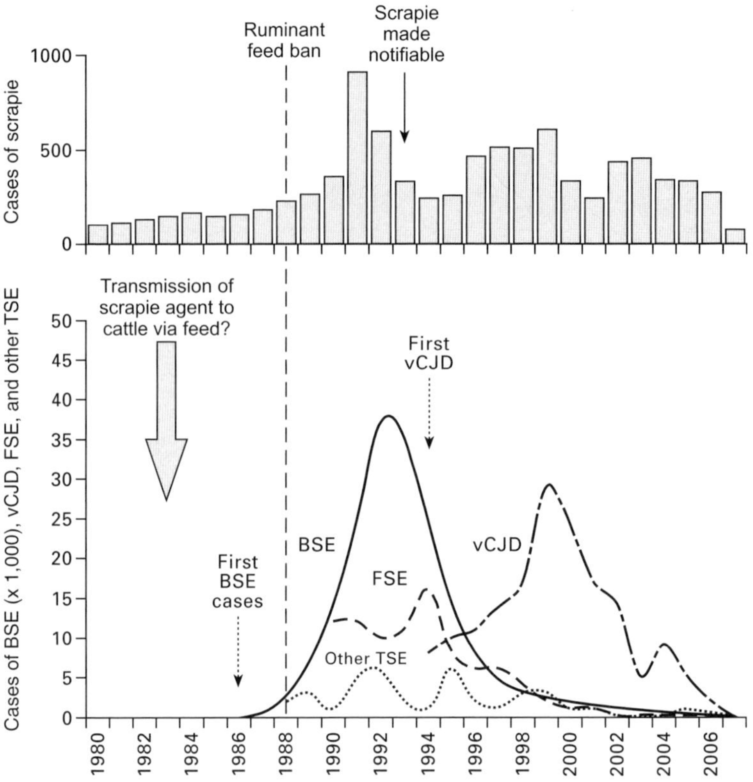

Fig. 5.5. Transmissible spongiform encephalopathies (TSEs) in the United Kingdom, 1980–2007

The histogram (upper graph) plots the annual count of scrapie cases in sheep. Note that scrapie became notifiable in 1993; the observed increase in cases in 1991–2 was associated with a bounty (£15 per head) offered to farmers for scrapie-infected sheep brains, used to form a pool of material to test various rendering processes for their ability to inactivate the scrapie agent. The line traces (lower graph) plot the annual count of cases of bovine spongiform encephalopathy (BSE) in cattle, feline spongiform encephalopathy (FSE) in domestic cats, variant Creutzfeldt–Jakob disease (vCJD) in humans, and other TSEs in species of exotic ruminant (including bison, nyala, gemsbok, oryx, and eland). Counts of vCJD include definite or probable cases by year of symptom onset. Cases of BSE have been scaled by a factor of 1,000. The date of implementation of the ruminant feed ban (1988) is indicated for reference. All data for 2007 relate to the period to July.

Sources: Drawn from information collated by the Department for Environment, Food, and Rural Affairs, London (http://www.defra.gov.uk), and the National Creutzfeldt–Jakob Surveillance Unit, Edinburgh (http://www.cjd.ed.ac.uk).

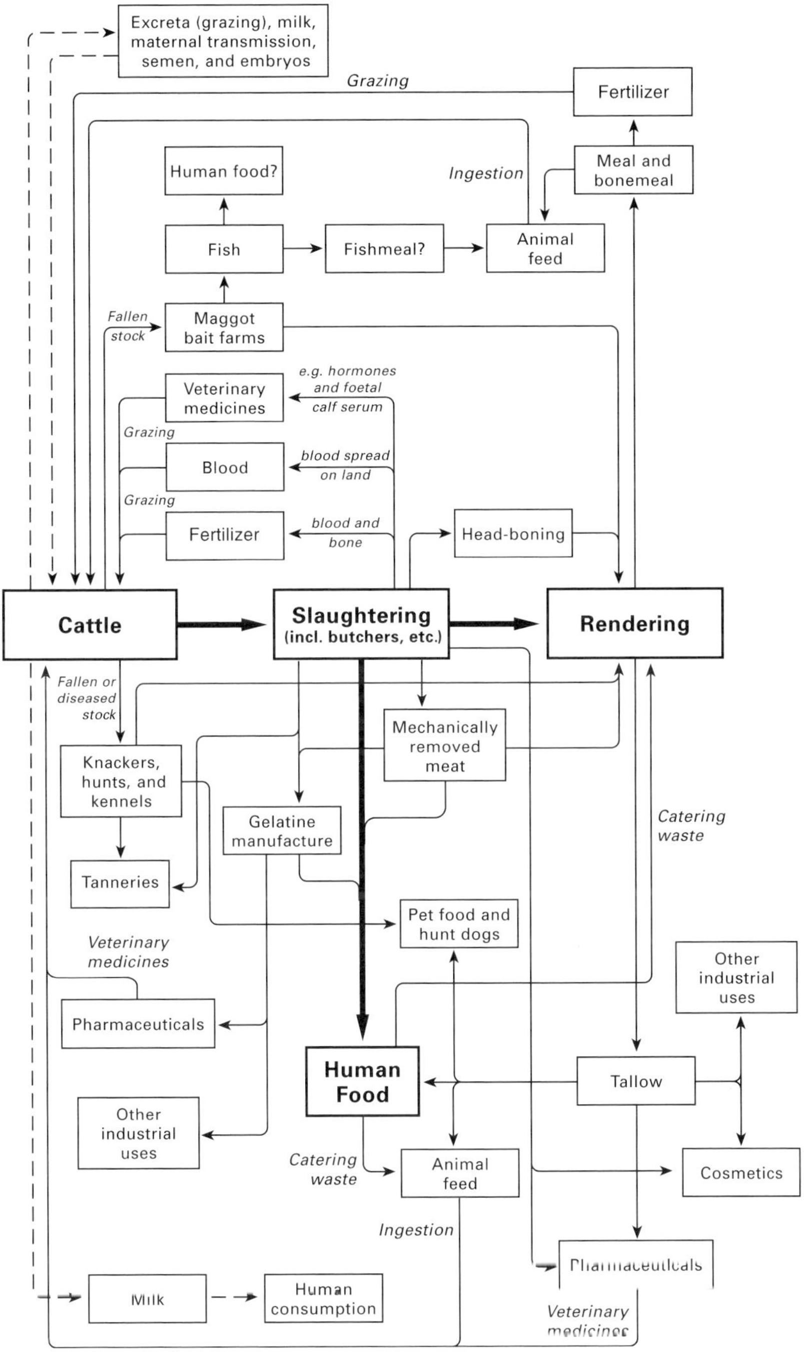

Fig. 5.6. The cattle carcass: routes of use in the late 1980s

Source: Redrawn from Phillips (2000, vol. 16, fig. 4.1, p. 72).

as part of the rendering process (Figure 5.6) is believed to have contributed to the persistence of the disease in cattle. The imposition of a ban on the inclusion of ruminant offal in cattle feed in July 1988, coupled with the pre-emptive slaughter of some 4.5 million head of cattle, heralded a pronounced decline in the BSE epizootic from the mid-1990s (Figure 5.5).

BSE, the Human Food Chain, and vCJD

The role of the food chain as a possible source of human exposure to BSE-infected tissues was recognized at an early stage of the BSE epizootic (Figure 5.6). Concerns were underscored as other species (including domestic cats and exotic ruminants in zoos) began to display signs of BSE-like diseases (Figure 5.5), with the food chain implicated as the likely source of infection (Pattison 1998).[6] To limit the human risk, a ban on the use of certain specified bovine offal (including brain, spinal cord, tonsil, and spleen) in human food was introduced in late 1989, while, to monitor for the occurrence of human disease, surveillance for CJD was reinstituted in the United Kingdom in 1990. In 1996—a full decade after the recognized onset of the BSE epizootic—the first cases of vCJD were reported in the human population (Figure 5.5). Subsequent studies have demonstrated the close similarities between the agents of BSE and vCJD, with the consumption of beef products contaminated with BSE-infected nervous system tissue regarded as the most likely source of human infection (Pattison 1998).

Available evidence suggests that the main period of hazard of BSE to the human food supply in the United Kingdom was 1984–9 (Collee *et al.* 2006), with the carcasses of an estimated 700,000 or more BSE-incubating cattle having entered the food chain in the interval to 1995 (Anderson, Donnelly, *et al.* 1996). Many of these animals were young (<30 months) and at an assumed phase of low infectivity. As Figure 5.5 shows, the annual incidence of vCJD peaked at 28 cases in 2000, eight years after the peak of the BSE epizootic. Post-peak projections of the likely future course of the vCJD epidemic in the United Kingdom provide a best estimate of 40–100 deaths in the interval 2003–80 (Ghani *et al.* 2003).

GEOGRAPHICAL PATTERNS OF VCJD IN THE UNITED KINGDOM

Figure 5.7 plots, by place of residence at the time of symptom onset, the geographical distribution of definite and probable cases of vCJD reported to the United Kingdom's National CJD Surveillance Unit by 31 December 2005. While vCJD cases are distributed throughout the country (Figure 5.7A), vCJD standardized incidence ratios (SIRs) for the 11 statistical

[6] Contaminated bovine offal in commercially produced pet foods is considered to be the most likely source of infection in domestic cats, while exotic ruminants are likely to have been infected through the consumption of the same contaminated dietary supplements that were fed to cattle. See Pattison (1998).

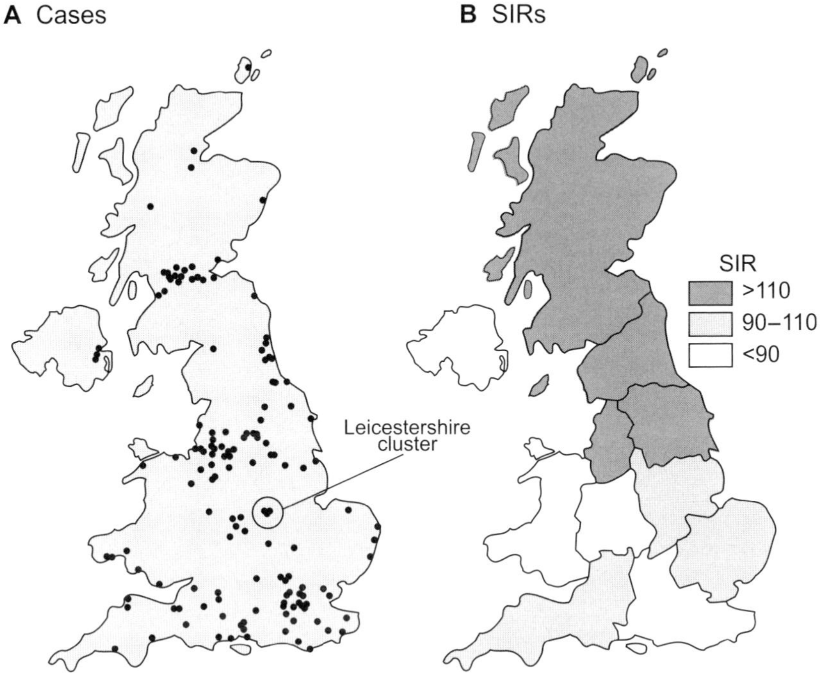

Fig. 5.7. Geographical distribution of vCJD, United Kingdom, 1994–2005
(A) Place of residence at onset of symptoms for definite or probable cases. The location of the Leicestershire cluster is indicated. (B) Standardized incidence ratios (SIRs) by statistical region of residence in 1991 for definite or probable cases.
Source: Adapted from National CJD Surveillance Unit (2006, figs 10, 11, pp. 18, 21).

regions of the United Kingdom reveal a tendency for the highest ratios (>110) to occur in more northerly regions (Figure 5.7B). As the National CJD Surveillance Unit (2006) observes, individuals living in northern areas of the United Kingdom in the early 1990s were 1.5 times more likely to develop vCJD than their southern counterparts. Although the factors that may have contributed to the geography of vCJD in the United Kingdom are uncertain, Cousens *et al.* (2001) report a statistically significant and positive spatial correlation between (i) reported disease activity and (ii) levels of consumption of meat and meat products other than carcass meat, bacon, and poultry.

vCJD Clusters

Analysis of the case distribution in Figure 5.7A reveals evidence of only one statistically significant spatial cluster of vCJD: five cases in the Charnwood district and environs of north Leicestershire (National CJD Surveillance Unit 2006). An investigation of the cluster, which included two cases in the

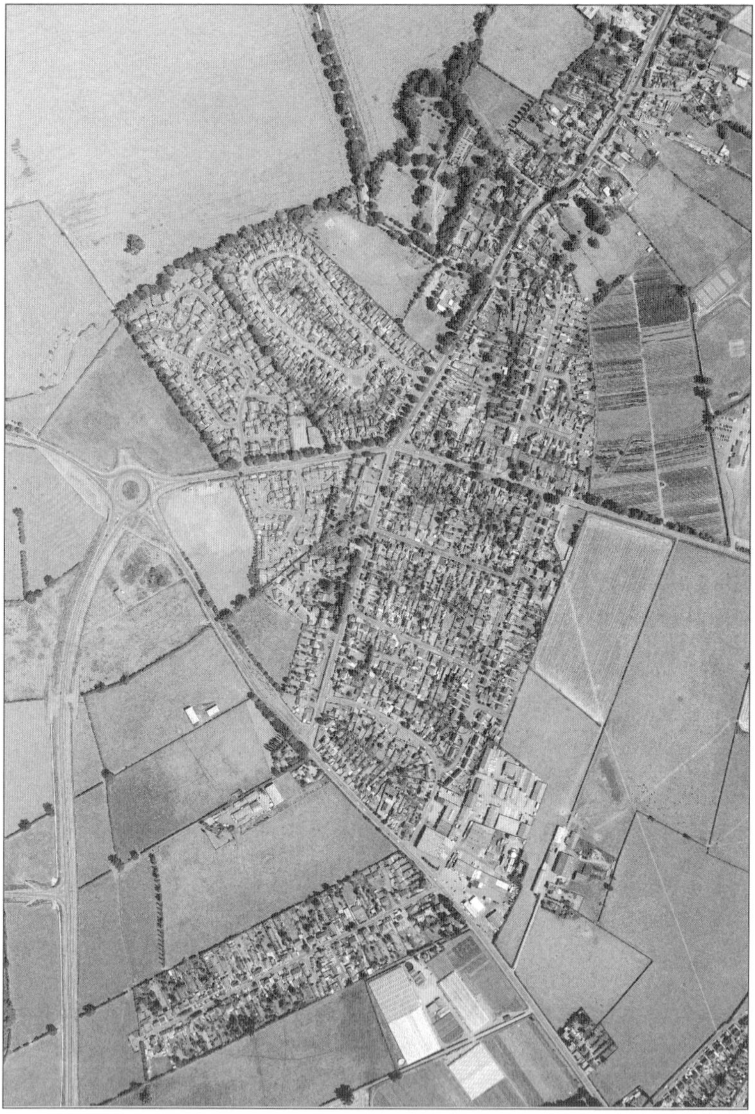

Pl. 5.2. Clusters of vCJD

Aerial photograph of the village of Queniborough, Leicestershire, the site of a small cluster of vCJD cases. The location of the cluster is indicated in Fig. 5.7A.

Sources: Cliff, Haggett, and Smallman-Raynor (2004, fig. 11.29, p. 178), from Cambridge University Collection of Air Photographs.

village of Queniborough (Plate 5.2), concluded that four of the patients may have been exposed to the BSE agent through the purchase and consumption of contaminated beef from local butchers' shops (Bryant and Monk 2001).

5.2.6 Summary

This section has shown the variety of ways in which changes in food production and processing technologies can create new ecological niches for human pathogens to occupy. In recent years, there has been a rapid expansion in the number of recognized foodborne pathogens of public health importance—some apparently wholly new (e.g. *E. coli* O157:H7), some known but only recently recognized as foodborne (e.g. *Campylobacter jejuni*), and some known as foodborne but not appreciated as seriously pathogenic until recently (e.g. *Listeria monocytogenes*). The rapid increase may be attributed to many causes including improved surveillance, international sourcing and centralized production of food for retail outlets (which means that a single-point breakdown in hygiene in a production unit can have geographically widespread consequences), and failures in food handling procedures. This multifactorial causality makes control difficult, and we have illustrated with examples from the United States and the United Kingdom the kinds of outbreak which can occur. These have ranged in scale from a general rise in the traffic of 'gastroenteritis', through to the much more intractable and serious outbreaks associated with *E. coli* O157:H7 and vCJD.

Just as old and new pathogens have occupied fresh niches to cause serious public health problems in the food processing industry, so new opportunities have been created by technological advances in industry more generally. As we noted earlier, the type example is the emergence of Legionnaires' disease, and it is this which we now consider.

5.3 Cooling and Plumbing Systems: Legionnaires' Disease

Legionnaires' disease (*ICD*-10 A49.1) provides the type example of a disease whose emergence is intimately associated with technological development. The disease was first recognized in the course of an outbreak that caused the deaths of 29 members of the American Legion who were attending a conference in Philadelphia in July 1976 (Plate 5.3). While the causative agent of Legionnaires' disease (*Legionella pneumophila*) is neither new nor localized, the increasing incidence of the disease underlines the way in which changes in the human environment (through the sophisticated modification of the micro environments of buildings) can provide new niches which previously existing

244 MORBIDITY AND MORTALITY WEEKLY REPORT August 6, 1976

Epidemiologic Notes and Reports

Respiratory Infection – Pennsylvania

A total of 152 persons associated with a state American Legion convention in Philadelphia July 21-24 have been hospitalized with respiratory infections. Onsets of illness were in the period July 22-August 3; the majority occurred from July 25 to July 31. Twenty-two of these patients have died. The deaths, reported over the past week, were primarily due to pneumonia.

Although information about the disease and its epidemiology is incomplete, it appears to be characterized by the acute onset of fever, chills, headache, and malaise, followed by a dry cough and myalgia. Some of the most seriously ill developed high fever and died in shock with extensive pneumonia. No etiologic agent has yet been incriminated. There is no information available concerning other Legionnaires who may be ill with less severe symptoms.

The patients, among several thousand attending the convention, stayed in at least 3 or 4 hotels while in Philadelphia. There is no evidence of increase in respiratory disease in Philadelphia residents, nor has there been any confirmed secondary spread to family members or other contacts. There have been several reports of similar disease in non-conventioneers who were in Philadelphia at the same time as the convention.

Reported by RG Sharrar, MD, City of Philadelphia Dept of Public Health; WE Parkin, DVM, Acting State Epidemiologist, Pennsylvania State Dept of Health; the Bur of Epidemiology and the Bur of Laboratories, CDC.

U.S. DEPARTMENT OF HEALTH, EDUCATION, AND WELFARE
PUBLIC HEALTH SERVICE / CENTER FOR DISEASE CONTROL
ATLANTA, GEORGIA 30333

Director, Center for Disease Control, David J. Sencer, M.D.
Director, Bureau of Epidemiology, Philip S. Brachman, M.D.
Editor, Michael B. Gregg, M.D.
Managing Editor, Anne D. Mather, M.A.

OFFICIAL BUSINESS FIRST CLASS

U.S. MAIL

POSTAGE AND FEES PAID
U.S. DEPARTMENT OF HEW
HEW 399

AIR MAIL

Dr F T Perkins 475/421s
Ch, Biological Standardization
World Health Organization
Ave Appia
1211 Geneva 27, Switzerland

HEW Publication No. (CDC) 76-8017

Pl. 5.3. First report of the outbreak of Legionnaires' disease in Philadelphia, 1976
A brief note by two Pennsylvania physicians calling attention to respiratory infections among members attending the July 1976 American Legion convention, published in CDC's *Morbidity and Mortality Weekly Report*, 35/30 (1976), 244.

bacteria can colonize. The natural habitat of *L. pneumophila* appears to be aquatic bodies including rivers, lakes, streams, and thermally polluted waters. It is also known as 'legionellosis' or 'Legionnaires' pneumonia'. Pontiac fever (*ICD*-10 A48.2) is a closely related non-pneumonic form of the disease.

5.3.1 Nature of Legionnaires' Disease

The severity of illness in Legionnaires' disease ranges from asymptomatic infection to life-threatening pneumonia. In clinical cases, a typical incubation period of 5–6 days (range 2–10 days) is followed by the acute onset of malaise, muscle aches, and slight headache. A rapidly rising temperature, accompanied by shaking chills, is observed within 24–48 hours. Lower respiratory tract symptoms, including a non-productive cough and dyspnoea, develop over the next few days, with the disease progressing to pneumonia with hypoxaemia and shock in severe cases. Case-fatality rates of 5–30 per cent have been recorded in outbreaks (Butler and Breiman 1998; Heymann 2004: 292–5).

Within their primarily aqueous reservoirs, *L. pneumophila* bacilli can survive a wide range of environmental conditions: temperatures from freezing to 63°C; pH from 5.0 to 8.5; and dissolved oxygen from 0.2 to 150 mg/L. Human infection is believed to occur through the inhalation of aerosolized water particles, and, although other modes of transmission are possible, none has been proven conclusively. Susceptibility and resistance to *L. pneumophila* is complex. Illness occurs most frequently with increasing age; most cases are among individuals aged $\geq$50 years. Patients who smoke, have diabetes mellitus, chronic lung disease, end-stage renal disease, or malignancy are at heightened risk of severe disease. Resistance is also low among the immunosuppressed. Treatment with a single antibiotic (usually erythromycin) or with combined antibiotics (for example, erythromycin and rifampin in severe cases) is effective. For further details, see Butler and Breiman (1998) and Heymann (2004: 292–5).

5.3.2 Technology and the Emergence of Legionnaires' Disease

As Breiman (1996: 4) observes, 'Legionnaires' disease is a model infectious disease for demonstrating the effects of technology, because a variety of man-made devices have provided ideal settings for the multiplication of the etiologic agent while also providing effective means for disseminating the organism to humans.' While *Legionellae* live in low numbers in most natural aquatic settings, the bacteria can only amplify in waters with temperatures 25–42°C. Such conditions are unusual in nature, but technological innovations include a number of devices that utilize and maintain water at these temperatures. For example, cooling towers and evaporative condensers used in air cooling systems for buildings and for the cooling of water for industrial purposes generally maintain sizeable water reservoirs at 25–35°C. Likewise, whirlpool spas, hot tubs, and showers also maintain water temperatures within the required range, as do room-air humidifiers, ice-making machines, misting equipment, architectural fountains, and plumbing systems in some large buildings. Many of these devices produce fine droplets of water (1–5 μm in diameter) which can carry *Legionellae* and which, if inhaled, may result in infection of the respiratory tract (Breiman 1996).

5.3.3 Past Patterns in the United States

THE PHILADELPHIA OUTBREAK, 1976

Between 21 and 24 July 1976, the Pennsylvania branch of the American Legion—a fraternal organization of military veterans—held its annual meeting at the Bellevue Stratford Hotel in downtown Philadelphia (Plate 5.4). Within a few days of the end of the convention, reports began to reach the Legion's headquarters that several of those who had attended the Philadelphia convention had subsequently developed severe pneumonia of undetermined aetiology. An investigation by the state epidemiological service supported by CDC followed. The investigation identified 221 cases in Legionnaires who had attended the convention and others who had been in or near the headquarters hotel. As Figure 5.8 shows, the earliest case had onset

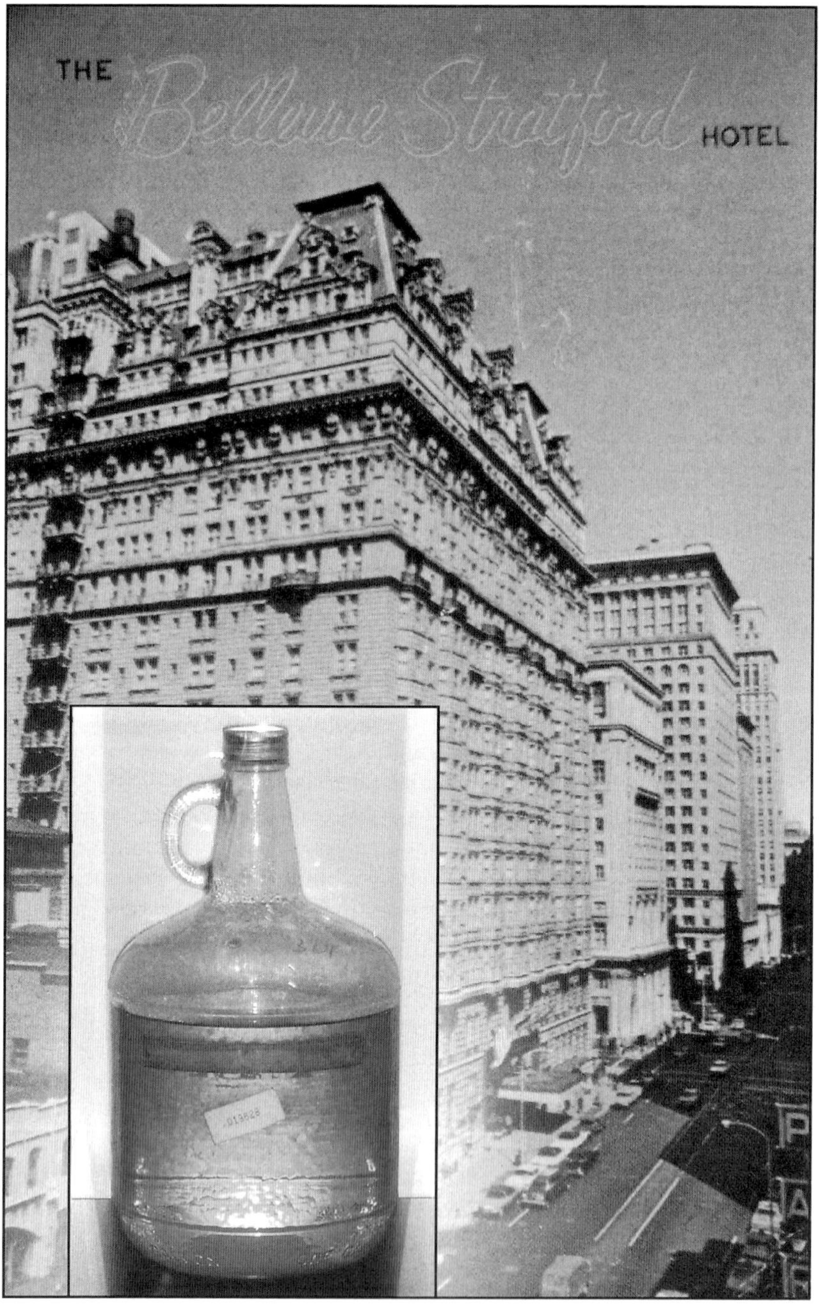

Pl. 5.4. Legionnaires' disease investigation, Philadelphia, 1976. I
The Bellevue Stratford hotel, Philadelphia, and a carboy of the chiller water from the hotel's cooling system from which Joseph McDade isolated the causative agent of Legionnaires' disease, *Legionella pneumophila*. The water cooling plant is visible on the roof of the hotel.

Source: CDC museum, Atlanta, with permission.

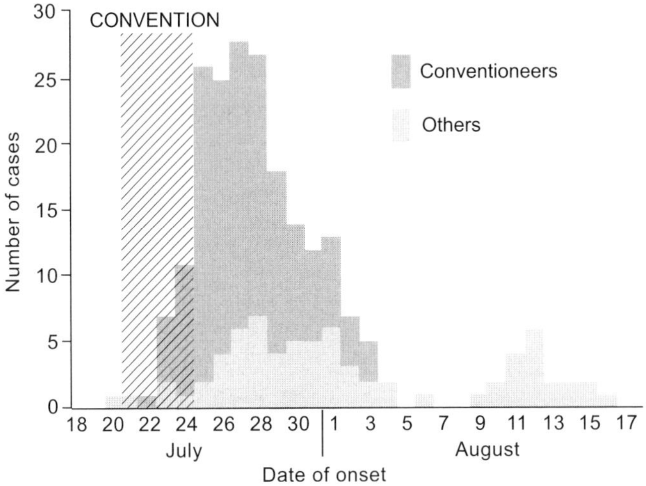

Fig. 5.8. Graph of the Philadelphia outbreak of Legionnaires' disease, July–August 1976 The log-normal shaped distribution of cases in the Philadelphia epidemic was typical of an outbreak arising from a common source. It rose rapidly from 22 July through to 25 July and then declined more slowly. The relation between the dates of the convention and the onset of illness suggests that the incubation period of Legionnaires' disease ranged from 2–10 days. Cases among people attending the convention and others are shown separately.

Sources: Redrawn from Cliff, Haggett, and Smallman-Raynor (2004, fig. 11.6, p. 169), originally from Brock (1990, fig. 2.2, p. 15).

on 20 July. Peak occurrence extended from 24 July–1 August, with decreasing numbers of cases through to mid-August. In all, 90 per cent of case-patients developed pneumonia and 15 per cent died (Fraser *et al.* 1977).

The investigation proved frustrating because standard diagnostic laboratory tests for all known agents of pneumonia were negative. Epidemiological studies pointed to an airborne spread of the agent. Plate 5.5 shows a map made at the time of the investigation. Rooms in which American Legion members stayed are marked, along with their health status. The air handling system for a typical floor is also plotted. Risk of infection grew with the length of time spent in the lobby of the hotel and on the nearby sidewalk, while those who drank water at the Bellevue Stratford also had a higher risk. There was no evidence of person-to-person transmission of the disease (Fraser *et al.* 1977). It was five months later that Joseph McDade at the CDC laboratories in Atlanta isolated a bacillus (subsequently named *L. pneumophila*) as the causative agent of Legionnaires' disease in a water sample taken from the rooftop evaporative condenser plant which supplied the hotel's room air cooling system (Plate 5.4). The condenser plant not only

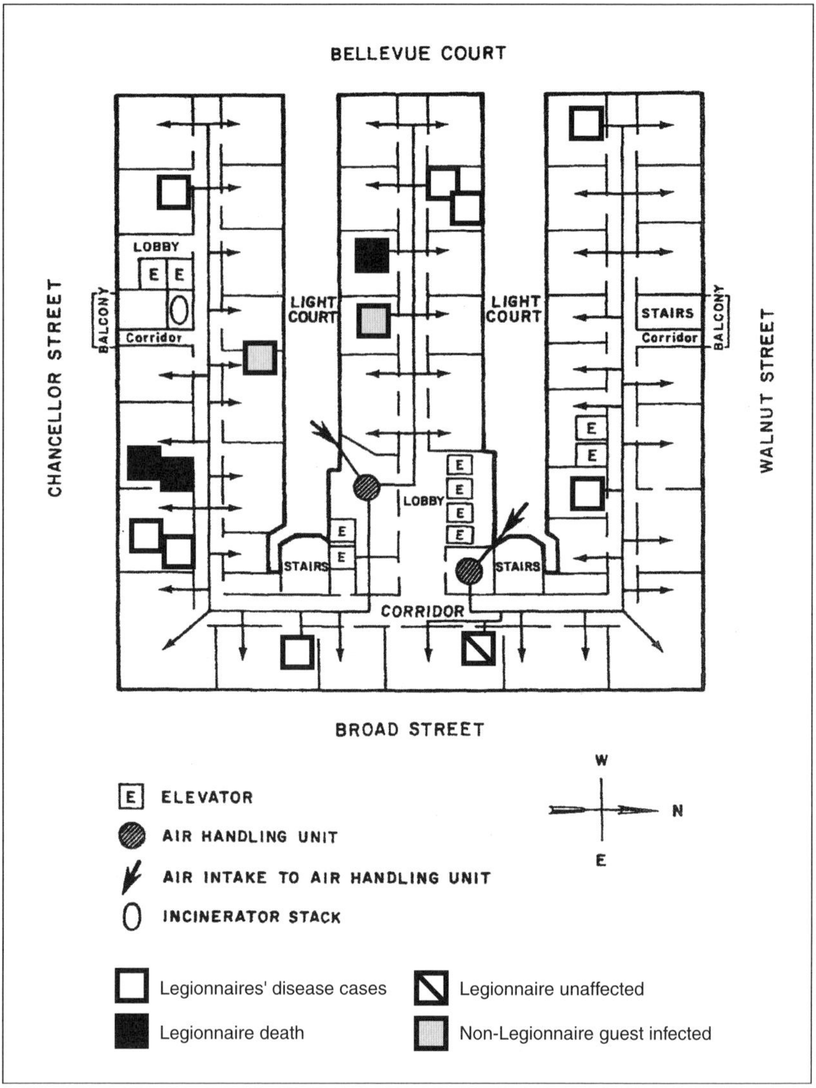

Pl. 5.5. Legionnaires' disease investigation, Philadelphia, 1976. II
Sketch plan made from data collected at the time of the 1976 investigation of the second-floor rooms at the Bellevue Stratford with health status of American Legion occupants indicated. The air circulation system on a typical floor is also shown.
Sources: CDC museum, Atlanta, and Dr S. B. Thacker, US Centers for Disease Control and Prevention.

provided ideal conditions for the agent to multiply but it also blew the contaminated air through the hotel. The bacillus had been missed in earlier pneumonia tests because of its (i) weak staining capacity and (ii) inability to grow in the usual cultures (Butler and Breiman 1998; Cliff, Haggett, and Smallman-Raynor 2004).

Retrospective Studies: Evidence of L. pneumophila Prior to 1976

Once isolated, serological studies retrospectively identified *L. pneumophila* (or a closely related organism) as the cause of unsolved outbreaks of pneumonia at a convention of the Independent Order of Odd Fellows held at the Bellevue Stratford Hotel, Philadelphia, in 1974 (Terranova *et al.* 1978), a psychiatric hospital in Washington, DC, in 1965 (Thacker, Bennett, *et al.* 1978) and a meat packing plant in Austin, Minnesota, in 1957 (Osterholm *et al.* 1983). In addition, McDade *et al.* (1979) provide evidence that *L. pneumophila* was circulating and causing disease as early as 1947, while Glick *et al.* (1978) identify *L. pneumophila* as the cause of an outbreak of a non-pneumonic febrile disease (Pontiac fever) in a health department building in Pontiac, Missouri, in 1968.

EPIDEMIOLOGICAL TRENDS IN LEGIONNAIRES' DISEASE

Epidemiological overviews of Legionnaires' disease in the United States in the years since its first recognition in 1976 appear in Benin *et al.* (2002) and Fields *et al.* (2002). *Legionella* infections are responsible for an estimated 8,000–18,000 hospital admissions each year. The majority of these are attributable to *L. pneumophila*, with cohort studies attributing 2–15 per cent of hospitalized cases of community-acquired pneumonia to Legionnaires' disease.

Evidence from Reported Cases

As Fields *et al.* (2002) warn, many cases of Legionnaires' disease go undiagnosed or unreported each year in the United States and accurate data for the assessment of disease trends are not available. For a total of 6,757 cases of Legionnaires' disease reported nationally to CDC in the period 1980–98, Benin *et al.* (2002) observe the following patterns:

(i) the median annual number of cases was 360, with no evidence of a temporal trend in case incidence per 100,000 population over the 19-year observation period;
(ii) 35 per cent of all cases were attributable to nosocomial transmission, with nosocomial cases accounting for between 25 per cent (1997) and 45 per cent (1986) of the annual disease count;
(iii) the case-fatality rate decreased from a high of 34.0 per cent (1985) to 11.5 per cent (1998), with a marked reduction in the case-fatality for both nosocomial and community-acquired cases over the 19-year observation period;

(iv) 21 per cent of all cases met the definition of travel-associated Legionnaires' disease, varying from 14 per cent (1983) to 25 per cent (1994–6).

Factors that may account for the decrease in observed mortality may include improved diagnosis, leading to the identification of less severely ill patients, and developments in the antibiotic therapy of patients admitted to hospital with pneumonia.

EPIDEMIC INTELLIGENCE SERVICE (EIS) OUTBREAK INVESTIGATIONS, 1976–2005

The histogram in Figure 5.9 is based on the records of the US Epidemic Intelligence Service (EIS; Section 3.4) and plots the annual count of domestic (shaded) and international (unshaded) legionellosis and suspected legionellosis outbreak investigations undertaken in the period 1976–2005. Of the 67 investigations, 62 were domestic and five were international (including cruise ships). On average, two investigations were undertaken in each year, but with an

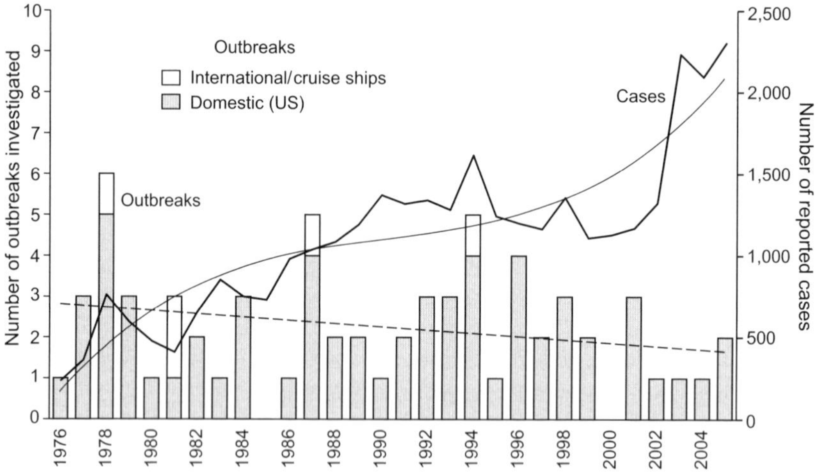

Fig. 5.9. Trends in legionellosis in the United States, 1976–2005
The histogram plots the annual count of domestic (US) and international (including cruise ships) outbreaks of legionellosis investigated by the US Epidemic Intelligence Service. For reference, the heavy line trace plots the annual count of legionellosis cases reported to the US National Notifiable Diseases Surveillance System. Trends are depicted by the linear (outbreak investigations) and polynomial (case count) regression lines, fitted to the respective data sets by ordinary least squares.

Sources: Drawn from the records of the US Epidemic Intelligence Service (outbreak investigations) and the Centers for Disease Control and Prevention's annual *MMWR Summary of Notifiable Diseases* (Atlanta: CDC).

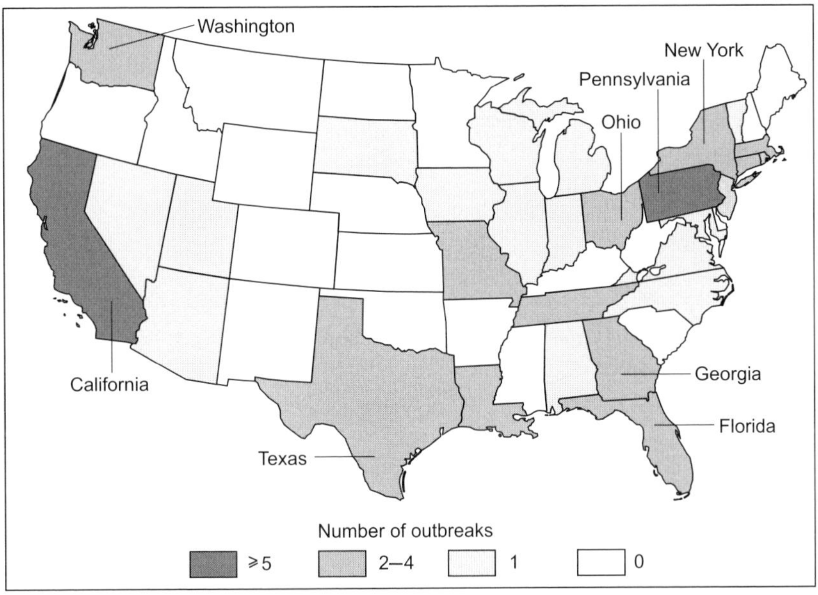

Fig. 5.10. Legionellosis and suspected legionellosis outbreak investigations in the conterminous United States
The map plots the number of outbreak investigations conducted by the US Epidemic Intelligence Service by state, 1976–2005. The distribution excludes one travel-related outbreak involving the states of New Jersey, New York, Pennsylvania, and Vermont.
Source: Drawn from the records of the US Epidemic Intelligence Service.

underpinning negative trend.[7] Of the domestic investigations, California (7) and Pennsylvania (5) accounted for one-fifth of all investigations undertaken (Figure 5.10). Consistent with Benin *et al.* (2002), the EIS studies showed that outbreaks of Legionnaires' disease are of three main types: nosocomial, community-acquired, or associated with multistate travel. By way of illustration we give one example of each.

(1) Possible nosocomial transmission, Burlington, Vermont (1977). Broome, Goings, *et al.* (1979) describe an EIS investigation of a Legionnaires' disease outbreak focused on the Medical Center Hospital in Burlington, Vermont. Over an 8-month period, 1 May–31 December 1977, 69 laboratory-confirmed cases of Legionnaires' were recorded. The possible site(s) of exposure of the patients to *L.*

[7] A countervailing (positive) trend in the annual count of legionellosis cases reported to the US National Notifiable Diseases Surveillance System is indicated by the heavy line trace in Figure 5.9. The exact reasons for this observed increase are unclear, although possible explanations include an actual increase in disease incidence, greater use of diagnostic testing, and/or improvements in surveillance (Centers for Disease Control and Prevention 2007*a*).

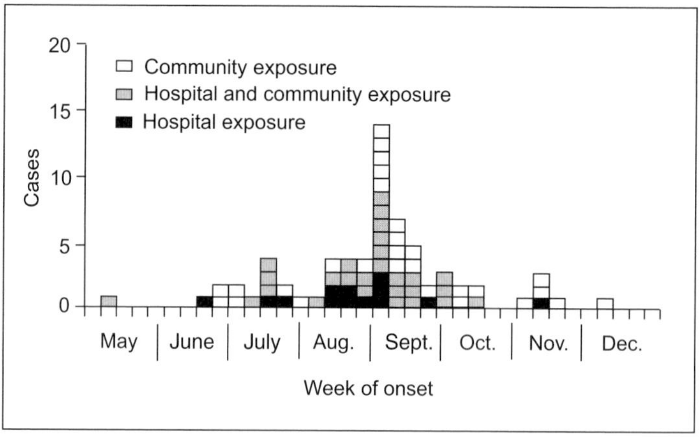

Fig. 5.11. Legionnaires' disease in Burlington, Vermont, May–December 1977
Cases are plotted by week of onset and inferred site of exposure. Cases are classified according to a three-category division of exposure: (1) cases that had been hospitalized throughout the 10-day period (presumed incubation period) prior to onset of symptoms ('hospital exposure'); (2) other cases that had some form of contact with hospitals in the 10-day period prior to onset of symptoms ('hospital and community exposure'); and (3) cases that had no contact with hospitals prior to onset of symptoms ('community exposure'). Note that one case has been omitted from the time series owing to lack of information on date of onset.

Source: Redrawn from Broome et al. (1979, fig. 1, p. 574).

pneumophila are shown by week of disease onset in Figure 5.11 and include (i) hospital exposure (13 patients), (ii) hospital and community exposure (28 patients), and (iii) community exposure (28 patients). No common source of exposure for the epidemic was identified, although nosocomial transmission was presumed in the 'hospital exposure' cases. The 69 cases included 25 immunocompromised patients, indicative of the raised susceptibility to infection and disease in these individuals.

(2) Community-acquired infection, Manhattan, New York (1978). Cordes *et al.* (1980) report an EIS investigation of a Legionnaires' disease outbreak in the garment district of Manhattan, New York City, 1978, centred on 'Building A' at the intersection of 35th Street and Seventh Avenue; see Figure 5.12C. Seventeen confirmed and 21 presumptive cases of Legionnaires' occurred in the period 1 August–11 September (Figure 5.12A), with the work locations of patients clustered in the vicinity of Building A. Additional cases of illness, coincident with the outbreak of Legionnaires' disease, and some with evidence of seropositivity to *L. pneumophila*, were recorded in the employees of one business in Building A (Figure 5.12B). Environmental sampling resulted in the isolation of *L. pneumophila* from water specimens taken from the cooling towers of a 10-storey building opposite to Building A but not in Building A itself.

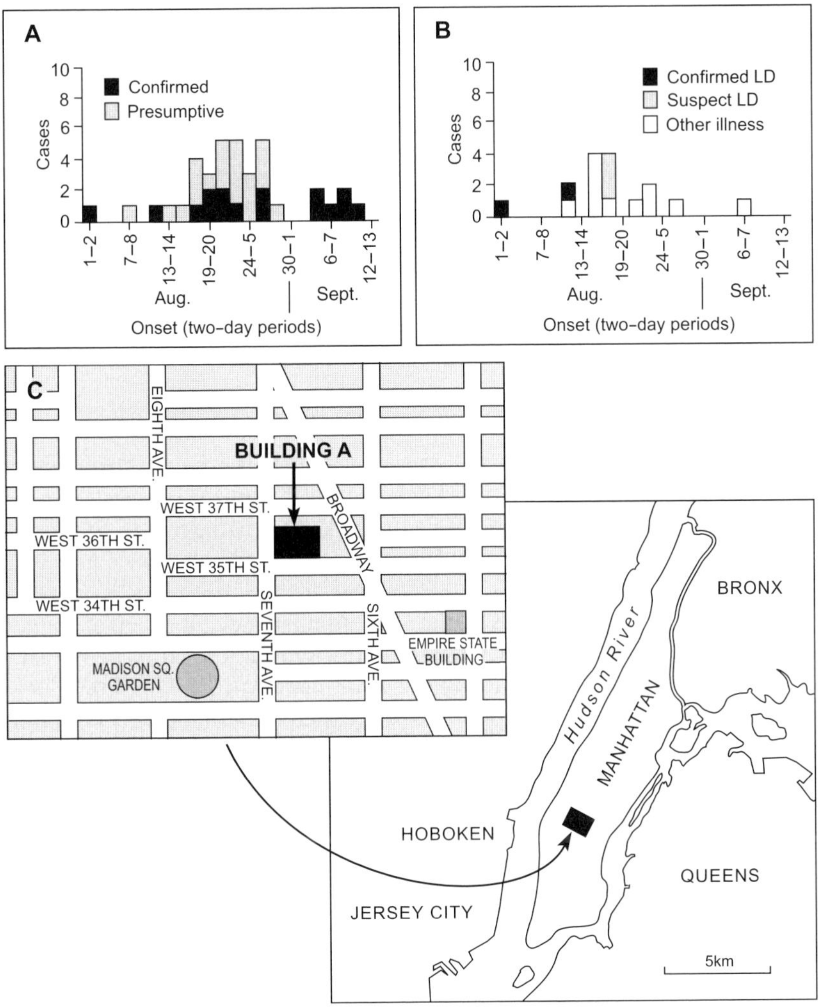

Fig. 5.12. Outbreak of Legionnaires' disease in the garment district of Manhattan, New York City, August–September 1978
(A) Confirmed and presumptive cases of Legionnaires' disease in the garment district, by two-day period of onset. (B) Illnesses recorded in a business located in building A of the garment district, by two-day period of onset. (C) Map showing the garment district of Manhattan, with the location of building A indicated. LD = Legionnaires' disease.

Source: Graphs A and B redrawn from Cordes *et al.* (1980, figs 1, 3, pp. 472, 474); map C drawn from Cordes *et al.* (1980).

(3) Multistate travel-associated outbreak linked to Vermont (1987). Mamolen *et al.* (1993) summarize the results of an EIS investigation of a multistate outbreak of Legionnaires' disease linked to Vermont. The outbreak centred on members of nine tour groups of elderly persons, originating from three states (Pennsylvania, New Jersey, and New York), who visited Vermont in late October 1987. The 17 case-patients (including three deaths) were epidemiologically linked to two ski lodges (located within 600m of each other), with overall attack rates for the tour members of 6.4 per cent (lodge A) and 3.1 per cent (lodge B). The two outbreaks were caused by a single outbreak strain of *L. pneumophila* serogroup 1. The strain was isolated in water specimens taken from the skimmer in a swimming pool and standing water in the boiler room at Lodge A, and from a whirlpool spa at Lodge B.

5.3.4 Summary

The example of Legionnaires' disease, like the foodborne pathogens, illustrates the old adage that nature abhors a vacuum. Wherever a vacant ecological niche is created, a pathogen will eventually follow. In the case of Legionnaires', the niche was created by the widespread occurrence of various air handling and similar units, often in inaccessible, out-of-sight locations like rooftops, basements, and outhouses. Almost inevitably, given human nature, standards of maintenance slip and eventually local environmental conditions become ripe for pathogen development. *Legionella* is now known to be widespread. For example, it was isolated in half of all US cooling towers inspected in 1980. It probably causes up to 2 per cent of the pneumonia cases in the United States (perhaps 50,000 cases) annually. Studies of stored serum and tissue samples revealed the pathogen to have been the cause not only of outbreaks of pneumonia-like disease in Los Angeles, Washington DC, and Pontiac, Michigan, but also in Nottingham (England) and Benidorm (Spain). The examples we have chosen illustrate the three main ways in which *Legionella* infection is acquired—nosocomially, in the community, and in association with travel. These are repeating factors in the emergence and re-emergence of infectious diseases.

5.4 Conclusion

This chapter has examined the role of technology and industry in creating conditions in which new pathogens can emerge. The food processing and cooling and plumbing industries have been used to provide illustrative examples of the law of unintended consequences. New advances and changes in industrial processes can inadvertently create ecological niches which are eventually occupied by pathogens harmful to humans. In other chapters of this book, further examples of unintended consequences appear—for example, in Section 11.3.2, where vaccine failure led to 158 notified cases of paralytic and 46 cases of non-paralytic poliomyelitis. These side-effects of technological advances and industry are at best difficult to anticipate. They make the case for continual vigilance through surveillance and for predictive models which can provide early warning of problems, topics which we consider in Chapters 10 and 11.

Among the many technological advances which have facilitated the emergence of diseases, changes in transport technology stand supreme. In the last two centuries, journey times from one part of the world to another have collapsed so that now it is possible to circumfly the globe in less than two days. Since this is less than most disease incubation times, infected people can travel undetected from one continent to another, thus opening the potential for disease emergence in new locations. It is to the role of changing transport technology as an engine for disease emergence that we now turn in Chapter 6.

6

Population Changes: Magnitude, Mobility, and Disease Transfer

6.1 Introduction

The human population of the earth took the whole of its existence until 1800 to build to 1 billion. By 2000 it had exceeded 6 billion, more than doubling in the twentieth century alone. In 1800, the time taken to navigate the globe by sailing ship was about a year. Today, no two cities served by commercial aircraft are more than a couple of days apart. Since this is less than most disease incubation times, infected people can travel undetected—a concern noted from the early days of commercial air travel (Table 6.1). Within

Table 6.1. Travel times (days) by ship and air in relation to the incubation period of selected communicable diseases, 1933

Disease	Incubation period (maximum)	Infected countries trafficking with UK	Journey time to UK by sea	Journey time to UK by air
Plague	6	India	20	6
		Iraq	18	5
		Egypt	10	3
		East Africa	20	5
		West Africa	10	3
		South America	17	5
Cholera	5	India, Iraq	As above	As above
Yellow fever	6	West Africa, South America	As above	As above
Smallpox	14	India, Iraq, Egypt, West Africa, South America	As above	As above

Notes: All figures show that the incubation periods of the quarantine diseases were longer than journey times by air even in the early days of commercial air travel, thus permitting disease carriers to arrive infected but undetected at their destination. This was not the case for ships.

Source: Massey (1933: 6).

developed countries, the rate of individual circulation (in terms of average distances travelled) has increased 1,000-fold in the last 200 years.

While the processes of population growth and geographical churn have been at work for the whole of human history, it is in the last two centuries that the momentum of change has gathered increasing pace. As described in Section 2.1, McMichael (2004) recognizes four separate stages.

(i) Early human settlements from *c.*5,000 to *c.*10,000 years ago enabled enzootic pathogens to enter *Homo sapiens* populations. Some of these encounters led to the emergence of many of today's textbook infections: influenza, tuberculosis, cholera, typhoid, smallpox, measles, malaria, and many others.

(ii) Eurasian military and commercial contacts *c.*1,500 to *c.*3,000 years ago with swapping of dominant infections between the Mediterranean and Chinese civilizations. As described in Section 2.2, the plagues and pestilences of classical Greece and Rome date from this period.

(iii) European exploration and imperialism from *c.*1500 with the trans-oceanic spread of often lethal infectious diseases. The impact on the Americas, on Australasia, and on remote island populations is well known; ships' crews and passengers were the devastating vectors.

(iv) The fourth great transition is today's globalization, acting through demographic change and accelerating levels of contacts between the different parts of the world to facilitate disease emergence, re-emergence, and spatial transfer. Global warming, the destabilization of

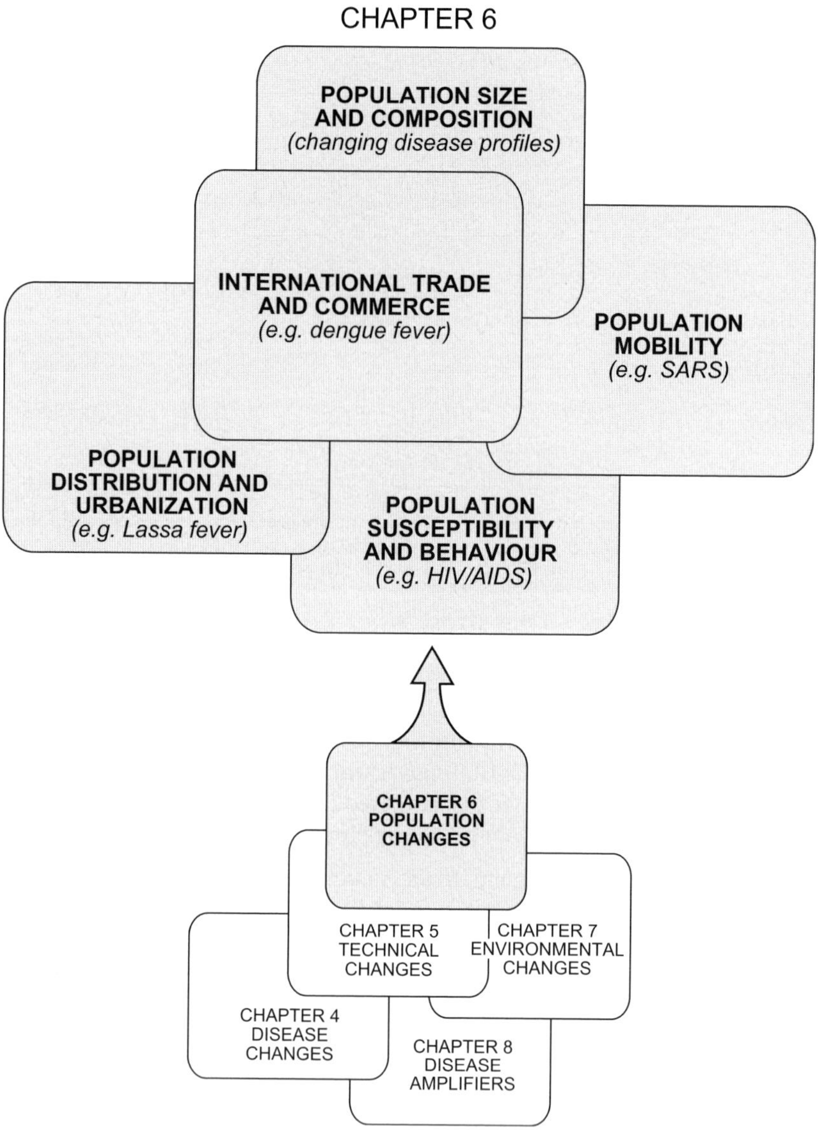

Fig. 6.1. (Upper) Venn diagram showing the facilitating factors for disease emergence and re-emergence associated with human demographic change
The lower diagram is redrawn from Fig. II.1 and shows the position of human demographic change (shaded box) within the suite of macro factors associated with the processes of disease emergence and re-emergence. SARS = severe acute respiratory syndrome.

environments, the unparalleled movement of peoples rapidly across the globe through air transport, are all part of an evolving host–microbe relationship (cf. Section 1.3.1).

In this chapter we look at the ways in which the rapid growth of the earth's human population and the accelerating collapse of long-distance geographical space have affected the emergence and geographical transfer of human infectious diseases. We look first in Section 6.2 at changes in the size and spatial concentration of the total population. Second, we look at the changes in its spatial mobility brought about by innovations in land and sea transport (6.3) and, crucially, in air transport (6.4). Figure 6.1 summarizes the facilitating factors for disease emergence and re-emergence associated with demographic change and travel.

6.2 Magnitude Changes in the Human Population

In this section we consider the manner in which the geography of the human population has changed over recent time. Emphasis is placed on (i) the way that population has arranged itself into ever-larger spatial clusters, (ii) how the distribution of these clusters across the world's land surface has shifted, and (iii) the epidemiological significance of these changes for disease emergence.

6.2.1 Changes in Cluster Size

The Neolithic revolution in agriculture 10,000–12,000 years ago is thought by archaeologists to be the key change which permitted the human population to live in permanent settled clusters rather than roaming in small bands, sustaining themselves by hunting and gathering. Over the succeeding millennia the total of *Homo sapiens* has increased by roughly three orders of magnitude from 10^7 to now approaching 10^{10}. The earlier totals are inevitably rough but a figure of 250 million humans at the start of the Christian Era, doubling to 500 million by AD 1650, would be widely supported. With the advent of national population censuses from the late eighteenth century, the world figures also become more reliable. The world total of 0.98 billion in 1800 had increased to 1.65 billion by 1900, and to 6.08 billion by 2000.

From the viewpoint of disease evolution, the changes in overall host totals, striking though they are, have less significance than the concentration of that population into a hierarchy of high-density clusters (villages, towns, metropolitan areas). The links between the growing size of human settlements and epidemic behaviour was investigated in a series of classic papers by the statistician Maurice Bartlett (Bartlett 1957, 1960*a*). He investigated the relationship between the periodicity of measles epidemics and population size for a series of urban centres on both sides of the Atlantic. His findings for British cities are summarized in Figure 6.2. The largest cities have an endemic pattern with periodic eruptions (Type I), while cities below a certain size threshold have an epidemic pattern with fade-out of infection between eruptions. Bartlett found the size threshold to be around a quarter of a million in (then) unvaccinated populations:

> The critical community size for measles (the size for which measles is as likely as not to fade out after a major epidemic until reintroduced from outside) is found for the United States to be about 250,000 to 300,000 in terms of total population. These figures agree broadly with the English statistics, provided notifications are corrected as far as possible for unreported cases. (Bartlett 1960*a*: 37)

A spatial version of this model is developed later in Section 10.2.

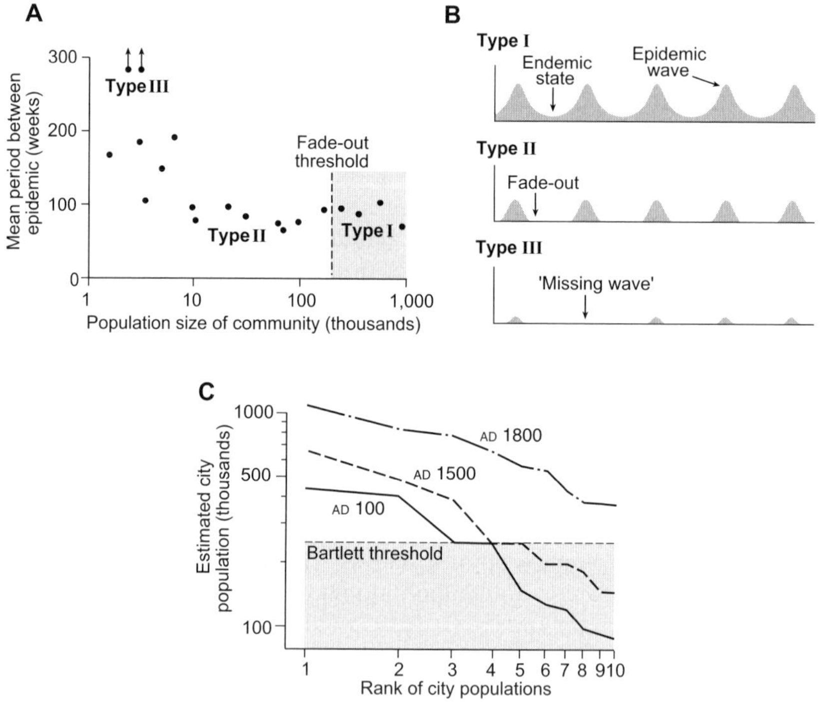

Fig. 6.2. Bartlett's findings on the epidemiological consequences of changing settlement size
(A) Relationship between the spacing of measles epidemics and population size for 19 English settlements. (B) Characteristic epidemic profiles for the three types indicated in A. (C) Log–log plots of estimated population size against rank for the largest 10 cities at AD 100, AD 1500, and AD 1800 in relation to the Bartlett threshold.

Sources: Haggett (2000, fig. 1.8, p. 23). Data on city population size in C based on tables in Chandler (1987).

Figure 6.2C plots the size distribution of the world's ten largest cities at a series of dates up to the present. Note that if both population size and rank are plotted on logarithmic scales, the distribution tends to form a characteristic Zipf curve (Haggett *et al.* 1977: 27–9). The population sum of the top 10 settlements rose from 1.8 million in AD 100 to 2.96 million by 1500, and 5.85 million by 1800. This threefold increase in the world's largest clusters over the period was over twice the rate at which world population as a whole increased; well before 1800, the urbanization trend had set in.

Subsequent research has shown that the threshold for measles, or indeed for any other infectious disease, is likely to be rather variable, with the threshold influenced by population densities and vaccination levels. But nevertheless, the threshold principle demonstrated by Bartlett remains intact (Cliff, Haggett, and Smallman-Raynor 2000: 85–118).

The impact of population growth in providing clusters in the host population where an infectious disease can be maintained endemically is illustrated in Figure 6.3 for a single country. This shows the growing number of cities within the conterminous United States that meet the 250,000–300,000 Bartlett threshold for measles endemicity over a 120-year period. In Map A, the number of cities in 1870 was only six, four along the Atlantic seaboard plus Chicago and St Louis in the Midwest. Subsequent maps show the steady growth in number and geographical spread at intervals of roughly a human generation (30 years). By 1990 (Map E) the number had increased 10-fold to 63 and the geographical spread was coast to coast with heavy concentrations in the southern states. The American story of increasing numbers of 'endemic cities' is repeated worldwide, and they have also shifted in location; it is that spatial shift to which we now turn.

6.2.2 Geographical Shifts in Clusters

Thanks to the work of the United Nations Population Bureau, it is possible to track with some confidence the global pattern of urban growth. International comparison of cities is notoriously difficult (see the arguments in Frey and Zimmer 2001). Despite some heroic attempts to provide standard definitions (e.g. Davis 1969), and the growing role of remote-sensing and Geographical Information Systems (GIS) in defining urban settlements more precisely, the task of establishing useful urban comparators from one country to another remains a contested enterprise. The results presented here are thus inevitably best estimates.

The spatial distribution of the world's largest cities over recent decades is shown in Figure 6.4. Each dot on the world map represents a massive human settlement, a city or metropolitan area with a population estimated to be not less than 5 million people (i.e. 20 times greater than the measles threshold used on the United States maps in Figure 6.3). The maps show the growth of the urbanized world at four cross-sections over a 60-year period, 1955–2015.

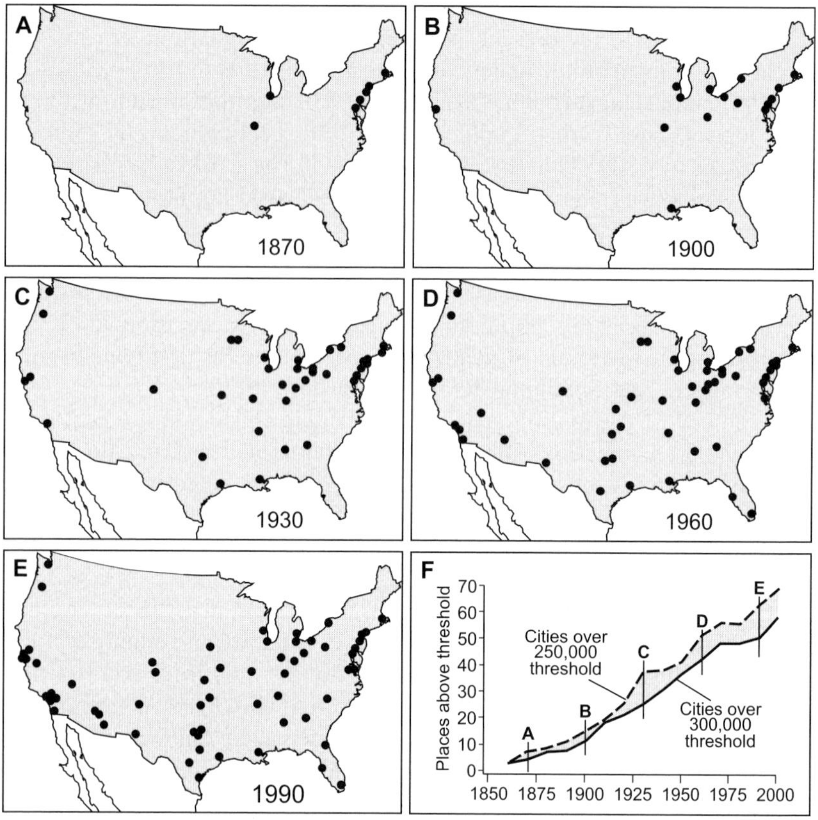

Fig. 6.3. Changes in the number of settlements meeting the Bartlett threshold for measles endemicity in the conterminous United States
(A)–(E) Maps at 30-year intervals over the period 1870–1990. (F) Graph of changing number of cities meeting the threshold, 1850–2000.
Source: 'United States Bureau of the Census: Tables for Population of the 100 Largest Urban Places, 1850–1990', in Gibson (1998).

Just after World War II, the world had only 11 of these megacities. As Map A indicates, they were predominantly Northern Hemisphere and mid-latitude in location, with Tokyo, Japan (13.7 million), as the largest. Together the megacities totalled 80 million and made up less than 3 per cent of an estimated world population of 2.7 billion.

Over the next 20 years the 1975 pattern shifted only a little (Map B with 18 megacities and a combined population of 170 million). There had been especially high growth in Latin America and South Asia. By 1995, the number of megacities had doubled in number (Map C) and the total population in them had also doubled to 343 million. Again, growth was especially

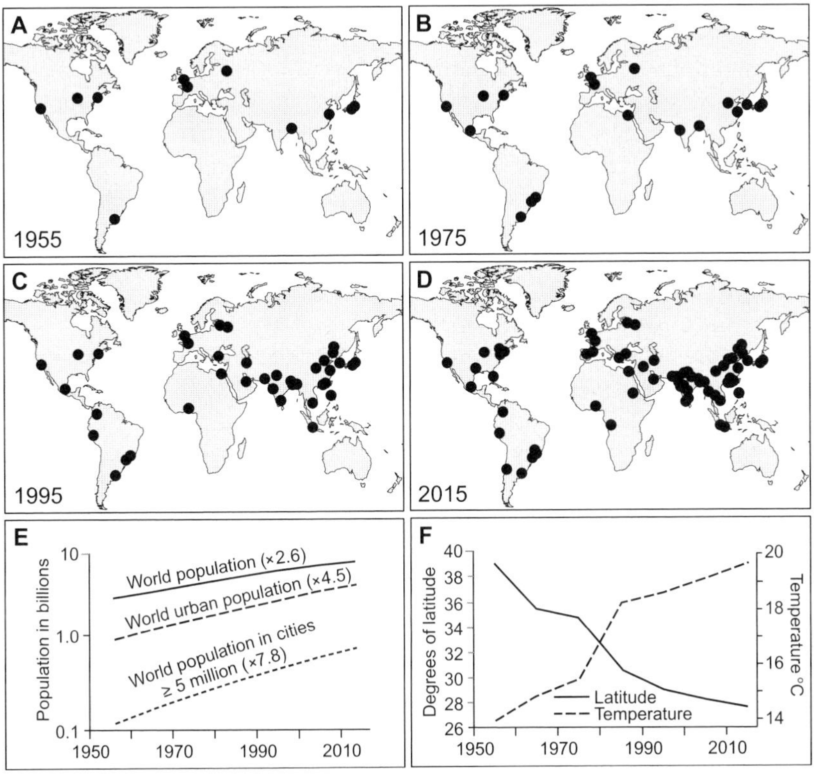

Fig. 6.4. Global changes in the world distribution of megacities
Maps A–D show the location of cities with 5 million or more inhabitants in 1955, 1975, 1995, and 2015. (E) Graph of population changes over the period 1955–2015. (F) Graph of changes in the average location of megacities in terms of latitude and temperature over the period.
Source: Data on city sizes from United Nations Population Division.

rapid in Latin America, but now Africa, India, and China were also expanding very quickly. Growth in megacities has continued apace since 1995. The world passed the 50 cities mark in 2005, and it is well on track to have 60 such cities by 2015 (Map D). Together they will have a combined population of 624 million, comprising 8.6 per cent of an estimated global population of 7.2 billion. In other words by 2015, one in eleven of the world's people are expected to live in one of its megacities.

The changes over the 60 years are shown in a time framework in Figure 6.4E. The number of megacities increased × 5.5, but their combined population increased × 7.8 while the world's urbanized population grew × 4.5, and the total world population × 2.6. The last three indicators are plotted on a logarithmic scale in Figure 6.4E, so that the three trend lines show how the world is not only growing and becoming ever more urbanized—but even more metropolitanized as that urban population crowds into ever larger agglomerations of 5 million or more people.

From an epidemiological viewpoint the most striking trends are shown in the last graph, Figure 6.4F. This looks at the shifting pattern of megacities in terms of their changing geography as measured by latitude and average year-round temperature. On latitude, megacities range from St Petersburg, Russia (60°N), as the most poleward, to Jakarta, Indonesia (6°S), as the most equatorward. Over the 60 years, the average location of megacities has shifted equatorwards by 11 degrees of latitude, from 39° (equivalent to that of Madrid) to 28° (that of Delhi).

If we now take the average temperature of cities over a year, this ranges from Moscow, Russia (4°C), to Khartoum, Sudan (29°C). Over the 60 years, the average for all megacities has shown an increase of 5.7°C—from 13.9°C (typical of Istanbul, Turkey) in 1955 to 19.6°C (typical of Lima, Peru) by 2015. To put this in a global perspective, this shift of nearly 6°C needs to be seen against the global warming trend over the same period of about 0.5°C. In other words, the relative geographical shift in population has outpaced global warming some 12-fold as a source of 'population warming'.

6.2.3 Implications for Disease Emergence

One implication of the above findings is that the battle against epidemic diseases will be increasingly fought in urban (and tropical urban) rather than rural arenas. But the disease implications of urbanization are complex. Positive effects from improved sanitation or better access to healthcare facilities have to be set against the negative effects from increased risk of disease contacts through crowding and pollution. Where rural–urban migration in developing countries results in peri-urban shanty settlements, then high rates of intestinal parasitic infections (notably amoebiasis and giardiasis) can result. Each is passed from human to human by the faecal–oral route. They pose an increasing health burden as the share of urban populations in developing countries rises towards one half of all population.

In the last four decades, the world's population has more than doubled. But that fast growth has largely occurred in developing countries still on Stage II to III of the demographic cycle. Figure 6.5A plots as a histogram the present latitudinal distribution of population along a pole-to-pole latitude continuum. It shows a marked concentration in the northern mid-latitudes. But that situation is changing. It is expected that some 94 per cent of population growth over the next 20 years will occur in the developing countries (Figure 6.5C). Present and future growth will shift the balance of world population towards the tropics and low latitudes with their wider range of diseases.

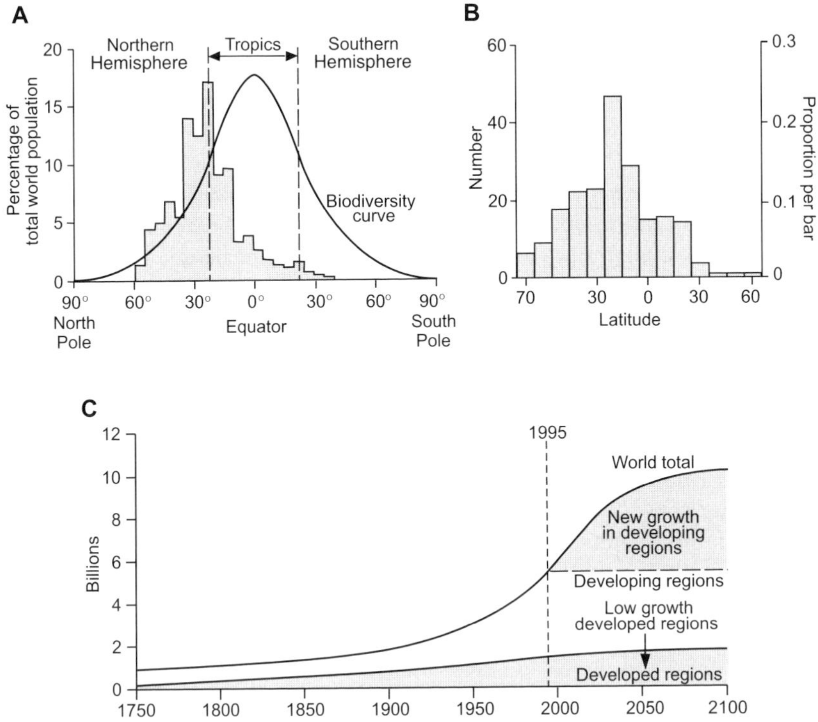

Fig. 6.5. Global population growth in relation to latitude
(A) Geographical distribution of population (shaded histogram) by 5-degree latitudinal bands north and south of the Equator. The biodiversity curve is approximate and does not make allowance for the global distribution of humidity. (B) Latitudinal variation in the number of infectious diseases. (C) Course of global population growth for the period from 1750 projected forward to 2100.
Sources: Haggett (2000, fig. 3.7, p. 85); Cliff, Haggett, and Smallman-Raynor (2000, fig. 7.1, p. 296).

This redistribution will also increase the average temperature of the global population by around +1°C, from 17°C to 18°C (even assuming no increase from global warming). This concentration will place more people than at any time in the world's previous history in areas of high microbiological diversity, potentially exposing a greater share of the world's population to conventional tropical diseases. In a previous study, we investigated the latitudinal distribution of infectious diseases as recorded by Wilson (1991) in her monumental *World Guide to Infections* (Cliff, Haggett, and Smallman-Raynor 2000: 294–301). From the records there we constructed a matrix of 269 infectious diseases recorded across 205 countries. Figure 6.5B plots the number of infections by 10-degree bands of latitude to give a curve paralleling the more generalized biodiversity curve in (A).

This biological diversity of viruses and bacteria is partly temperature-dependent, and it is much greater in lower latitudes than higher latitudes. Conditions of higher temperature would favour the expansion of malarious areas, not just for the more adaptable *Plasmodium vivax* but also for *P. falciparum*. Rising temperatures might also allow the expansion of the endemic areas of other diseases of human importance: these include, for example, leishmaniasis and arboviral infections such as dengue and yellow fever. Higher temperatures also favour the rapid replication of food-poisoning organisms. Warmer climates might encourage the number of people going barefoot in poorer countries, thereby increasing exposure to hookworm, schistosome, and Guinea worm infections. But not all effects would be negative. Warmer external air temperatures might reduce the degree of indoor crowding and lower the transmission of influenza, pneumonias, and 'winter' colds.

It is important to be cautious in interpreting the implications between climate factors and human disease, and we examine this link in some detail in Section 7.5. Here we note that McMichael *et al.* (2004) have conducted an exhaustive review of the impact of global warming as part of a WHO study on the quantification of health risks. They estimate a small proportional decrease in cardiovascular and respiratory disease mortality attributable to climatic extremes in tropical regions and a slightly larger benefit in temperate regions caused by warmer winter temperatures. They see an increase in mortality from diarrhoeal diseases and relatively large changes in the risk of falciparum malaria on the edge of the current distribution.

6.3 Changes in the Spatial Mobility of Human Populations I: Seaborne and Overland Movements

In the next two sections, we try to establish the main trends in the contraction of geographical space brought about by the changing patterns of travel. For both the conventional technologies of water-based and land-based travel (Section 6.3) and for the new technology of mass air travel (Section 6.4), we look first at the nature of these changes and then at their impacts on disease invasion and spread. As with the demographic changes, we touch only briefly on long-term historical changes (important though they were in the first three of McMichael's transitions discussed above) and concentrate on examples from the last two centuries.

6.3.1 Seaborne Movements

For most of human history, long-distance travel, whether within countries (using streams and rivers, later canals, and coastal shipping) or between continents (using seaborne shipping), was dominantly water-dependent. Inland waterways were the channels through which European explorers and traders brought in common infectious diseases; Ray's (1974) study of the role of fur traders in Canada from the seventeenth century on is a classic example. Away from navigable streams, travel overland up to the railroad revolution of the nineteenth century was slow and costly by comparison. We therefore take sea transport first and look briefly at the nature of the changes in sea transport since 1800 and then at their epidemiological impact.

NATURE OF THE CHANGES

The succession of technological changes in ships which generally made them faster, larger, and safer has been summarized by Fletcher (1910) and Rowland (1970). For the nineteenth century the story is largely one of the development of steam navigation and its succession over sail. Although the practical use of steamships can be traced to the early years of the century, the prototypes were slow, inefficient, and largely designed for river and canal transport. A number of fundamental advances from 1860 increased dramatically the speed and efficiency of ocean-going steamers. These included the commercial adoption of the compound steam engine, the succession of steel over iron hulls, introduction of the screw propeller and production of twin-screw vessels, development of the triple expansion steam engine, and, from the 1890s, the steam turbine.

The impact of these improvements on voyaging times is shown in Figure 6.6. This plots the changes in travel times by sea over two major oceans. Graph A shows crossing times from Europe across the North Atlantic over a 120-year

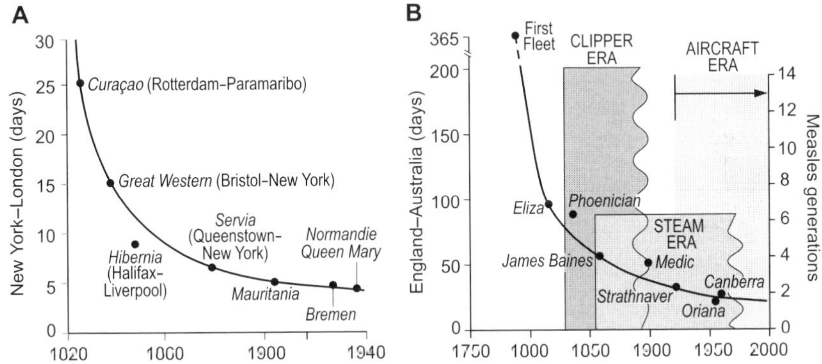

Fig. 6.6. Time changes in intercontinental travel by sea transport
(A) Transatlantic travel between Europe and North America, 1820–1940. (B) Travel between England and Australia, 1788–2000. The solid lines show the exponential decline in travel times. A measles generation is defined as 14 days.
Sources: Davies (1964, fig. 91, pp. 508–9); Cliff and Haggett (2004, fig. 1A, p. 89).

period. A three-week journey by sailing ship in 1820 had been reduced to a four-day crossing by passenger liner by 1940. Graph B shows the time in days for sea travel from Britain to Australia from the sailing of the First Fleet in 1788. The vertical axes of the graph have two scales, measuring travel times in days (left-hand vertical axis) and—as an epidemiological exemplar—measles generations (right-hand vertical axis). We define a measles generation (or serial interval) as 14 days, the average time between the observation of symptoms of measles in one case and the observation of symptoms in a second case directly infected from the first.

The solid lines on both graphs in Figure 6.6 depict an exponentially declining trend in voyage times. As the early decades of the nineteenth century passed, so the size and speed of ships on both routes increased. On the England–Australia run, the periods encompassing the clipper era (1830s–1890s) and the steam era (from the 1850s) are indicated for reference. By 1840, clippers had reduced the voyage time to 100 days, and, by the first decade of the twentieth century, steamers had halved the voyage time again. In terms of measles virus generations, the reduction was from six to three, greatly increasing the chance of infections surviving on board and of infectives causing outbreaks in Australia.

The breakdown of Australia's epidemiological isolation has been studied in great historical detail by Australia's pioneering Director of Health J. H. L. Cumpston, for influenza (Cumpston 1919), diphtheria, scarlet fever, measles, and whooping cough (Cumpston 1927), and for intestinal infections and typhus fever (Cumpston and McCallum 1927). Australian trends over the next four decades for a still wider set of infections were studied by H. O. Lancaster (Lancaster 1967, 1990).

EPIDEMIOLOGICAL IMPACTS OF SEA TRAVEL

Medical literature abounds with examples of the ways in which infectious diseases were shared as sea travel expanded. Increasing contacts with the Levant at the time of the Crusades, the New World contacts following the Columbus voyages, and Muslim pilgrimages to Mecca in the nineteenth century all brought major consequences for disease distribution. In the nineteenth century the exponential growth in international shipping and the technological changes which allowed greater speed and size in ocean-going vessels greatly increased the risks from ship-imported diseases. In the United States, the fear lead to the passing of the 1878 Quarantine Act, specifically 'An Act to Prevent the Introduction of Contagious or Infectious Diseases into the United States'. The statistical records which sprang from this Act and the network of surveillance reports from United States consulates in port cities overseas have been studied in Cliff, Haggett, and Smallman-Raynor (1998). Case studies of disease imports from international shipping abound for a wide range of infectious diseases. Here we select just two widely spaced in both space and time: (i) measles imports into Fiji from the late nineteenth century and (ii) cholera into the Andaman Islands in the early years of the present century.

Measles Invasions of Fiji (1879–1920)

The history of the first importation of measles into Fiji in January 1875 and the devastating impact on the native population over the ensuing six months is one of the classic cases of a 'virgin-soil' outbreak and has been widely studied (McArthur 1967; Cliff and Haggett 1985). In the anxious years that followed, the islands provided what was essentially a test case in the use of quarantine to prevent further invasions of the measles virus (cf. Section 11.2).

Fijian sugar plantations provide an example of the way in which a change in transport technology—from sailing ship to steamship—brought about the end of natural isolation as a defensive barrier to disease importation. In the late nineteenth century, Fiji in the Pacific was one of a series of tropical islands (others included Trinidad in the Caribbean and Mauritius in the Indian Ocean) whose climate and soils were ideal for growing sugar cane, a crop in soaring demand in Europe. But all three islands were short of suitable local labour. In the post-slavery period, the import of slave plantation labour from Africa was banned. A new source area (India) and a new form of bondage (indentured labour) provided a solution.

Between 1879 and 1920, Indian immigrant ships made 87 voyages to Fiji carrying nearly 61,000 indentured emigrants. The main routes followed are mapped in Figure 6.7A. This illustrates an important distinction between voyages by sailing ships (used between 1879 and 1904) and steamships (used between 1884 and 1916). To take advantage of prevailing winds, sailing ships followed the route south of Australia and took about 70 days for the voyage. Steamships used the more direct Torres Strait north of Australia and halved the sailing ship times; they were also able to carry a larger number of immigrants.

The health and welfare of the immigrants were the responsibility of the Surgeon-Superintendent who accompanied each ship and whose report was incorporated into the Annual Reports on Indian Immigration published regularly as official papers of Fiji's Legislative Council. These papers show how the transition from sail to steam dramatically altered the ways in which infectious diseases were transmitted between India and Fiji.

Since measles was an endemic disease in India, it is not surprising that cases were recorded on departure, although there were checks in the camps at both Calcutta and Madras (the two exit ports) before embarkation: the evidence in the Fijian annual reports shows a 1:3 probability of measles being detected on board on departure from India, and this proportion of 'infected' voyages remained constant over the period. These are shown in Figure 6.7B, in which each voyage is plotted in terms of the time taken and the passenger size of each vessel.

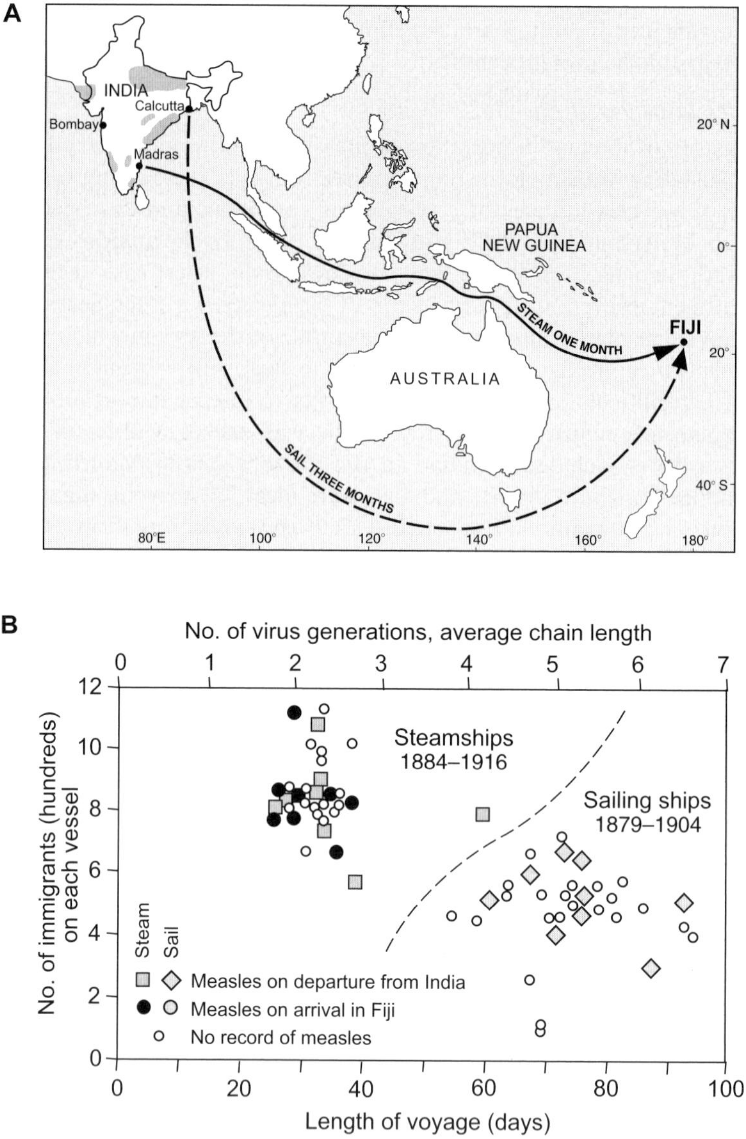

Fig. 6.7. Measles transfer from India to Fiji
(A) Routes from India to Fiji via sailing ships and steamships. (B) Vessels carrying indentured immigrants between India and Fiji, 1879–1916, categorized by length of voyage in days and in measles virus generations (14-day periods), type of vessel, and measles status.

Sources: Based on archival research by Cliff and Haggett (1985; see also 2004, fig. 4, p. 94).

For the smaller and slower sailing ships, around one-third of the vessels carrying labourers left India with infectives on board, but the measles virus did not survive the journey. By the end of the voyage those infected had either recovered or died and the long chain of measles generations needed to maintain infection (up to six on slower voyages) was broken. But for the faster and larger steamships, Figure 6.7B shows the situation was different. Ships on one in three voyages still carried infectives on departure and, in 11 instances, the virus continued to thrive on arrival in Fiji. The larger susceptible population and shorter travel times (as few as two generations on the fastest voyages) ensured the virus persisted to pose a potential threat at the receiving end. Only intensive quarantine guaranteed that the experience of the disastrous 1875 measles epidemic in Fiji was not repeated.

El Tor Cholera: Local Spread in the Andamans (2002)

Another island group presents an example of seaborne spread a century later. The Andaman and Nicobar Islands in the Bay of Bengal are sufficiently remote to have been missed by the seventh global cholera pandemic which swept from the island of Sulawesi in Indonesia and moved to affect the Indian subcontinent and later other countries in the third quarter of the twentieth century (see Section 9.2.2). But, in October 2002, an outbreak of diarrhoea (described by Sugunan *et al.* 2004) occurred in 16 of the 45 inhabited villages in the Nakowry island group (see Figure 6.8). It had an attack rate of 12.8 per cent and a case-fatality ratio of 1.3 per cent and was identified as the O1 El Tor strain of *Vibrio cholerae*. The tribal community in the Nancowry Islands lives in small villages along the shoreline. These villages are not connected to one another by road and, in most, the only access to transportation is by sea. The experience at Dering village, where the index case was a person who travelled to another village where the outbreak was ongoing, indicates that the movement of people between villages played a role in the spread of the infection.

The dates of onset of the outbreak are shown in Figure 6.8 for different villages in the three islands (Nancowry, Kamorta, and Trinket). The outbreak started at Tapong on 5 October, and, within the next few days, it spread to the villages on the northern part of Nancowry Island and then to villages on the southern edge of Kamorta Island. The outbreak then spread northward on both the eastern and western coasts of Kamorta Island.

No conclusive evidence on how the organism gained access to these remote islands could be obtained. One possibility is that the organism was introduced to the marine environment as a result of discharge of effluents from ships that sailed between Andaman and Nicobar and mainland India, as well as between the islands of the territory. It has been shown that *V. cholerae* El Tor can survive in untreated seawater for up to a week. McKarthy and Khambaty (1985) have shown that even ballast water carried by large ships may act as a vehicle of transmission of cholera across long distances. For

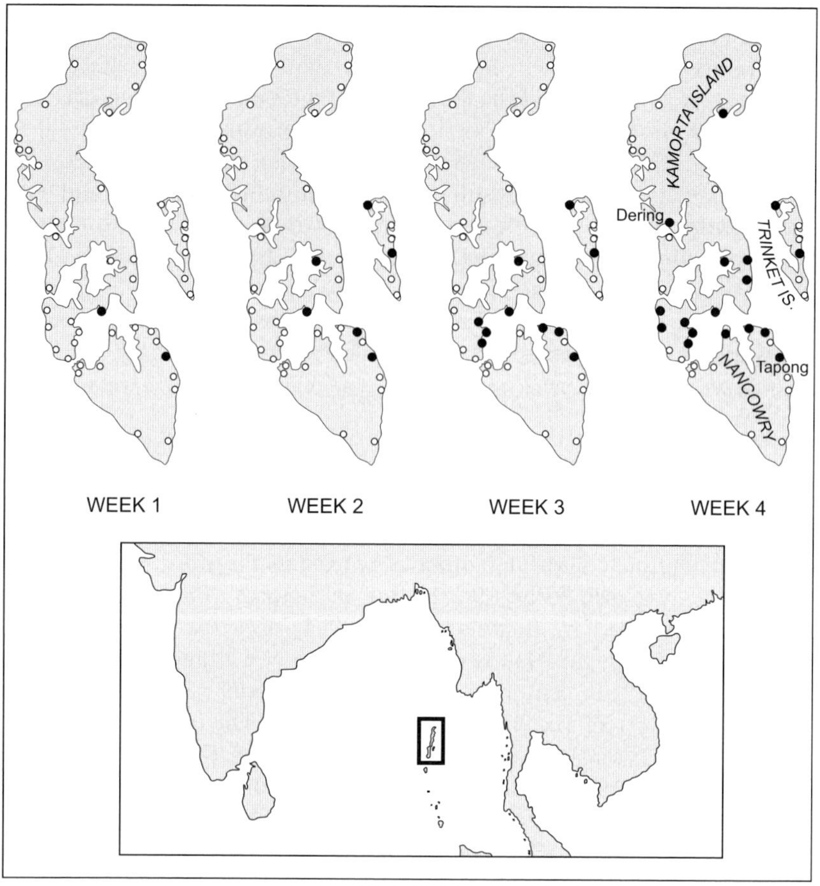

Fig. 6.8. Cholera epidemic in the southern Andaman Islands in 2002
The map sequence shows as black circles the week, measured from the start of the epidemic, in which the outbreak started in each village. Unaffected villages are shown as open circles.
Source: Adapted from Sugunan *et al.* (2004, figs 1 and 2, p. 823).

example, discharge of bilge water from contaminated long-distance ships was the probable cause for the introduction of cholera to the west coast of Latin America (Levine 1991). The pandemic potential of cholera is shown by this case; once reintroduced on that continent in 1991 after a century of absence, it caused more than 1 million cases in the next four years.

Shipboard Epidemics

Not only have ships historically transported diseases between places, but they can also be foci of on-board disease outbreaks. In the latter half of the twentieth century, passenger and cruise ships have achieved some notoriety in this regard, particularly for foodborne infections. The intermingling of passengers and crew, often from several nations, for extended periods of time in semi-enclosed environments presents an especial risk for infection. Shipboard activities increase the level of contact between passengers and crew. Shared sanitation facilities, exposure to common food and water supplies, the chance of legionella-contaminated air conditioning systems and other water sources, and the onshore consumption of food under conditions of low food safety standards, all add to the disease risk. The demographic profile of passengers on cruise ships, including a preponderance of the elderly and others with underlying health problems, also serves to enhance the likelihood of outbreaks (Miller, Tam, *et al.* 2000; Rooney *et al.* 2004; Ferson and Ressler 2005). By way of illustration, we look first at US and then at international data.

United States: EIS outbreak investigations. The histogram in Figure 6.9 plots the annual count of outbreak investigations on passenger and cruise

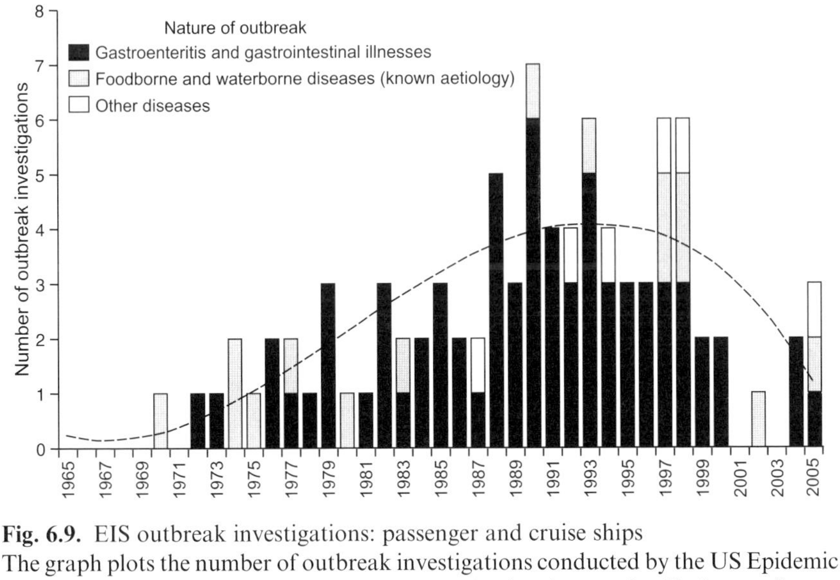

Fig. 6.9. EIS outbreak investigations: passenger and cruise ships
The graph plots the number of outbreak investigations conducted by the US Epidemic Intelligence Service (EIS) by year, 1965–2005. Outbreaks are classified according to EIS report titles as (1) gastroenteritis and gastrointestinal diseases, (2) foodborne and waterborne diseases of known aetiology (cyclosporiasis, *Escherichia coli*, hepatitis, shigellosis, salmonellosis, staphylococcal food poisoning, and typhoid fever), and (3) other diseases (legionellosis, rubella, tuberculosis, and varicella). A polynomial trend line, fitted to the data by ordinary least squares, is shown for reference.

Source: Drawn from the inventory of epidemic assistance investigations (Epi-Aids) undertaken by the US Epidemic Intelligence Service.

ships undertaken by the US Epidemic Intelligence Service (Section 3.4), 1965–2005. Of the 91 outbreak investigations included in Figure 6.9, the overwhelming majority (85) were associated with gastroenteritis and gastrointestinal illness, including foodborne and waterborne diseases of specified aetiology (shaded bars). The balance consisted of outbreaks of legionellosis, rubella, and tuberculosis (unshaded bars). Overall, the graph depicts a rising trend in the number of outbreak investigations in the 1970s and early 1980s, reaching a peak in the late 1980s and early 1990s. Recent work by CDC's National Calicivirus Laboratory suggests that the data may seriously underestimate the actual number of cruise ship outbreaks.[1] As Rooney *et al.* (2004) observe, the factors that contribute towards cruise ships as sources of foodborne outbreaks include: (i) large quantities of raw food from a variety of sources (depending on ports of call), (ii) centralized preparation and serving of meals, (iii) increased varieties of food used, and (iv) a rapidly changing workforce.

Gastroenteritis and the US Vessel Sanitation Program (VSP): Emergence of the recognition of norovirus as a cause of cruise-related gastroenteritis. In 1975, the Vessel Sanitation Program (VSP) of the National Center for Environmental Health, CDC, was established to assist the cruise ship industry in minimizing the risk of diarrhoeal diseases among passengers and crew sailing into the United States with ≥13 passengers. The programme includes twice-annual, routine unannounced inspections of ships with international itineraries that call at US ports. In association with the programme, the overall incidence of diarrhoeal disease on ships declined from 29.2 cases per 100,000 passenger days (1990) to 16.3 per 100,000 passenger days (2000). Outbreak-related diarrhoeal disease declined from 4.2 (1990–5) to 3.5 (1996–2000) per 100,000 passenger days. However, between 2001 and 2002, the annual count of gastroenteritis outbreaks increased from 2 to 29. Since then norovirus has emerged as a frequent cause of illness at sea (Widdowson, Cramer, *et al.* 2004; Isakbaeva *et al.* 2005; Cramer *et al.* 2006).

Foodborne disease outbreaks: International patterns, 1970–2003. Rooney *et al.* (2004) present an international review of 50 outbreaks of foodborne illness on passenger and cruise ships, 1970–2003. Of the 50 sample outbreaks, 44 were associated with cruise ships; one-fifth were reported on Caribbean cruise ships. The principal pathogens associated with outbreaks were *Salmonella* spp. (15 outbreaks), *Shigella* spp. (8), and enterotoxigenic *Escherichia coli* (8). The 50 outbreaks were associated with 10,000 hospitalized cases and one death. The principal food vehicles were seafood (14 outbreaks) and salad/buffet/fruit (7), with inadequate temperature control (7 outbreaks) and infected/suspected infected food handlers (5) as the main contributing factors.

[1] See <http://www.cdc.gov/mmwr/preview/mmwrhtml/mm5633a2.htm>.

6.3.2 Overland Movements

Until the coming of the railways in the early nineteenth century, transport overland was generally slow and costly. We look here at the changing role of land transport in disease transmission and give illustrative examples of the processes involved.

NATURE OF THE CHANGES

Some idea of the revolution in passenger travel overland is given in Figure 6.10. Graph A plots for the 300-mile distance between London and Scotland the reduction in travel time over two centuries. The 11-day stagecoach journey was progressively reduced as turnpike roads led to better surfaces. But it was not until 1850 that rail travel reduced the travel time to less than a day. A different order of geographical scale is analysed in graph B, the 3,000-mile transcontinental journey from the eastern to the western seaboard of the United States. Here, the 21-day stagecoach journey of 1850 was revolutionized by the completion of the transcontinental Union Pacific railroad in 1869. But it would be the 1930s before air travel (the Boeing 247) allowed the journey to be completed within a single day.

IMPACT OF LAND TRANSPORT CHANGES

Improvements in surfaces following toll road construction from the 1750s had only marginal effects upon the rate of disease spread when compared with a combination of coastal transport and subsequent riverine movements

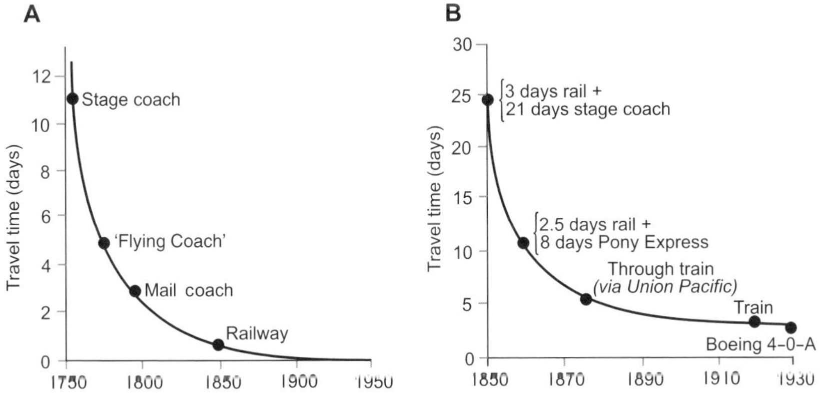

Fig. 6.10. Historical time changes in land transport at two geographical scales (A) London to Scotland, 1750–1950. (B) Transcontinental eastbound across the United States from New York to California, 1850–1930. The solid lines show the exponential decline in travel times.

Source: Based partly on Davies (1964, fig. 91, pp. 508–9).

into the interior of countries. From the mid-eighteenth century, rivers were reinforced by canal building in industrializing nations. But, despite the comparative slowness of overland movement, the tracks of imported diseases confirm that roads still played a central part in the spatial propagation of infection. Examples span the movement of bubonic plague from south coast ports into the heart of fourteenth-century England (Shrewsbury 1970) to the spread of AIDS along interstate highways in the United States (Gould 1993: 66–70) or along major trucking routes in East Africa (Smallman-Raynor, Cliff, and Haggett 1992: 152–3) at the end of the twentieth century. As illustrated later in Figure 7.6, logging roads cut into virgin tropical forest with subsequent pioneering farm settlement has been implicated in the spread of malaria through the Rondonia province of Brazil's Amazon basin (Mahar 1989). Examples of diseases being spread along the routes of railways abound. Railways across continental Russia allowed the 1889–90 influenza pandemic to spread rapidly from St Petersburg on the Baltic (October 1889) to Vladivostok on the Pacific (May 1890) (Clemow 1903). Similarly, rapid spread along railways was recorded for the same pandemic across the North American prairies, the South American pampas, and the Australian Murray–Darling basin. In each of these, railways had been constructed to exploit the rich grassland resources of a continental interior. Russian transcontinental railways were involved again in the huge typhus pandemics of 1918–22 in the Soviet Union.

We give here four examples of the transmission process which provide contrasts in disease, transport mode, geographical location, and historical time.

Cholera: Switch from Sea to Land Transport in the United States (1832–1866)

The nineteenth century saw six major pandemics in which cholera exploded from its base in the Indian subcontinent into other parts of Eurasia (Section 2.3.4). The increased volume of shipping and the falling travel times across the Atlantic made it all but inevitable that the United States and Canada would not escape the pandemics that were engulfing Europe. In fact they were affected by three, with the disease introduced in (i) June 1832 (a six-month-long outbreak), (ii) December 1848 (nine months), and (iii) May 1866 (five months). Pyle (1969) has plotted the progress of the three waves, city by city, charting the day of first reporting of the disease in each place. Over the 35-year period, the North American transport system was revolutionized, with canal transport being largely replaced by the rapidly expanding railroad system.

Figure 6.11A gives a generalized diagram of Pyle's results. Wave I (1832) had three spatial components, all involving water transport, (A) a Canadian pulse (starting in the St Lawrence Valley and moving via the Great Lakes), (B) an interior waterways pulse (starting at New York City and moving via the Hudson into the Ohio river system), and (C) a coastal waterways pulse (also starting at New York City but moving up and down the eastern

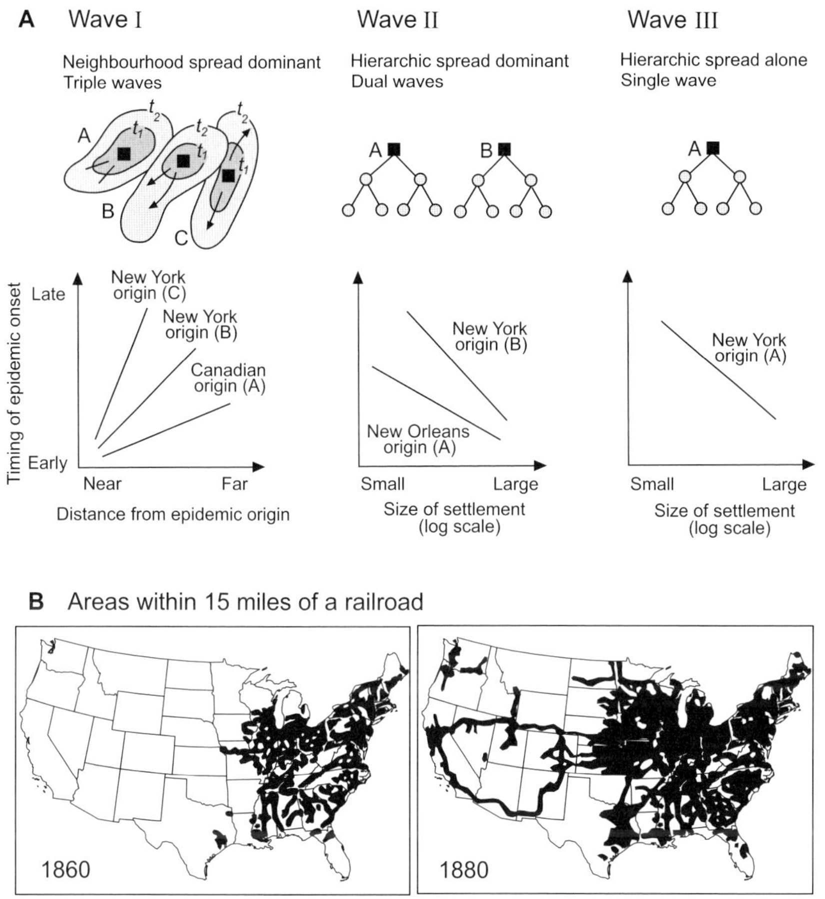

Fig. 6.11. Schematic diagram of Pyle's (1969) ideas on the changing spread of cholera in the United States, 1832–1866
(A) Wave I (1832) spread in three pulses mainly by contagious diffusion from two points of introduction. Wave II (1848–9) spread in two pulses mainly by hierarchical diffusion from two centres; it was reinforced by local contagious diffusion. Wave III spread in a single pulse by hierarchical diffusion from a single centre. (B) Areas (black) within 15 miles (24 km) of a railroad, 1860 and 1880.
Source: Cliff and Haggett (2004, fig. 6, p. 96).

seaboard). In contrast Wave II (1848–9) was also water-based but had a simpler twofold spatial structure: an interior waterways pulse based on cholera imported into New Orleans (A), and an eastern seaboard pulse fuelled by cholera imported into New York City (B). By the time of Wave III (1866), the pattern of spread was simpler still, with a single national system emanating from New York City (A).

Pyle was able to demonstrate that the shifts in the way cholera spread in the three epidemics reflected the evolving economic and political structure of the United States. The trend lines show the positive correlation between cholera arrival dates and nearness to the origins of the epidemic in Wave I (cities nearer to the origin recorded cholera first), the inverse correlation in Wave II between city size and outbreak timing (larger cities were hit first), although separate corridors of spread persisted, and the total dependence upon city size in the third wave. In the 34-year interval between the first and third cholera epidemics, the railroad mileage in the United States increased $\times 9$, with the wave of building pushing west of the Mississippi into the western states which showed a $\times 50$ increase in mileage over the same period (Modelski 1987; Figure 6.11B). As the railways (with their dominantly east–west grain) replaced the inland waterways (with their south–north grain) and the political economy became more integrated (a reunited United States replaced the Confederate South and Unionist North), so cholera diffusion became less dependent upon local and regional contact (transport) networks. Within three years the transcontinental network had linked the eastern US with California on the Pacific coast (the famous Golden Spike event at Promontory Summit, Utah, in May 1869); from now on disease spread would be ever more driven through intercity links in the urban metropolitan hierarchy.

Bubonic Plague: Railways and Spread in India (1897–1906)

The role of rail communication in the spread of bubonic plague in India at the turn of the twentieth century has been studied by Yu and Christakos (2006); see Figure 6.12. As described in Section 9.2.1, the onset of a century-long global pandemic of plague can be traced to China in 1855, but it was only after it reached the ports of Hong Kong and Canton in 1894 that it attracted international attention. Two years later it was introduced into Bombay, from which it spread inland 'like a cloud of varying size, depending on the geographical area' (Yu and Christakos 2006: 2).[2] As had happened in previous years, Bombay city suffered an epidemic attack during the spring. But the behaviour of Nagpur differed from that of its region. It held a key location as the capital of the Central Provinces and the major trade centre of middle India; it was then also one of the few cities connected with the Great Indian Peninsular Railway (GIP) system.

At this time, India was divided into two parts: (i) British India (Bombay Presidency, Punjab, United Provinces, Bengal Presidency, etc.) and (ii) the native Indian states (Hyderabad, Mysore, Central India, etc.). The GIP railway system offered good connections for most of British India but the native states were more difficult to reach. Yu and Christakos concluded that the prevailing transportation infrastructure provides some insight on why British India generally suffered more from bubonic plague than native India (compare Figures 6.12A and C). The railway also increased the speed of

[2] The cloud analogy aims to describe an epidemic propagation advancing but at the same time disappearing and reappearing in infected areas.

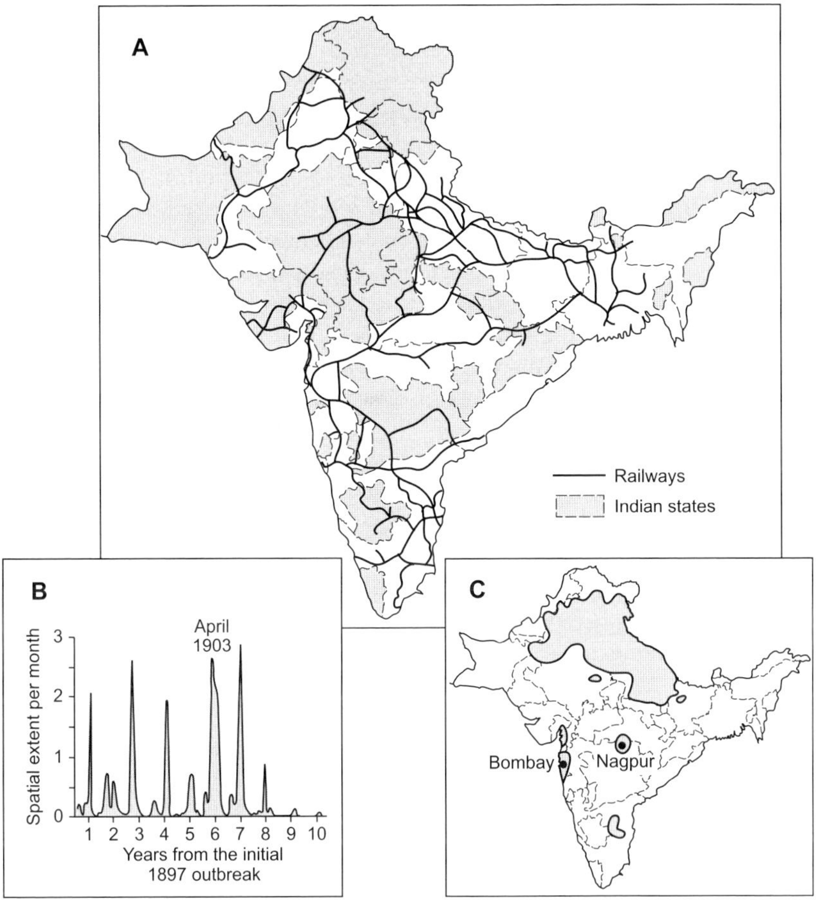

Fig. 6.12. The role of railways in the spread of bubonic plague in India
(A) Main routes of the Great Indian Peninsular Railway (GIP) in 1893 with native states shaded. (B) Time series of plague in India over the ten years from 1897. (C) Geographical distribution of the outbreak in Apr. 1903 (shaded areas), closely associated with the routes of the GIP serving British India.

Source: Adapted from Yu and Christakos (2006, figs 2, 5, pp. 3, 7).

spread of the bubonic plague during 1902–3. They instance the cases of Cawnpore (a railway junction in the United Provinces) and Bhagalpur (the administrative and marketing centre in Bihar, also with a railroad connection) as suffering more severely than the less accessible parts of the region.

Influenza: Railway Flows in France (1985)

Although rail transportation is often considered a nineteenth-century technology, it has continued as an organizing force in population interactions over medium distances. In 1988, a French group led by Flahault (Flahault,

Letrait, *et al.* 1988) utilized a model which we describe in Section 6.4.2 to simulate the spread of a 1985 influenza epidemic between 22 French metropolitan districts, using the mean annual passenger traffic flows by rail for 1972 to drive the diffusion process. Of the 231 potential links between the districts, flows on two-thirds were zero while at the other extreme two links (Paris: Centre and Paris: Haute-Normandie) each had over a million passengers.

The influenza parameters for the spread model were based on observations from 270 sentinel GP practices spread across France. These estimated a value of 0.55 for the contact rate (the number of people with whom an infectious individual will make contact daily, sufficient to pass infection) and 2.49 for the infectious period (the number of days in which the infective is able to make contact). The known spread of the 1985 influenza epidemic in France was compared with simulated spread. Since the location of the actual origin of the 1985 outbreak was unknown, the simulation assumed two simultaneous onsets in two separate locations (Aquitaine and Nord Pas-de-Calais).

Figure 6.13 shows the real and simulated patterns of outbreak for Weeks 7, 8, and 9 of the epidemic. The general shape of the two waves is consistent and in some cases the 'fit' between the epidemic curves for individual regions is rather close (e.g. for Auvergne and for Nord Pas-de-Calais). But in others the fit was rather poor, with the predicted peak occurring a month later than the real peak (Bretagne and Île-de-France).

Foot and Mouth Disease (FMD): Roads as Barriers at the Micro Scale to Disease Transmission in the UK (2001)

With the evident emphasis on roads and railways aiding and accelerating the rate of disease spread, it is worth noting that at the micro scale the reverse effect may occasionally be observed. Savill *et al.* (2006) studied the topographic determinants of foot and mouth disease (FMD) transmission in the UK 2001 epidemic using detailed tracking of vehicle, personnel, milk tankers, farm equipment, and livestock. They paid special attention to the geographical features that can act as barriers to FMD movement. These were found to include lakes, rivers, and estuaries but also major transport arteries (railway lines, motorways, and major arterial roads) across which infection between adjacent farms, but on opposite sides of the route, was highly unlikely. Crossing a motorway with cattle is illegal and the specially built cattle bridges

Fig. 6.13. Use of railway passenger data between 22 French metropolitan districts to calibrate flows in an influenza prediction model
(A) French metropolitan districts with the assumed locations of originating cases shown. (B) Comparison between observed and patterns estimated by simulation for weeks 7, 8, and 9 of the outbreak. Shading shows the number of cases per general practitioner. (C) Example of a fairly good fit to the observed epidemic curve (Auvergne) and a poor fit (Bretagne).
Source: Adapted from Flahault, Letrait, *et al.* (1988, fig. 2, p. 1151).

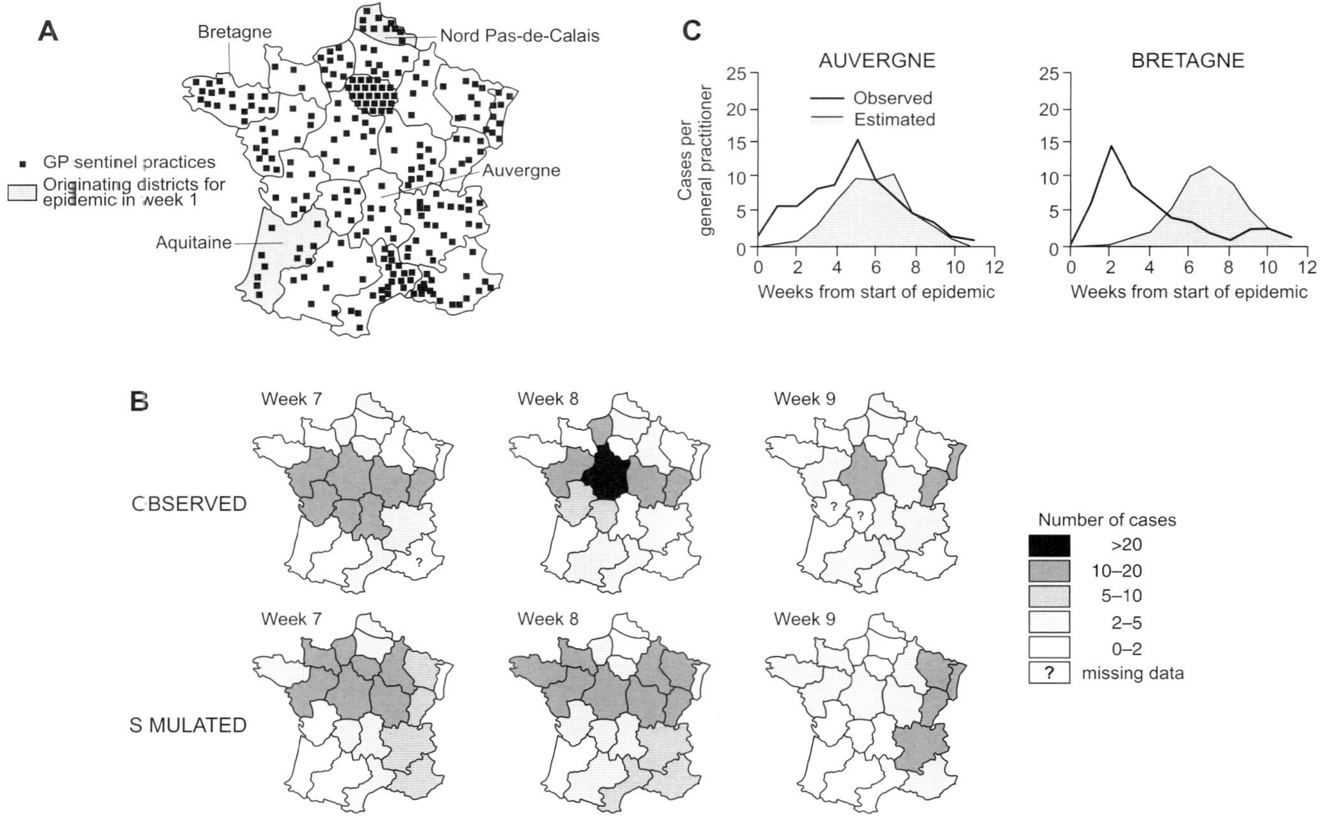
A
Bretagne
Nord Pas-de-Calais
GP sentinel practices
Originating districts for epidemic in week 1
Auvergne
Aquitaine
C
AUVERGNE
Observed
Estimated
Cases per general practitioner
25
20
15
10
5
0
0 2 4 6 8 10 12
Weeks from start of epidemic
BRETAGNE
25
20
15
10
5
0
0 2 4 6 8 10 12
Weeks from start of epidemic
B
Week 7
Week 8
Week 9
OBSERVED
?
Week 7
Week 8
Week 9
SIMULATED
Number of cases
>20
10–20
5–10
2–5
0–2
?
missing data

and tunnels were easily blocked. The study concluded that the dense network of minor roads facilitated spread except where farms were close to barriers.

6.4 Changes in the Spatial Mobility of the Human Population II: The Air Transport Revolution

Although the principles of 'heavier-than-air' flight had been worked out by Cayley by 1850 and the first experimental flights had been started by the Wright brothers by 1903, it was World War I that launched the air transport industry. Not only were aircraft used for military reconnaissance and conflict, but Britain, France, Italy, Germany, and Austro–Hungary each developed small airline networks for mail and movement of key personnel. The war had scarcely ended before the first civil mail networks were established in Europe and North America, and, within a decade, airlines were being pioneered on all continents and the first intercontinental air travel links were being forged. The history of this process is documented by Davies (1964). In this section we look at (i) the nature of air transport, (ii) its spatial representation through graph theory, and (iii) the epidemiological impact of air travel.

6.4.1 The Nature of Air Transport

If steamships accelerated global interaction in the second half of the nineteenth century, parallel inventions for aircraft were to do the same again in the second half of the twentieth century. Spurred on by the technological advances that accompanied World War II, notably the development of high-precision navigational aids and the gas turbine (jet) engine, passenger aircraft increasingly replaced ships as the international carrying medium. Figure 6.14 charts the decline in passenger flight times at two geographical scales. Graph A shows the change in transcontinental flight times across the United States (approximately 3,000 miles). A crossing which took two full days in the late 1920s had been reduced to half a day by 1960. Graph B shows even more striking changes in the 12,000-mile England–Australia run since 1925. In both cases the exponential decline in travel times is shown by a solid line, comparable in shape to the distance-decay curves for sea transport (Figure 6.6) and land transport (Figure 6.10).

Like travel times by sea, the graphs tell a similar story of exponentially diminishing journey times, with exponentially increasing speeds and growing carrying capacities. However, the collapse of geographical space has not been uniform. It is the distance between major centres, notably the world's great cities, that has been cut most dramatically. The ability of long-distance aircraft to 'overfly' intermediate locations (which previously served as necessary refuelling places along the route) has now made these places relatively

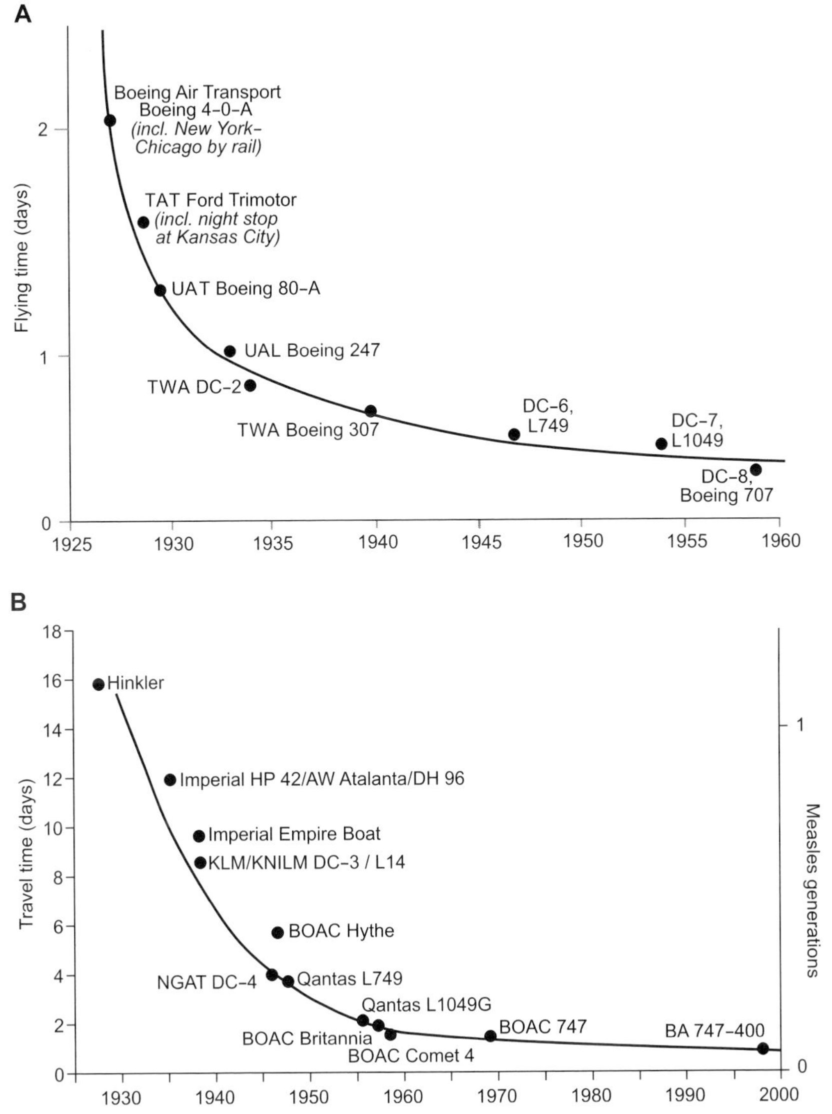

Fig. 6.14. Historic changes in travel times by air transport
(A) Transcontinental in the United States eastbound New York–California, 1925–60.
(B) Intercontinental between Europe and Australia, 1925–2000. The solid lines show the exponential decline in travel times. A measles generation is defined as 14 days.

Sources: Adapted from Davies (1964, fig. 91, pp. 508–9) and Cliff and Haggett (2004, fig. 1B, p. 89).

less accessible. Thus, the shrinking world is marked by (i) reducing travel times between major centres, balanced by (ii) unchanging or reducing accessibility for minor centres off the well-beaten transport tracks.

In addition to increased speed, the increasing size in terms of passenger numbers also needs to be taken into account. Bradley (1989) postulates a hypothetical situation in which the chance of one person in the travelling population having a given communicable disease in the infectious stage is 1 in 10,000. Assume that, with a 200-seat aircraft, the probability of having one infected passenger on board (x) is small, say 0.02, and the number of potential contacts (y) is 199. If we assume homogenous mixing, this gives a combined risk factor (xy) of 3.98. If we double the aircraft size to 400 passengers, then the corresponding figures are $x = 0.04$, $y = 398$, and $xy = 15.92$. In other words, *ceteris paribus*, doubling the aircraft size increases the risk from the flight fourfold, although in practice such probabilities would be modulated by the air circulation technology used. Thus, new generations of wide-bodied jets present fresh possibilities for disease spread, not only through their flying range and their speed, but also from their size.

A realistic example of the spread of SARS within an aircraft is given in Figure 6.15 based on research by Olsen, Chang, *et al.* (2003) and Whaley (2004). This shows the location of passengers on China Airlines flight 112 from Hong Kong to Beijing on 15 March 2003. The aircraft was a Boeing 737–300, which can typically carry up to 126 passengers; on this flight there were 112 with eight crew members. The 72-year-old index case, who had stayed at the Metropole Hotel in Hong Kong and was returning home, was unwell with well-developed SARS. Subsequent tracking confirmed that 22 fellow passengers and two crew members were infected by this index case, four of whom eventually died. WHO studies of other flights with SARS cases on board showed within-plane virus spread on only four of 35 flights, so CA 112 looks like an extreme event on the virus spreading scale.

The potential for rapid onward spread of the virus is underlined by the presence on Flight CA 112 of passengers going on to Taipei, Singapore, Bangkok, and Inner Mongolia. As Figure 6.16 shows, this onwards spread did occur, and, by May 2003, cases of SARS were occurring worldwide, driven by international air travel. The global pattern of cases and deaths by July 2003 is mapped in Figure 6.17.

6.4.2 Airline Links as Transmission Networks

The complex connection patterns provided by air transport have created ever more rapid and complete routes for disease transmission over long distances. We look here at the basic structure of such networks, the ways in which disease transmission has been modelled on them, and the increasing use of global airline networks for pandemic studies.

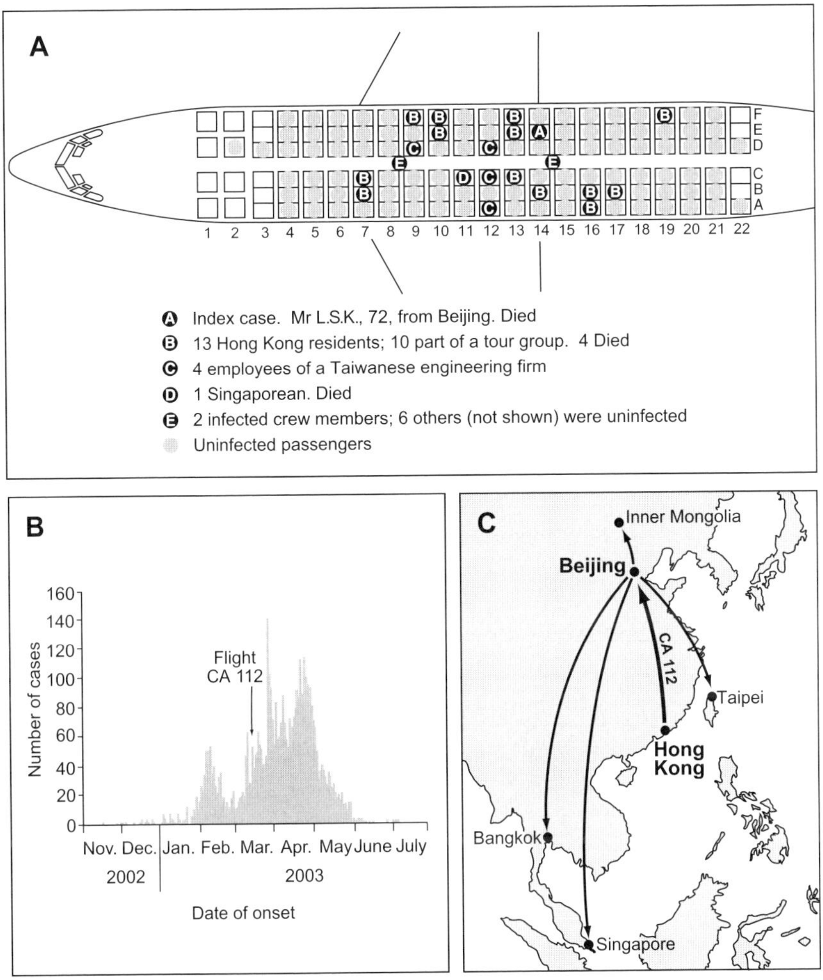

Fig. 6.15. Pattern of SARS spread, 2003, by aircraft
(A) Contacts within an aircraft cabin. SARS infections on flight CA 112 from Hong Kong to Beijing, 15 Mar. 2003. (B) SARS epidemic curve, Nov. 2002–July 2003 showing fuelling of the curve by flight CA 112 and its sequelae. (C) Subsequent movement of infected passengers.
Source: Whaley (2006, fig. 15.1, p. 150).

NETWORKS AS GRAPHS

The complexity of airline networks can be usefully approached through the branch of combinatorial mathematics termed graph theory. This treats a network as a topological graph made up of nodes (vertices), connected by links (edges). A very simple example is provided by Figure 6.18, which shows

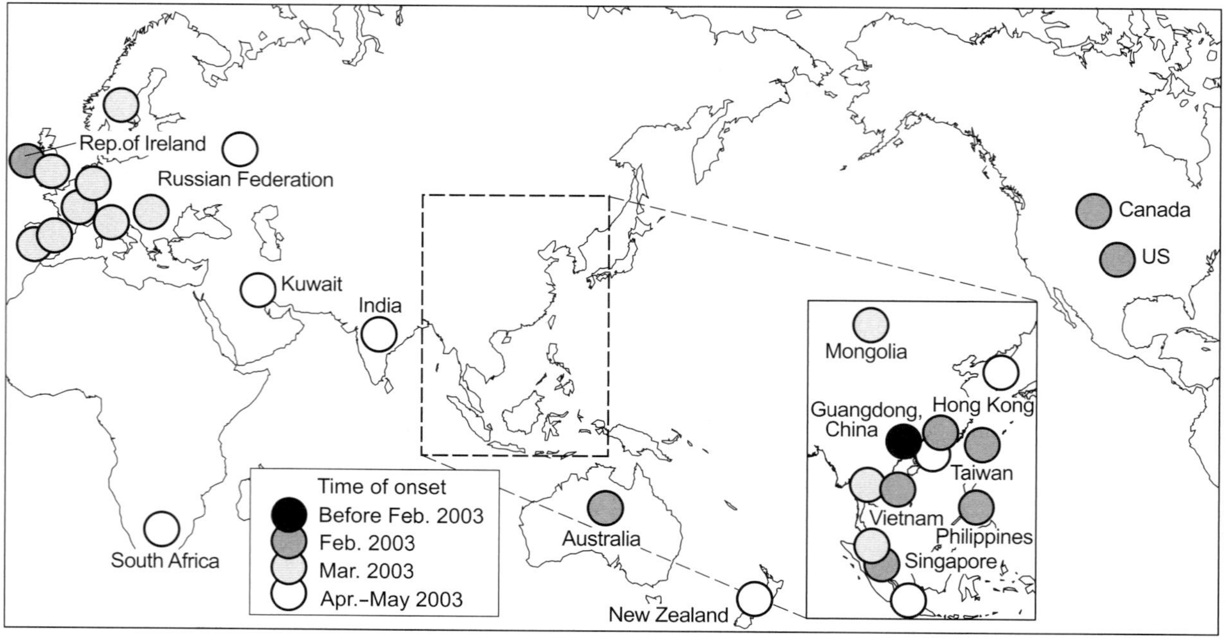

Fig. 6.16. Global spread of SARS, November 2002–May 2003
Sequence of appearance of probable SARS cases in 29 countries and major administrative regions, Nov. 2002–May 2003. Timings are based on the date of onset of the first recorded case in a given geographical area.

Source: Based on World Health Organization (2005*f*).

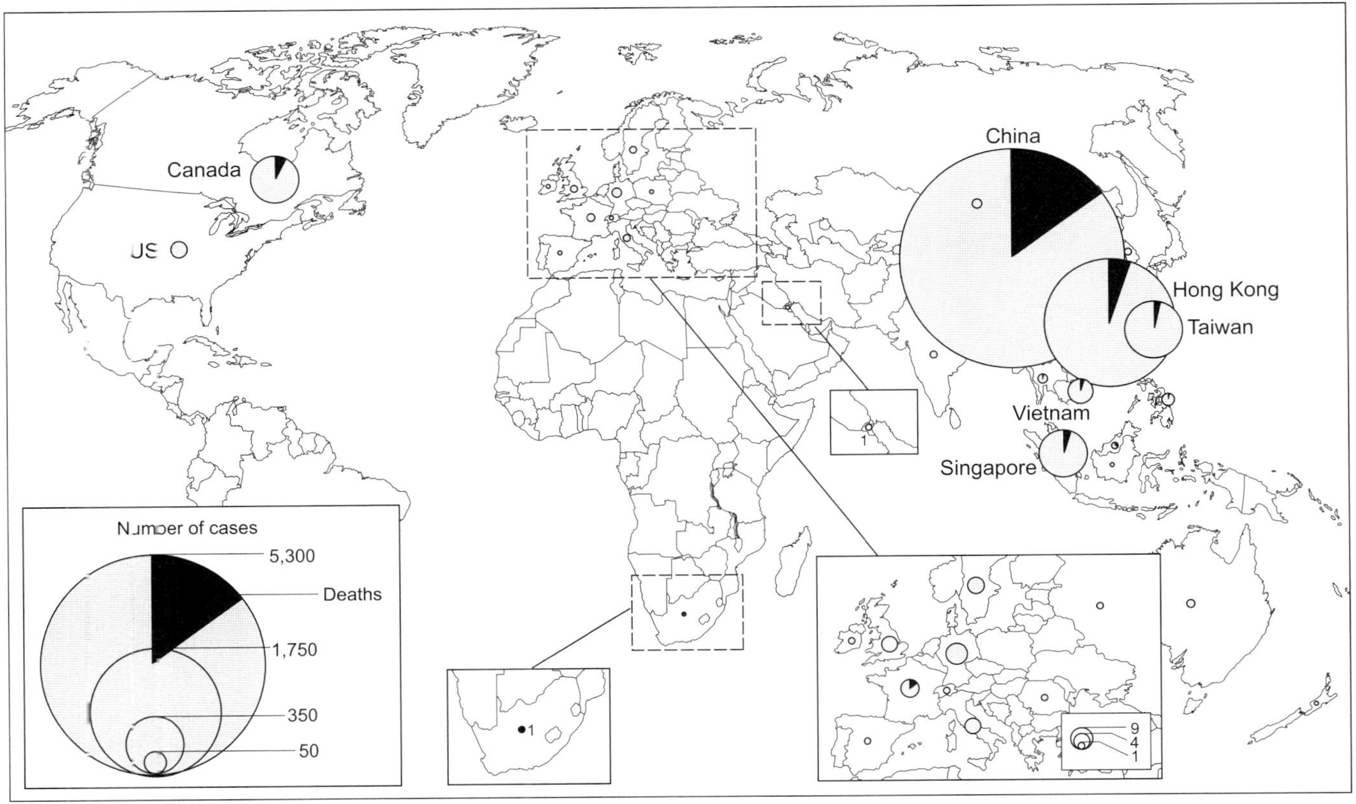

Fig. 6.17. Global distribution of SARS, 1 November 2002–31 July 2003
Circle areas are drawn proportional to the number of probable cases of SARS by country. Shaded sectors indicate, as a proportion of all probable cases, the number of SARS-related deaths.
Source: World Health Organization (2005*f*).

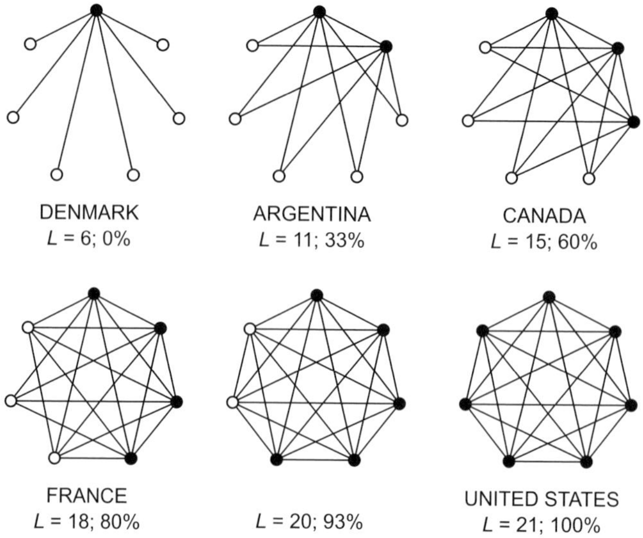

Fig. 6.18. Increasing connectivity of national airline networks
Nodes are the largest seven cities within the country while links are direct scheduled airline services between pairs of cities. Data are historical and show the position in 1978; since then, sample countries shown have tended to move towards fully connected networks on the United States pattern.
Source: Cliff, Haggett, and Ord (1979, fig. 13, p. 305).

a set of graphs, each made up of seven nodes. The number of links varies from $E = 6$ in the first graph (a minimally spanning tree) to $E = 21$ in the last (a fully connected graph), with intermediate graphs showing increasing stages of connectedness.

We can translate the abstract topology of the graphs into national airline networks by (i) equating the nodes to the largest seven cities in a given country and (ii) equating a link to a scheduled direct airline service. At the time of the study (Cliff, Haggett, and Ord 1979), Denmark had a minimal airline structure with all services centred on the capital city, Copenhagen, while the United States major cities were all fully connected. From an epidemiological viewpoint, it is important to note that airline development over time has progressively moved countries into increasingly connected structures where passenger movements (and thus micro-organism movements) have an ever greater valency, i.e. the range of directions in which rapid spread can occur has increased.

The basic measures for describing the connectedness of such networks and the centrality of individual nodes within them were developed four decades ago by Kansky (1963) and Haggett and Chorley (1969). The realization of the key role of graph networks as frameworks for studying disease transmission has led to a flurry of recent work revising and extending the early findings. Draief (2006) has provided a review of probabilistic work of epidemic flows on complex networks and has confirmed the effect of topology on the spread of epidemics. In Europe, Barrat *et al.* (2004) have provided metrics for analysing weighted networks (weighting of both nodes for flow generation and links for flow capacity), linking these to the basic topological complexity of the network. The vulnerability of weighted networks and defensive strategies for network interruption (potentially a part of a global pandemic spread initiative) has also been studied by Dall'Asta *et al.* (2006). In North America, similar work by Guimera *et al.* (2005) has concentrated on identifying the varying centrality of nodes within the network and the contrasting transmission roles of different global cities.

DISEASE TRANSMISSION MODELLING ON SMALL NETWORKS

One breakthrough in modelling disease spread through networks came from Russia in the 1970s with the work of Baroyan and Rvachev on influenza outbreaks. They modified the susceptible–infected–removed (SIR) model, which we discuss later in Section 10.2, to incorporate geographically separate areas (i and j) linked by a migration or traffic term (M_{ij}). The earliest study analysed the spread of influenza from Leningrad to five other Russian cities, comparing predicted with observed daily influenza morbidity. The original Russian work is difficult to consult, but a summary is provided in Cliff, Haggett, and Ord (1986: 35–44).

A further step came in joint work with Longini in the United States (Rvachev and Longini 1985), extending the applications to a larger canvas of 52 major cities with a worldwide distribution (Figure 6.19A). They modelled retrospectively the global spread of a new strain of influenza (H3N2) from its 1968 Hong Kong origin to major cities in other parts of the world. This virus type spread around the world in less than two years, and the underlying assumption was that air travel was the main route of international dispersion.

The general contours of predicted pandemic spread are shown in Figure 6.19B. Most cities were forecast with some accuracy in that their actual peak morbidity came within a month of the predicted peak. One city (Tokyo) was under-predicted in that the peak came more than a month before its predicted timing; conversely, five cities were over-predicted in that the peak came more than a month after its predicted timing (Caracas, Lima, Santiago, Cape Town, and Warsaw).

The Rvachev–Longini model has been further extended by Flahault, Deguen, *et al.* (1994) in a study of potential influenza spread between a small network of west European cities (Amsterdam, Berlin, Budapest, Copenhagen, London, Madrid, Milan, Paris, and Stockholm). Model parameters were estimated from French data. The location of the cities is

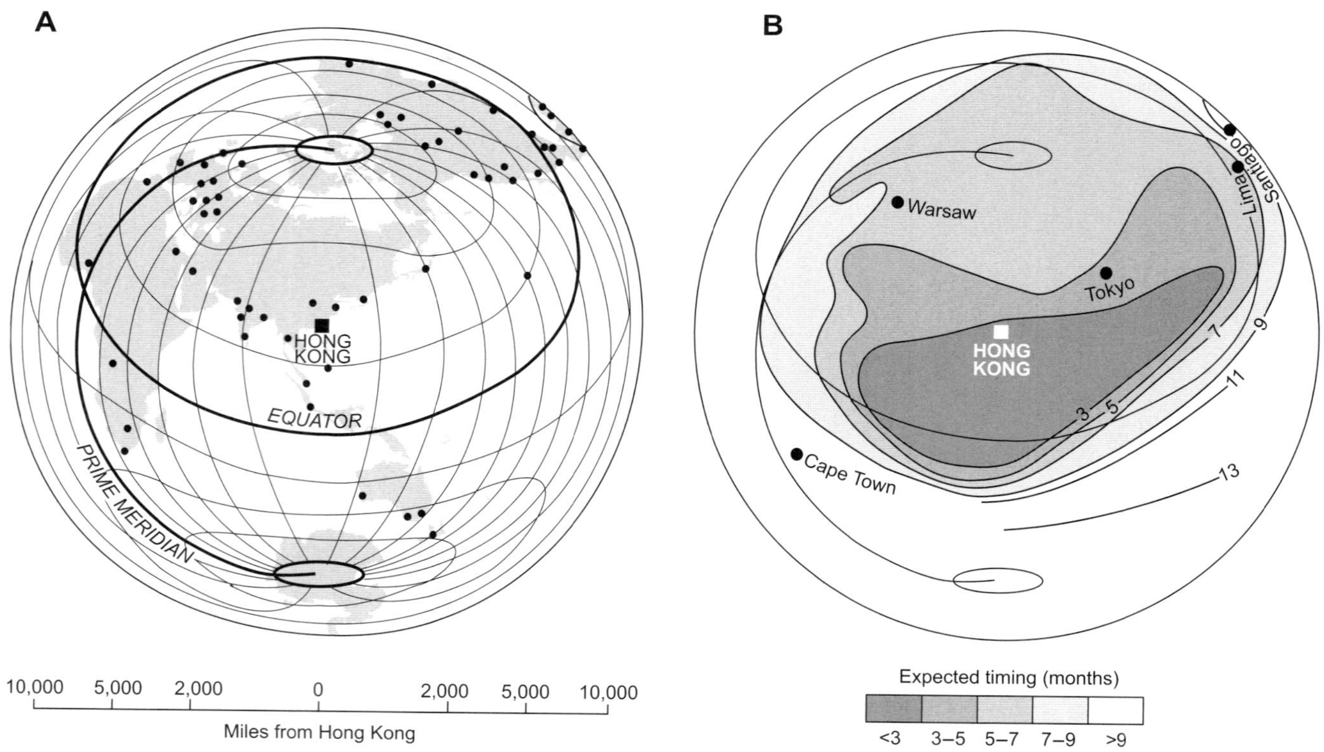

Fig. 6.19. Rvachev–Longini model of the global spread of Hong Kong influenza (1968–1969) by air transport (A) Location of world cities included in the model. (B) Isochrone map of predicted timing of the peak of the influenza pandemic in months from the start of the outbreak where Hong Kong is $t = 0$. Cities referred to in the text are labelled. Both world maps are drawn on an azimuthal projection centred on Hong Kong with distances measured on a logarithmic scale.

Source: Cliff, Haggett, and Ord (1986, fig. 2.15, pp. 41–2).

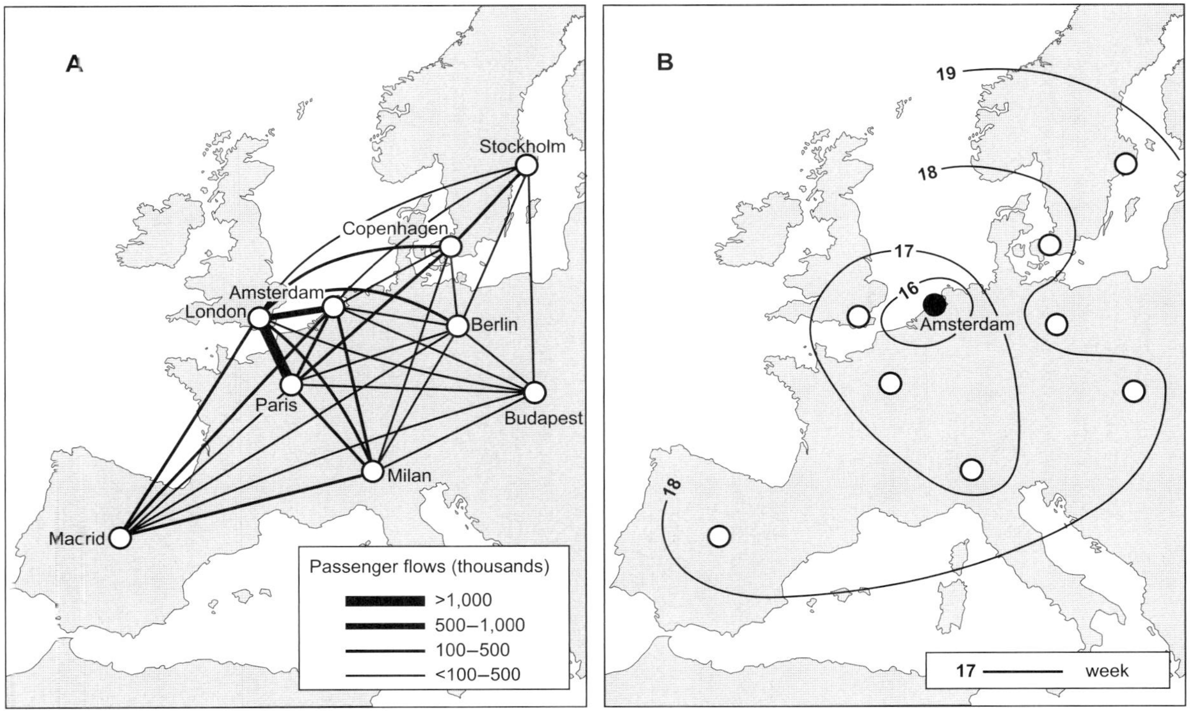

Fig. 6.20. Simulating the spread of a new strain of influenza in Europe
The strain was assumed to originate in Amsterdam and its spread to eight other European cities was modelled with a standardized incidence ratio (SIR) model using airline data. (A) Estimated annual passenger flows by airlines between nine cities. (B) Map of simulated epidemic peaks in weeks after the Amsterdam start.
Source: Adapted from part of Flahault, Deguen, and Valleron (1994, figs 4 and 5, pp. 473–4).

shown in Figure 6.20A, with the mean number of airline passengers flying between them based on data from the International Civil Aviation Organization.

Their simulation assumed that an influenza epidemic started in Amsterdam in a population with one in four susceptible to the new strain of the virus. The contact rate was assumed to be eight persons per week, along with an incubation time of 0.42 weeks and a length of illness of 0.714 weeks. The isochrone map showing the simulated timing of epidemic peaks appears in Figure 6.20B. In the starting city (Amsterdam) the peak was reached in the sixteenth week of the epidemic; in London, Paris, and Milan in the seventeenth week; in Budapest, Copenhagen, and Madrid in the eighteenth; and finally Berlin and Stockholm in the nineteenth. The results of the model show that the time lag for action within Europe is probably short (about one month) after the first detection of a new epidemic focus.

DISEASE TRANSMISSION MODELLING ON GLOBAL NETWORKS

One impact of SARS and the increasing concern about another 1918-style influenza pandemic from the H5N1 virus has been to focus on global modelling of spread on very large and very complex networks. The International Air Transport Association (IATA) now makes available a world list of airport pairs connected by direct flights and the number of available seats. This worldwide air transport network (WAN) is growing, but as of 2002 consisted of 3,880 airports (Figure 6.21). In terms of graph theory, the network may be thought of as a weighted graph with V=3,880 vertices which are connected by E=18,810 edges, each with a weight w_{ij} related to passenger flow between airports i and j. Flows along some links are very small so that the network can be pruned to 3,100 airports and 17,182 links while retaining 99 per cent of total flow. Colizza *et al.* (2006*a*) show that the distribution of airport sizes (the main urban area the airport is serving, i.e. Washington DC for Dulles) and of link flows form highly skewed and heavy-tailed distributions. In other words, a relatively small number of airports and pairs make up a very large share of the total traffic; conversely, a large number of small airports and lightly used links make up only a small fraction of WAN activity.

A number of epidemiologists in the United States have studied the WAN as a spatial framework for predicting the potential spread of infectious diseases from foreign sources along airline routes into the homeland. The basic Rvachev and Longini deterministic SIR model using 1968 data has been modified to update population levels, incorporate more recent travel patterns, adjust seasonality parameters, add stochasticity, and incorporate far more cities, both foreign and domestic (US). In general these models found that epidemics would now spread faster and that the order of cities would change as compared with 1968. Simulation of intervention strategies by imposing travel restrictions within the network have given mixed results;

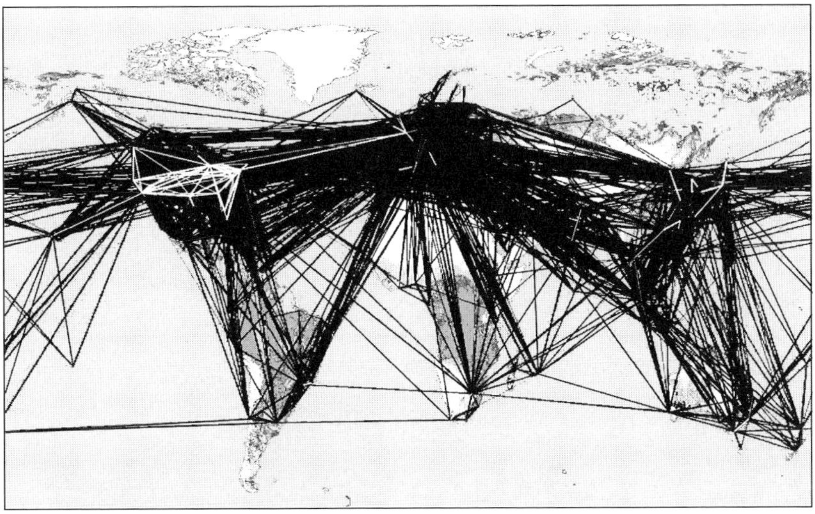

Fig. 6.21. The World Airline Network (WAN) at the millennium
A simplified representation of the global aviation network at the start of the present century showing direct civil aviation routes between the world's largest 500 international airports, as measured by passenger traffic. Each line on the map represents a direct connection between airports. Although the map shown represents only one in eight of international airports, it captures over 95 per cent of international civil aviation traffic.
Source: Hufnagel *et al.* (2004, fig. 1, p. 15125).

Colizza *et al.* (2006*a*,*b*, 2007) suggest the procedure is worthwhile, but Cooper *et al.* (2006) concluded that international travel restrictions do little to reduce the rate of spread globally. Rather, they suggest that local interventions at source aimed at reducing transmission are more likely to reduce the rate of spread. These views are supported by Hollingsworth *et al.* (2006), using a simplified global model. Figure 6.22 provides a typical example of the kind of spread predictions, although a number of papers now present results in a video form where maps and graphs are set in a dynamic time-frame.

Epstein *et al.* (2007) concluded from their modelling of pandemic influenza that air travel restrictions could be useful less in ameliorating the pandemic than in buying time to develop and deliver vaccines and in developing other protective measures (e.g. public education, social distancing among susceptibles, emergency hospital arrangements); see Sections 11.2 and 11.3, where control strategies are discussed in detail. They also found that travel restrictions could be harmful in circumstances where the delay achieved through travel restriction simply pushed the peak into a high epidemic season where local transmission is likely to be greater. The increasing range and capacity of computer simulation models to 'mimic' the behaviour of epidemic waves on a spatially intricate world and national stage now means that quite

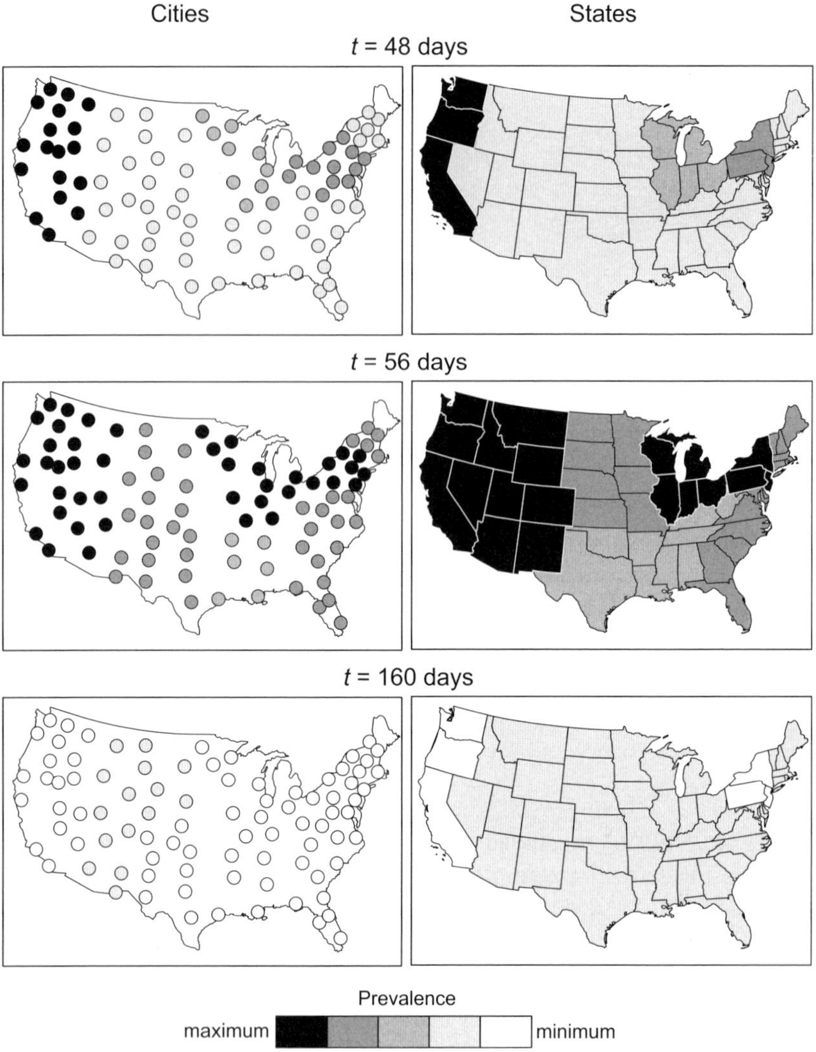

Fig. 6.22. Simulation of influenza epidemic spread on an airline network
Maps of the simulated evolution of influenza prevalence for an epidemic starting in Hong Kong at $t = 1$ and entering the conterminous United States via the world airline network (WAN) after only a few days. The progress is shown for cities and states with shading related to the prevalence level at $t = 48$, $t = 56$, and $t = 160$ days after the initial Asian outbreak. For the sake of easier visualization, only the 100 city airports with the largest traffic are shown, although the original data related to 2,100 airports.
Source: Redrawn from part of Colizza *et al.* (2006*b*, fig. 4, p. 1905).

sophisticated strategies for dealing with potential pandemic events can be tested and revised. That some results are clearly counter-intuitive (e.g. some plausible intervention strategies actually exacerbate morbidity rates) underlines the need for continuing work in this area. Grais *et al.* (2003), in their simulation studies of the spread of a Hong Kong type of influenza through a network of 52 global cities, emphasize how short the time can be for public health intervention.

6.4.3 Historical Studies of the Epidemiological Impact of Air Travel

While simulation on airline networks is a powerful investigative tool, it needs to be backed up by specific epidemiological studies of the actual movement of infected passengers. We know, for example, that the country-wide dispersal of HIV-1 in the United States in the early 1980s can be attributed to the activities of the initial case, so-called 'Patient 0', an HIV-positive airline steward (see Figure 6.23), while the rapidity of the spread of AIDS between Africa and the Soviet Union was facilitated by HIV-infected Russian technicians moving to and fro between the origin and destination areas (Smallman-Raynor, Cliff, and Haggett 1992). At a population-wide rather than individual level, Brownstein *et al.* (2006) have presented evidence that the grounding of aeroplanes in the United States after 11 September 2001

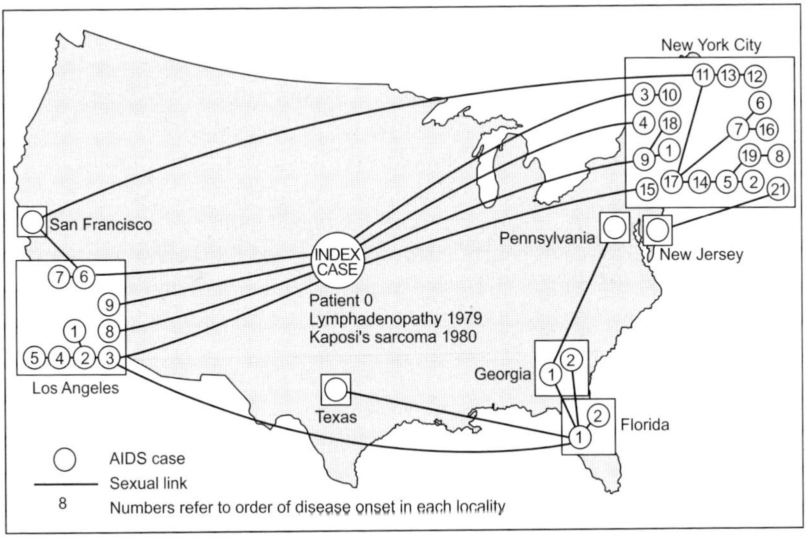

Fig. 6.23. Contact network of 'Patient 0' in the early stages of the US HIV/AIDS epidemic

Each circle represents an AIDS case, with the known links between cases indicated. Numbers refer to the order of disease onset in each location.

Source: Redrawn from Smallman-Raynor, Cliff, and Haggett (1992, fig. 4.2A, p. 147).

delayed the dynamics of influenza during the 2001–2 season by approximately two weeks. This conclusion has been challenged by Viboud, Miller, *et al.* (2006).

We choose here two detailed examples to illustrate the impact of airline traffic upon disease spread: (i) the 1967 Marburg fever outbreak and, in contrast, (ii) the historical impact over several decades of air transport on the behaviour of measles epidemics in Iceland.

Marburg Fever: Air Travel from Africa (1967)

In recent decades, the tropical haemorrhagic diseases have provided some striking instances of the rapid transport of infections from low-latitude to mid-latitude countries. The history of one of these is illustrated in Figure 6.24. In July 1967 a total of 200 African green monkeys (*Cercopithecus aethiops*) wild-caught in the Lake Kyoga region of Uganda, Central Africa, were flown in two batches from Entebbe to Europe. As the map shows, one batch was shipped to the German cities of Marburg and Frankfurt (via London) and the other to Belgrade in (the then) Yugoslavia (Smallman-Raynor, Cliff, and Haggett 1992: 132–3).

Soon after the arrival at a vaccine/sera plant at Marburg, a monkey handler developed a sudden fever, from which he died. Within days the disease appeared in other laboratory workers. In total, 23 definitive cases of the disease were identified (both from primary contact with the monkeys and from secondary contacts with partners and medical staff). Smaller similar outbreaks occurred in Frankfurt and Belgrade, bringing the total cases to 32 (with seven deaths). Serological examination proved the common presence of a rodlike virus (subsequently termed the Marburg virus), which could be traced to the imported monkeys. Subsequent veterinarian investigation in the Kyoga source region showed high prevalence rates (20–36 per cent) of Marburg virus infection in newly caught batches of green monkeys. Subsequent occurrence of Marburg fever in humans has been reported from Central Africa (Section 9.3.2), but no imported outbreaks on the scale of the original Marburg–Frankfurt–Belgrade event have yet been recorded.

Measles: Air Transport Impacts on Epidemics in Iceland Post-1945

A striking example of how infectious diseases respond to transport changes is provided by the sub-Arctic island of Iceland. Because of its exceptional epidemiological records, Iceland has been intensively studied by epidemiologists (see the reviews by Cliff, Haggett, and Smallman-Raynor 2000). Over the 150-year period from 1840 to 1990, some 93,000 cases of measles were recorded in Iceland. Over 99 per cent of these occurred in 19 distinct epidemic waves. The Icelandic doctors kept detailed written accounts of the geographical pattern of spread of many of these epidemics. The early waves frequently diffused from one community to another as infectives travelled coastwise by boat. In addition, Iceland has always had too small a population to maintain

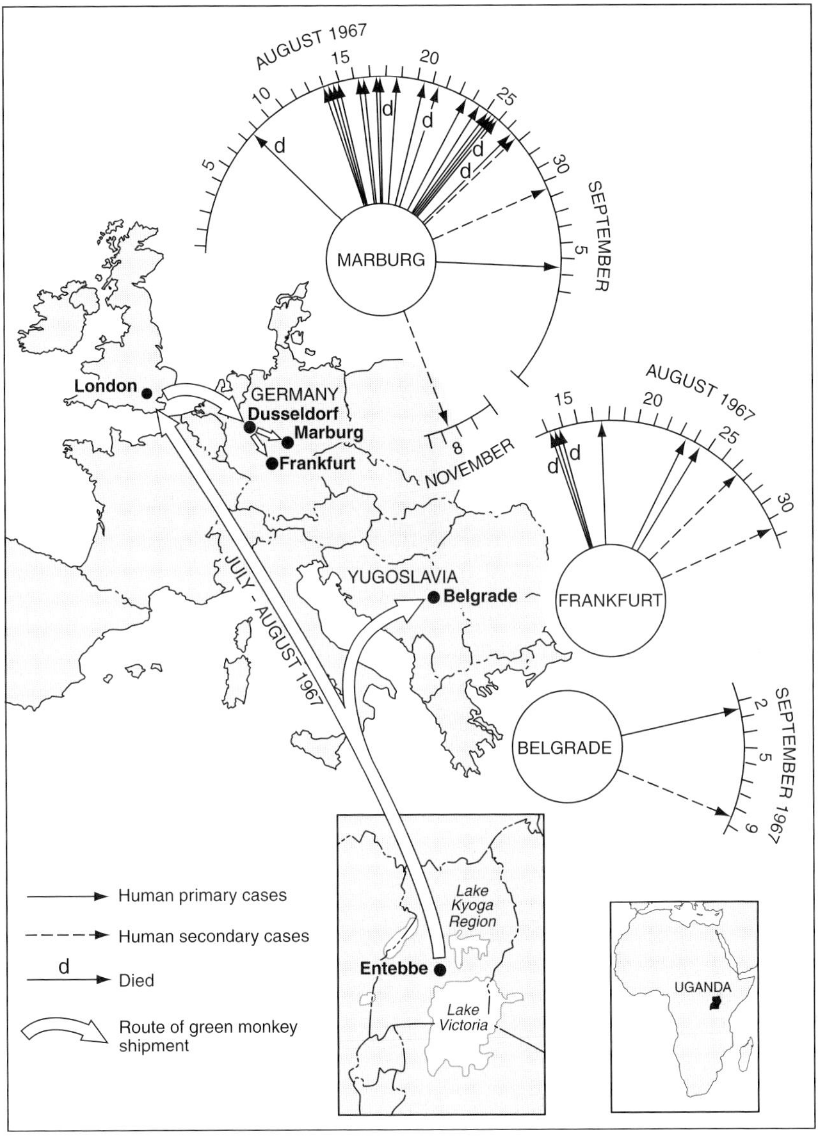

Fig. 6.24. History of the 1967 Marburg fever outbreak in Europe
The map shows the movement as air cargo of green monkeys from Uganda to laboratories in Germany and Yugoslavia. The circular charts show the subsequent dates of cases and deaths from Marburg fever.
Source: Smallman-Raynor, Cliff, and Haggett (1992, fig. 3.4A, p. 133).

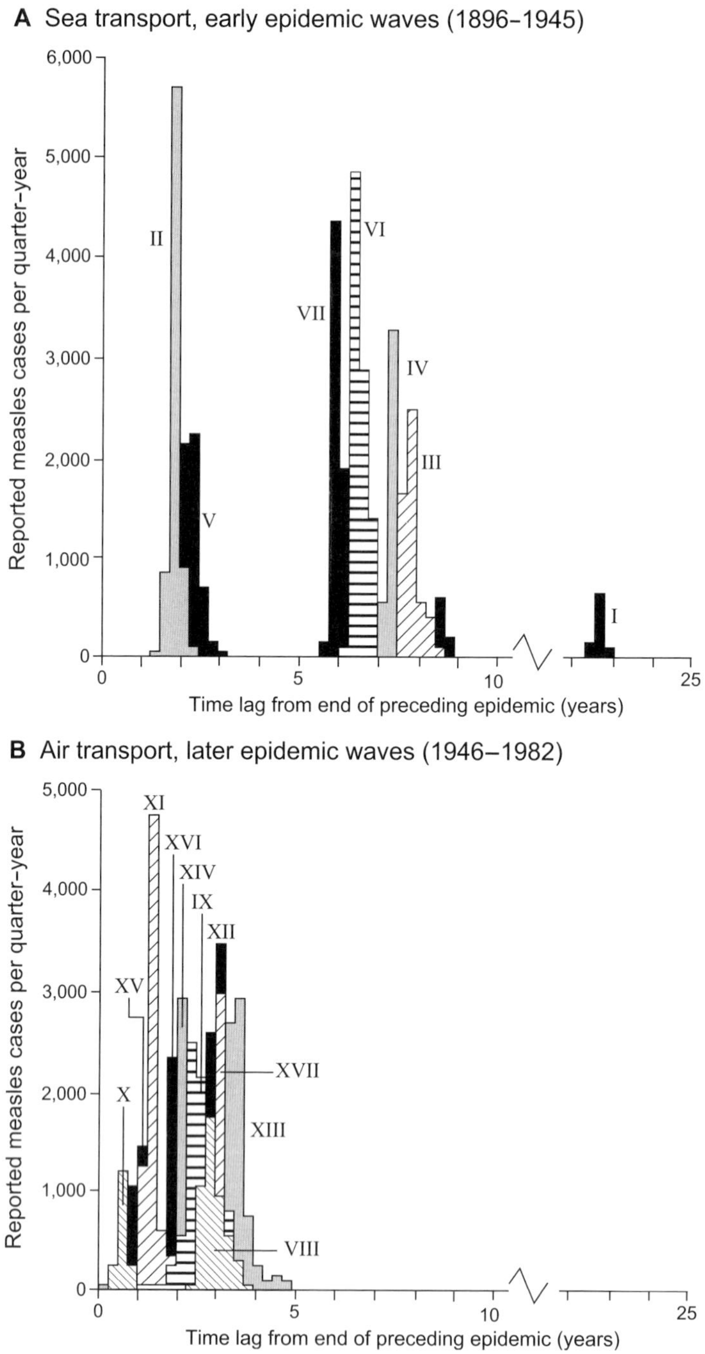

Fig. 6.25. Time intervals between epidemic measles waves in Iceland, 1896–1982
The diagram shows spacing contrasts between earlier and later measles epidemics between 1896 and 1982. The horizontal axis gives the time in months since the preceding epidemic wave. The waves which occurred in the 87-year time window are numbered I (earliest) to XVII (last).

Source: Cliff and Haggett (2004, fig. 5, p. 95).

measles permanently, and introductions of the disease into Iceland at the start of each wave was, until the end of World War II, exclusively by ship. After 1945, both measles introductions and the subsequent spread of the disease within Iceland became dominated by movements of infectives by air rather than by boat. Virus introductions also became more frequent as population flux in Iceland increased.

The impact of more frequent virus introductions is shown in Figure 6.25. The spacing of Iceland's measles waves became shorter over time as the island's population grew and contacts with the outside world became more frequent. The average gap between waves in the period 1896 to 1945 was more than 5 years; from 1946 to 1982 it had fallen to a year and a half. More frequent virus introductions also meant there was less time for the susceptible population to increase and so epidemics became smaller as well as more closely spaced.

6.5 Combined Impacts of Mobility

6.5.1 Combined Movement

In Sections 6.2–6.4 we have tried to illustrate the epidemiological impacts of changes in individual transport modes. But, since we typically use a number of different modes to move around, it is important to put these together in some indicator of combined movement. We then illustrate the disease impacts of such combined movement.

The broad statistical trend for movement over the last 200 years for an individual country is given in Figure 6.26. This plots for France since 1800 the average kilometres travelled daily by people (i) by particular transport mode and (ii) by all modes. For the former we see how one mode reaches a peak and declines to be overtaken by a successor but the combined movement total keeps on growing. Since the vertical scale is logarithmic, the graph demonstrates that, despite changes in the mode used, average travel increased exponentially over the period, broken only by the two world wars—a rise of over 1,000-fold in mobility. Over this same 200 years the fall in long-distance travel times for another country has been dramatic. If we combine the Australian data in Figures 6.6 and 6.14, they show the England–Australia travel time dropping from one year in 1788 to around one day at the millennium.

Historical changes in travel patterns have been shown in a different but equally interesting way by Bradley (1989). He compared the travel patterns of four successive generations of the Bradley family: his great-grandfather, his grandfather, his father, and himself (see Figure 6.27). The lifetime travel track of his great-grandfather around a village in Northamptonshire, England, could

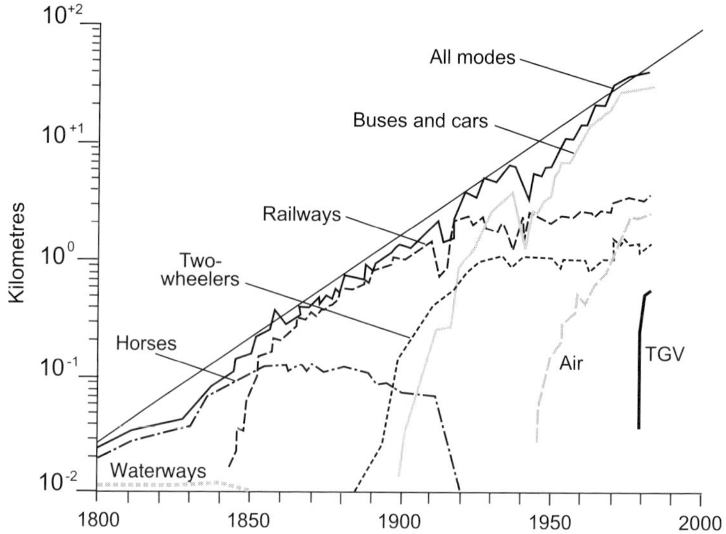

Fig. 6.26. Increased spatial mobility of the population of France over a 200-year period, 1800–2000

The vertical scale is logarithmic so that increases in average travel distance by all transport modes is shown to be increasing exponentially over time. TGV = high-speed train (train à grande vitesse).

Source: Haggett (2000, fig. 3.10, p. 94).

be contained within a square of only 40 km side. His grandfather's map was still limited to southern England, but it now ranged as far as London and could be contained within a square of 400 km side. If we compare these maps with those of Bradley's father (who travelled widely in Europe) and Bradley's own sphere of travel, which has been worldwide, then the enclosing square has to be widened to sides of 4,000 km and 40,000 km, respectively. In broad terms, the spatial range of travel has increased 10-fold in each generation so that Bradley's own range is 1,000 times wider than that of his great-grandfather.

The precise rates of population flux or travel both within and between countries are difficult to catch in official statistics. But most available evidence suggests that the flux over the last few decades has risen at an accelerating rate. While the world population growth rate since the middle of the twentieth century has been running at between 1.5 and 2.5 per cent per annum, the growth in international movements of passengers across national boundaries has been between 7.5 and 10 per cent per annum. One striking example is provided by Australia: over the last four decades, its resident population has doubled, whereas the movement of people across its international boundaries (that is, into and out of Australia) has increased nearly 100-fold.

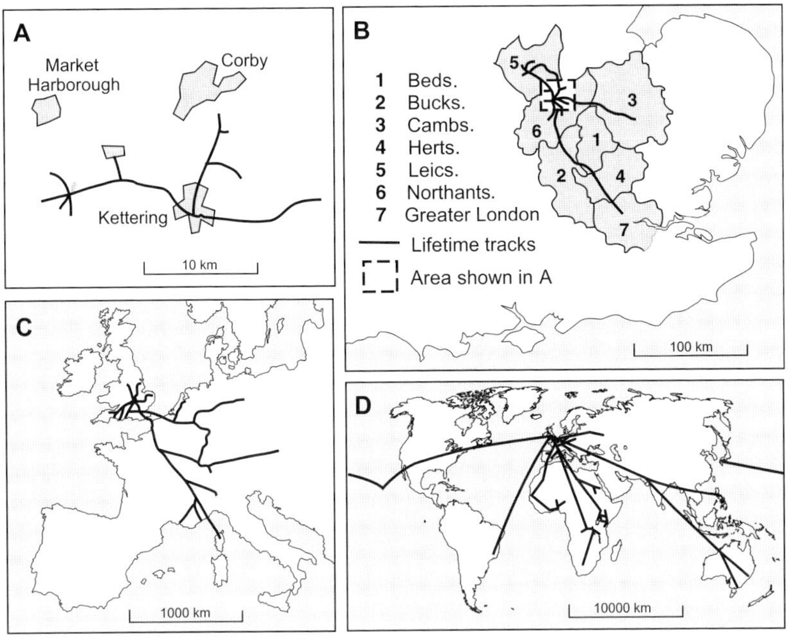

Fig. 6.27. Bradley's record of increasing travel over four male generations of the same family
(A) Great-grandfather. (B) Grandfather. (C) Father. (D) Son. Each map shows in a simplified manner the individual's 'lifetime tracks' in a widening spatial context, with the linear scale increasing by a factor of 10 between each generation.
Source: Cliff and Haggett (2004, fig. 2, p. 91).

The implications of increased travel are twofold: short-term and long-term. First, an immediate and important effect is the possible exposure of the travelling public to a greater range of diseases than they might meet in their home country. The relative risks encountered in tropical areas by travellers coming from Western countries (data mainly from North America and western Europe) have been estimated by Steffen (World Health Organization 1995) and are given in Figure 6.28. These suggest a spectrum of risks from unspecified traveller's diarrhoea (a high risk of 20 per cent) to paralytic poliomyelitis (a very low risk of less than 0.001 per cent).

On a longer time-scale, increased travel brings some possible long-term genetic effects. With more travel and longer-range migration, there is an enhanced probability of partnerships being formed and reproduction arising from unions between individuals from formerly distant populations. As Khlat and Khoury (1991) have shown, this can bring advantages from the viewpoint of some diseases. For example, the probability of occurrence of multifactorial conditions such as cystic fibrosis or spinal muscular atrophy is

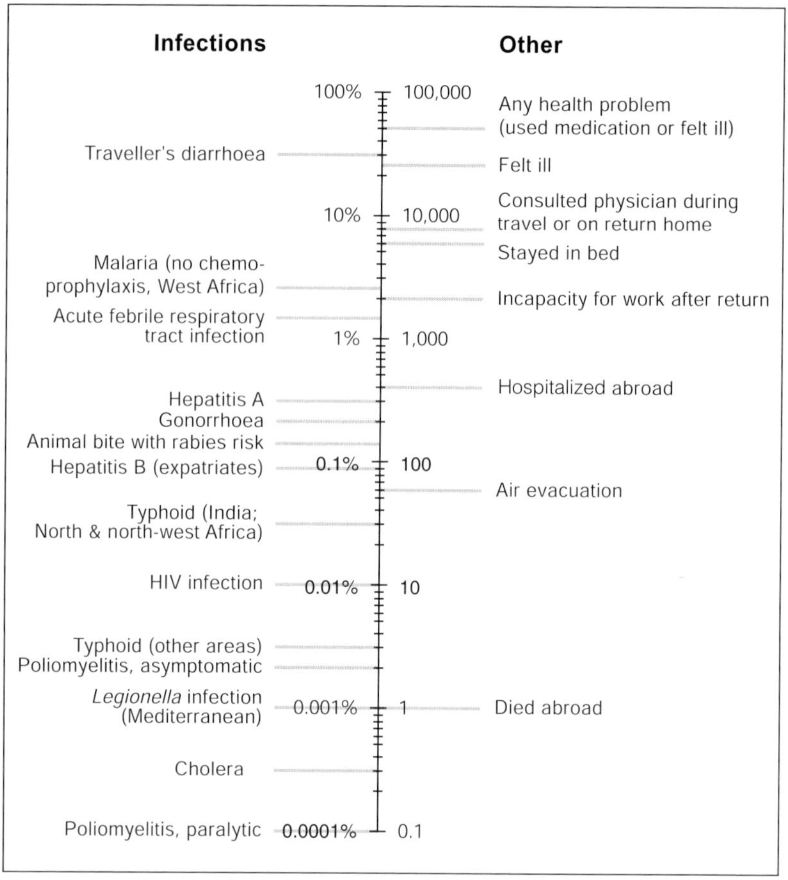

Fig. 6.28. WHO estimates of relative disease threats to travellers in tropical areas The scale is logarithmic.
Source: Cliff and Haggett (2004, fig. 7, p. 97).

reduced; the risk of these conditions is somewhat higher in children of consanguineous unions. Conversely, inherited disorders such as sickle cell anaemia might become more widely dispersed.

6.5.2 Combined Movement and Human Disease Agents

The above discussion implies that the potential for existing diseases to be introduced into new geographical locations as a consequence of the exponentially growing churn of humans at all spatial scales, and with access to multiple transport modes, is enormous. Here we explore some examples which are known to have occurred, taking a human agent in this subsection and non-human agents in the next.

NEISSERIA MENINGITIDIS SEROGROUP W135 AND THE HAJ

In the years following its description in 1968, *N. meningitidis* W135 was considered a minor meningococcal serogroup of little clinical importance. However, in the early 1980s, this organism was described as a fully pathogenic strain, recognized as an emerging cause of disease in Africa (Section 9.3.2), and as an important new cause of disease in Europe and North America. The first cases of W135 disease in pilgrims were described in 1993 in Saudi Arabia (Aguilera *et al.* 2002), with the first worldwide outbreak recorded in association with the haj of 2000 (Lingappa *et al.* 2003). Prior to the 2000 outbreak, W135 meningococcal disease was uncommon and accounted for <2 per cent of meningococcal cases worldwide (Lingappa *et al.* 2003).

Multinational Outbreak of W135, Europe (2000)

Spread of W135 to Europe in association with the 2000 haj (15–18 March) is examined by Aguilera *et al.* (2002). Between 18 March and 31 July, 90 cases of meningococcal infection were reported from nine countries—UK (42 cases), France (24 cases), Netherlands, Germany, Finland, Sweden, Belgium, Switzerland, and Norway. Most early cases were in pilgrims (12 cases), but spread onwards to their household and non-household contacts (52 cases) and, subsequently, to those with no contacts with pilgrims (26 cases). Figure 6.29 plots cases of invasive W135 disease identified in the period March–July 2000 in Europe as a whole (Figure 6.29A; $n = 90$ cases) and England and Wales (Figure 6.29B; $n = 38$ cases). Cases are categorized according to their known association with the haj: (i) pilgrims, (ii) close contacts of pilgrims, and (iii) no known contact with pilgrims. Overall, the outbreak in Europe peaked two to three weeks after the first return of pilgrims from the haj, with cases decreasing thereafter. All cases in pilgrims were reported in the four weeks after the haj, with peak activity two weeks after the haj; peak activity in contacts occurred three weeks after the haj and among non-contacts eight weeks after (Figure 6.29A). The same basic pattern occurred in England and Wales (Figure 6.29B), where sustained transmission occurred mainly among Muslim communities; of the 51 cases recorded up to the start of the 2001 haj, 8 were pilgrims, 22 were contacts of pilgrims, and 21 had no identifiable connection with the haj (Hahné *et al.* 2002).

Following the outbreak, European countries recommended quadrivalent vaccine for travellers to the 2001 haj. Notwithstanding this advice, coverage of the pilgrim population with quadrivalent vaccine in 2001 was estimated at just 47 per cent, and another outbreak of W135 occurred in pilgrims and their contacts, with cases recorded in the UK (25) and France (10) in the period 28 March–29 June 2001 (Aguilera *et al.* 2002).

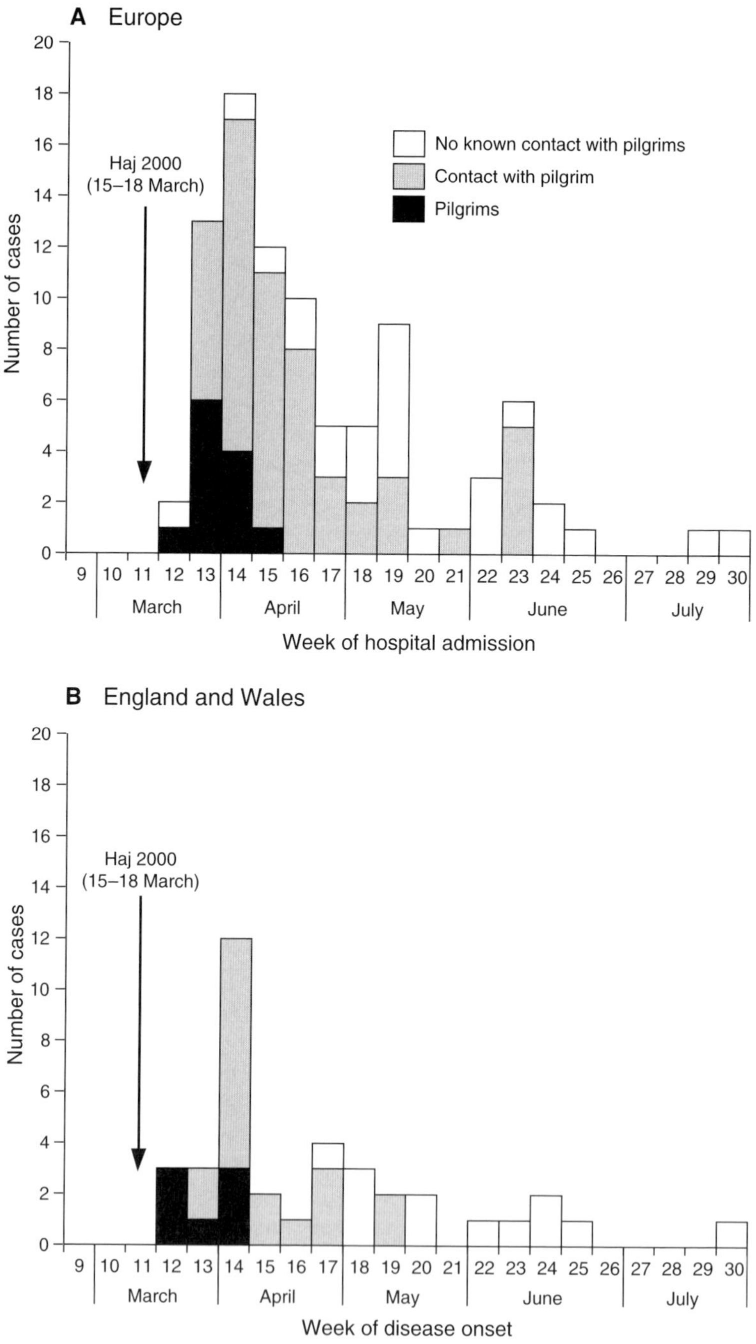

Fig. 6.29. Weekly count of cases of W135 invasive meningococcal disease, March–July 2000

(A) Europe. (B) England and Wales. Cases are categorized according to their known association with haj 2000.

Sources: Drawn from Aguilera *et al.* (2002, fig. 3, p. 763) and Hahné *et al.* (2002: 582).

6.5.3 *Combined Movement and Non-Human Disease Agents*

Although the emphasis in this chapter has been on the movement of infected passengers, with implications for subsequent person-to-person disease spread, the acceleration of travel also applies with some force to the combined movement of non-human disease-causing agents via sea, land, and air. Tens of millions of wild animals are shipped around the world each year, mainly from subtropical to temperate regions. As we saw in Section 6.4.3, examples include the air shipment of green monkeys for laboratory use in the original Marburg fever outbreak. The import of 800 small mammals from Ghana in West Africa to Texas in April 2003 has been implicated in subsequent outbreaks of monkeypox within both native rodents and humans. As we saw in Sections 4.2.3 and 4.2.4, the deepening concern over highly pathogenic avian influenza (H5N1) in South-East Asia has highlighted the role of land-based poultry movements as well as airborne wild bird movements in the spread of the disease.

WEST NILE VIRUS

In another group of cases, pathogens are thought to have 'hitch-hiked' their way onto aircraft. The North American outbreak of West Nile disease from 1999 is an example; prior to August 1999, West Nile virus had not been recorded in the Western Hemisphere, and so the outbreak was a classic example of a newly emerging disease.

West Nile is a single-stranded RNA virus belonging to the genus *Flavivirus*, family *Flaviviridae*, and forms part of the complex that includes St Louis, Murray Valley, Japanese, and Rocio encephalitis virus. It infects a large number of vertebrates, including humans, domestic animals, and several species of birds. Birds are the reservoir. Oniphilic mosquitoes of the genus *Culex* serve as the vector in virus transmission to other species, including humans. In humans, the incubation period of the disease is 2–14 days. About 20 per cent develop a mild febrile disease, but about 1 in 150 develop meningitis or encephalitis, with neurological symptoms being more frequent in those aged >50 years. With neurological involvement, severe muscle weakness is common. In some cases, symmetrical flaccid paralysis has been documented (Johnson 2003).

Onset of the Epidemic in New York, 1999

On 23 August 1999, the New York City Department of Health received notice of two patients with apparent neurological infections with severe weakness and who had been attended by physicians at Flushing Hospital, northern Queens. Within a week, investigation of hospital records had revealed the existence of eight cases of encephalitis resident in a ~40 km^2 area of northern Queens.[3] While no common exposures could be deduced for

[3] As described by Asnis *et al.* (2000), the first recognized patients had begun to present at Flushing Hospital, New York City, in mid-Aug.; one patient was admitted with fever, weakness, and nausea

Table 6.2. Reported outbreaks of West Nile virus in humans, Israel, 1941–2000

			West Nile virus cases	
Year	Location	Type of locality	Number of cases studied	Number of deaths
1941	Central Israel & Tel Aviv	Urban & rural	500	0
1950	Hadera & coastal plain	Army camps & communal settlement	105	0
1951	Haifa	Agricultural settlement	123	0
1950–3	Military hospital	Army camps	400	0
1953	Tel Hashomer Hospital	Army camps	70	0
1953–4	Central & northern Israel	Army camps	300	0
1957	Hadera area	Army camps	300	0
		Urban & rural	65	0
		Nursing homes	49	4
1980	Negev Desert	Army camps	32	0
2000	Countrywide	Urban & rural	417	35

Source: Weinberger *et al.* (2001, table 1, p. 689).

the eight patients, all had spent evening hours outdoors in activities that included gardening and smoking on the porch. This finding—which suggested the role of mosquito activity—resulted in the detection of mosquito larvae in open containers, old tyres, and a partially drained swimming pool in the neighbourhood. On 2 September, mosquito control began in the city. In a seemingly unrelated incident in earlier August, bird deaths (especially crows) had been recorded in the Bronx, while a number of exotic birds in the Bronx zoo had died of encephalitis. The recovery of West Nile virus from these birds marked the first record of West Nile virus in the Western Hemisphere. Current evidence suggests that West Nile virus was first introduced to New York in 1999 (Nash *et al.* 2001; Johnson 2003).

The exact origin of the virus in New York is unknown. However, the recovered viruses were found to be closely related to a virus isolated from the brain of a dead goose in Israel in 1998. This suggests that the epidemic in North America may have been sparked by the introduction of a virus circulating in the Middle East (Lanciotti *et al.* 1999; Giladi *et al.* 2001), possibly imported via a mosquito in an aircraft (Johnson 2003). West Nile fever is endemic in Israel, with several outbreaks of the disease in the period from the 1940s to the 1980s (Table 6.2). The majority of the patients have been young soldiers in training and who contracted the infection in army camps. No

of three days' duration on 12 Aug., followed by a case of fever, headache, weakness, and diarrhoea on 15 Aug. Further cases were admitted on 18, 20, 23, 27, and 31 Aug. These were documented as the first cases of West Nile virus infection on the North American continent.

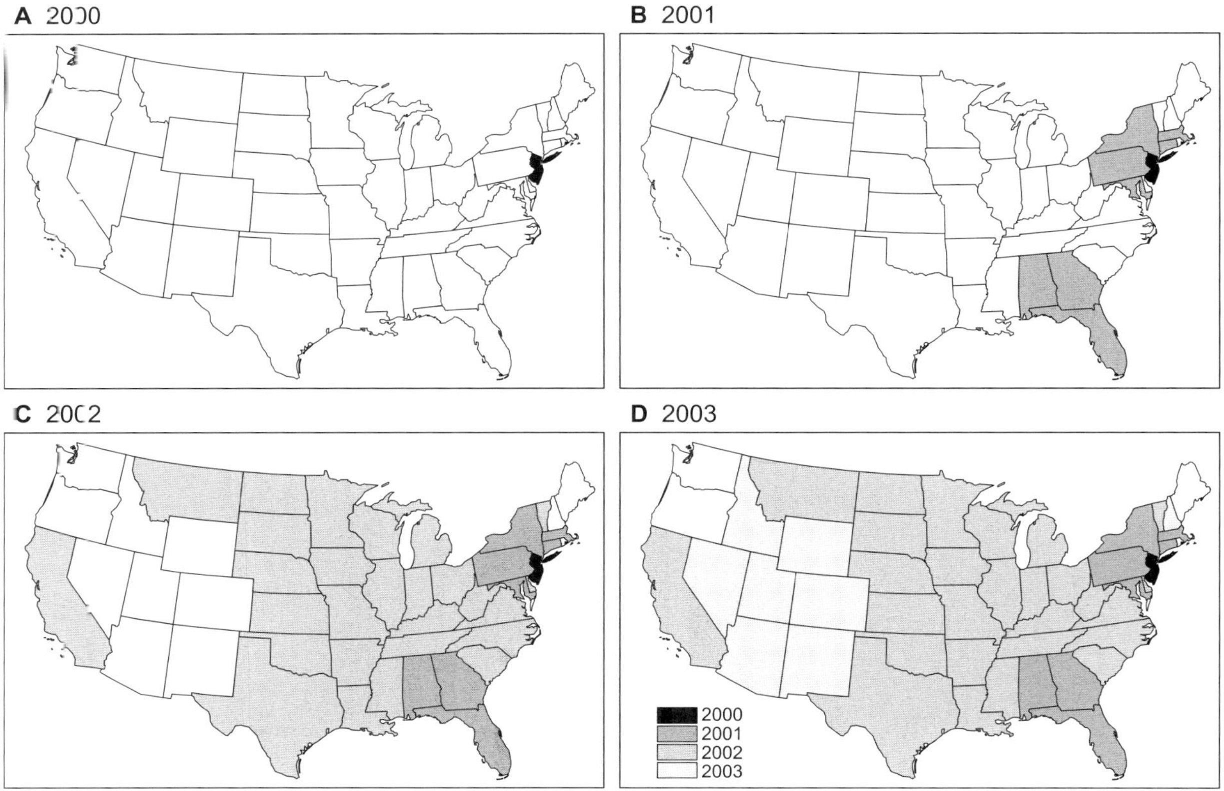

Fig. 6.30. Spread of West Nile virus in the United States, 1999–2003
States reached by (A) 2000, (B) 2001, (C) 2002, (D) 2003.

human cases of the disease were reported in Israel in the period 1990–8, but three human cases were recognized in 1999. Thus, the human epidemic of 2000 marked a re-emergence of the disease in Israel (Weinberger *et al.* 2001).

The geographical distribution of patients hospitalized with West Nile virus infection in New York City and environs during the 1999 outbreak is given in Table 6.3. Estimates suggest that the outbreak ultimately consisted of 8,200 (range 3,500–13,000) West Nile virus infections, including ~1,700 febrile infections (Mostashari *et al.* 2001). Subsequent serosurveys in Queens indicated that <1 per cent of those infected with West Nile developed encephalitis. The virus was identified in a variety of mosquito species, but with *Culex pipiens* as the prime vector (Nash *et al.* 2001; Johnson 2003). The virus successfully overwintered in 1999 and, within three years, spread to reach the Pacific seaboard (Figure 6.30).

AIRPORT YELLOW FEVER AND MALARIA

Another indicator of the way in which international aircraft from the tropics can inadvertently cause the spread of disease to a non-indigenous area is seen in the occasional outbreaks of tropical diseases around mid-latitude airports and the steps taken to prevent them. For example, Plate 6.1 (Binson 1936; Pridie 1936) shows the controls taken at Juba, Sudan, in the mid-1930s because of concerns that yellow fever would be spread by the stopover there by Imperial Airways on its route between London and Cape Town. In a similar vein, Table 6.4 summarizes the number of outbreaks of so-called 'airport malaria' recorded in mid-latitude countries over a 30-year period from 1969. Cases occurred in late summer, when high temperatures allowed the in-flight survival of infected anopheles mosquitoes which had been

Table 6.3. Geographical distribution of patients hospitalized with West Nile virus infection in New York City and environs, 1999

Place of residence	Population at risk (million)	Number of patients[1]	Clinical attack rate (per million population)
New York City			
Brooklyn	2.3	3	1.3
Bronx	1.2	9	7.5
Manhattan	1.5	1	0.7
Queens	2.0	32	16.4
Staten Island (Richmond)	0.4	0	0.0
New York State			
Nassau County	1.3	6	4.7
Westchester County	0.9	8	9.1
TOTAL	9.5	59	6.2

Note: [1]Hospitalized patients only.
Source: Nash *et al.* (2001, table 1, p. 1810).

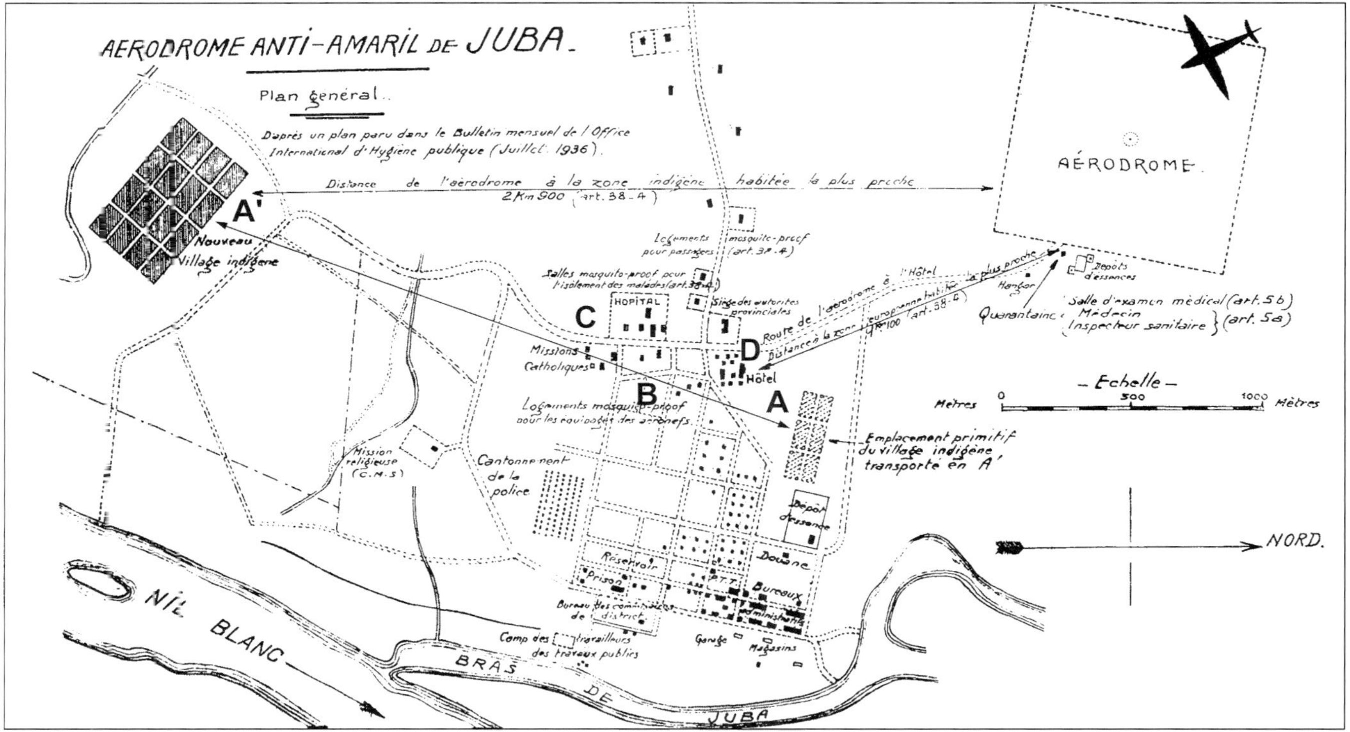

Pl. 6.1. Inter-war plan of the anti-amaril aerodrome at Juba, Sudan

The putative identification of yellow fever virus (amaril) activity in southern Sudan in the mid-1930s necessitated remedial action if the aerodrome at Juba was to remain operative as a stopover on the Imperial Airways route between London and Cape Town. As implemented under part III (chapter II) of the International Sanitary Convention for Aerial Navigation (1935), 'Measures Applicable in Case of Yellow Fever', steps taken included the relocation of the indigenous village of Juba from site A (1.1 km to the south-east of the aerodrome) to site A′ (2.9 km due south of the aerodrome), beyond the flight range of potentially infective mosquitoes. Other measures included the construction of mosquito-proof residences for air crew (B), isolation rooms for patients (C), and a hotel for passengers (D), all located within approximately 1 km of the aerodrome.

Sources: Binson (1936), originally from Pridie (1936, opp. p. 1296).

Table 6.4. Confirmed or probable cases of mid-latitude airport malaria, 1969–1999[1]

Country	Cases
France	26
Belgium	17
United Kingdom	14
Switzerland	9
Luxembourg	5
Italy	4
US	4
Germany	4
Netherlands	2
Spain	2
Israel	1
Australia	1
TOTAL	89

Note: [1] To Aug. 1999.
Source: Gratz *et al.* (2000, table 2, p. 998).

inadvertently introduced into aircraft while at airports in malarious areas. The infected mosquitoes escape when the aircraft lands to cause malaria cases among local residents.

New Zealand

The most comprehensive assessment of the risks posed by mosquito importation is that undertaken by Derraik (2004) for New Zealand, 1925–2004. Prior to the arrival of humans about 800 years ago, New Zealand had only 12 indigenous mosquito species. Since the arrival of humans, the New Zealand environment has been plagued by the invasion of a large number of exotic species. The potential threat of invading vector mosquitoes to New Zealand's public health has been recognized since at least the 1950s. While outbreaks of mosquito-borne infectious diseases have not yet been recorded in New Zealand, the situation could change with the tide of species introductions, and the potential risks for arboviral diseases such as Ross River and dengue in New Zealand have recently been highlighted by Maguire (1994) and Weinstein *et al.* (1995).

Under these circumstances, Derraik (2004) has undertaken a comprehensive review of recorded mosquito interceptions in association with aircraft and ships in the period 1925–2004, yielding information on 171 mosquito interceptions over the 80 years. Of these, 97 were associated with unidentified and already established exotic mosquito species in New Zealand, while 74 interceptions were exotic (non-established) species. The latter interceptions were associated with 27 species.

Time series of mosquito interceptions. Figures 6.31A and B plot by 10-year period the distribution of mosquito interceptions (unidentified, already established exotic, and non-established exotic species) for 1925–2004. The main graphs give the number of interceptions by inferred region of origin (South, Pacific, Asia, and other). Further geographical detail is provided by the inset graphs, which plot the number of interceptions by inferred country of origin. Several features of A and B are noteworthy:

(i) Figure 6.31A: aircraft interceptions have largely been associated with sources in the South Pacific, especially Australia, Fiji, and, to a lesser extent, New Caledonia;
(ii) Figure 6.31B: the recorded number of ship interceptions grew markedly from the mid-1980s, with the majority originating in Asia. The pattern is dominated by Japan.

Figures 6.31C and D refer to non-established exotic mosquito species. The same broad pattern described for Figures 6.31A and B is repeated. Japan has become the main documented source of exotic mosquitoes since the 1990s, accounting for over one-third of all interceptions from January 1990 to 2004, associated with used machinery and tyres imported to New Zealand in ships (Derraik 2004).

Potential pathogens. Figure 6.32 is again based on information from Derraik (2004) and plots, for the periods 1925–74 (graph A) and 1975–2004 (graph B), the number of non-established exotic mosquito species intercepted on aircraft and ships. For a given time period, the inset graphs give the number of interceptions by mosquito species, while the main graphs give the number of interceptions according to the pathogens (arboviruses and others) known to be associated with the intercepted species. Several features are notable:

(i) The graphs draw a sharp distinction between the early period (1925–74; graph A), when the majority of documented interceptions were associated with aircraft, and the late period (1975–2004), when the majority of documented interceptions were associated with ships. This shift, from aircraft to ships, has been highlighted by Derraik (2004).
(ii) Associated with the change in transport medium, the inset graphs demonstrate a shift in the dominant species of intercepted mosquito, from *Culex* spp. (1925–74) to *Aedes* spp. and *Ochlerotatus* spp. (1975–2004). As noted above, these changes are associated with the used machinery and tyres trade with Japan.
(iii) The change in dominant intercepted species has been associated with a shift in the pathogens of public health significance that may be introduced with the invading species; the post-1975 period has seen a significant increase in mosquitoes associated with West Nile and yellow fever viruses, Chikungunya, Eastern equine encephalitis, Japanese encephalitis, and La Crosse encephalitis viruses.

As Derraik (2004: 442) notes:

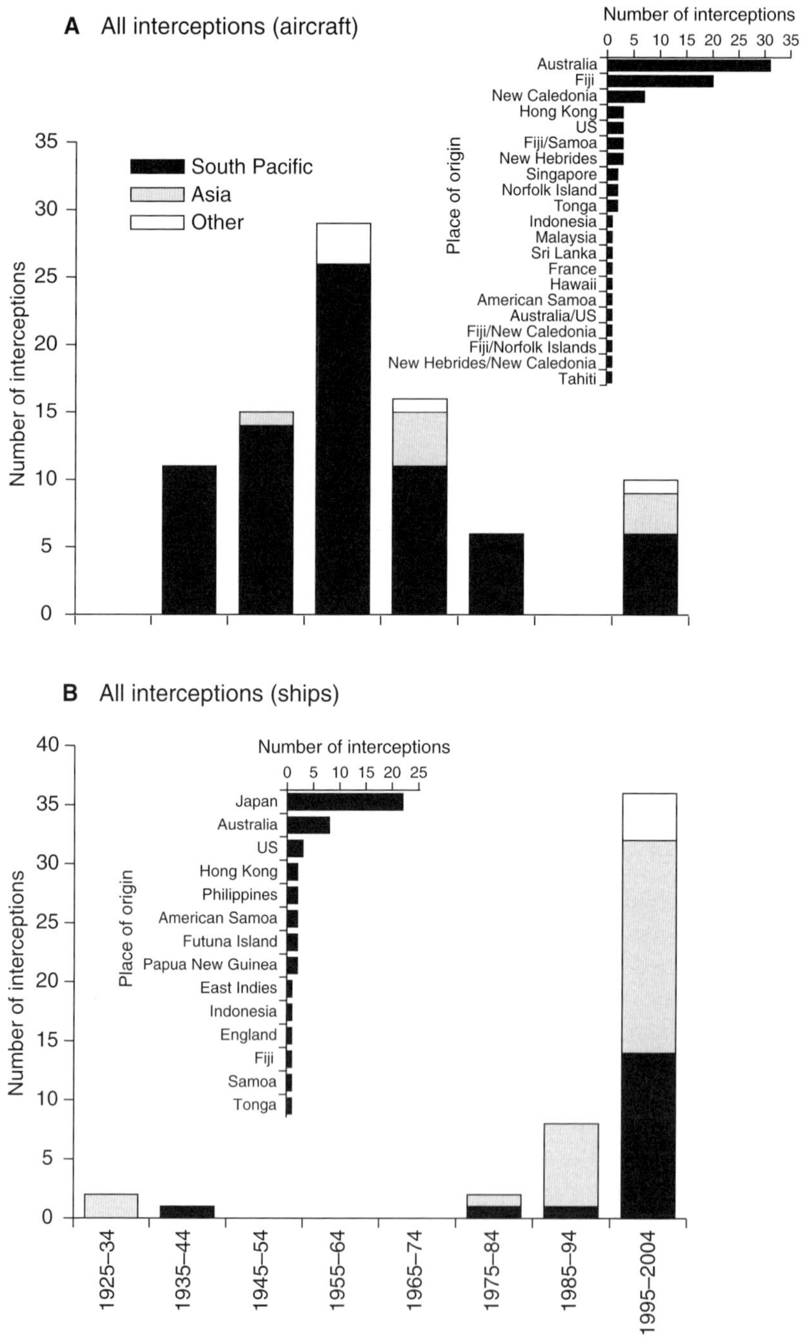

Fig. 6.31. Interceptions of mosquito species on aircraft and ships, New Zealand, 1925–2004

All interceptions of mosquito species (unidentified, exotic established, and exotic non-established species) in association with aircraft (A) and ships (B). Interceptions of exotic (non-established) mosquito species in association with aircraft (C) and ships (D).

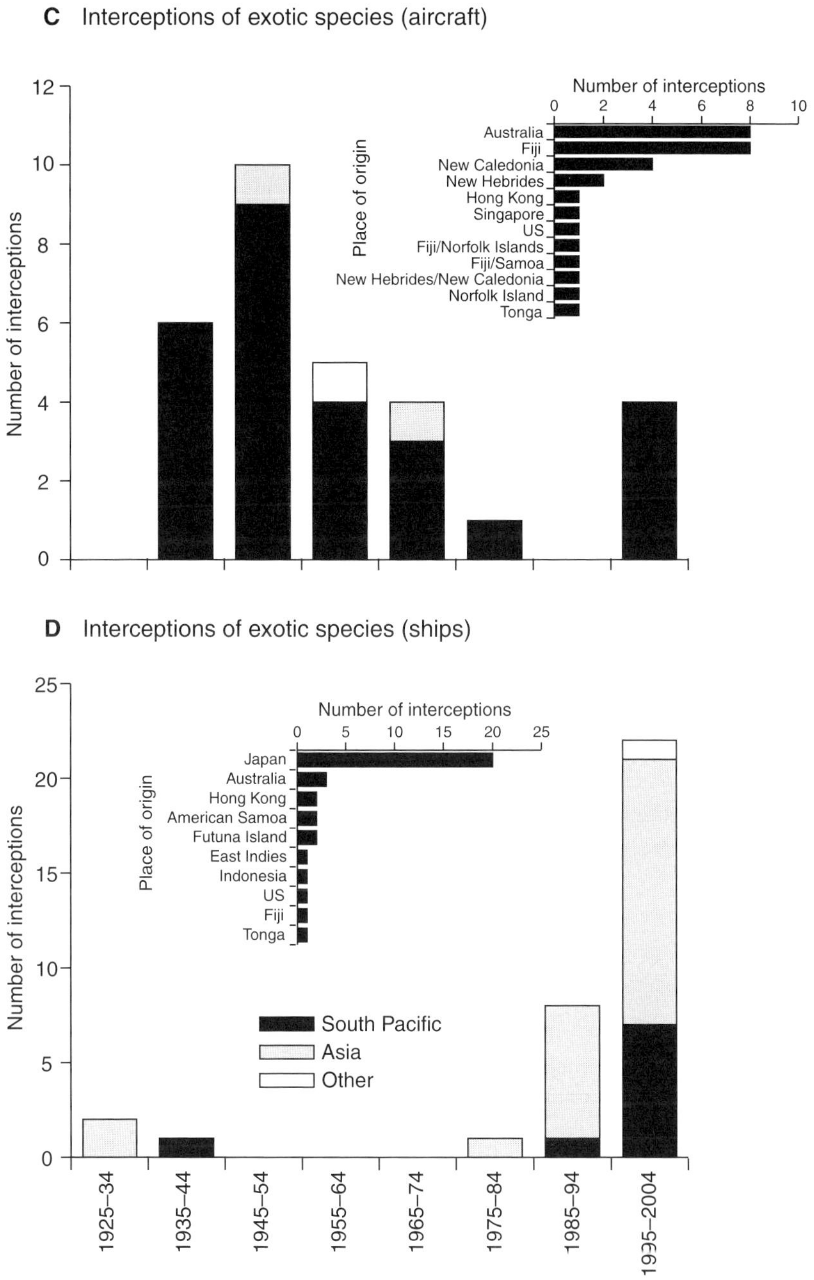

Fig. 6.31. (Continued)
Main graphs show the number of interceptions by 10-year period according to the inferred region of geographical origin (South Pacific, Asia, and other). Inset graphs show the place of origin of each subset of interceptions. In forming the graphs, the 10-year intervals 1955–64 and 1975–84 include interceptions for which the time brackets are recorded in Derraik (2004) as 1955–65 and 1973–8, respectively.

Source: Drawn from data in Derraik (2004, tables 2, 3, pp. 435–6, 438–9).

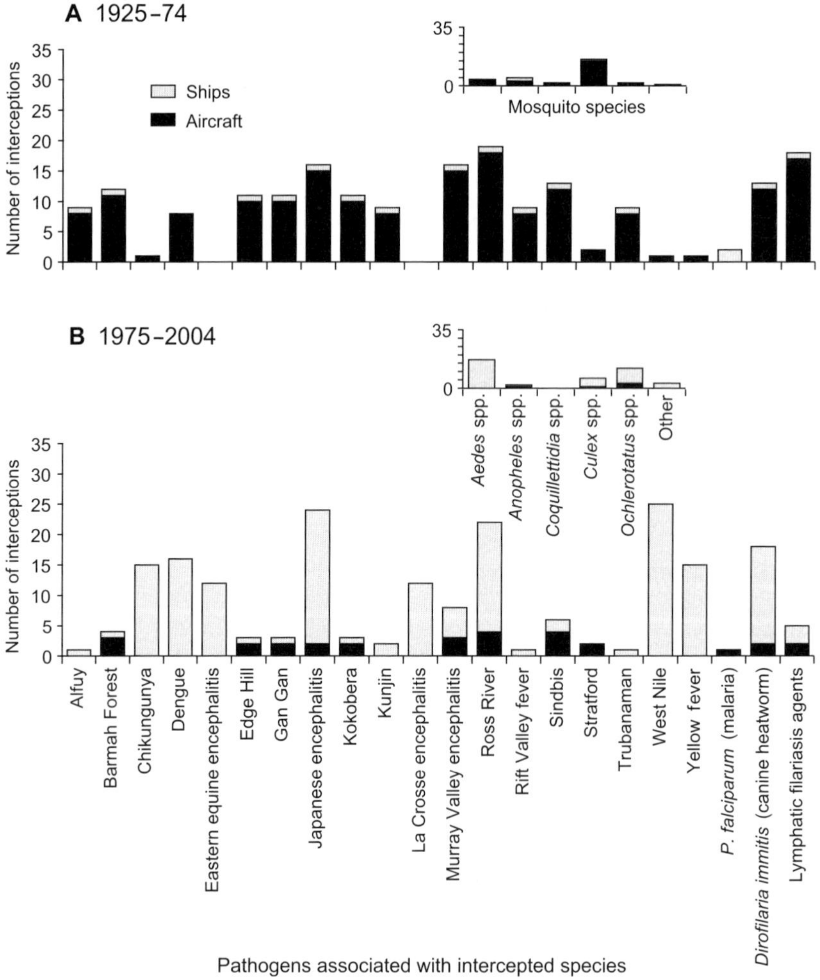

Fig. 6.32. Temporal changes in recorded interceptions of exotic (non-established) mosquito species on aircraft and ships, New Zealand, 1925–2004
(A) 1925–74. (B) 1975–2004. For each time period, graphs plot the number of interceptions by mosquito species (inset graph) and pathogen(s) known to be associated with intercepted species (main graph).
Source: Drawn from data in Derraik (2004, table 3, pp. 438–9).

New Zealand is under a serious risk of arboviral infection outbreaks, and it is predicted that human-induced climatic change will further facilitate the survival and establishment of new exotic disease vectors in the country. Under these circumstances, adequate monitoring and border surveillance, and inspections of all incoming goods and crafts are of utmost importance to safeguard the public health of New Zealand's population.

Gibbs (2005) has estimated that, although three-quarters of emerging diseases are zoonotic, animal and public health responses are separated by culture and organization and more integrated surveillance and protection are needed. We return to the question of protection and control in Chapter 11.

6.6 Conclusion

We have seen in this chapter that, over the last 200 years, the earth's human population has grown sevenfold from less than a billion to over 6 billion. Half of that increase has come in the last 40 years. Striking as this is, still more impressive has been the growth in the spatial mobility of the expanding population as transport barriers have been reduced. In Western countries this has increased mobility 1,000-fold with half the rise coming since 1960. If we combine the two increases of population numbers ($\times 7$) and mobility (up to $\times 1{,}000$), we arrive at a 3,000- to 7,000-fold increase in population flux in just two centuries.

This increase in world population, coupled with the collapse of distance brought about by changes in transport technology over the last 200 years, has been shown here to influence the transfer of communicable diseases. The geographical extent of many diseases has increased; they appear more frequently in different locations. Some also generally occur today as small outbreaks rather than as the massive epidemics witnessed in the nineteenth and early twentieth centuries. In addition, greater international population flux carries genetic implications for population mixing as well as enhancing the opportunities for new diseases to emerge.

7

Environmental Changes: Ecological Modifications

7.1 Introduction

Diseases originate, spread, and persist or wither, within a specific environmental context. For the entire time during which humans have lived on the earth, this environmental context has changed and, viewed from the beginning of a new millennium, all the available evidence suggests that the environment is set to change further and faster than at any other time in human history. In this chapter, we explore aspects of the changing environmental terrain in which diseases spread, and how these changes have served to promote the emergence and resurgence of infectious agents.

Table 7.1. Infectious diseases and disease agents with the strongest evidence for known or suspected links to environment and land use change

Vector-borne and/or zoonotic diseases	Soil	Water	Human	Other
Dengue	Anthrax	Cholera	Influenza	Foot and mouth
Filariasis	Coccidioidomycosis	Cryptosporidiosis	Tuberculosis	Rice blast
Haemorrhagic fevers	Hookworm	Leptospirosis		Trachoma
Hantavirus	Melioidosis	Rotavirus		
Japanese encephalitis		Salmonellosis		
Kyasanur Forest fever		Schistosomiasis		
Leishmaniasis		Shigellosis		
Lyme disease				
Malaria				
Meningitis				
Nipah virus				
Onchocerciasis				
Plague				
Rabies				
Rift Valley fever				
Trypanosomiasis				
Yellow fever				

Source: Adapted from Patz *et al.* (2004, table 1, p. 1093).

ENVIRONMENTAL CHANGES AND INFECTIOUS DISEASES

Anthropogenic environmental changes and ecological modifications that promote the emergence and resurgence of infectious diseases are numerous and include deforestation and reforestation, road construction, agricultural development, dam building, irrigation and water control schemes, coastal zone degradation and wetland modification, mining and urbanization, and macro- and micro-climate change and variability (Morse 1995; Patz, Graczyk, *et al.* 2000; Patz, Daszak, *et al.* 2004; McMichael 2004). As Patz, Daszak, *et al.* (2004: 1092) observe, these changes and modifications can, in turn, provoke a 'cascade effect' of habitat fragmentation, ecosystem degradation, and biodiversity loss, pollution, poverty, and human migration that serve to amplify the risks of disease emergence and spread. Examples of infectious diseases that are known or suspected to be especially prone to the effects of environmental and land use change are given in Table 7.1.

STRUCTURE OF CHAPTER

Of the many environmental and land use changes that can facilitate the processes of infectious disease emergence and resurgence, we have selected the five interlinked factors in Figure 7.1 for study here. We illustrate each factor with special reference to one or more examples drawn from the sample diseases and regions listed in Table 7.2. Our examples include: agricultural

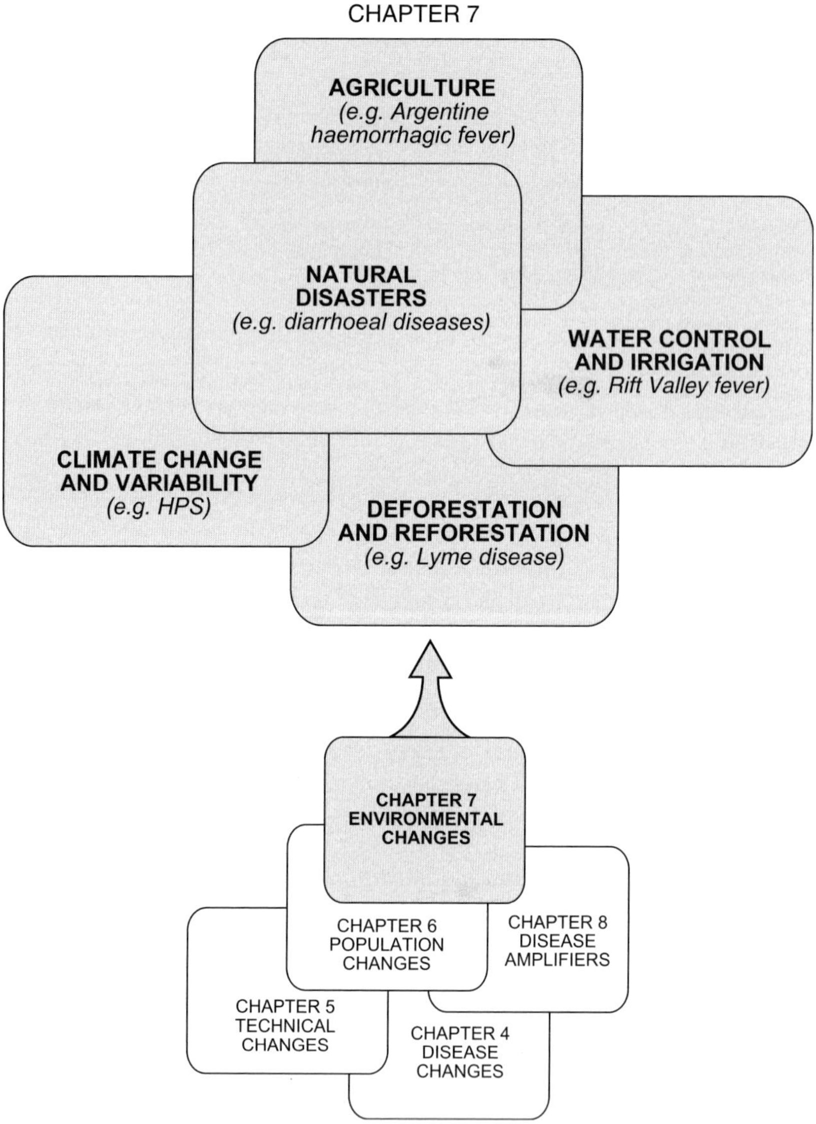

Fig. 7.1. (Upper) Venn diagram showing the facilitating factors for disease emergence and re-emergence associated with environmental changes
The lower diagram is redrawn from Fig. II.1 and shows the position of environmental changes (shaded box) within the suite of macro factors associated with the processes of disease and emergence and re-emergence. HPS = hantavirus pulmonary syndrome.

Table 7.2. Environmental changes and disease emergence

Facilitating factor	Sample diseases	Sample geographical regions
Agricultural development	Argentine haemorrhagic fever (AHF)	Americas (South)
	Korean haemorrhagic fever (KHF)	Western Pacific
Water control and irrigation	Dracunculiasis	Africa
	Filariasis	Africa/eastern Mediterranean
	Japanese encephalitis	Western Pacific
	Malaria	Africa
	Onchocerciasis	Africa
	Rift Valley fever	Africa/eastern Mediterranean
	Schistosomiasis	Africa/eastern Mediterranean/western Pacific
Deforestation and reforestation	Lyme disease	Americas (North)/Europe
	Malaria	Americas (South)
	Nipah viral disease	Western Pacific
Climate change and variability	Cholera	Africa/South-East Asia
	Dengue	Americas (South)/South-East Asia/western Pacific
	Hantavirus pulmonary syndrome (HPS)	Americas
	Malaria	Americas (South)/South-East Asia
	Nipah viral disease	Western Pacific
Natural disasters	Diarrhoeal diseases	Americas (North)/South-East Asia
	Malaria	South-East Asia

Sources: Based on Morse (1995) and McMichael (2004).

development and Argentine haemorrhagic fever in South America (Section 7.2); water control schemes and Rift Valley fever in Africa and the eastern Mediterranean (Section 7.3); deforestation and Nipah viral disease in the western Pacific (Section 7.4.1); reforestation and Lyme disease in North America (Section 7.4.2); climate variability and hantavirus pulmonary syndrome in North America (Section 7.5); and natural disasters and disease in North America and South-East Asia (Section 7.6). In making our selection, we emphasize that the processes involved are not discrete and that a given example could be used to illustrate aspects of more than one of the overlapping themes in Figure 7.1—a reflection of the complexity of the ecosystems in which diseases emerge and spread (McMichael 2004).

7.2 Agricultural Development

Agricultural development is one of the key ways by which people alter their environment, and it is a prominent driver of disease emergence and resurgence—not least by increasing the risk of human exposure to the pool of disease agents harboured by both wild and domestic animals (Morse 1995; McMichael 2004; Patz, Daszak, *et al.* 2004). In parts of Asia, for example, post-war developments in rice production have favoured an increase in Hantaan virus-carrying rodents (*Apodemus agrarius*), with a corresponding increase in the incidence of Korean haemorrhagic fever in farmworkers (see Section 8.2.1). Likewise, certain types of agricultural system in South-East Asia have been posited as sources of human exposure to avian influenza A viruses, raising the spectre of the emergence of new human pandemic strains of the virus (see Section 4.2). Intersecting with other themes in Figure 7.1, the implementation of crop irrigation systems (Section 7.3), the replacement of forests with farmland (Section 7.4), and climate-induced shifts in agricultural production systems (Section 7.5) can all result in new habitats that are supportive of disease microbes, their vectors and reservoirs. Thus, there have been documented increases in the incidence of lymphatic filariasis (Harb *et al.* 1993), malaria (Sogoba *et al.* 2007), Rift Valley fever (Wilson 1994), and schistosomiasis (Malek 1975) in association with the development of crop irrigation schemes in Africa. The spread of Lyme and other tick-borne diseases has been associated with the implementation of agricultural land set-aside policies in the European Union (Süss *et al.* 2008) and, as described in more detail here, the emergence of Argentine haemorrhagic fever with the establishment of crop cultivation in South America (Morse 1995).

7.2.1 Argentine Haemorrhagic Fever

BACKGROUND TO THE DISEASE

Argentine haemorrhagic fever (AHF) (*ICD*-10 A96.0) is an acute febrile disease that occurs in a geographically circumscribed area of the Argentine pampas in South America. The aetiological agent is Junín virus, a single-stranded RNA virus of the genus *Arenavirus* in the family *Arenaviridae* (Plate 7.1). The virus belongs to the New World (Tacaribe) arenavirus complex, of which Guanarito virus (Venezuelan haemorrhagic fever), Machupo virus (Bolivian haemorrhagic fever), and Sabía virus (Brazilian haemorrhagic fever) are also known to be pathogenic for humans (Table 7.3). The reservoirs of these viruses are rodents of the family *Cricetidae*, each with an ecologically determined range that limits the geographical distribution of the associated diseases (Downs 1993). The currently recognized endemo-epidemic areas of the diseases are indicated in Figure 7.2.

Nature of AHF

As described by Jahrling (1997), AHF presents a clinical syndrome that includes manifestations of renal, cardiovascular, haematological, and neurological involvement. A typical incubation period of 7–14 days gives way to

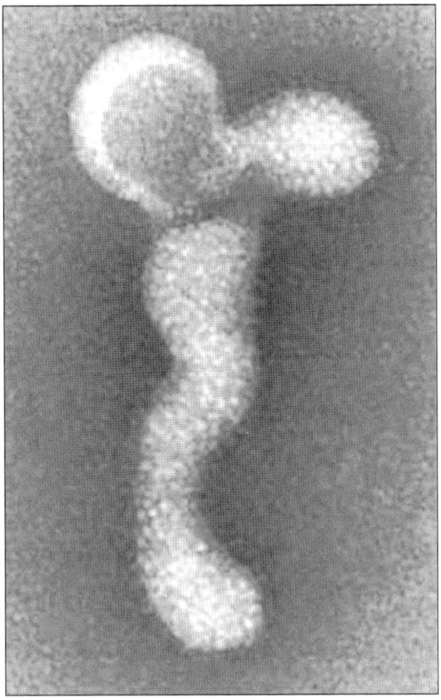

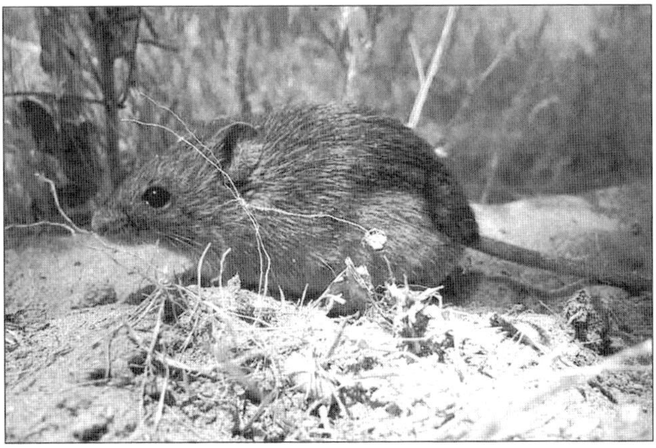

Pl. 7.1. Argentine haemorrhagic fever (AHF)
The aetiological agent of AHF is Junín virus, a single-stranded RNA virus of the genus *Arenavirus* in the family *Arenaviridae*. *Arenavirus* particles range in size from 50–300 nm, with a mean of 100–30, and in shape from mainly spherical to highly pleomorphic, as with the negatively stained Junín virus shown in the transmission electron micrograph. The principal rodent host is the corn mouse or drylands vesper mouse, *Calomys musculinus*.

Sources: Micrograph: Geisbert and Jahrling (2004, fig. 1, p. S112). *Calomys musculinus*: M. Asher, http://www.cricyt.edu.ar/institutos/iadiza/ojeda/mamnacu.htm.

Table 7.3. Arenaviruses known to cause acute disease in humans

		Associated human disease		
Virus	Natural (rodent) host	Disease	First clinical description	Geographical distribution
Old World (LCMV[1]-Lassa) arenavirus complex				
Lymphocytic choriomeningitis virus	*Mus musculus*	Acute aseptic meningitis	?[2]	Europe, Americas
Lassa virus	*Mastomys* spp.	Lassa fever	1969	West Africa
New World (Tacaribe) arenavirus complex				
Junín virus	*Calomys musculinus*, *C. laucha*	Argentine haemorrhagic fever	1953	Argentina
Machupo virus	*C. callosus*	Bolivian haemorrhagic fever	1959	Bolivia
Guanarito virus	*Sigmodon alstoni*, *Zygodontomys brevicauda*	Venezuelan haemorrhagic fever	1989	Venezuela
Sabía virus	Not known	Brazilian haemorrhagic fever	1990	Brazil

Notes: [1] Lymphocytic choriomeningitis virus.[2] Virus first isolated in 1933.

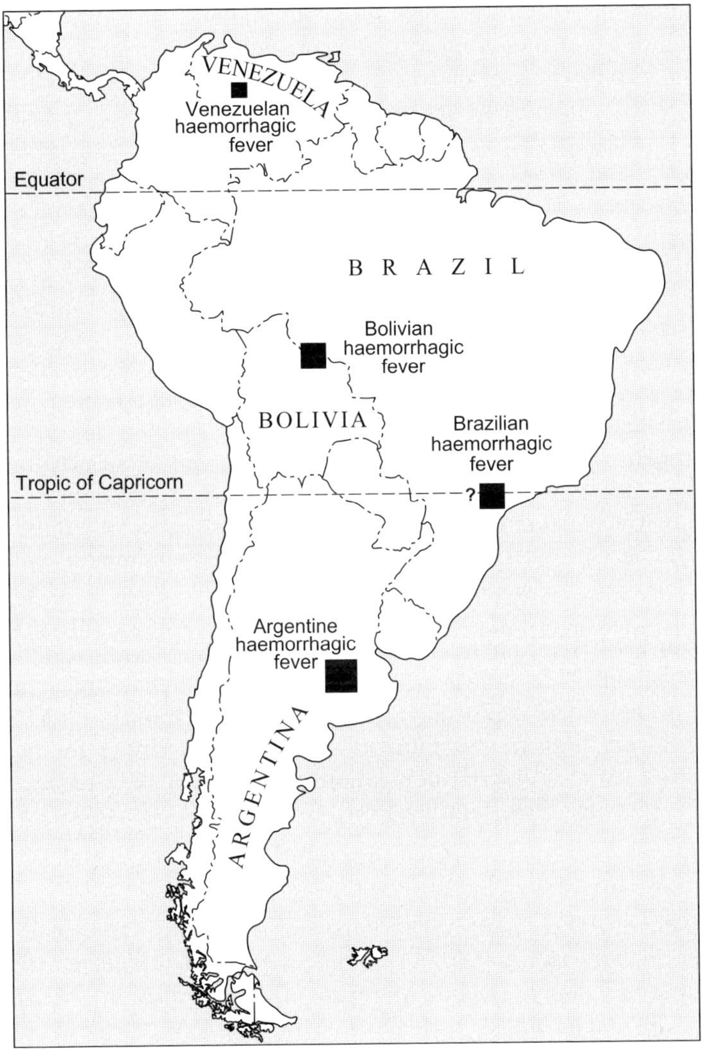

Fig. 7.2. Currently recognized endemo-epidemic areas for haemorrhagic fevers due to arenaviruses in South America

The map plots the geographical distributions of Argentine, Bolivian, and Venezuelan haemorrhagic fevers. The distribution of Brazilian haemorrhagic fever, first identified in São Paulo state in 1990, is currently unknown.

Sources: Based on Pan American Health Organization (1994; 2003: 66–7), Manzione *et al.* (1998), and García *et al.* (2000).

the gradual onset of fever, malaise, chills, fatigue, and dizziness. Many patients also experience conjunctival congestion, retro-orbital pain, nausea, vomiting, constipation, or diarrhoea. In mild cases, the disease resolves after about 6–7 days. In more severe cases, clinical manifestations continue for up to 15 days and may include haemorrhaging, muscular tremors, confusion or excitability, and, occasionally, convulsive seizures. The case-fatality rate is 15–30 per cent in untreated cases (Jahrling 1997; Heymann 2004: 26–8).

The main reservoirs of Junín virus in nature are the corn mouse (*Calomys musculinus*) and the small vesper mouse (*C. laucha*) (Plate 7.1). The virus is shed in the secretions and excretions of infected rodents, and the principal route of transmission to humans is by inhalation of contaminated aerosol particles. Other potential transmission routes include the ingestion of contaminated products and the exposure of skin abrasions to contaminated materials. Human-to-human transmission is believed to be uncommon (Jahrling 1997).

The rodent reservoirs of Junín virus are opportunistic species that place low demands on habitat quality and thrive in disturbed environments such as croplands (Carballal *et al.* 1988). Cultivated fields—especially those associated with maize production—form the principal place of human exposure to Junín virus, and, historically, epidemics of AHF have been concentrated in agricultural workers. The disease is highly seasonal, with outbreaks peaking in the Southern Hemisphere autumn (April–June) and terminating with the onset of winter. This pattern reflects the seasonal rhythms of agricultural activity in the endemo-epidemic area, with the peak months of AHF cases coinciding with both (i) the influx of transient farm labour for the maize harvest and (ii) the seasonal population maximum of the *Calomys* rodent reservoirs (Mettler 1969; Jahrling 1997).

THE GEOGRAPHY OF AHF

The first detailed account of AHF was provided by R. A. Arribalzaga (1955), who described the clinical features of an apparently new epidemic disease in the pampas of northern Buenos Aires province, Argentina, in 1953 and 1954 (Figure 7.3A).[1] The highest incidences of the disease were recorded in farm labourers, with the earliest patients being potato harvesters who had worked on the outskirts of the towns of Bragado and Alberti. With anecdotal evidence of further cases of the disease in the index area in 1955–7, AHF finally garnered public attention in 1958:

> It so happened that the Minister of Public Health, a physician with knowledge of the problem, had landholdings in the endemic area. The epidemic that year was more severe than ever, and it received wide publicity through newspapers, radio, and television. All these circumstances combined to press the public health authorities into action. (Mettler 1969: 3)

[1] A disease closely resembling AHF ('malignant grippe') had been observed in the contemporary endemo-epidemic area of AHF as early as 1943; see Mettler (1969).

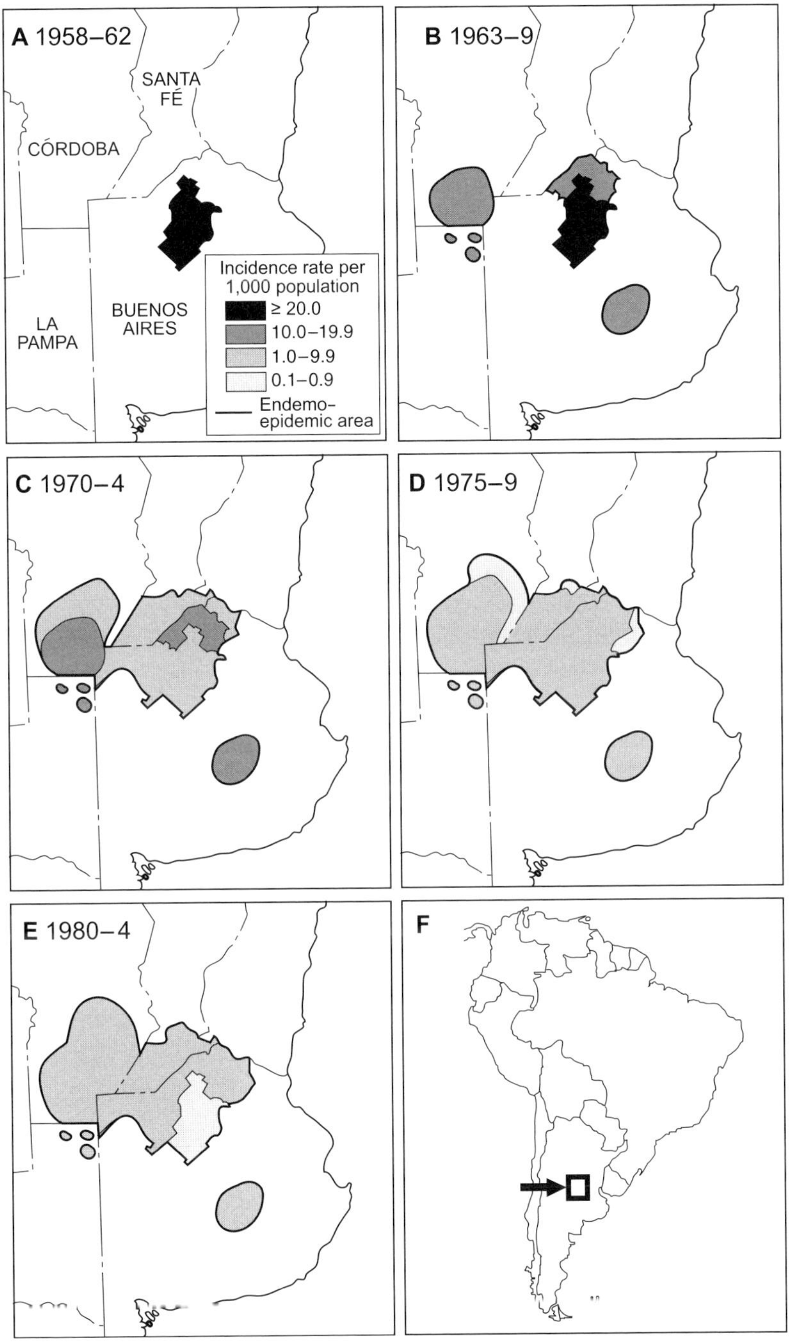

Fig. 7.3. Argentine haemorrhagic fever (AHF): geographical expansion of the recognized endemo-epidemic area, 1958–1984

The maps plot the geographical extent of the recognized endemo-epidemic area in (A) 1958–62, (B) 1963–9, (C) 1970–4, (D) 1975–9, and (E) 1980–4. Infected areas are shaded according to the AHF incidence rate (per 1,000 population) in a given time period.

Source: Drawn from Maiztegui *et al.* (1986, fig. 1 and table 1, pp. 150–1).

With the impetus afforded by these developments, the search for the aetiological agent of AHF resulted in the recovery of a novel virus from patient materials collected at Junín Regional Hospital in 1958. Subsequent investigations traced the natural reservoir of the newly named Junín virus to wild *Calomys* rodents (Mettler 1969; Jahrling 1997).

The Endemo-Epidemic Area

The currently recognized endemo-epidemic area of AHF lies between latitudes 33° and 37° S and longitudes 59° and 65° W, extending across a large and heavily cultivated area of the Humid Pampas in northern Buenos Aires and La Pampa provinces and southern Córdoba and Santa Fé provinces. As the map sequence in Figure 7.3 shows, the endemo-epidemic area has expanded markedly since the first descriptions of the disease in the 1950s. In the late 1950s and early 1960s, AHF was limited to a 16,000 km^2 area in northern Buenos Aires province (Figure 7.3A). Further endemic areas were identified in central Buenos Aires, southern Córdoba, and northern La Pampa in the mid- to late 1960s (Figure 7.3B), with the total endemo-epidemic area expanding to over 120,000 km^2 by the mid-1980s (Figures 7.3C–E); see Mettler (1969), Maiztegui (1975), and Maiztegui *et al.* (1986). Further expansion, concentrated along the north-central perimeter of the zone in Figure 7.3E, has subsequently been documented by Enria *et al.* (2008).

Morbidity Patterns

During the period 1958–84, over 20,000 cases of AHF were recorded in the endemo-epidemic area. An uninterrupted series of annual epidemics—ranging in size from a few hundred to a few thousand cases—occurred in this interval, with the highest case count (>3,000) in 1964 (Mettler 1969; Maiztegui *et al.* 1986). As the choropleth shading in Figure 7.3 shows, AHF incidence rates were generally highest in the 5–10 years following the first appearance of the disease in a given part of the endemic area, with a gradual reduction in levels of recorded disease activity in subsequent time periods. While the adoption of crop substitution and rotation techniques provided an ecological check on AHF activity in the 1980s (Maiztegui *et al.* 1986), control of the disease took a major step forward with the introduction of a live attenuated Junín vaccine (Candid #1) in 1990 (Ambrosio *et al.* 2006). A pronounced decrease in the annual incidence of AHF has been recorded since that time (Enria *et al.* 2008).

AGRICULTURE AND THE EMERGENCE OF AHF

The emergence and spread of AHF is intimately associated with the adoption of agricultural activities that favour the rodent reservoirs of Junín virus, and which bring the rodents and their excreta into contact with humans. High rodent densities in the endemo-epidemic area are correlated with the cultivation of grains (especially maize), with the concentration of AHF among grain harvesters so well recognized that the condition is colloquially referred to as 'stubble disease' (Mettler 1969). Against this background, Viglizzo *et al.* (2004) note that the pampas has a relatively short farming history, having remained as native grassland until the latter part of the nineteenth century. In the twentieth century, the extensive conversion of grassland to maize cultivation provided an environment in which *Calomys* rodents could flourish, increasing the opportunities for the zoonotic transmission of Junín virus and the emergence of an apparently 'new' viral disease in the human population (Morse 1995; McMichael 2001; Hui 2006).

While changes in land use account for the appearance of AHF in the human population, additional factors have been invoked to explain the progressive expansion of the endemo-epidemic area in Figure 7.3. Based on genetic evidence, González Ittig and Gardenal (2004) hypothesize that the introduction of agriculture in the Humid Pampas resulted in explosive increments in the density of *C. musculinus*. The resulting population pressure, in turn, forced a range expansion of the rodent and the microbes that it carries. If correct, the apparent slowdown in the expansion of the endemo-epidemic area in more recent times (see Figures 7.3C–E) is suggestive of some as yet undetermined limiting mechanism in the range expansion of the rodent (González Ittig and Gardenal 2004).

7.3 Water Control and Irrigation

Man-made water control projects are closely associated with the emergence and resurgence of a range of infectious diseases that are transmitted by water-breeding vectors such as mosquitoes, flies, and aquatic snails (Table 7.2). The construction of dams, reservoirs, agricultural irrigation systems, and drainage schemes can result in the expansion of vectors, their larvae, and their associated parasites. Excavation pits, generated during the construction of dams and canals, can also provide breeding grounds for vectors, as can irrigation systems that result in raised water tables, seepage, and impounded water (Morse 1995; Patz, Graczyk, *et al.* 2000; Patz, Daszak, *et al.* 2004). The disease impacts of such developments have been documented in many regions of the world, as Saker *et al.* (2004: 27) observe:

> Changes in the prevalence of vector-borne diseases associated with the construction of large dams have been reported from many regions and settings. Overall, most research suggests that the construction of large dams in tropical areas is associated with increases in prevalence of endemic vector-borne infections. . . Most reservoir and irrigation projects undertaken in malaria endemic areas have led to an increase in malaria transmission and disease, an increase which is more pronounced for dams below 1900 metres altitude than for those above. In Africa, the development of many reservoirs has been associated with big rises in malaria prevalence . . . in Latin America

and Asia also, malaria has been the biggest public health problem associated with large water projects. But it is not only malaria. Dramatic increases in schistosomiasis have followed the construction of dams in many African countries due to extensive colonization of the new reservoirs by the snail vectors ... while, in parts of the Middle East and Africa, filariasis prevalence has increased following the creation of reservoirs. Similarly, onchocerciasis has become more prominent in some areas of West Africa near to the spillways of newly constructed large dams ... while construction of reservoirs in the Siberian and Volga regions of the former USSR has led to dramatic increases in diphyllobothriasis ...

Globally, small-scale water control schemes—rather than their larger 'flagship' counterparts—may have had a greater aggregate impact on vector-borne infections due to the larger total surface area that they cover, their closer association with human settlements and the frequent lack of regulatory control of such schemes. Regardless of size, however, an increase in vector-borne diseases is not an inevitable consequence of water control schemes and, in some instances, ecological changes may result in a reduction in disease activity. (Saker *et al.* 2004)

Water Control Projects and Parasitic Disease: Schistosomiasis

Schistosomiasis (*ICD*-10 B65) has emerged as a particular concern in relation to water control projects in parts of Africa and Asia, with dams and irrigation systems providing aquaria for the intermediate hosts (aquatic snails) in the trematode lifecycle. In West Africa, for example, the construction of the Diama Dam, Senegal, in the 1980s resulted in river conditions that favoured the growth of freshwater snails, with the consequent introduction of *Schistosoma mansoni* to humans in the Senegal River basin (Harrus and Baneth 2005). Elsewhere, in Egypt, an increase in the prevalence of schistosomiasis has been correlated with the introduction of year-round agricultural irrigation that followed on the construction of the Aswan High Dam in the 1970s (Malek 1975). More recently, concerns have been expressed over the possible increase in schistosomiasis in consequence of the ecological changes arising from the construction of Three Gorges Dam on the Yangtze River, China (Li, Raso, *et al.* 2007).

7.3.1 Rift Valley Fever

Rift Valley fever (RVF) (*ICD*-10 A92.4) is an arthropod-borne disease of certain ruminants (buffalo, cattle, goats, and sheep), camels, and humans. The aetiological agent is RVF virus, a member of the genus *Phlebovirus* in the family *Bunyaviridae* (Plate 7.2). Little is known of the cycle of RVF virus in nature, although available evidence suggests that mosquitoes perform the role of both reservoir and vector. Mosquitoes perpetuate transmission both vertically (transovarially), from one mosquito generation to another, and horizontally (via blood meals) to and from vertebrates. The relative importance of vertical and horizontal transmission in the natural cycle of the virus remains speculative. The enzootic vectors of RVF are mosquitoes of the genus *Aedes*, although other genera (including *Culex*) have also been implicated in transmission during epizootics and epidemics. In addition, human infection may occur as a consequence of direct exposure to infected animals.

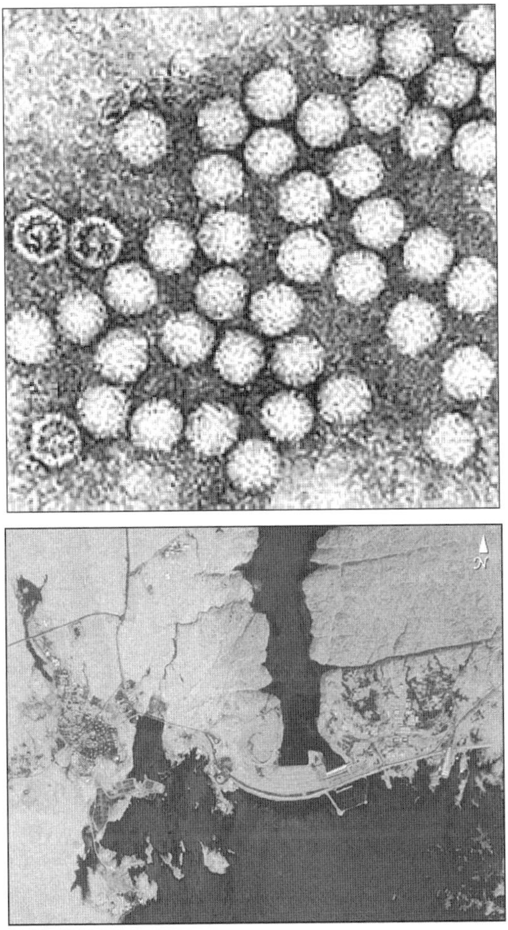

Pl. 7.2. Rift Valley fever (RVF) and water management projects
The aetiological agent of RVF is RVF virus, a member of the genus *Phlebovirus* in the family *Bunyaviridae*. The plate shows (top) an electron micrograph of the virus, (centre) a NASA satellite image of the Aswan High Dam (Egypt), and (bottom) a photograph of the Diama Dam (Senegal). The lakes created by these dams have provided ideal breeding grounds for *Culex* mosquitoes, the vector for RVF.

Sources: Micrograph: CDC public health image library. Aswan Dam: NASA photo ID STS102–303–17. Diama Dam: http://yalemedicine.yale.edu/ym_su05/dam.html.

Clinically, the disease in humans is associated with a broad spectrum of illness, from asymptomatic infection, through a benign febrile illness, to severe disease in a small proportion (<4 per cent) of cases. Although clinical manifestations are typically mild, and recovery is usually complete, ocular complications may occasionally result in loss of vision. More rarely, death (usually associated with haemorrhagic manifestations and meningoencephalitis) has been recorded in RVF patients during severe epidemics (Pan American Health Organization 2003: 276–83; Heymann 2004: 45–8).

HISTORICAL OCCURRENCE

Rift Valley fever virus was first isolated from sheep during an epizootic in farm animals in the East African Rift Valley, Kenya, in 1930. Since that time, major epizootics and epidemics of RVF have occurred at irregular intervals throughout the African continent (Figure 7.4). Following Sall *et al.* (1998), two modes of virus circulation can be identified: (i) local circulation in enzootic/endemic areas, as illustrated for East and West Africa by the circulation cells in Figure 7.4; and (ii) long-distance spread from enzootic/endemic areas in sub-Saharan Africa to apparently disease-free areas, as depicted by the transmission vectors in Figure 7.4. The earliest reports of RVF north of the Sahara were associated with explosive outbreaks of human and animal disease in Egypt in 1977–8. Thereafter, outbreaks were documented for the first time in West Africa (1987, 1998), Madagascar (1990–1), and the Arabian Peninsula (2000)—the latter development underscoring the potential of RVF to spread to extra-African locations (Pan American Health Organization 2003: 276–83).

THE RVF EMERGENCE COMPLEX: DAMS AND IRRIGATION PROJECTS

Wilson (1994: 173, table 2) identifies a gamut of ecological and environmental factors that have precipitated the emergence of RVF in recent decades. While these factors extend to include many of the themes covered in Part II of this book, particular importance attaches to the role of water in the emergence complex. The occurrence of excessively heavy seasonal rains and associated floods, resulting in an increase in the density of the mosquito vector population, has been implicated as a precipitating factor for the 1997–8 outbreaks in East Africa (Figure 7.4) (World Health Organization 1998*a*). Other outbreaks in ecological zones not formerly associated with enzootic/epizootic activity, including Egypt (1977–8) and Mauritania (1987), have pointed to the possible role of water control projects in the promotion of virus activity (World Health Organization 1982). In particular, Wilson (1994) observes that dam and irrigation schemes have contributed to the emergence of RVF by (i) increasing the endemic prevalence of RVF infection, (ii) increasing the epidemic intensity of RVF infection, and (iii) promoting the expansion of RVF activity into previously uninfected areas:

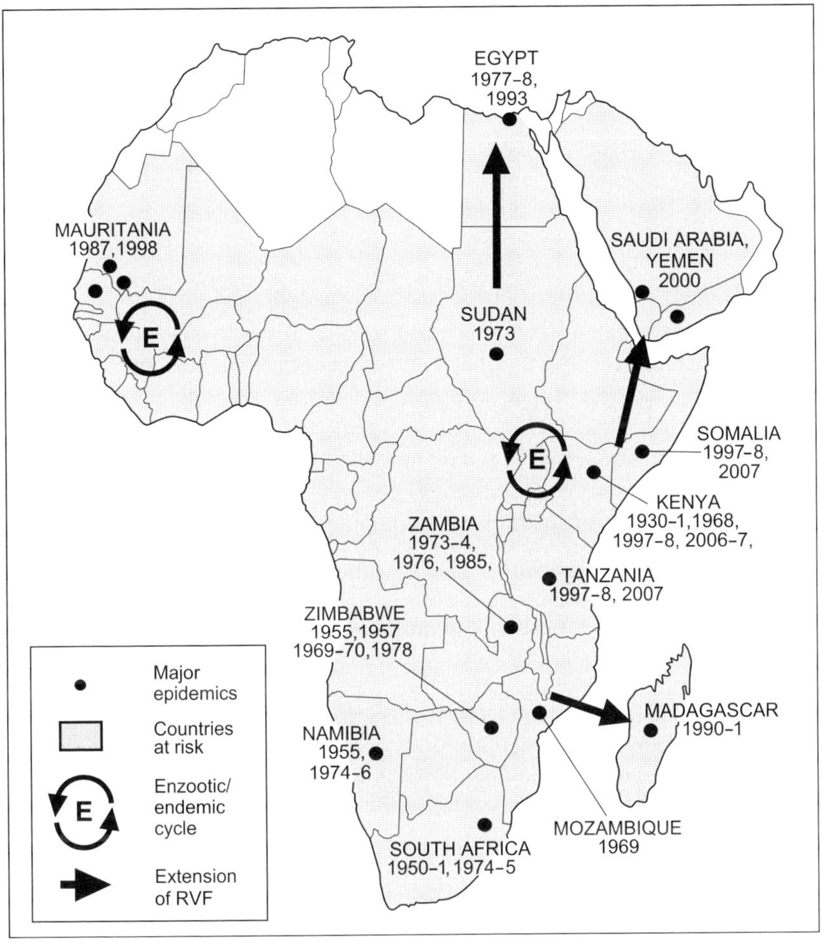

Fig. 7.4. Location of major epidemics of Rift Valley fever, 1930–2007
The map identifies countries in which major epidemics were recorded to Sept. 2007. Enzootic/endemic circulation cells in East and West Africa are indicated for reference. The likely routes of extension of the disease to Madagascar, North Africa (Egypt), and the Arabian Peninsula (Saudi Arabia and Yemen) are indicated by the vectors.
Sources: Based on World Health Organization Epidemic and Pandemic Alert and Response (2007), with supplementary information from Sall *et al.* (1998, fig. 2, p. 613).

Changing patterns of water storage and use that alter the breeding and larval development of vector species affect intensity of transmission. Particular patterns of standing water following damming of rivers and irrigation of surrounding land may encourage reproduction of certain *Culex* mosquitoes ... Thus, increased populations of *Culex* species that enhance transmission among animals and to humans would increase local endemic prevalence without impacting on the frequency of such epidemics. The intensity of epidemics, however, may be expanded as in the Mauritanian outbreak. Finally, damming and irrigation alone should not cause the distribution of RVF virus to change, although habitats could be created that support eventual virus introductions. (Wilson 1994: 174)

To illustrate the issues involved, we examine the role of dam construction and irrigation schemes as facilitating factors in the emergence of RVF in North Africa (Egypt, 1977–8) and West Africa (Mauritania, 1987).

NORTH AFRICA: EGYPT AND THE ASWAN HIGH DAM, 1977–1978

The 1977–8 epidemic of RVF in Egypt marked the northwards extension of a virus that, until that time, had been entirely confined to sub-Saharan Africa (Figure 7.4). The appearance and spread of the disease in a new and ecologically distinct area, yielding an outbreak of unprecedented magnitude (~200,000 cases) and severity (~600 recorded deaths) in the human population, was a signal event in the epidemic history of RVF. As Hoogstraal (1978: 129–30) observes, prior to the Egyptian epidemic:

> The virus had not been recorded in a climatically rainless zone where humans, domestic animals, and most insects and other arthropods thrive due to the beneficence of irrigation water. The virus was also unknown in a geographically extensive zone with the limited variety of small-size and large-size wild vertebrates, and with few species of mosquitoes and of most other hematophagous arthropods that faunistically characterize the irrigated areas of Egypt where RVF erupted in 1977. It is probably safe to say that RVF virus has not previously been recognized to circulate among such densely crowded human populations as that in Egypt, where so many people dwell so closely with domestic animals ... And lastly, there is little or no recorded precedent for the virus spreading like a firebolt through a rural area some 500 miles in length within a three-month period, as it did, to the best of our knowledge, from Aswan to the southeastern Nile Delta ... in August–October 1977.

Course of the Epidemic

Epidemiological and other aspects of the Egyptian RVF epidemic of 1977–8 are reviewed by El-Akkad (1978), Meegan (1979), Shope *et al.* (1982), and Ghoneim and Woods (1983). The area of disease activity is mapped in Figure 7.5. On 8 October 1977, the Egyptian Ministry of Health received a report from Sharqiya governorate of an acute febrile disease and a fatal haemorrhagic-like illness among villagers in the south-eastern Nile Delta region in northern Egypt (Meegan 1979). The appearance of the disease in humans was accompanied by raised mortality and abortion in sheep and other domestic animals—an epizootic which, in retrospect, could be traced several hundred kilometres south to Aswan governorate, where the disease had first manifested in July 1977 (World Health Organization 1978). Although the evidence is sketchy, Hoogstraal (1978) infers that RVF spread rapidly from its apparent index location in Aswan, northwards up the Nile Valley, and into the delta region, to infect animals and humans in adjacent agricultural areas in August,

September, and October. While attempts were made to limit virus transmission through the aerial insecticiding of mosquitoes, raised levels of RVF activity continued among humans in November and the first half of December. The epidemic eventually waned with the onset of colder winter weather in mid- to late December, for a modest resurgence in 1978 (Meegan 1979).

Geographical Foci of RVF Activity

Some impression of the geographical pattern of RVF activity can be gained from Figure 7.5, which plots, as pie charts, the results of serological studies to determine the prevalence of antibodies to the virus in sheep. The highest prevalences were identified in the Nile delta governorates of Sharqiya (52.0 per cent), Qalyubiya (37.0 per cent), and Giza (23.2 per cent), and the Nile Valley governorates of Asyut (40.5 per cent), Aswan (32.0 per cent), Minya (9.5 per cent), and Faiyum (9.4 per cent). Overall, the pattern corresponds with the primary foci of reported human cases in Sharqiya, Qalyubiya, Giza, Asyut, and Minya governorates (World Health Organization 1978), although the lack of reported cases in Aswan is noteworthy (Meegan 1979).

RVF and the Aswan High Dam

The appearance and spread of RVF has been linked to the construction of the Aswan High Dam in Upper Egypt; see Figure 7.5 and Plate 7.2. Completed in 1970, the dam created an 800,000-hectare water body (Lake Nasser) and stabilized water tables so that surface water provided breeding sites for mosquitoes (Gerdes 2004). Whether the mosquito population provided a corridor for RVF virus transmission from neighbouring Sudan—where the disease was epizootic in previous years (Figure 7.4)—has yet to be proven.[2] Whatever the source of the virus, however, RVF retreated from Egypt after the epidemic of 1977–8, only to reappear in Aswan governorate in the early summer of 1993 (Arthur *et al.* 1993).

WEST AFRICA: MAURITANIA AND THE DIAMA DAM, 1987

In 1987, concurrent with the completion of the Diama Dam on the Senegal River, an upstream outbreak of RVF was recorded in southern Mauritania (Figure 7.4 and Plate 7.2). Over 1,200 human cases and 250 deaths resulted. But, in contrast to Egypt, immunological studies showed RVF to be already endemic among people and livestock in a wide area of the Senegal River basin. Ecological changes favouring the vector and associated with dam building seem to be implicated in allowing both (i) invasion of the virus into a previously virgin population and (ii) severe flare-ups in a population with low-level endemicity (World Health Organization 1987; Cliff, Haggett, and Smallman-Raynor 2004).

[2] A variety of mechanisms have been proposed for the introduction of RVF virus to Egypt from Sudan in the summer of 1977, including wind-borne vectors (Sellers *et al.* 1982), viraemic camels (Hoogstraal *et al.* 1979), and the transportation, via Lake Nasser, of sheep from holding areas in north-central Sudan to animal markets in the vicinity of Aswan (Gad *et al.* 1986).

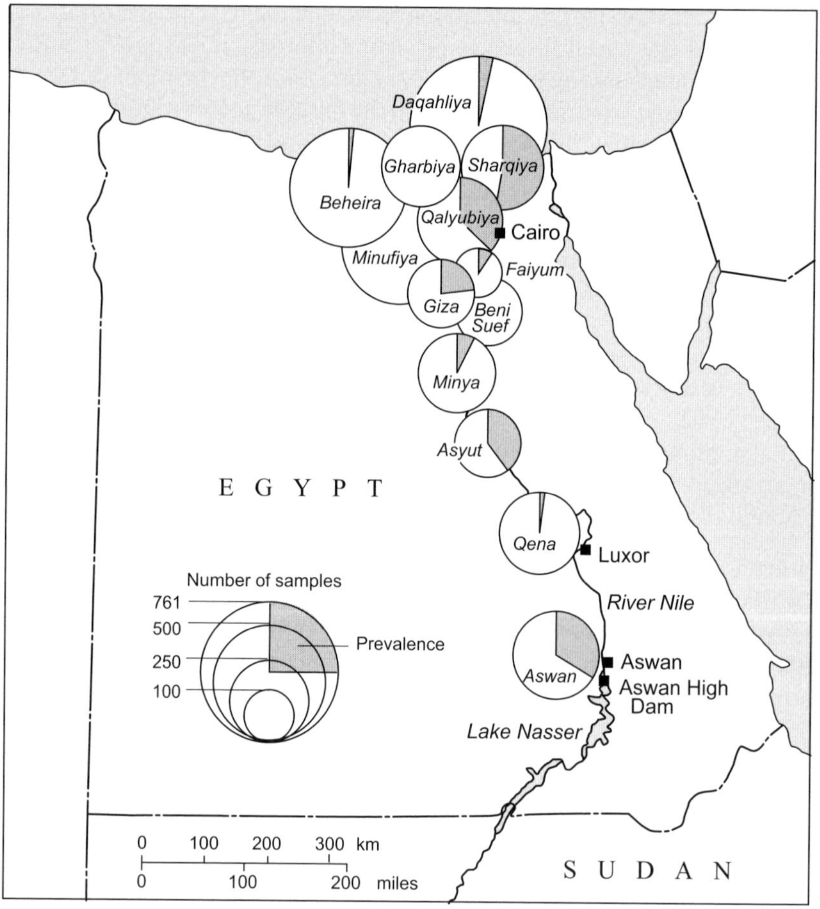

Fig. 7.5. Rift Valley fever (RVF) in Egypt, 1977–1978
For sample Egyptian governorates, the proportional circles show the percentage prevalence of antibodies to RVF virus in sheep. Lake Nasser and the Aswan High Dam are indicated for reference.
Source: Drawn from data in Meegan (1979, tables II and III, p. 621).

7.4 Deforestation and Reforestation

Changes in global forest cover are linked to disease changes in complex ways. Among the many interconnected factors, ecological changes that have followed on the massive deforestation of tropical and temperate areas over the last century—and which have heightened the risk of human exposure to the zoonotic pool (Section 1.5.1)—have been identified as key drivers of disease emergence and resurgence:

> Rates of deforestation have grown exponentially since the beginning of the 20th century. Driven by rapidly increasing human population numbers, large swathes of species-rich tropical and temperate forests... have been converted to species-poor agricultural and ranching areas. The global rate of tropical deforestation continues at staggering levels, with nearly 2–3% of forests lost globally each year. Parallel with this habitat destruction is an exponential growth in human–wildlife interaction and conflict. This has resulted in exposure to new pathogens for humans, livestock, and wildlife... Deforestation and the processes that lead to it have many consequences for ecosystems. Deforestation decreases the overall habitat available for wildlife species. It also modifies the structure of environments, for example, by fragmenting habitats into smaller patches separated by agricultural activities or human populations. Increased 'edge effect' (from a patchwork of varied land uses) can further promote interaction among pathogens, vectors and hosts... Evidence is mounting that deforestation and ecosystem changes have implications for the distribution of many other microorganisms and the health of human, domestic animal and wildlife populations. (Patz, Daszak, *et al.* 2004: 1093)

Deforestation, and the reverse process of reforestation, have been directly associated with the emergence and resurgence of several vectored and non-vectored infectious diseases (Table 7.2). Among the vector-borne conditions, high levels of malarial infection have been encountered by settlers who have followed the logging roads into Amazonia (Figure 7.6). As the ecology of an area changes, so the vector species may also change. Some vectors may convert from a primarily zoophylic to a primarily anthropophylic orientation as contact with humans increases, while those settlers new to an area may lack protective immunity to the local diseases and/or familiarity with the practices that would serve to limit the risks of pathogen transmission. In turn, as human population density increases, so the opportunity for exchange and transmission of disease micro-organisms rises (Patz, Graczyk, *et al.* 2000; Patz, Daszak, *et al.* 2004).

7.4.1 Tropical Deforestation: Nipah Viral Disease

Since the late 1980s, viruses of the family *Paramyxoviridae* have been associated with newly recognized diseases in a variety of mammalian species including seals (Osterhaus and Vedder 1988), porpoises (Kennedy *et al.* 1988), dolphins (Domingo *et al.* 1990), lions (Roelke-Parker *et al.* 1996), and humans (Murray, Selleck, *et al.* 1995; Chua *et al.* 2000). Among the latter, Hendra virus and Nipah virus are two zoonotic pathogens that were first identified when they manifested as severe respiratory and encephalitogenic diseases in the 1990s. The viruses are now classified as the first two members of a novel genus (*Henipavirus*) of the *Paramyxoviridae*. Here, we examine the emergence of Nipah viral disease as a pathogenic 'spillover' that has been linked to the depletion of the natural forest habitat of fruit bat species in parts of South-East Asia. The emergence of the related Hendra viral disease in Australia is reviewed in Section 9.4.2.

NATURE OF NIPAH VIRAL DISEASE

Nipah viral disease (*ICD*-10 B33.8) is a severe, frequently fatal, disease of humans and some domestic animals (notably pigs) arising from infection with Nipah virus (Plate 7.3). The main presenting features of the disease in humans are fever, headache, vomiting, respiratory symptoms, and altered level of consciousness, sometimes proceeding to coma and death. The observed case-fatality is approximately 50 per cent, with most deaths arising due to severe brain stem involvement. Persistent neurological deficits are

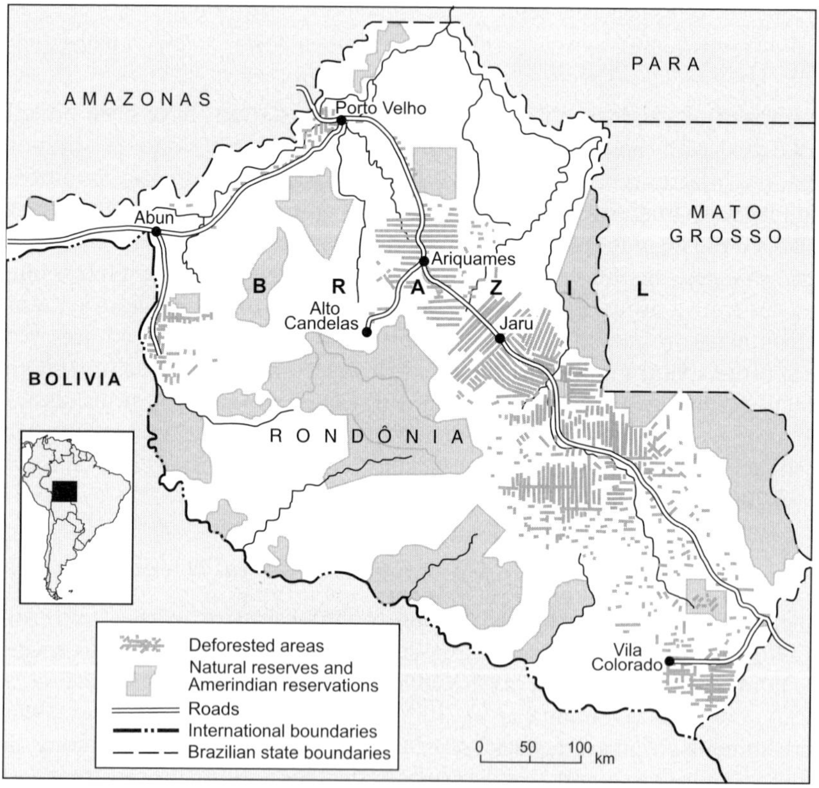

Fig. 7.6. Disease implications of the destruction of tropical rainforest in South America Deforestation in the Brazilian state of Rondônia, showing the intricate pattern of forest dissection by logging roads with associated clearing and farm settlement. The increases in 'edge' conditions along the forest boundary favour some mosquito vectors and add to the risk of malaria transmission.

Sources: Redrawn from Cliff, Haggett, and Smallman-Raynor (2004, fig. 12.5, p. 185), originally from Mahar (1989, fig. 4, p. 32).

witnessed in some survivors, while others make a complete recovery (Goh *et al.* 2000; Lam and Chua 2002; Heymann 2004: 245–7).

Virus Reservoirs and Transmission Routes

The primary reservoirs of Nipah virus in nature are Pteropid fruit bats of South and South-East Asia, including the Malayan flying fox (*Pteropus vampyrus*) and the Island flying fox (*Pteropus hypomelanus*) (Plate 7.3). Considerable uncertainty surrounds the mode of transmission of Nipah

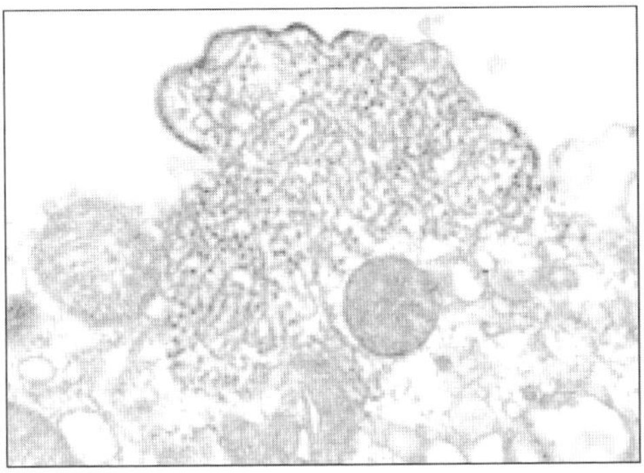

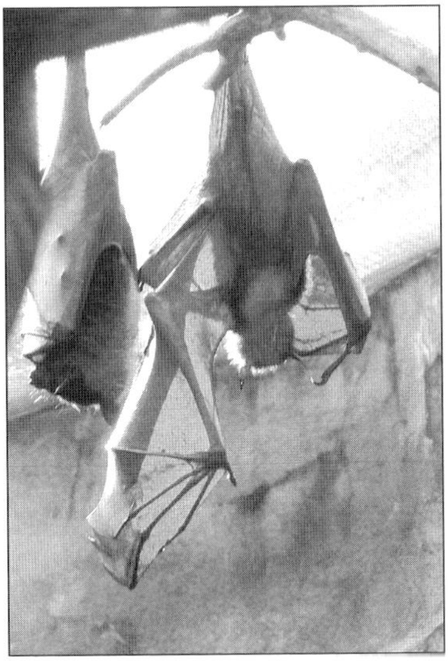

Pl. 7.3. Nipah virus and Pteropid fruit bats
(Upper) Electron micrograph of Nipah virus. Nipah viral disease is a severe, frequently fatal, disease of humans and some domestic animals (notably pigs). (Lower) The Malayan flying fox (*Pteropus vampyrus*), one of the primary reservoirs of Nipah virus.
Sources: Micrograph: CDC public health image library. *Pteropus vampyrus*: Wikimedia Commons.

virus from animal to animal and from animal to human, although available evidence suggests that close contact with contaminated tissue or body fluids is required. During the Malaysian outbreak of 1998–9, described below, domestic swine served as an intermediate host and the sequence of virus transmission was established as bats → swine → humans; no evidence of human-to-human transmission was documented. Subsequent outbreaks of Nipah viral disease in humans have occurred in the apparent absence of an intermediate animal host, and alternative routes of human exposure to the virus (including direct or indirect bat-to-human and human-to-human) have been inferred from the epidemiological evidence (see, for example, Chadha *et al.* 2006; Gurley *et al.* 2007).

THE FIRST RECORDED OUTBREAKS: MALAYSIA AND SINGAPORE, 1998–1999

Nipah viral disease was first recognized in the course of an epidemic of severe febrile encephalitis in peninsular Malaysia, September 1998–May 1999. The earliest human cases were linked to pig farms in the village of Ampang, some 8 km from Ipoh city, Perak state, in late September 1998; see Figure 7.7. The outbreak had been preceded by a respiratory illness and encephalitis in local pigs, and close contact with infected pigs was established as the immediate source of infection for the vast majority of human cases in the epidemic that followed. The epidemic spread routes, which tracked the transport movements of pigs from infected farms, are reconstructed in the main map of Figure 7.7; the associated graphs plot the number of human cases by week of onset in infected states of Malaysia (A–C) and in Singapore (D). As the map shows, by February 1999, the disease had been carried southwards from the index location in Perak to localities in Negri Sembilan, resulting in a major outbreak of the disease among pig farmers, workers, and others in Bukit Pelanduk and adjacent localities of Sungai Nipah and Sepang (graph 7.7C). In March, cases were recorded among abattoir workers in Singapore who had been in contact with pigs from infected regions of Malaysia, while, in May, the epidemic spread with the movement of pigs to Sungai Buloh in Selangor (Chua 2003; Henipavirus Ecology Collaborative Research Group 2005).

Recognition of the role of pigs in the spread of the epidemic, coupled with the recovery of the previously unknown Nipah virus from a case-patient in March 1999, prompted the Malaysian authorities to undertake a cull of some 1.1 million swine on 950 farms. By the end of the epidemic, in late May, a total of 265 human cases (including 105 deaths) had been recorded in Malaysia, with an additional 11 cases (including one death) in Singapore. Following a two-year surveillance period, when no further cases of disease due to Nipah virus were recorded, the livestock of Malaysia was officially declared free of the virus by the World Organization for Animal Health (OIE) in June 2001 (Chua 2003; Henipavirus Ecology Collaborative Research Group 2005).

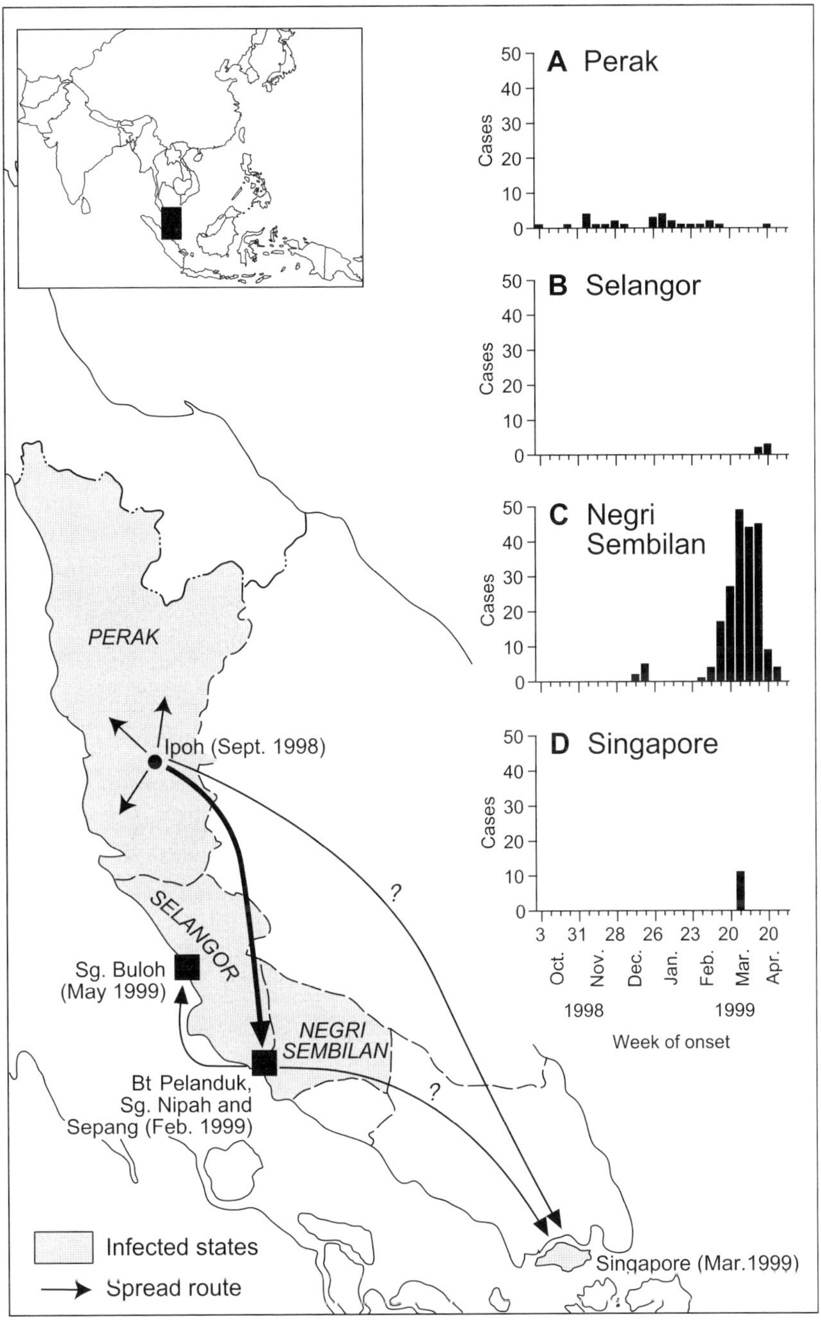

Fig. 7.7. Spread of Nipah virus in Malaysia and Singapore, September 1998–May 1999
Vectors show the spread of Nipah virus with the movement of infected pigs. Graphs plot the week of onset of documented human cases of illness due to Nipah virus in the three infected states of Malaysia (graphs A–C) and Singapore (graph D).

Sources: Based on Centers for Disease Control and Prevention (1999, fig. 1, p. 336) and Chua (2003, fig. 1, p. 267).

Pteropid Bats, Deforestation, and the Emergence of Nipah Virus: The Chua Model

The identification of Pteropid fruit bats as the wildlife reservoir of Nipah virus raises a number of questions regarding the events of 1998–9. In particular, what processes were associated with the spillover of the virus from bats to domestic pigs, with onwards spread to the human population? And why did this happen, apparently for the first time, in the late 1990s? Observations made at the index farms in the Malaysian village of Ampang provide some clues to the series of events involved. As described by the Henipavirus Ecology Collaborative Research Group (2005), the farms are interspersed with orchards, with fruit trees overhanging the open areas of pig pens. Fruit bats frequently drop partially eaten fruit from the trees, which is scavenged by the pigs, while the pigs are also exposed to bat urine. In turn, Nipah virus has been recovered from bat saliva on partially eaten fruit and from bat urine, and both fluids represent a potential source of infection for exposed animals. As for the timing of events at Ampang, the residents noted the sudden appearance of one known Nipah virus reservoir species—the Malayan flying fox (*P. vampyrus*)—in the vicinity of the village in 1997.

To account for the encroachment of forest-dwelling fruit bats on cultivated orchards in the late 1990s, with the resultant emergence of Nipah virus, K. B. Chua (2003) identifies the complex web of local, regional, and global interactions in Figure 7.8. At the heart of the Chua model, the ongoing destruction of vast areas of tropical rainforest in Malaysia has served to reduce the forest habitat of species such as fruit bats, presumably placing pressure on the food supply of these creatures. Whether or not the food situation had reached critical levels in the late 1990s is unknown, but aggravating factors relating to anthropogenic forest fires in Indonesia and El Niño–Southern Oscillation- (ENSO-)induced drought in southern Malaysia may have compounded the problem. As Chua (2003: 271–2) explains:

> In a nutshell, over the last two decades, the forest habitat of... fruitbats (flying-foxes) in Southeast Asia has been substantially reduced by deforestation for pulpwood and industrial plantation. In 1997/1998, slash-and-burn deforestation resulted in the formation of a severe haze that blanketed much of Southeast Asia in the months directly preceding the Nipah virus disease outbreak. This was exacerbated by a drought driven by the severe 1997–1998 El Niño Southern Oscillation (ENSO) event. This series of events led to an acute reduction in the availability of flowering and fruiting forest trees for foraging by flying-foxes in their already shrinking wildlife habitat. This culminated in an unprecedented encroachment of flying-foxes into cultivated fruit orchards in the initial outbreak area in the suburb of Ipoh, in 1997/1998. These anthropogenic events, coupled with the location of piggeries in orchards and the design of pigsties in the index farms allowed transmission of a novel paramyxovirus from its reservoir host to the domestic pig and ultimately to the human population and other domestic animals.

Since the events of 1998–9, several outbreaks of Nipah virus have been recorded elsewhere in Asia (Table 7.4). Whether the same processes of

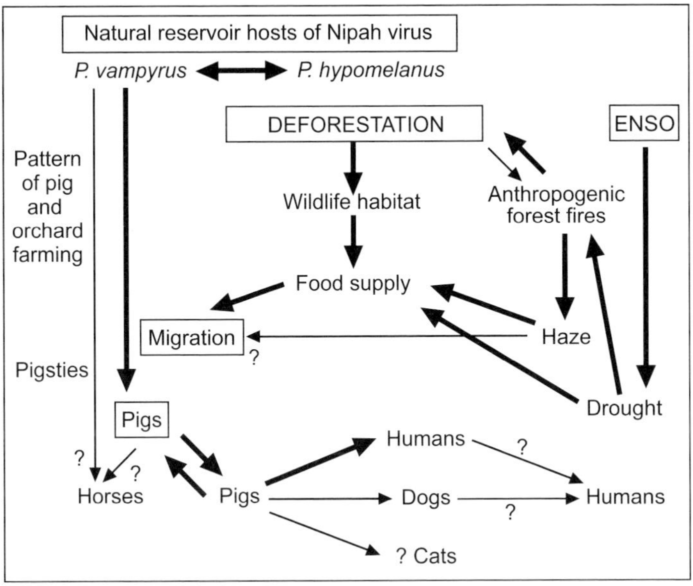

Fig. 7.8. Factors involved in the emergence of Nipah virus in Malaysia, 1998–1999 Vector widths are indicative of the relative importance of events in the emergence process. ENSO = El Niño–Southern Oscillation.

Source: Redrawn from Chua (2003, fig. 2, p. 272).

habitat loss and increased human–wildlife interaction have contributed to these more recent developments requires elucidation.

7.4.2 Temperate Reforestation: Lyme Disease

Lyme disease (*ICD*-10 A69.2, L90.4), also known as 'Lyme borreliosis' or 'tickborne meningopolyneuritis', provides an archetypal example of the role of reforestation as a facilitating factor in the emergence of a newly identified disease. First recognized in the United States in 1975, the appearance and spread of Lyme disease is intimately associated with a complex of ecological changes arising from the abandonment of farmland and the subsequent reforestation of large tracts of the north-eastern US in the twentieth century. Similar processes are believed to have driven the recent emergence of Lyme disease in Europe, while cases of the disease have also been documented in Australia, China, Japan, and countries of the former Soviet Union.

NATURE OF LYME DISEASE

Lyme disease is a tick-borne spirochaetal disease. Clinically, the disease manifests as a multisystem disorder that generally occurs in stages.

Table 7.4. Documented outbreaks of Nipah virus encephalitis in humans, September 1998–December 2004

Country	Date	Cases	Deaths
Malaysia	Sept. 1998–May 1999	265	105
Singapore	Mar. 1999	11	1
India	Jan.–Feb. 2001	66[1]	
Bangladesh	Apr.–May 2001	13[2]	9
	Jan. 2003	12[3]	8
	Jan.–Feb. 2004	23[4]	17[4]
	Mar.–Apr. 2004	30[4]	18[4]

Notes: [1] 74 per cent case-fatality for patients with known outcome.[2] Includes four confirmed and nine probable cases.[3] Includes four confirmed and eight probable cases.[4] Documented status as of 23 Apr. 2004.

Sources: Based on Paton *et al.* (1999), Chua (2003), Hsu *et al.* (2004), World Health Organization (2004*a*), and Chadha *et al.* (2006).

In early-stage infection, a mean incubation period of 7–10 days (range 3–32 days) gives way to the appearance of one or more characteristic cutaneous lesions (termed 'erythema migrans', EM) that expand slowly in an annular manner. Additional symptoms, including fever, headache, lethargy, and muscular pains, may also appear in the absence of antibiotic therapy. Within weeks or months, some untreated patients develop multiple EM, neurological and cardiac abnormalities, and, in about 60 per cent of cases, recurrent arthritic attacks of the knees and other large joints that occasionally take a chronic course. Finally, months or years after primary infection, patients may develop late-stage symptoms of infection, including degenerative skin disorders and neurological and articular changes. Prompt antibiotic treatment of early disease is usually curative; advanced disease can result in a level of physical disability, while, in rare instances, the disease may be fatal. For further information, see Heymann (2004: 315–20).

Agents, Vectors, and Transmission Cycle

Lyme disease is caused by certain bacteria of the genus *Borrelia. Borrelia burgdorferi* is the principal agent of Lyme disease in North America, while *B. burgdorferi*, *B. afzelii*, and *B. garinii* are implicated in European cases. The bacteria are transmitted to humans via the bite of species of tick belonging to the genus *Ixodes*. Evidence from the United States suggests that tick larvae and nymphs acquire infection with *B. burgdorferi* during blood meals from rodents and these small mammals maintain the enzootic transmission cycle in nature. Deer, in turn, serve as important maintenance mammalian hosts for adults of the vector species. Most cases of Lyme disease result from bites by infected nymphs, and the seasonal distribution of cases corresponds to periods of nymphal tick activity. The disease peaks in June and July in the Northern Hemisphere, but may occur in other seasons depending on the life

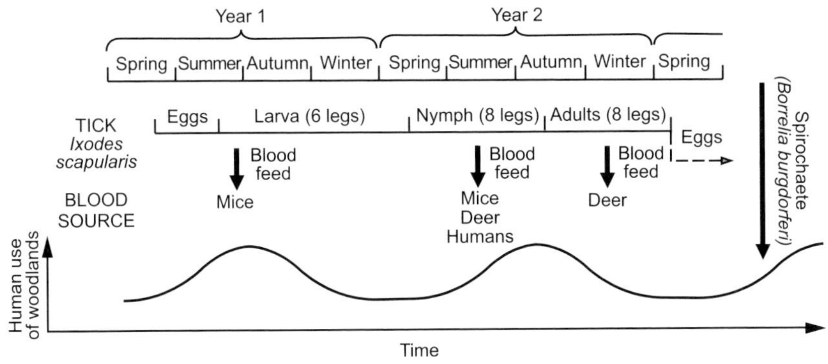

Fig. 7.9. Cycle of Lyme disease, illustrated with reference to the tick vector of *B. burgdorferi* in the north-eastern United States

Relationship between (*a*) the two-year life cycle of the tick (*Ixodes scapularis*) and (*b*) human summertime exposure by walking in the woods. Eggs are deposited in the spring and the larvae emerge several weeks later. They feed once during the summer, usually on the blood of small mammals such as mice. Larvae moult the following spring into slightly larger nymphs, which also feed once during the summer—on mice or larger mammals such as dogs, deer, or human beings—before moulting into adults in the fall. Adults attach themselves to a host, usually the white-tailed deer, where they mate.

Sources: Cliff, Haggett, and Smallman-Raynor (2004, fig. 11.10, p. 170), originally from Haggett (2001, fig. 20–23(*a*), p. 649).

cycle of the tick in different geographical areas. A picture of the transmission cycle, illustrated with reference to the tick vector *Ixodes scapularis* (formerly *I. dammini*) in the eastern and Midwestern United States, is given in Figure 7.9.

THE RECOGNITION OF LYME DISEASE

In 1975, the Connecticut State Health Department was informed of an unusual number of cases of childhood arthritis in the town of Old Lyme, Connecticut. An investigation by the Yale epidemiologist Allen Steere observed that the cases formed distinct clusters in rural, wooded areas and that a characteristic rash was displayed in a number of patients (Steere, Malawista, *et al.* 1977). The syndrome (named 'Lyme disease' to record the town in which it was first observed) was found to be more prevalent in areas west of the Connecticut River where much of the farmland had been allowed to revert to woodland and where deer were plentiful. Children commonly used the woods for recreation, particularly in the summer months. It was several years later, in 1982, that Burgdorfer and colleagues isolated a spirochaete (subsequently named *B. burgdorferi*) from the gut of *I. scapularis* ticks in the endemic area (Burgdorfer *et al.* 1982). Shortly thereafter, studies by Benach *et al.* (1983) and Steere, Grodzicki, *et al.* (1983) confirmed the spirochaetal aetiology of Lyme disease in humans.

The American work was subsequently linked to earlier European work. In 1909 a Swedish dermatologist had described a rash on a patient following a bite from an *Ixodes* tick. Later work associating the disease with tick bites had been conducted in Austria and France in 1913 and 1922. As early as 1951, penicillin was shown to be useful in treating the condition. As in the case of Legionnaire's disease (Section 5.3), recognition and labelling of the disease in the United States was the precursor to widespread retrospective recognition in other developed countries (Leff 1993).

THE GEOGRAPHY OF LYME DISEASE

Lyme disease has been documented in North America, Europe, Asia, Australia, and North Africa. Figure 7.10 maps the distribution of the disease and the geographical extent of major vectors in North America, Europe, and Australia. The distribution of the majority of cases coincides with the distribution of *I. scapularis* ticks in the eastern and Midwestern US, *I. pacificus* in western US, and *I. ricinus* in Europe. In addition, the map also delimits the geographical distribution of the Lone Star tick (*Amblyomma americanum*), associated with a Lyme-like illness known as southern tick-associated rash illness (STARI) in the southern United States.

Ecological Change: Reforestation and the Emergence of Lyme Disease

Since Lyme disease became notifiable in the United States in 1991, the number of reported cases has doubled to approximately 20,000 per annum (Figure 7.11) and it is now the most commonly recorded arthropod-borne disease in the country. The major foci of reported disease activity are mapped in Figure 7.12 and include: (i) the Atlantic coast from Massachusetts to Maryland; (ii) the upper Midwest, including Wisconsin and Minnesota; and (iii) the Pacific coast, intermittently from southern California to northern Washington.

Factors associated with the emergence of Lyme disease as a significant public health problem in the United States, and which would account for the primary foci of disease activity in Figure 7.12, are reviewed by Barbour and Fish (1993), Spielman (1994), and Steere (1998). In earlier centuries, demand for trees as fuel for domestic and industrial purposes, coupled with the extension of agricultural activities, rendered much of the eastern United States virtually treeless. From the early twentieth century, however, the transfer of agriculture to the Great Plains resulted in the reforestation of vast regions of the eastern United States. The abundance of deer—important as maintenance hosts for the tick vectors—increased in parallel with that of woodland. In turn, the invasion of reforested areas by *Ixodes* ticks initiated the appearance of Lyme disease. As Steere (1998: 222–3) explains:

> The emergence of Lyme disease in the United States in the late twentieth century is thought to have occurred primarily because of ecological conditions favorable for deer... As farmland in the northeast reverted to woodland, the habitat for deer

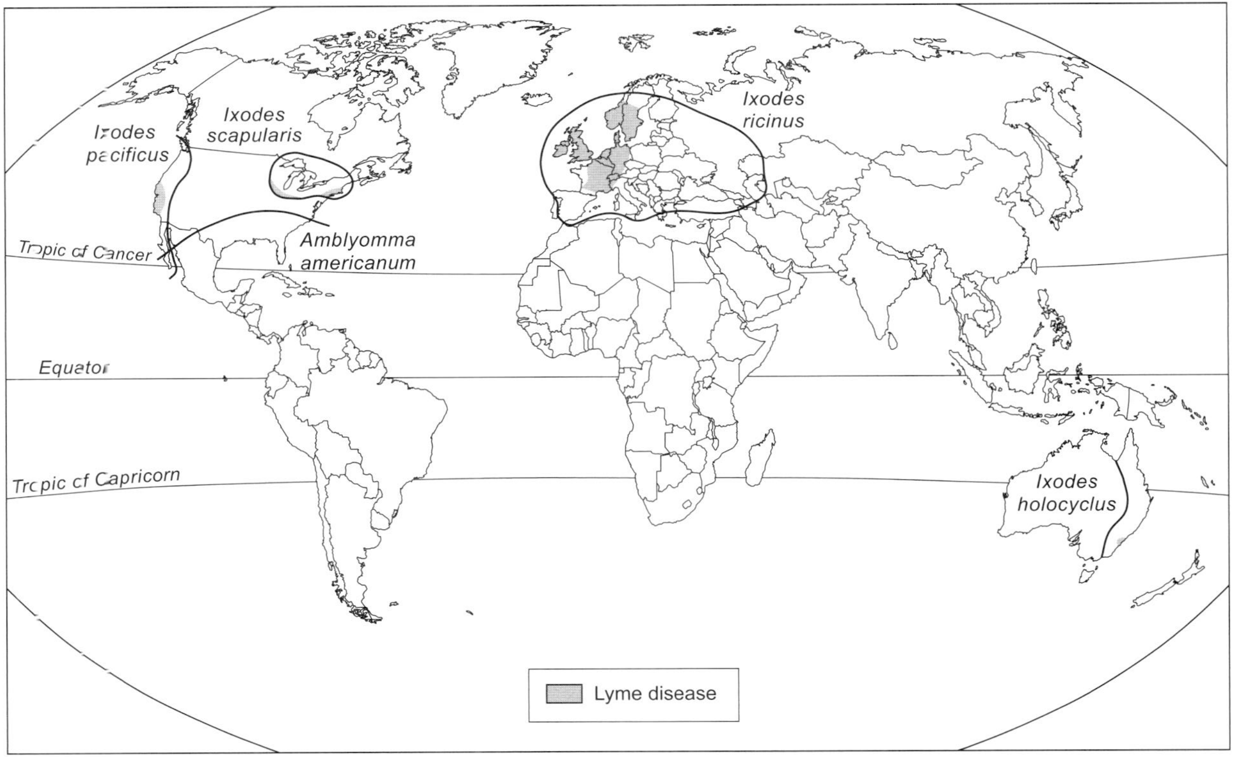

Fig. 7.10. World map of Lyme disease

Distribution of Lyme disease and its major *Ixodes* vectors in North America, Europe, and Australia. The geographical distribution of the Lone Star tick (*Amblyomma americanum*), associated with a Lyme-like illness in the southern United States, is also shown.

Sources: Cliff, Haggett, and Smallman-Raynor (2004, fig. 11.11, p. 171), originally from World Health Organization (1989, map 25, p. 68).

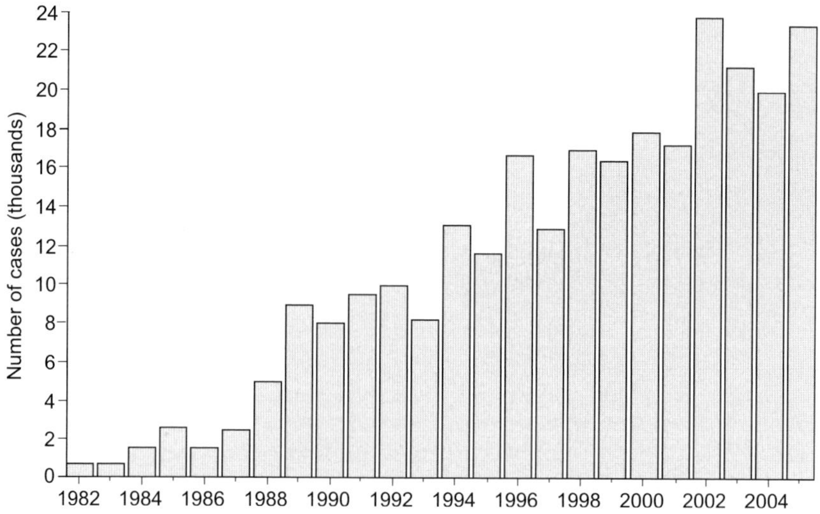

Fig. 7.11. Trends in Lyme disease in the United States
Annual time series of reported cases, 1982–2005.

Sources: Redrawn from Cliff, Haggett, and Smallman-Raynor (2004, fig. 11.13, p. 171), with additional information from Centers for Disease Control and Prevention (2007*a*, table 8, pp. 76–7).

improved: the natural predators were gone, the number of deer increased dramatically, they migrated to new areas, and federal programs protected them. With the advent of the automobile and super-highways, rural and suburban areas, where deer now lived, became populated with large numbers of susceptible urbanites who had never been exposed to the spirochete.

Similar processes of reforestation and increased deer abundance have been witnessed across the North Temperate Zone, resulting in the development of deer-infested stands, interspersed with houses, in North America and Europe:

> [the] pattern of spread of Lyme disease and its vectors in the northeastern United States and Europe derives from the recent proliferation of deer, and the abundance of deer derives from the process of reforestation now taking place throughout the North Temperate Zone of the world. Residential development seems to favor small tree-enclosed meadows interspersed with strips of woodland, a 'patchiness' much prized by deer, mice, and humans. As a result, increasingly large numbers of people live where risk of Lyme disease . . . is intense. (Spielman 1994: 154)

7.5 Climate Change and Variability

Climate is inextricably linked to human health. Extremes of climate—of cold or heat—can have direct impacts on the health of humans, typically

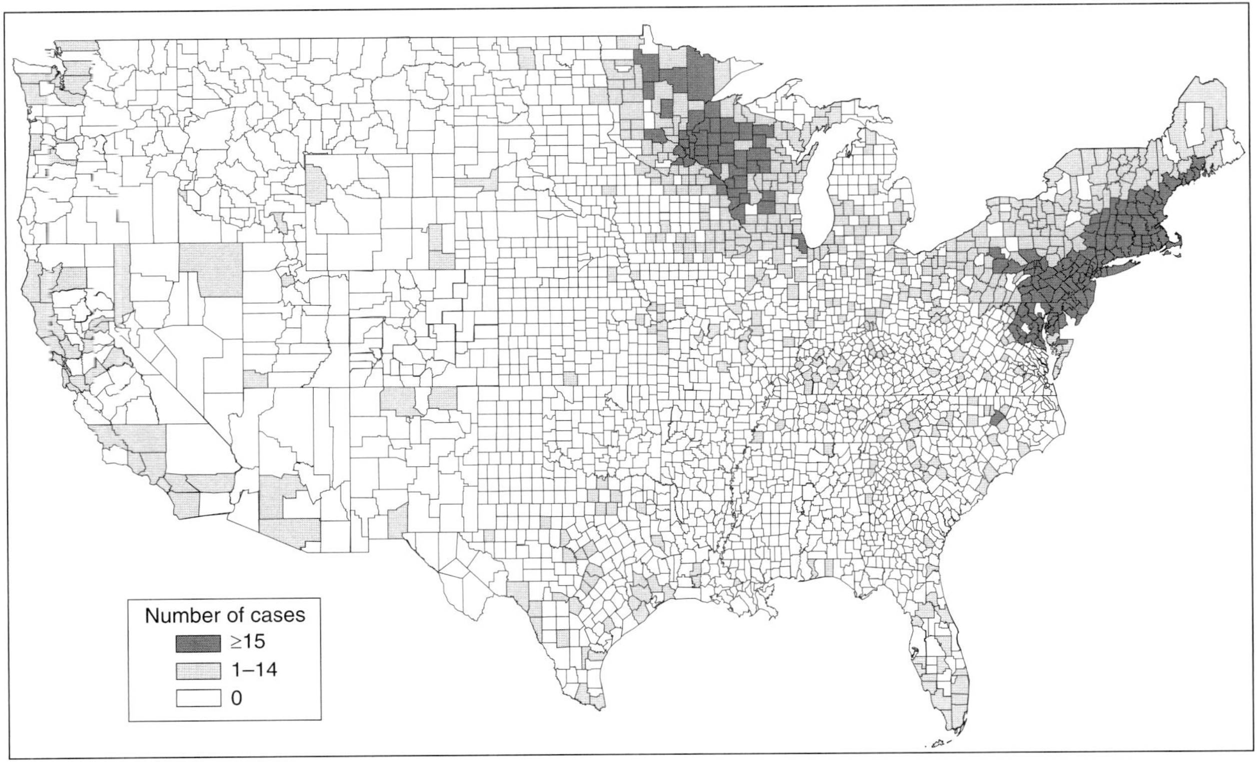

Fig. 7.12. Lyme disease in the United States, 2005
The map shades counties from which cases of Lyme disease were reported.
Source: Redrawn from Centers for Disease Control and Prevention (2007*a*: 59).

manifesting in temperate latitudes as excess morbidity and mortality from hypothermia (winter months) and heat stroke (summer months). But climate can also have indirect impacts by influencing such factors as levels of atmospheric pollution, the operation of agricultural and marine systems, the distribution of disease vectors and pathogens, and patterns of human activity and behaviour. Viewed in historical perspective, short-, medium-, and long-term swings in climate have had pronounced impacts on the geographical occurrence of many old human diseases. And, very occasionally, the same climatic swings have been implicated as precipitating factors in the appearance of previously unknown pathogens in the human population (Table 7.2).

The present section examines two types of climate condition as drivers of infectious disease emergence and resurgence: (i) *climate change*, denoting medium- and long-term shifts in the average values of meteorological variables over periods of decades; and (ii) *climate variability*, denoting short-term fluctuations in the values of meteorological variables over weeks, months, or years. We begin in Section 7.5.1 by reviewing the evidence of the Intergovernmental Panel on Climate Change on the observed and predicted impacts of climate change on global and world regional patterns of infectious disease activity. We then turn to the issue of climate variability, with special reference to the impacts of the quasi-periodic inter-annual El Niño–Southern Oscillation (ENSO) on infectious disease activity in general (Section 7.5.2) and the emergence of hantavirus pulmonary syndrome in particular (Section 7.5.3).

7.5.1 Climate Change and Human Health

Of the many global scenarios for disease and the environment under discussion in the late twentieth and early twenty-first centuries, it is the health implications of climate change that have caught the attention of scientists, governments, and the media. Major studies of the link between climate change and health have been undertaken in a number of countries, including the United States (Smith and Tirpak 1989), Australia (Ewan *et al.* 1990), and the United Kingdom (Bannister 1991; Department of Health and Health Protection Agency 2008), while the World Health Organization's (WHO's) Climate Change and Health Programme is dedicated to the global assessment of the issue.

DIMENSIONS OF CLIMATE CHANGE: THE IPCC *FOURTH ASSESSMENT REPORT* (2007)

The Intergovernmental Panel on Climate Change (IPCC) was established by the World Meteorological Organization (WMO) and the United Nations Environment Programme (UNEP) in 1988. Since inception, the remit of the IPCC has been to review the published scientific literature relating to the processes of human-induced climate change, the impact of these changes on human societies, and the responses that could be implemented to ameliorate the effects (Githeko and Woodward 2003). Among the principal conclusions of the fourth and most recent IPCC *Assessment Report*, published in 2007, the average surface temperature of the earth has warmed by 0.74°C since the early twentieth century (Figure 7.13), having risen above the upper limit of historical variability in the last 30 years. This warming has been accompanied by changes in the magnitude and/or frequency of a range of hydro-meteorological and oceanographic phenomena, including wind intensity, drought, heavy precipitation and flood events, hurricane intensity, and sea level rises (Intergovernmental Panel on Climate Change 2007*a*). Future scenarios for climate change are speculative, although the IPCC project a global surface air warming of 1.1–6.4°C during the twenty-first century (Figure 7.13)—a rate of warming that is well beyond any natural increase in the last 10,000 years (McMichael 2003).

POTENTIAL HEALTH IMPACTS OF GLOBAL WARMING

Climate change can have diverse impacts on human health via multiple pathways (Figure 7.14) (McMichael, Campbell-Lendrum, Corvalan, *et al.* 2003). According to volume ii of the IPCC *Fourth Assessment Report*, the currently recognized (early) effects of climate change on health are relatively minor and include changes in the distribution of some species of disease vectors, altered seasonal distributions of some allergenic pollen species, and

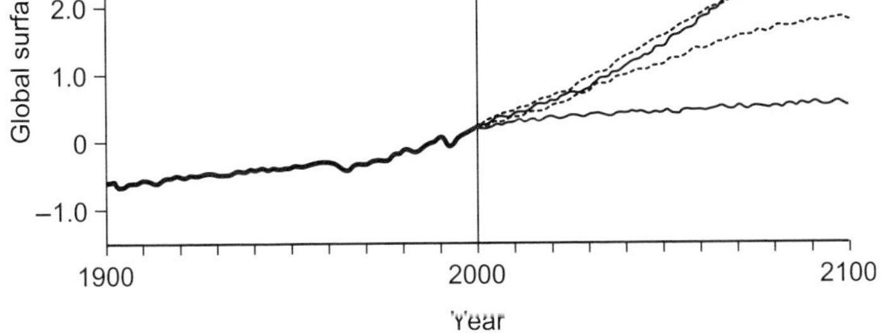

Fig. 7.13. Projections of global surface warming according to the Intergovernmental Panel on Climate Change *Fourth Assessment Report*, 2000–2100
Graph plots projected global averages of surface warming (relative to 1980–99) for a range of scenarios relating to the concentration of greenhouse gases. Surface temperatures in the 20th century are shown for reference.
Source: Adapted from Intergovernmental Panel on Climate Change (2007*a*, fig. 10.4, p. 762).

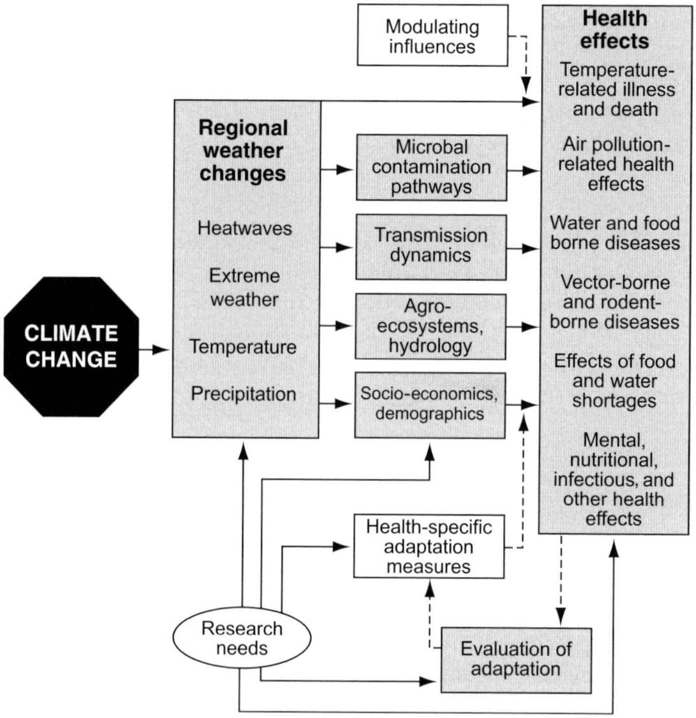

Fig. 7.14. The health effects of climate change
Conceptual diagram of the pathways by which climate change may impact on human health.
Source: Redrawn from World Health Organization (2007*c*).

increased levels of death during heatwaves. The effects, however, are projected to increase with time in all countries and world regions. As we noted in Section 6.2.3, while climate change can be expected to have some positive health impacts (for example, a reduction in cold-related mortality in temperate latitudes), the IPCC predict that 'the balance of impacts will be overwhelmingly negative' (Intergovernmental Panel on Climate Change 2007*b*: 407); see Table 7.5.

Geographical Assessments

Although the impacts of climate change will be felt everywhere, the health consequences are anticipated to be most pronounced in low-income countries (Intergovernmental Panel on Climate Change 2007*b*). By way of illustration, Table 7.6 draws on the analysis of Campbell-Lendrum *et al.* (2003) and gives regional estimates of disability-adjusted life years (DALYs) for sample health outcomes (malnutrition, diarrhoea, malaria and the consequences of floods) that are identified by the IPCC as being

Table 7.5. Intergovernmental Panel on Climate Change: projected trends in selected climate-change-related exposures of importance to human health, and associated confidence levels attached to the projected outcome

Projected trend	Confidence level
Mixed effects on malaria; in some places the geographical range will contract, elsewhere the geographical range will expand and the transmission season may be changed	Very high
Increased malnutrition and consequent disorders, including those relating to child growth and development	High
Increased number of people suffering death, disease, and injury from heatwaves, floods, storms, fires, and droughts	High
Continued change in the range of some infectious disease vectors	High
Increased cardio-respiratory morbidity and mortality associated with ground-level ozone	High
Some benefits to health, including fewer deaths from cold, although it is expected that these will be outweighed by the negative effects of rising temperatures worldwide, especially in developing countries	High
Increased burden of diarrhoeal diseases	Medium
Increased number of people at risk of dengue	Low

Source: Intergovernmental Panel on Climate Change (2007*b*: 393).

especially sensitive to climate change. All estimates are for the year 2000. When judged in terms of DALYs per million population, by far the greatest burden of climate-change-sensitive conditions falls on Africa (3,071.5), South-East Asia (1,703.5), and the eastern Mediterranean (1,586.5). Within these regions, diarrhoea, malaria, and malnutrition are likely to account for a

Table 7.6. Year 2000 estimates of the impact of climate change in terms of disability-adjusted life years (DALYs) associated with sample health conditions

World region	DALYs (000s)					DALYs per million population
	Malnutrition	Diarrhoea	Malaria	Floods	Total	
Africa	616	414	860	4	1,894	3,071.5
Eastern Mediterranean	313	291	112	52	768	1,586.5
Latin America & Caribbean	0	17	3	72	92	188.5
South-East Asia	1,918	640	0	14	2,572	1,703.5
Western Pacific[1]	0	89	43	37	169	111.4
Developed countries[2]	0	0	0	8	8	8.9
Global total	2,847	1,460	1,018	192	5,517	920.3

Notes: [1] Excluding Australia and New Zealand.[2] Including Australia, Canada, Cuba, New Zealand, US, and the countries of the WHO European region.

Source: Campbell-Lendrum *et al.* (2003, table 7.9, p. 152).

substantial proportion of the climate-change-induced pattern of ill health in future years (Campbell-Lendrum *et al.* 2003).

CLIMATE CHANGE AND VECTOR-BORNE DISEASES

Within the scientific literature, special attention has focused on the possible impact of climate change on vector-borne diseases; see Githeko *et al.* (2000), Gubler *et al.* (2001), Kovats, Campbell-Lendrum, *et al.* (2001), Reiter (2001), Molyneux (2003), Patz, Githeko, *et al.* (2003), Sutherst (2004), and Rogers and Randolf (2006), among others. Although the effects of climate on the physical and biotic controls on vectors, pathogens, and vertebrate hosts are complex, the IPCC anticipates that increased mean temperatures and changes in precipitation will serve to alter (primarily, to extend) the geographical range of a number of vector-borne diseases, including dengue, Lyme disease, malaria, and tick-borne encephalitis (Table 7.7). An illustration of the projected effects on one of these diseases (dengue) is provided by Patz, Martens, *et al.* (1998), who use three climate general circulation models (GCMs) to generate the estimated changes in dengue-transmission potential shown in Figure 7.15. Each circulation model provides evidence of a projected increase in biting-mosquito numbers, but, as the maps show, there is considerable variation in the specific spatial pattern of increase.

7.5.2 Inter-Annual Climate Variability: The El Niño–Southern Oscillation (ENSO)

Climate variability on temporal scales of days, seasons, and years is an inherent characteristic of climate, regardless of whether or not the system is subject to long-term climate change. The El Niño–Southern Oscillation (ENSO) is the name given to quasi-periodic inter-annual climate variability that arises from changes in sea temperature (El Niño) and atmospheric pressure (Southern Oscillation) in the Pacific basin. ENSO events are linked to worldwide weather changes (Plate 7.4). During an ENSO event, a typical increase in the average global temperature of 0.5°C is accompanied by heterogeneous effects on regional patterns of precipitation. As Figure 7.16 shows, past ENSO events have been associated with droughts in parts of Central and South America, southern Africa, South and South-East Asia, and the western Pacific. Conversely, areas at risk of excess rainfall—with the associated danger of flooding—have been observed in parts of North and South America, Central and East Africa, and South Asia. Although the potential impact of long-term global climatic change on ENSO events remains uncertain, it is anticipated that such developments will result in greater extremes of dry weather and heavy rainfall, thereby increasing the risk of ENSO-related droughts and floods (Kovats 2000; Kovats, Bouma, *et al.* 2003).

Table 7.7. Selected projections of the impact of climate change on sample vectored diseases at global, world regional, and national levels

Disease	Geographical area	Results	Source
Malaria	Global	Estimates of the additional population at risk for >1 month transmission range from >220 million to >400 million	van Lieshout *et al.* (2004)
	Africa	By 2100, 16–28 per cent increase in person-months of exposure, including 5–7 per cent increase in (mainly altitudinal) distribution, with limited latitudinal expansion. Countries with large areas that are close to the climatic thresholds for transmission show large potential increases in malaria transmission	Tanser *et al.* (2003)
	Africa	Decreased transmission in 2020s in south-east Africa. By 2050s and 2080s, localized increases in highland and upland areas, and decreases around the Sahel and south central Africa	Thomas *et al.* (2004)
	Great Britain	Increase in risk of local malaria transmission of 8–15 per cent; highly unlikely that indigenous malaria will be re-established	Kuhn *et al.* (2002)
	India	By 2050s, geographical range projected to shift away from central regions towards south-western and northern states. The duration of the transmission window is likely to widen in northern and western states and shorten in southern states	Bhattacharya *et al.* (2006)
Dengue	Global	By 2085, with both population growth and climate change, global population at risk 5–6 billion; with climate change only, global population at risk 3.5 billion	Hales *et al.* (2002)
	New Zealand	Potential risk of dengue outbreaks in some regions under the current climate. Climate change projected to increase risk of dengue in more regions	de Wet *et al.* (2001)
Lyme disease	Canada	Northwards expansion of approximately 200 km by 2020s, and up to 1,000 km northwards by 2080s	Ogden *et al.* (2006)
Tick-borne encephalitis	Europe	From low to high degrees of climate change, tick-borne encephalitis is pushed further north-east of its present range, only moving westwards into southern Scandinavia. Disease remains in central and eastern Europe by the 2050s only under certain scenarios	Randolph and Rogers (2000)

Source: Abstracted from Intergovernmental Panel on Climate Change (2007*b*, table 8.2, pp. 409–10).

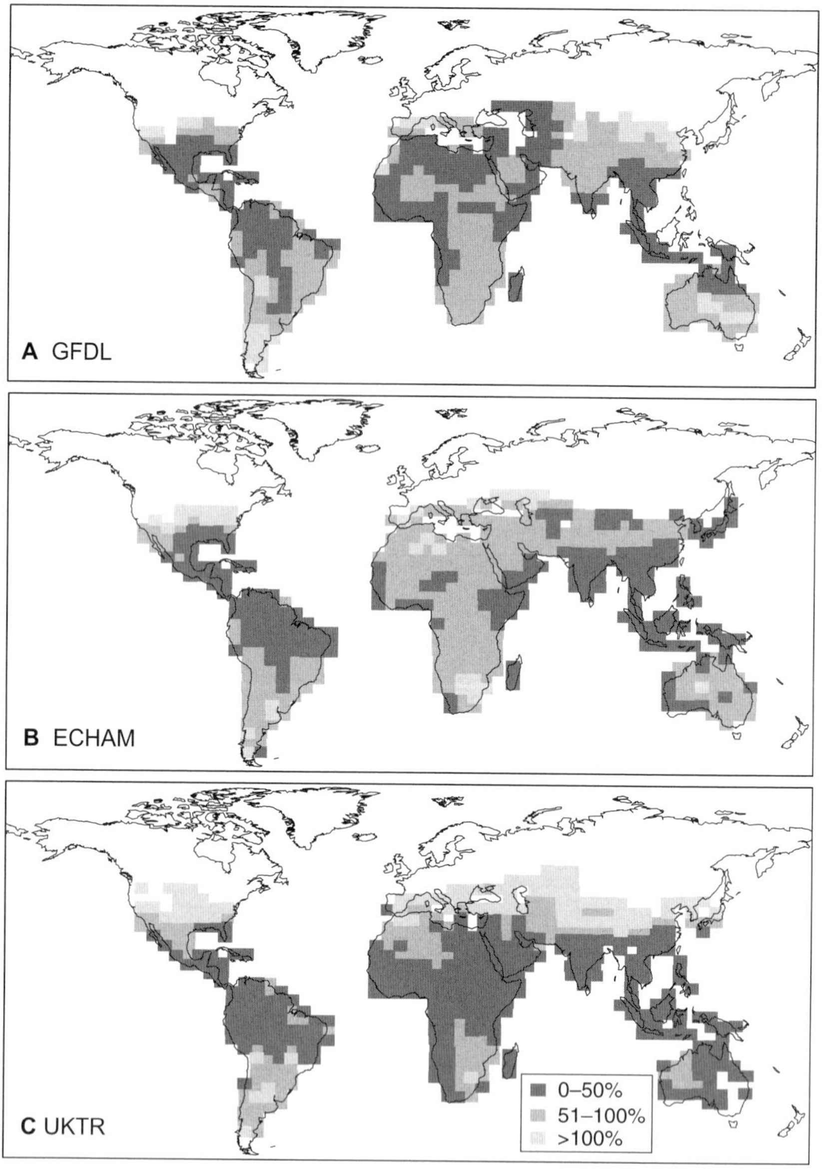

Fig. 7.15. Global climate change models and potential dengue expansion
Results of the application of three general circulation models (GCMs) of climate to estimate the increase in dengue average annual epidemic potential due to global warming. The GCMs were developed by research groups working in (A) the United States (GFDL), (B) Germany (ECHAM), and (C) the United Kingdom (UKTR). Maps of projected changes in dengue-transmission potential, presented as percentage increases on baseline values, are illustrated for each model. All three models predict substantial increases based on a temperature rise of 1.16°C, but the specific geographical distribution of these increases differs from model to model.

Sources: Redrawn from Cliff, Haggett, and Smallman-Raynor (2004, fig. 12.7, p. 186), originally from Patz, Martens, *et al.* (1998, fig. 3, p. 151).

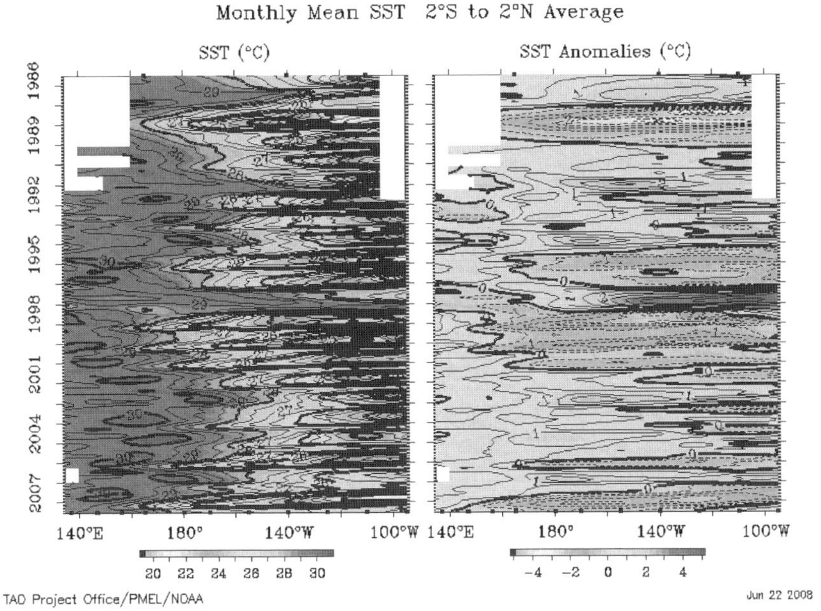

Pl. 7.4. El Niño events, 1986–1998
Mean and anomalies of sea surface temperature (SST) showing El Niño events of 1986–7, 1991–2, 1993, 1994, and 1997–8, when warm water penetrated eastwards (darker colours). The anomalies show the amount by which the SST differs from the normal value in that month. On both images, darker colours represent higher temperatures or greater positive anomalies, but note temperature contours are in black.
Source: NOAA Operational El Niño–Southern Oscillation (ENSO) Observing System web site (http://www.pmel.noaa.gov/tao/elnino/.noaa/enso.html).

ENSO events occur on an irregular cycle of 2–7 years and vary in terms of their time of onset, duration, and intensity. Since 1950, there have been 16 ENSO events of greater or lesser magnitude, with the events of 1972–3, 1982–3, 1987–8, and 1997–8 being of particular note on account of their strength (Kovats 2000; Kovats, Bouma, *et al.* 2003).

IMPACT ON INFECTIOUS DISEASES

ENSO-related changes in temperature and precipitation can affect the abundance and distribution of pathogens, arthropod vectors, and intermediate hosts, and the pattern of human and arthropod behaviour and land use. Rarely, however, is there a simple association between changes in these variables and disease incidence. In a review of the scientific literature, 1980–2002, Kovats, Bouma, *et al.* (2003) identified 21 reports of a temporal relationship between ENSO and human infectious diseases (including Barmah forest virus disease, cholera, dengue, malaria, plague, Rift Valley fever,

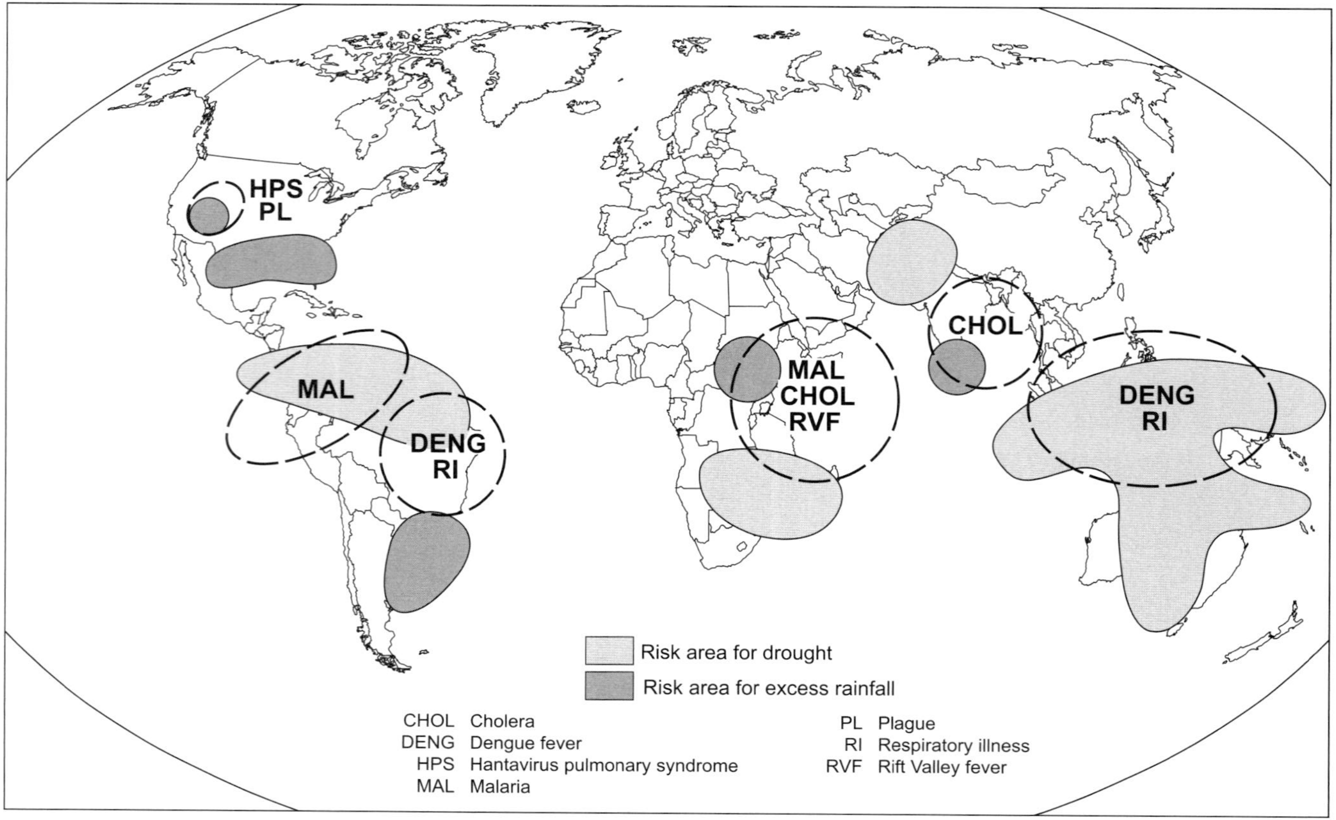

Fig. 7.16. El Niño–Southern Oscillation (ENSO) and global disease patterns
Shaded areas are based on averages of previous ENSO events and identify regions at risk for excess rainfall and drought. Sites of elevated disease risk associated with a predicted 2006–7 ENSO event are indicated.

Sources: Adapted from Kovats, Bouma, *et al.* (2003, fig. 1, p. 1482) and Anyamba *et al.* (2006, fig. 5, unpaginated).

Table 7.8. Sample countries/localities in which El Niño–Southern Oscillation (ENSO) has been implicated in the increased activity of certain vectored and non-vectored diseases

Vectored diseases				Non-vectored diseases
Malaria	Dengue	Other arboviruses	Visceral leishmaniasis	Cholera
Africa				
Kenya				Uganda
Rwanda				
Uganda				
Americas				
Colombia	Colombia		Brazil	
Guyana	French Guiana			
Peru	Surinam			
Venezuela				
Eastern Mediterranean/South-East Asia				
India	Indonesia			Bangladesh
Pakistan				India
Sri Lanka				
Western Pacific				
	Pacific islands	Australia[1,2]		

Notes: [1] Barmah Forest virus disease. [2] Ross River virus disease.
Source: Based, in part, on Kovats, Bouma, *et al.* (2003: 1484).

Ross River virus disease, and visceral leishmaniasis) in countries of the WHO Africa, Americas, Eastern Mediterranean, South-East Asia, and Western Pacific regions. Certain vectored (dengue, malaria, and other arboviral diseases) and non-vectored (cholera) diseases were linked to ENSO in multiple locations (Table 7.8), with a consistent and positive association for malaria in coastal Colombia and Venezuela and cholera in Bangladesh. On the basis of the accumulated evidence, areas of elevated risk for sample diseases in association with the predicted ENSO event of 2006–7 are plotted in Figure 7.16.

ENSO and Arthropod-Borne Diseases: The Example of Malaria

Evidence for an association between ENSO events and heightened levels of malaria transmission is particularly strong (Table 7.9 and Figure 7.16)—especially in fringe areas where precipitation and/or temperature are the main limiting factors in disease transmission. The association, however, is complex and several longitudinal studies have pointed to the existence of an annual lag in the climate–disease system (Table 7.9).

Following Kovats (2000), Kovats, Bouma, *et al.* (2003), and Hales, Edwards, *et al.* (2003), ENSO-related increases in malaria activity have variously been associated with (i) increased rainfall and temperature and (ii) droughts and post-drought periods.

Table 7.9. Malaria: high-risk years in relation to the El Niño–Southern Oscillation (ENSO) cycle

Country (district)	Study period	Timing
Americas		
Colombia	1960–92	Year after El Niño
	1959–93	Year after El Niño
Venezuela	1910–35	Year after El Niño
Venezuela (Carabobo)	1975–90	Year after El Niño
South-East Asia		
India (Rajasthan)	1982–92	El Niño year
India and Pakistan (Punjab)	1867–1943	Year after El Niño
Sri Lanka (south-west)	1870–1945	El Niño year

Source: Kovats (2000, table 3, p. 1131).

(i) *Increased temperature and rainfall.* In Central and East Africa, where ENSO events are associated with increased rainfall (Figure 7.16), short-term increases in malaria transmission have been documented for highland areas of Rwanda (Loevinsohn 1994) and Uganda (Lindblade *et al.* 1999). In Kenya, the heavy rains and floods that occurred in association with the 1997–8 ENSO event were followed by a major epidemic of *P. falciparum* malaria (Hales, Edwards, *et al.* 2003), although, in neighbouring Tanzania, the same event is believed to have reduced the malaria risk by washing away the breeding sites of mosquitoes (Lindsay, Bodker, *et al.* 2000). Elsewhere, in South Asia, ENSO-related increases in temperature have been associated with heightened levels of malaria activity in the highlands of northern Pakistan (Bouma *et al.* 1996).

(ii) *Droughts and post-drought periods.* ENSO events have been linked to malaria transmission in a number of the drought-risk areas identified in Figure 7.16 including Irian Jaya, Indonesia (Bangs and Subianto 1999), Venezuela (Bouma and Dye 1997), and Colombia (Poveda *et al.* 2001). In the latter two countries, malaria transmission is usually highest in the year following an ENSO event (Table 7.9). Factors that could account for post-drought outbreaks are outlined by Kovats, Bouma, *et al.* (2003) and include the more rapid re-establishment of mosquito populations than their predators in the aftermath of dry years.

7.5.3 ENSO And Hantavirus Pulmonary Syndrome in the United States

In this subsection, we illustrate the complex relationship between climate variability and disease emergence with reference to the appearance and spread of the rodent-borne hantavirus pulmonary syndrome (HPS) in the south-western United States. In so doing, we demonstrate how the hypothesized links between the environmental trigger (quasi-periodic ENSO events) and the human disease response (outbreaks of HPS) are mediated through a chain-like sequence of reactions encapsulated in the *trophic cascade model* of HPS emergence.

HANTAVIRUSES AND HANTAVIRUS PULMONARY SYNDROME

Viruses of the genus *Hantavirus* in the family *Bunyaviridae* are found on all continents and are associated with two principal types of human disease: haemorrhagic fever with renal syndrome (HFRS), an Old World disease; and hantavirus pulmonary syndrome (HPS), a New World disease (Schmaljohn and Hjelle 1997). Rodents are the natural reservoirs of hantaviruses, with the primary route of human exposure via contact with rodents and their excreta—a transmission process analogous to that described for Argentine haemorrhagic fever in Section 7.2.1. Hantaviruses known to be pathogenic for man are given with their Old/New World status, associated diseases, rodent reservoirs, and documented geographical distributions in Table 7.10.[3]

Hantavirus Pulmonary Syndrome

Hantavirus pulmonary syndrome (HPS) (*ICD*-10 B33.4) is usually the most severe of the hantaviral diseases. The disease presents as a prodromal febrile phase (chills, myalgia, headache, abdominal pain) followed by a pulmonary phase (coughing and rapid development of respiratory deficiency). The crude fatality rate is 40–50 per cent. Geographically, the risk of HPS extends across the New World, with sporadic cases and outbreaks due to one or more HPS-causing viruses (Table 7.10) having been reported in countries of both North and South America (Table 7.11). For further details of the nature and distribution of HPS in the Western Hemisphere, see Pan American Health Organization (2003: 98–109) and Heymann (2004: 243–5).

THE GEOGRAPHY OF HPS IN THE UNITED STATES

HPS was first described in the spring of 1993 when it manifested as an outbreak of fatal respiratory illness in the Four Corners region of the south-western United States; the states that constitute the index region (Arizona, Colorado, New Mexico, and Utah) are identified by the heavy border in Figure 7.17A. The earliest recognized cases were recorded among Native Americans in New Mexico, with investigations in neighbouring states and elsewhere yielding evidence of a total of 42 cases (including 26 deaths) by October 1993. The case distribution, with a primary focus on the Four Corners region, is represented by the proportional circles in Figure 7.17A. Early suspicions that a virus was involved in the aetiology of the disease were confirmed when a novel hantavirus, later named Sin Nombre virus, was

[3] See Section 8.2.1 for a consideration of HFRS due to Hantaan virus in Korea (Korean haemorrhagic fever).

Table 7.10. Members of the genus *Hantavirus*, family *Bunyaviridae*, associated with human disease

Species	Disease[1]	Principal reservoir(s)	Geographical distribution of virus
Old World			
Hantaan	HFRS	*Apodemus agrarius* (striped field mouse)	China, Korea, Russia
Dobrava-Belgrade	HFRS	*Apodemus flavicollis* (yellow-neck mouse), *Apodemus agrarius* (striped field mouse)	Balkans, central and north-eastern Europe
Seoul	HFRS	*Rattus norvegicus* (Norway rat)	Worldwide
Puumala	HFRS	*Clethrionomys glareolus* (bank vole)	Europe, Russia, Scandinavia
New World/Americas			
Sin Nombre	HPS	*Peromyscus maniculatus* (deer mouse)	Canada, US
New York	HPS	*Peromyscus leucopus* (white-footed mouse)	US
Black Creek Canal	HPS	*Sigmodon hispidus* (cotton rat)	US
Bayou	HPS	*Oryzomys palustris* (rice rat)	US
Andes	HPS	*Oligoryzomys longicaudatus* (long-tailed pygmy rice rat)	Argentina, Chile, Uruguay
Araraquara	HPS	Unknown	Brazil
Bermejo	HPS	*Oligoryzomys chacoensis* (Chacoan pygmy rice rat)[2]	Bolivia
Choclo	HPS	*Oligoryzomys fulvescens* (fulvous pygmy rice rat)	Panama
Lechiguanas	HPS	*Oligoryzomys flavescens* (fulvous pygmy rice rat)	Argentina
Laguna Negra	HPS	*Calomys laucha* (vesper mouse)	Bolivia, Paraguay
Oran	HPS	*Oligoryzomys longicaudatus* (long-tailed pygmy rice rat)[2]	Argentina
HU39694	HPS	Unknown	Argentina
To be named	HPS	*Calomys laucha* (vesper mouse)	Paraguay

Notes: [1] HFRS = haemorrhagic fever with renal syndrome; HPS = hantavirus pulmonary syndrome. [2] Suspected (unconfirmed).
Source: Pan American Health Organization (2003, table 1, p. 100).

Table 7.11. Hantavirus pulmonary syndrome in the region of the Americas, 1993–2004[1]

Country	Cases	Deaths
Argentina	592	11
Bolivia	36	17
Brazil	321	71
Canada	88	0
Chile	331	124
Panama	35	3
Paraguay	99	13
Uruguay	48	13
US	362	132
TOTAL	1,912	384

Note: [1] Reported status as of 26 Apr. 2004.
Source: Pan American Health Organization (2005).

isolated from case-patients (Plate 7.5). Environmental investigations yielded evidence of the same virus in deer mice (*Peromyscus maniculatus*) in the outbreak area, and the deer mouse is now recognized as the natural reservoir of Sin Nombre virus (Table 7.10) (Hughes *et al.* 1993; Centers for Disease Control and Prevention 2008*a*).

Since the isolation of Sin Nombre virus in 1993, three further hantaviruses have been implicated in the occurrence of HPS in the United States: Bayou virus (reservoir: rice rat), Black Creek Canal virus (cotton rat), and New York-1 virus (white-footed mouse) (Table 7.10). The maps in Figure 7.18 plot the known range of the rodent reservoirs, along with the distribution of reported cases of HPS due to the corresponding viruses through May 2006. As the maps show, the distribution of HPS is skewed to the western United States, with the vast majority of cases due to infection with Sin Nombre virus (Figure 7.18A).

Disease Time Series

Cases of HPS have been recorded on a near-continuous basis since the first recognition of the disease in 1993. Figure 7.19 plots the time series by month of onset in the Four Corners states (black bars) and other US states (grey bars), 1993–2006. A cumulative total of 465 cases (including 165 deaths) was recorded from across the Union (Figure 7.17B), with periodic spring/summer outbreaks in the Four Corners states forming a prominent feature of the disease curve (Figure 7.19).

EXPLAINING EMERGENCE: ENSO, TROPHIC CASCADE, AND HPS IN THE UNITED STATES

The foregoing observations raise a series of intrinsically geographical questions concerning the appearance and spread of HPS in the United States.

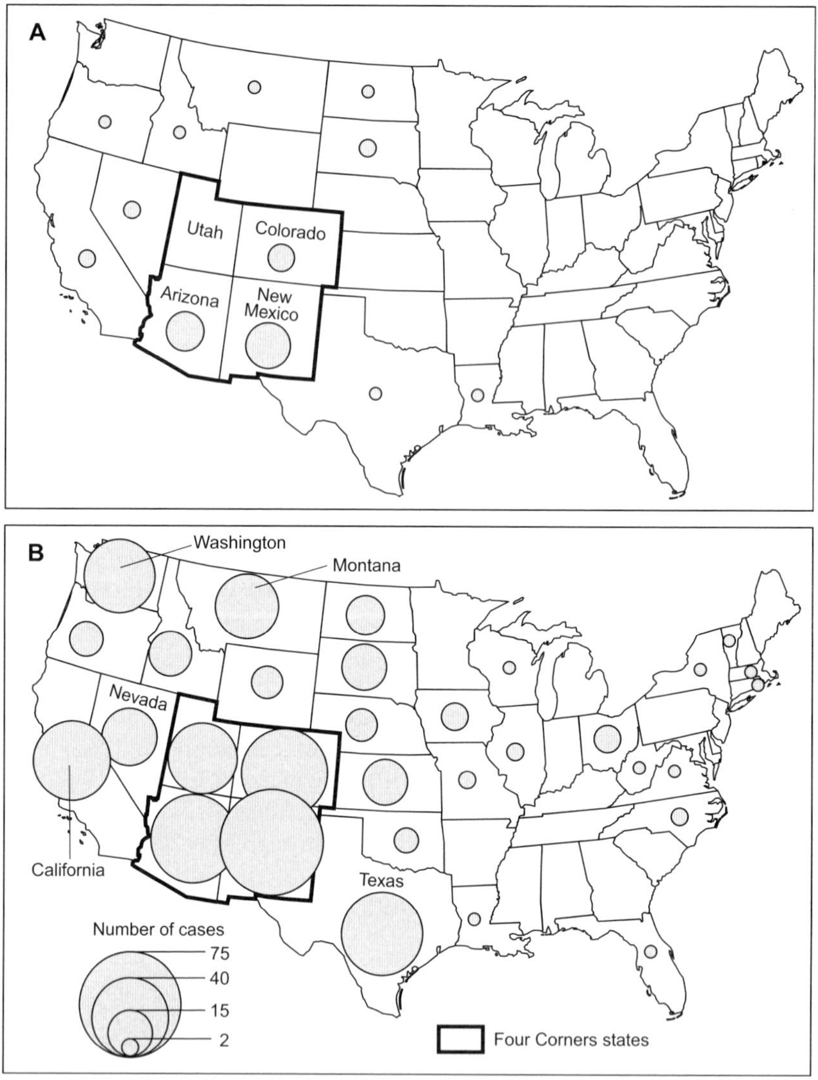

Fig. 7.17. Cases of hantavirus pulmonary syndrome (HPS) by reporting state, United States
Cumulative cases to (A) 21 Oct. 1993 and (B) 26 Mar. 2007. The Four Corners states (Arizona, Colorado, New Mexico, and Utah) are indicated.
Sources: Drawn from maps in Centers for Disease Control and Prevention (1993*b*, fig. 1, p. 816; 2008*a*).

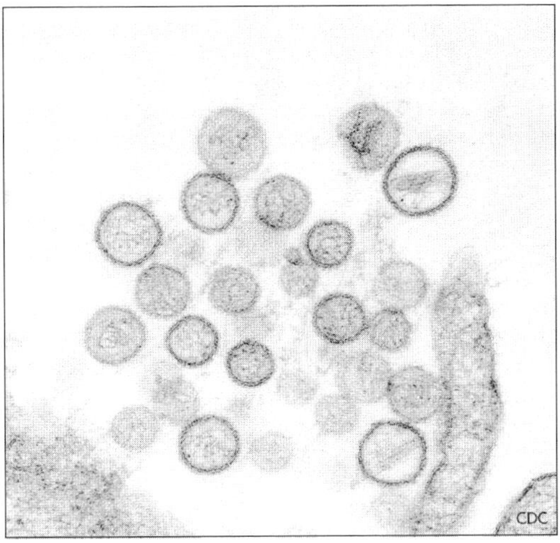

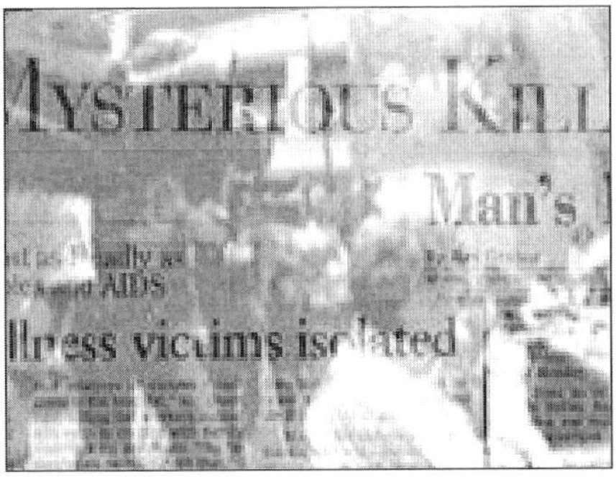

Pl. 7.5. Hantavirus pulmonary syndrome (HPS)
(Upper) Thin section electron micrograph of Sin Nombre virus isolate, a causative agent of HPS, from the 1993 outbreak of HPS in the Four Corners region of the south-western United States. (Lower) Sample media coverage of the 1993 outbreak.
Source: CDC public health image library.

Why did the disease emerge, apparently for the first time, in the Four Corners region in the spring of 1993? And what factors could account for the periodic outbreaks of HPS in the index region in subsequent years? Possible answers to these questions can be found in the hypothesized link between HPS activity and ENSO-related patterns of climate variability.

ENSO and the Trophic Cascade Model of HPS Emergence

The hypothesized links between ENSO and the emergence of HPS in the Four Corners region are outlined by Epstein (1995) and Engelthaler *et al.* (1999) and are summarized in the trophic cascade model in Figure 7.20. The model hinges on the observed tendency for ENSO events to yield excess levels

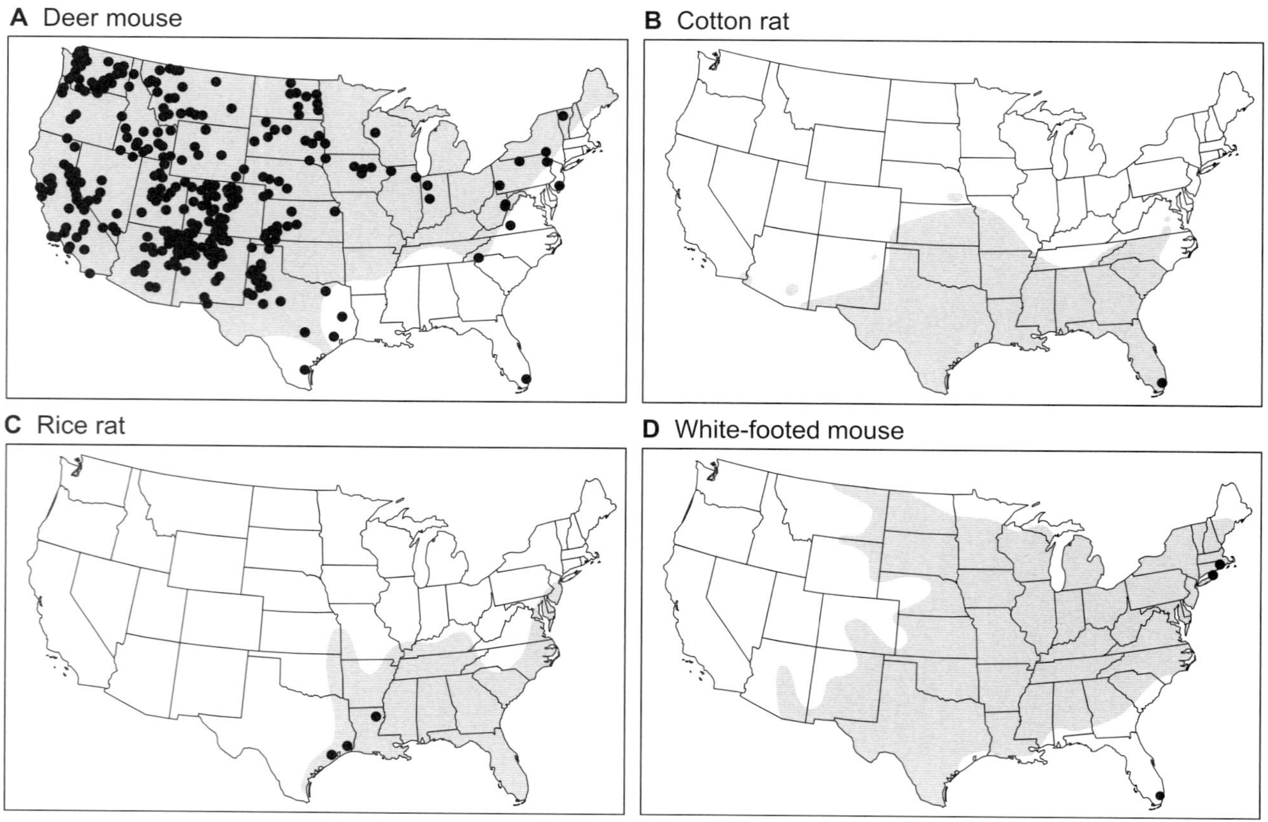

Fig. 7.18. Hantavirus pulmonary syndrome (HPS) in the United States
The shaded areas of the maps show the distribution of rodent carriers of HPS-causing hantaviruses; circles mark the locations of virus-specific cases of HPS to 9 May 2006. (A) Deer mouse (*Peromyscus maniculatus*), carrier of Sin Nombre virus. (B) Cotton rat (*Sigmodon hispidus*), carrier of Black Creek Canal virus. (C) Rice rat (*Oryzomys palustris*), carrier of Bayou virus. (D) White-footed mouse (*Peromyscus leucopus*), carrier of New York-1 virus.
Source: Redrawn from Centers for Disease Control and Prevention (2008*a*).

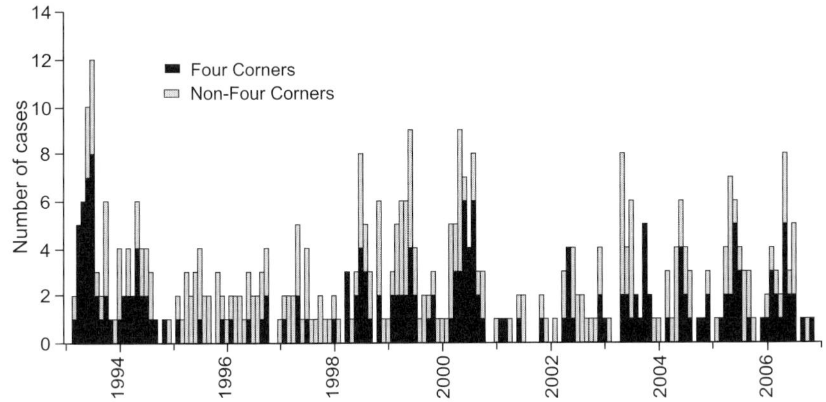

Fig. 7.19. Time series of hantavirus pulmonary syndrome (HPS) cases by month of onset, United States, January 1993–December 2006
Cases reported as of 26 Mar. 2007. Cases reported from the Four Corners states (Arizona, Colorado, New Mexico, and Utah) are indicated by the black shading. A total of 32 cases with onset before Jan. 1993 have been excluded from the graph.
Source: Redrawn from Centers for Disease Control and Prevention (2008*a*).

of rainfall in the south-western United States (Figure 7.16). From this starting point, Figure 7.20 depicts a chain-like sequence of events in which the environmental trigger (the ENSO event of 1991–3) resulted in a short-term climate response (above average precipitation, December 1992–March 1993) and an associated rodent habitat response (increased vegetation and food) that favoured an explosive increase in local populations of deer mice. As Engelthaler *et al.* (1999: 88) explain, these developments may have

> increased the likelihood of more rodent-to-rodent contact, rodent-to-human contact, and viral transmission . . . In addition, as rodent populations surpassed the carrying capacity of their local environments and precipitation plummeted, available food may have been depleted, resulting in rodent population stress. Increased stress likely increased rodent-to-rodent contact, as rodents competed for food and water, and increased rodent-to-human contact, as rodents moved into new, potentially less stressful environments, such as homes and peridomestic structures.

It is hypothesized that these developments precipitated the emergence of HPS in the region in 1993. Hjelle and Glass (2000) have subsequently provided evidence for ENSO as a driver of ongoing HPS activity in the index region (Figure 7.19).

EXAMINING THE TROPHIC CASCADE MODEL

To examine statistically the climate–disease associations invoked by the trophic cascade model in Figure 7.20, information for indices relating to each of three meteorological parameters (ENSO, precipitation, and drought)

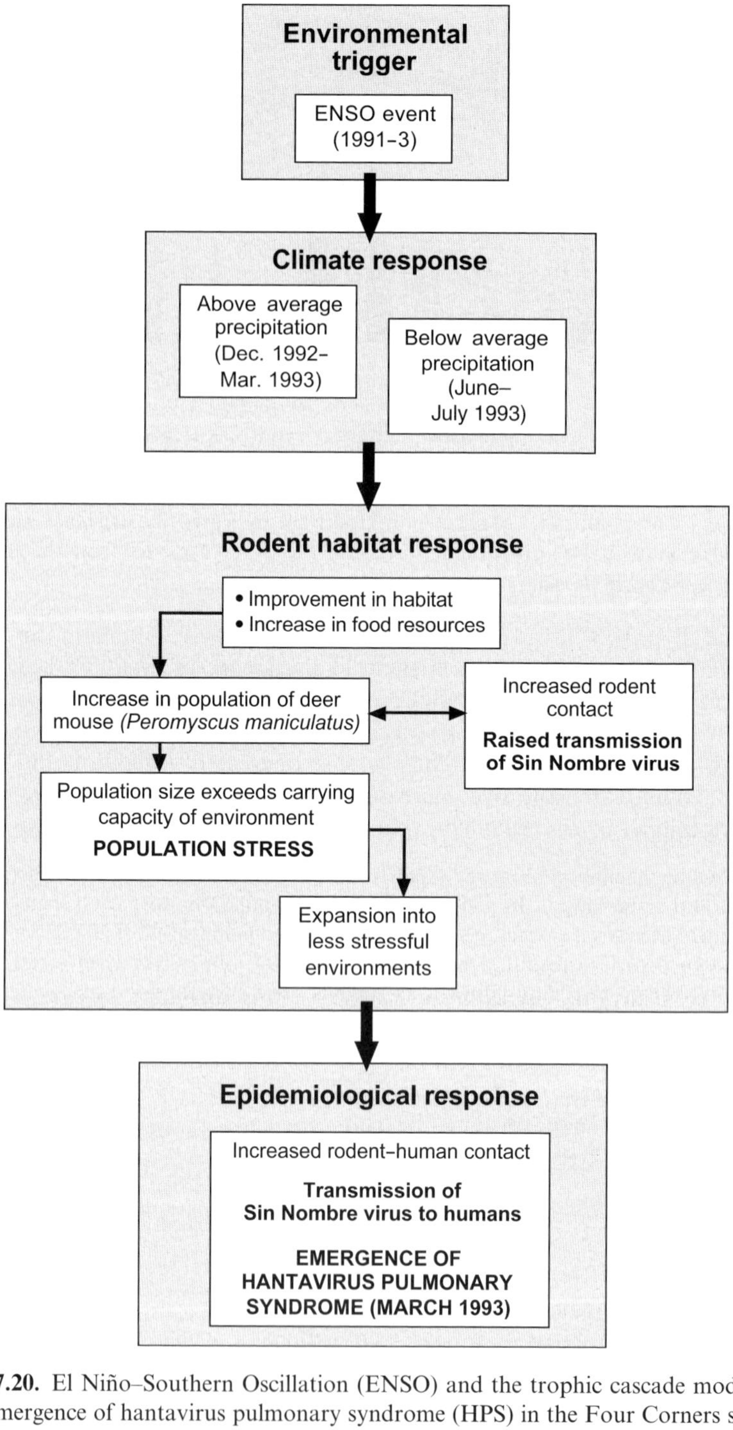

Fig. 7.20. El Niño–Southern Oscillation (ENSO) and the trophic cascade model of the emergence of hantavirus pulmonary syndrome (HPS) in the Four Corners states of the United States, 1993

was accessed from the National Oceanic and Atmospheric Administration (2008*a*,*b*) for a 16-year observation period, 1991–2006. These indices were:

(1) *the Multivariate ENSO Index (MEI)*, formed as a (running) bi-monthly weighted measure of six hydro-meteorological parameters in the tropical Pacific and serving as a global index of ENSO activity (Wolter and Timlin 1998). Positive MEI scores (MEI > 0) correspond to the warm ENSO phase (El Niño), while negative MEI scores (MEI < 0) correspond to the cold ENSO phase (La Niña);
(2) *monthly precipitation*, measured in inches for the US Southwest region;
(3) *the Palmer 'Z' Drought Index (PZDI)*, formed for the US Southwest region as a monthly measure of departure from normal of the moisture climate (National Oceanic and Atmospheric Administration 2008*b*). Positive PZDI scores (PZDI > 0) mark degrees of wetness, while negative PZDI scores (PZDI < 0) mark degrees of drought.

While index (1) is a universal measure of ENSO activity, indices (2) and (3) are aggregate measures of precipitation and drought for the Four Corners states (= US Southwest region). The line traces in Figure 7.21 plot, by quarterly period, average monthly/bimonthly values of the Multivariate ENSO Index (graph A), precipitation (graph B), and the Palmer 'Z' Drought Index (graph C), 1991–2006.[4] For reference, the histograms on each graph are based on information in Figure 7.19 and plot the quarterly count of HPS cases in the Four Corners states.

Time Series Analysis

To examine whether the temporally lagged system responses of the trophic cascade model (environmental trigger → climate response → rodent habitat response → epidemiological response) are reflected in the phase relationships of the meteorological and epidemiological time series in Figures 7.21A–C, techniques of cross-correlation were applied. Following Box *et al.* (1994), cross-correlation analysis proceeds by computing the correlation coefficient, r_k, between any pair of time series which are k time lags (in the present analysis, quarters) apart. The value of k at which the maximum correlation occurs is conventionally taken as the lead or lag of one time series with respect to another. Specifically, let x_{it} denote the value of meteorological variable i in quarterly period t and y_t denote the corresponding number of HPS cases. Then the cross-correlation at lag k, r_k, is given by

$$r_k = \mathrm{corr}[x_{it}, y_{t+k}]$$
$$= \sum_t [(x_{it} - \bar{x}_i)(y_{t+k} - \bar{y})] \Big/ \left[\sum_t (x_{it} - \bar{x}_i)^2 \sum_t (y_t - \bar{y})^2\right]^{1/2} \quad (7.1)$$

[4] Average quarterly values of the running bimonthly MEI were formed by averaging all bimonthly scores that intersected in part or whole with a given calendar quarter.

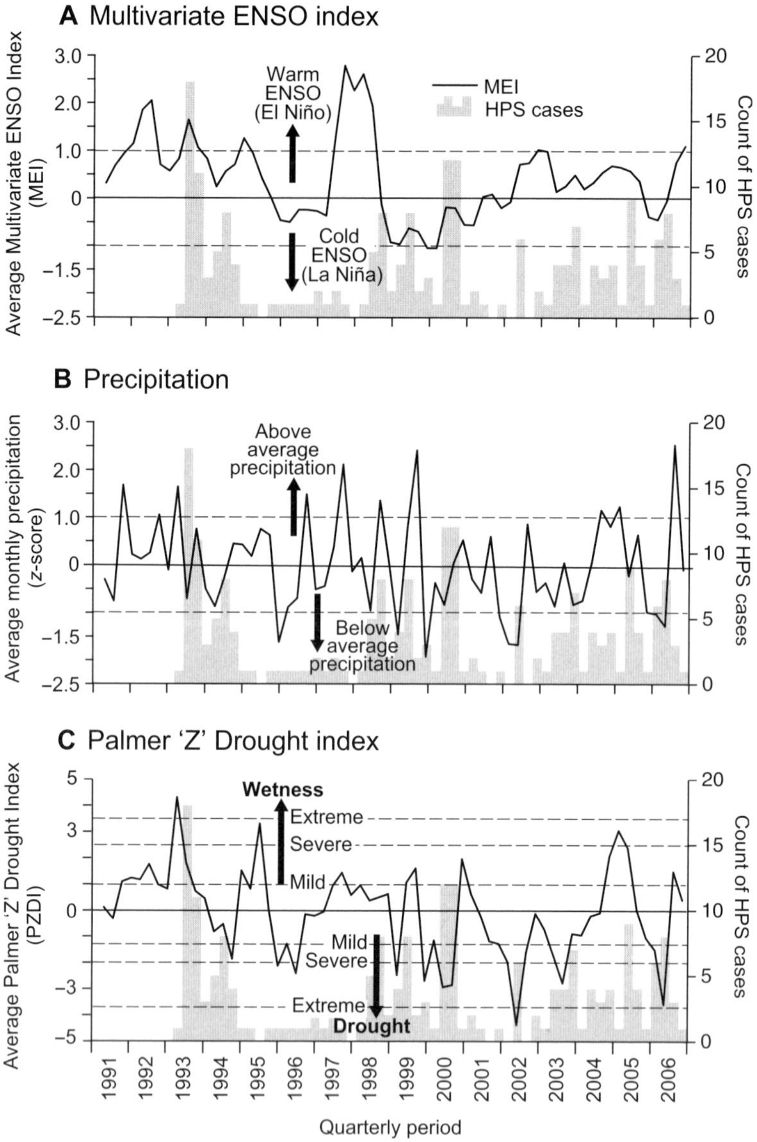

Fig. 7.21. US National Oceanic and Atmospheric Administration (NOAA) indices of the El Niño–Southern Oscillation (ENSO) and climatic variability in the Four Corners states of the United States, 1991–2006
(A) Average values of the bimonthly Multivariate ENSO Index (MEI) by quarterly period. The MEI is formed as a weighted average of the principal ENSO features over the tropical Pacific as measured by six variables (sea-level pressure, the east–west and north–south components of the surface wind, sea surface temperature, surface air temperature, and total amount of cloudiness). MEI scores >0 correspond to the warm

where $\bar{x}_i$ and $\bar{y}$ are the means of the time series. In the notation of equation 7.1, the $\{x_{it}\}$ are termed the reference series and the $\{y_t\}$ the comparison series. If $k = 0$, the reference and comparison series are said to be in phase; $+\ k\ (k > 0)$ signifies that the comparison series lags the reference series, and $-k\ (k < 0)$ that the comparison series leads the reference series. A plot of the correlation coefficient, r_k, against the lag k yields the cross-correlation function (CCF). Finally, cross-correlation analysis assumes that the data under analysis are time-stationary, which is reasonable for the length of series considered here.

Equation 7.1 was used to compute the CCFs between the quarterly time series of HPS cases and each of the three quarterly time series of meteorological indices in Figure 7.21. The results of the analysis appear in Figure 7.22. A striking feature of all three CCFs is the occurrence of the maximum cross-correlation at $k = +\ 4$ quarters, indicating that peaks in HPS activity lag the meteorological impulses by one year. This finding is consistent with the observations of Glass *et al.* (2002), who identified an approximate 12-month lag between the end of an ENSO event and an increase in Sin Nombre virus prevalence among deer mice in the south-western United States.

Wet–Dry Periods

Interpretation of Figure 7.22C is complicated by the fact that positive values of the Palmer 'Z' Drought Index mark periods of *relative wetness*, while negative values mark periods of *relative drought*. Thus, the maximum correlation at $k = +4$ quarters signals the role of wetness rather than drought in the epidemiological complex. To disentangle the effects of wet and dry periods, the original series of the Palmer 'Z' Drought Index was reduced to five series of dummy variables in which quarters of mild/severe wetness (PZDI $\geq$ 1.00) and severe wetness (PZDI $\geq$ 2.50), and quarters of mild/severe/extreme drought (PZDI ≤ -1.25), severe/extreme drought (PZDI ≤ -2.00), and

ENSO phase (El Niño), while MEI scores >0 correspond to the cold ENSO phase (La Niña). (B) Average values of monthly precipitation by quarterly period. Precipitation is expressed in standard Normal score (z-score) form; $z > 0$ marks periods of above average precipitation and $z < 0$ marks periods of below average precipitation. (C) Average values of the monthly Palmer 'Z' Drought Index by quarterly period. The Palmer 'Z' Drought Index is a measure of departure from normal of the moisture climate for a given month. Positive index scores mark periods of mild–moderate (1.00–2.49), severe (2.50–3.49), and extreme ($\geq$3.50) wetness. Conversely, negative index scores mark periods of mild–moderate (-1.25 – -1.99), severe (-2.00 – -2.74) and extreme (≤ -2.75) drought. Meteorological data in (B) and (C) relate to the Four Corners states (Arizona, Colorado, New Mexico, and Utah). The count of hantavirus pulmonary syndrome (HPS) cases in the Four Corners region, by quarterly period of disease onset, is represented on each graph as a bar chart.

Sources: Based on data from the National Oceanic and Atmospheric Administration (2008*a*,*b*) and Centers for Disease Control and Prevention (2008*a*).

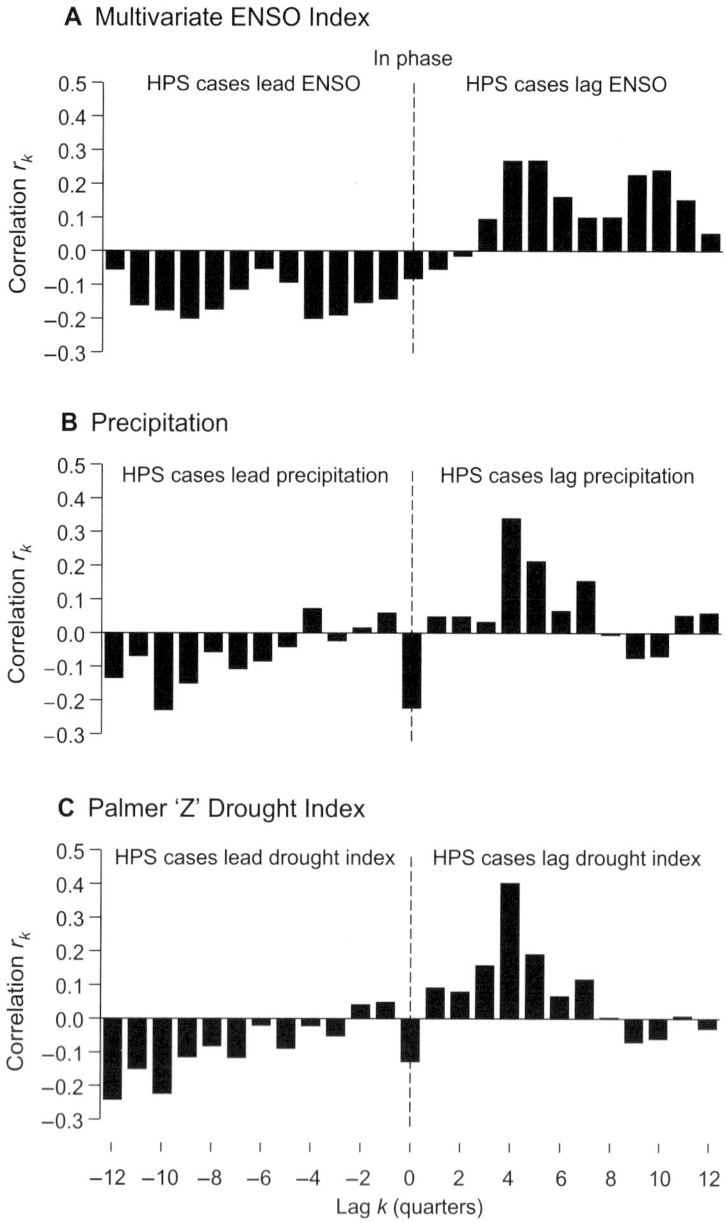

Fig. 7.22. Cross-correlation functions (CCFs) of quarterly series of hantavirus pulmonary syndrome (HPS) cases and indices of climatic variability
(A) Multivariate ENSO Index. (B) Precipitation. (C) Palmer 'Z' Drought Index.

extreme drought (PZDI ≤ −2.75) were coded 1, and all other quarters were coded zero. Here, the categories of wetness and drought follow the conventions of the Palmer 'Z' Drought Index as described by the National Oceanic and Atmospheric Administration (2008*b*) and summarized in the caption to Figure 7.21.

Figure 7.23 plots the CCFs between the quarterly series of HPS cases and the corresponding series of dummy variables for the two categories of wetness (graph A) and the three categories of drought (graph B). The highest CCF values are observed for mild/severe wetness (leading HPS cases by four quarters; graph A) and extreme drought (in phase with HPS cases; graph B). These findings are consistent with the dual operation of a time-lagged meteorological impulse (mild/severe wetness at one year prior to the HPS outbreak) and an immediate meteorological trigger mechanism (extreme

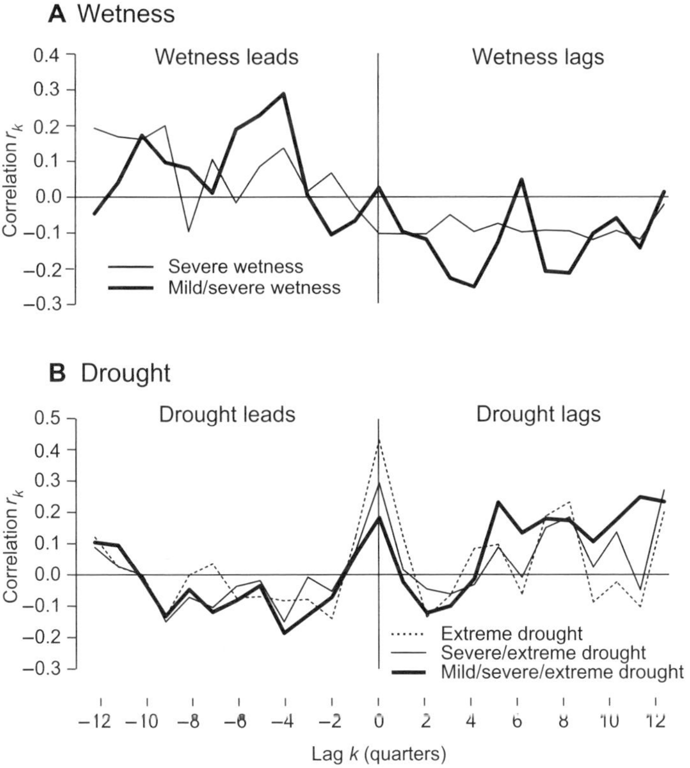

Fig. 7.23. Cross-correlation functions (CCFs) of quarterly series of hantavirus pulmonary syndrome (HPS) and measures of wetness and drought

Measures of wetness (A) and drought (B) have been defined according to values of the Palmer 'Z' Drought Index.

drought) invoked in the climate/habitat/epidemiological response components of Figure 7.20.

Regression Analysis

To examine further the time-lagged associations implied by the CCFs in Figure 7.23, the regression model

$$y_t = \beta_0 + \beta_1 x_{1,t-4} + \beta_2 x_{2,t} + e_t \qquad (7.2)$$

was postulated. Here, y_t denotes the number of recorded cases of HPS in quarter t of the observation period 1991–2006, $x_{1,t-4}$ is the dummy variable measure of mild/severe wetness at $t-4$ quarters,$x_{2,t}$ is the dummy variable measure of extreme drought, e_t is an error term, and β_0, β_1, and β_2 are parameters to be estimated. Model fitting was by ordinary least squares using a stepwise algorithm. The results are summarized in Table 7.12. Entry of $x_{2,t}$ in step 1 of the model confirms the primary importance of extreme drought as an immediate trigger mechanism in the appearance of HPS, with $x_{1,t-4}$ in step 2 underscoring the importance of mild/severe wetness a year in advance as an initiating factor in the trophic cascade.

Summary

Studies of the 1993–4 and 1998–9 outbreaks of HPS in the Four Corners region of the south-western United States have highlighted the possible role of ENSO-related climate variability as an environmental trigger of disease activity. Based on evidence for an extended period of 16 years, 1991–2006, our analysis has confirmed that ENSO events (Figure 7.22A) and associated increases in precipitation (Figures 7.22B and 7.23A) presaged HPS outbreaks in Four Corners by an average of one year. The same analysis has also demonstrated an in-phase relationship between extreme drought and HPS cases (Figure 7.23B)—a finding consistent with the hypothesized role of below average precipitation in the post-ENSO period as an immediate trigger mechanism for (i) heightened rodent population stress and (ii) the consequent spread of Sin Nombre virus to the human population (Figure 7.20).

Table 7.12. Results of stepwise multiple regression analysis to examine the time-lagged response of hantavirus pulmonary syndrome (HPS) to measures of wetness and drought in the Four Corners states of the United States, 1991–2006

Independent variable, slope coefficient (t-statistic)		
Step 1	Step 2	R^2 (F-ratio)
$x_{2,t}$, 6.38 (4.38*)	$x_{1,t-4}$, 3.48 (3.46*)	32.49 (13.59*)

Notes: * Significant at the $p = 0.01$ level (two-tailed test). Variables: x_1 = mild/severe wetness; x_2 = extreme drought.

7.6 Natural Disasters

Natural disasters are catastrophic environmental events that bring the human socio-economic system into crisis.[5] Disaster phenomena include avalanches, cyclones and hurricanes, droughts, earthquakes and tsunamis, extreme temperatures, floods, forest and scrub fires, lightning strikes, mud-slides and landslides, storm surges, tornadoes, volcanic eruptions, wind-storms, and—within some classifications—insect infestations. Natural disasters can have slow or rapid onset; they can range in scale from highly localized to global incidents; and they can result in devastating social, economic, and health outcomes for those involved. The International Federation of Red Cross and Red Crescent Societies' *World Disasters Report 2007* lists 3,670 natural disasters in the decade to 2006, resulting in the death of almost 1.11 million people and adversely affecting the lives of hundreds of millions more (Table 7.13). Geographically, the overwhelming majority of those affected (>98 per cent) resided in countries classified as 'medium' or 'low' on the UN Development Programme's Human Development Index—a reflection, in part, of the limited resources, infrastructure, and disaster response systems in these locations (International Federation of Red Cross and Red Crescent Societies 2007).

Table 7.13. Natural disasters recorded by the International Federation of Red Cross and Red Crescent societies, 1997–2006

Disaster phenomenon	Number of disasters	Number of people reported: Killed	Number of people reported: Affected (000)	Estimated costs of damage (US$m.[1])
Hydro-meteorological				
Avalanches/landslides	188	8,513	2,684	1,511
Droughts/food insecurity	294	459,447	1,106,191	30,925
Extreme temperatures	204	90,263	5,764	22,993
Floods	1,486	88,042	1,155,139	193,165
Forest/scrub fires	165	429	530	32,641
Windstorms	942	63,196	365,483	386,642
Other[2]	25	2,586	57	147
Geophysical				
Earthquakes/tsunamis	307	395,384	39,983	119,500
Volcanic eruptions	59	263	1,312	190
TOTAL	3,670	1,108,123	2,677,143	787,714

Notes: [1] 2006 prices. [2] Includes insect infestations and waves/surges.

Source: International Federation of Red Cross and Red Crescent Societies (2007, annex, tables 9–12, pp. 193–6).

[5] For a consideration of the nature and definition of natural disasters, see Alexander (1997).

7.6.1 Epidemiological Dimensions of Natural Disasters

Deaths associated with natural disasters are primarily due to blunt trauma, crush-related injuries, or drowning; large-scale mortality due to communicable diseases is—contrary to popular perception—a relatively uncommon sequel to such events (de Ville de Goyet 2000; Floret *et al.* 2006; Watson *et al.* 2007). The presence of large numbers of cadavers rarely poses an epidemic hazard to disaster survivors and, according to the WHO's Communicable Diseases Working Group on Emergencies (CD-WGE), the main risk of infectious disease outbreaks is associated with the size and characteristics of any ensuing population displacement. Factors that have a direct bearing on the latter include: the availability of potable water and functioning latrines; nutritional status; levels of immunity to vaccine-preventable diseases; and access to healthcare services. Natural disasters that do not result in population displacement are seldom associated with infectious disease outbreaks (de Ville de Goyet 2000; Communicable Diseases Working Group on Emergencies 2006; Floret *et al.* 2006; Watson *et al.* 2007).

COMMUNICABLE DISEASES ASSOCIATED WITH NATURAL DISASTERS

The principal disease risks in the aftermath of natural disasters are reviewed by Ligon (2006) and Watson *et al.* (2007) and include (i) water- and food-related diseases, (ii) diseases associated with crowding, and (iii) vector-borne diseases. Examples of disaster-related outbreaks associated with each of the three disease categories are given in Table 7.14.

(i) *Water- and food-related diseases.* Natural disasters can result in the disruption of sanitation systems, with a concomitant risk of contamination of water and food supplies. Outbreaks of diarrhoeal diseases due to a spectrum of infectious agents (including *Escherichia coli*, norovirus, and *Vibrio cholerae*) have been associated with recent flood events in India (1998), Bangladesh (2004), and the United States (2005). Other diseases, including hepatitis A and E, leptosporosis, rotavirus, shigellosis, typhoid fever, and a range of parasitic conditions (amoebiasis, cryptosporidiosis, cyclosporiasis, and giardiasis) are also recognized as potential risks in disaster settings.

(ii) *Diseases associated with crowding.* Crowding in temporary and makeshift camps increases the risk of transmission of many common communicable diseases in disaster-displaced populations. Outbreaks of measles in the Philippines (volcanic eruption, 1991) and measles, meningococcal disease, and acute respiratory infections in Indonesia (tsunami, 2004) and Pakistan (earthquake, 2005) are illustrative of the problem.

(iii) *Vector-borne diseases.* Natural disasters, especially hydro-meteorological events such as floods and hurricanes, can result in environ-

Table 7.14. Infectious diseases and infectious disease outbreaks in association with sample natural disasters, 1991–2005

Disaster		Epidemiological study		
Type of event	Date	Location	Sample findings	Source
Volcanic eruption	June 1991	North-western Philippines	Measles outbreak associated with 349 cases in 12 weeks; diarrhoea; respiratory tract infections	Centers for Disease Control and Prevention (1992)
Earthquake	Apr. 1991	Atlantic region, Costa Rica	Increases in the incidence of malaria as high as 1,600 per cent and 4,700 per cent above the average monthly rate for the pre-earthquake period	Saenz *et al.* (1995)
Earthquake	Jan. 1994	California, US	Outbreak of 203 coccidioidomycosis cases, including 3 fatalities	Schneider *et al.* (1997)
Flood	July 1998	West Bengal, India	Severe outbreak of cholera due to *Vibrio cholerae* O1	Sur *et al.* (2000)
Hurricane	Oct.–Nov. 1998	Villanueva, Nicaragua	Significant increase in incidence of acute diarrhoea and respiratory tract infections in comparison with pre-disaster data	Campanella (1999)
Flood	Jan.–Mar. 2000	Gaza state, Mozambique	Incidence of malaria increased by four to five times over non-disaster periods	Kondo *et al.* (2002)
Flood	July 2004	Dhaka, Bangladesh	Outbreaks of diarrhoea due to enterotoxigenic *Escherichia coli* and *Vibrio cholerae* O1	Qadri *et al.* (2005)
Tsunami	Dec. 2004	Aceh, Indonesia	Measles outbreak associated with 35 cases; acute respiratory infections; tetanus (clusters); meningococcal disease	World Health Organization (2005*b*), Watson *et al.* (2007)
Typhoon	July 2005	Taiwan	Outbreak of 54 melioidosis cases	Su *et al.* (2007)
Flood	July 2005	Mumbai, India	Incidence of leptospirosis increased by eight times over the pre-disaster period	Maskey *et al.* (2006)
Earthquake	Oct. 2005	Northern Pakistan	Measles (sporadic cases and clusters); acute respiratory infections; tetanus; meningococcal disease	Watson *et al.* (2007)
Hurricane	Aug. 2005	Southern states, US	Norovirus outbreak (evacuees in a 'megashelter', Houston, Texas)	Yee *et al.* (2007)

mental changes that are conducive to the proliferation of mosquitoes and other disease vectors. Documented instances of vector-borne diseases in the wake of disasters include malaria in Costa Rica (earthquake, 1991) and Mozambique (flood, 2000), while disaster-related cases of dengue and dengue haemorrhagic fever have also been documented (Pradutkanchana *et al.* 2003).

Among the other diseases in Table 7.14, cases of tetanus due to wound contamination with *Clostridium tetani* have been recorded in numerous disaster settings. More rarely, outbreaks of coccidioidomycosis and melioidosis have been documented in the aftermath of disasters.

7.6.2 Geophysical Phenomena

In an epidemiological review of >600 geophysical disasters (including 516 earthquakes, 89 volcanic eruptions, and 16 tidal waves and tsunamis), 1985–2004, Floret *et al.* (2006) identify only three recorded outbreaks of communicable diseases: measles (>18,000 reported cases) after the June 1991 eruption of Mt Pinatubo, Philippines; *Plasmodium vivax* malaria (>3,500 reported cases) after the April 1991 earthquake and heavy rains in Atlantic Region, Costa Rica; and coccidioidomycosis (>200 reported cases) after the January 1994 earthquake in Northridge, California. The epidemiological evidence does not lend support to the general notion that geophysical disasters provide short-term risk for epidemics (Floret *et al.* 2006). However, some geophysical events—such as the Asian tsunami of December 2004—occur on such a massive scale, and engender such complex and wide-ranging social and environmental disruptions, that continued monitoring for the emergence and spread of communicable diseases is a major public health priority.

THE ASIAN TSUNAMI (DECEMBER 2004)

At 00.58.53 UTC on 26 December 2004, the Sumatra–Andaman earthquake occurred with an epicentre off the west coast of northern Sumatra, Indonesia. Measuring 9.1–9.3 on the Richter scale, it was the second-largest earthquake ever recorded on a seismograph. The event triggered a series of tsunamis that, in the hours that followed, inundated the Asian and African coastlands that surround the Indian Ocean. With an estimated total power of 5 megatons of TNT, a wave height at landfall of up to 30 metres, and reaching 2 km or more inland at some locations, the tsunamis resulted in the extensive destruction of coastal regions of India, Indonesia, Malaysia, Maldives, Myanmar, Sri Lanka, Thailand, and Somalia (Figure 7.24) (Kohl *et al.* 2005).

Communicable Diseases

The information in Table 7.15 relates to eight of the most severely affected countries in Figure 7.24 and gives, at four weeks into the emergency

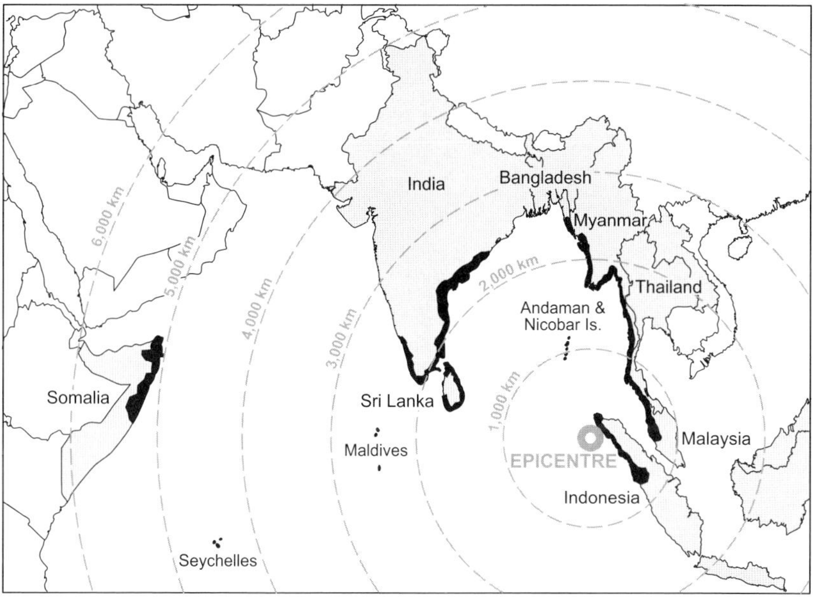

Fig. 7.24. Location map of areas affected by the Sumatra–Andaman earthquake and the Asian tsunami, 26 December 2004
Countries affected by the tsunami are identified by the grey shading; the worst-affected areas are highlighted in black. The epicentre of the earthquake, located off the west coast of northern Sumatra (3.30° N, 95.78° E), is indicated.

(23 January 2005), summary details of the estimated demographic and epidemiological impact of the Asian tsunami. Notwithstanding the large number of dead (>200,000) and displaced (>1.5 million), Table 7.15 shows that the reported epidemiological effects of the disaster were largely restricted to sporadic cases of diarrhoea and viral fevers, tetanus, and wound infections. No major outbreaks of communicable diseases were documented.

Local disease studies I: Epidemic-Prone Diseases in Aceh, Indonesia. The Indonesian province of Aceh, situated at the northern tip of Sumatra and close to the epicentre of the Andaman–Sumatra earthquake, was the place most severely affected by the tsunami (Table 7.15). During the first 12 weeks of the emergency, a WHO-sponsored disease surveillance/early warning and response network (EWARN) recorded a cumulative total of 40,706 cases of epidemic-prone diseases among *in situ* and displaced populations. Acute respiratory infections (25,212 cases), acute watery diarrhoea (9,483 cases), and fever of unknown origin (4,589 cases) accounted for the majority of illnesses. Among the other diseases, several case clusters (tetanus, dengue,

Table 7.15. Demographic and disease impact of the Asian tsunami, December 2004: reported status as of 23 January 2005

		Demographic impact			Communicable diseases	
Country	Affected area(s)	Dead	Missing	Displaced	Major outbreaks	Sporadic infections
India	Andaman and Nicobar Islands, Tamil Nadu, Andhra Pradesh, Kerala, Union Territory of Pondicherry	>10,000	5,551	647,556	None reported	None reported
Indonesia	Northern and western parts of island of Sumatra, especially Aceh province	166,760	6,222	452,845	None reported	Melioidosis (2 suspected cases); tetanus (91 cases); shigellosis (11 cases); dengue (1 suspected case)
Malaysia	North-west coast	68	6	8,000	None reported	None reported
Maldives	All 20 atolls	82	26	10,578	None reported	Diarrhoea (680 cases); acute respiratory infections (10 cases); viral fevers (86 cases); fever and vomiting (4 cases)
Myanmar	Townships in Ayeyawaddy, Tanintharyi, and Yangon divisions, and Rakkhine state	61	3	—	None reported	None reported
Somalia	Hafun Peninsula, Bender Beyla, Baargaal, and Eyl, regional state of Puntland	~150	—	~4,000	None reported	None reported
Sri Lanka	Ampara, Hambantota, Trincomalee, Batticaloa, and Galle	30,955	5,637	403,245	None reported	None reported
Thailand	South-western and coastal areas	5,374	3,132	—	None reported	Diarrhoea, pneumonia, influenza, dengue fever, and wound infections[1]

Note: [1] Total of 3,685 cases of disease.
Sources: World Health Organization (2005*e*) and Lawrence (2005).

bloody diarrhoea, typhoid, scrub typhus, hepatitis A and E) and one outright epidemic (measles) were also identified (World Health Organization 2005*b*).

Local Disease Studies II: Ecological Changes and Malaria Risk in South Andaman. Framed by more general concerns over the spread of vector-borne diseases in tsunami-affected areas (Wilder-Smith 2005), Krishnamoorthy *et al.* (2005) reviewed the ecological alterations favourable to the epidemic transmission of malaria in one severely affected Indian Ocean island (South Andaman) of the Andaman and Nicobar group; see Figure 7.24 for location. At the time of the survey (March 2005), South Andaman was still experiencing the recurring phenomenon of sea water intrusion, either directly from the ocean or through networks of creeks. Low-lying paddy fields and fallow, now with high salinity levels, were identified as new sites for the profuse breeding of the local malaria vector (the brackish water breeder *Anopheles sundaicus*), while pools and puddles of salt water offered further potential breeding grounds for the mosquito. Given the endemic nature of *Plasmodium falciparum* and *P. vivax* malaria, and with evidence of a sharp increase in the malaria slide positivity rate in the aftermath of the tsunami, the study of Krishnamoorthy and colleagues underscores the potentially profound impact of disaster-related ecological disruptions on vector-borne diseases.

7.6.3 Hydro-Meteorological Phenomena

Hydro-meteorological phenomena are the most common types of natural disaster, adversely affecting the lives of many millions of people each year in both developed and developing countries (Table 7.13). Although the health impacts vary according to the type of event and population affected, epidemics are better documented in the wake of floods (Ahern *et al.* 2005) and tropical cyclones (Shultz *et al.* 2005) than geophysical phenomena of the type described in Section 7.6.2. Examples of infectious disease outbreaks in association with hydro-meteorological events are given in Table 7.14. Here, we take the final example in the table—Hurricane Katrina (August 2005)—to illustrate the impact of a hurricane-associated flood event on recorded patterns of infectious disease activity in one developed country (United States).

HURRICANE KATRINA

On 24 August 2005, Tropical Depression 12 (TD #12)—having formed in the south-eastern Bahamas the previous day—was upgraded to Tropical Storm Katrina. Intensifying to a category 1 hurricane as it tracked westwards across southern Florida and into the Gulf of Mexico, and to a category 5 hurricane as it swung northwards towards the coast of Louisiana and Mississippi,

Hurricane Katrina finally made landfall near Buras, Louisiana, as a category 3 hurricane on 29 August (Figure 7.25). With sustained winds of 125 mph and a minimum central pressure of 920 mb, it was one of the deadliest hurricanes to strike the coastal United States in 100 years (Plate 7.6).[6] Storm damage extended over some 230,000 km^2 of Louisiana, Mississippi, Alabama, and Florida, disrupting basic utilities and infrastructure and resulting in the displacement of many thousands of people. The cities of New Orleans, Mobile, and Gulport bore the brunt of the storm. In New Orleans, the destructive force of the hurricane was magnified by storm surge conditions and the low-lying nature of the land, with breaches of the local levee system resulting in catastrophic flooding of the city. The situation was compounded on 24 September when a second category 3 hurricane (Hurricane Rita) forced the temporary suspension of response activities in New Orleans and elsewhere along the Gulf coast (Figure 7.25) (Centers for Disease Control and Prevention 2006*b*).

The exact death toll due to Hurricanes Katrina and Rita will never be known with certainty. Almost one year after the event, the number of hurricane-related deaths in Louisiana was officially placed at 1,464. An additional 220 or more are believed to have died in Mississippi, Florida, and neighbouring states (Centers for Disease Control and Prevention 2006*b*; Louisiana Department of Health and Hospitals 2006).

Communicable Diseases in Evacuation Centres

Some 750 evacuation centres in at least 18 states were established to accommodate >200,000 evacuees from Katrina-affected areas.[7] The results of enhanced surveillance for infectious conditions in these facilities are summarized for the first three weeks of the emergency (late August to mid-September 2005) in Table 7.16. Among the diseases reported, an outbreak of methicillin-resistant *Staphylococcus aureus* (MRSA) infection was identified at a facility in Dallas, Texas. Wound infections due to *Vibrio vulnificus* and *V. parahaemolyticus* were observed at facilities in several states, while, among the numerous cases of diarrhoeal disease, a large outbreak of norovirus gastroenteritis was recorded at the Reliant Park 'megashelter' in Houston, Texas (Centers for Disease Control and Prevention 2005*b*,*c*; Yee *et al.* 2007).

Ongoing Surveillance in Louisiana Evacuation Centres. Figure 7.26 is based on information relating to approximately 500 evacuation centres in the state of Louisiana, and plots, on a daily basis, the total number of evacuees under

[6] Hurricane Katrina weakened after landfall, eventually to lose hurricane strength some 160 km inland, near Jackson, Mississippi. Katrina was downgraded to a tropical depression near Clarksville, Tennessee, as it continued to track northwards to the eastern Great Lakes.

[7] For maps of the distribution of evacuation centres, see Centers for Disease Control and Prevention (2006*f*).

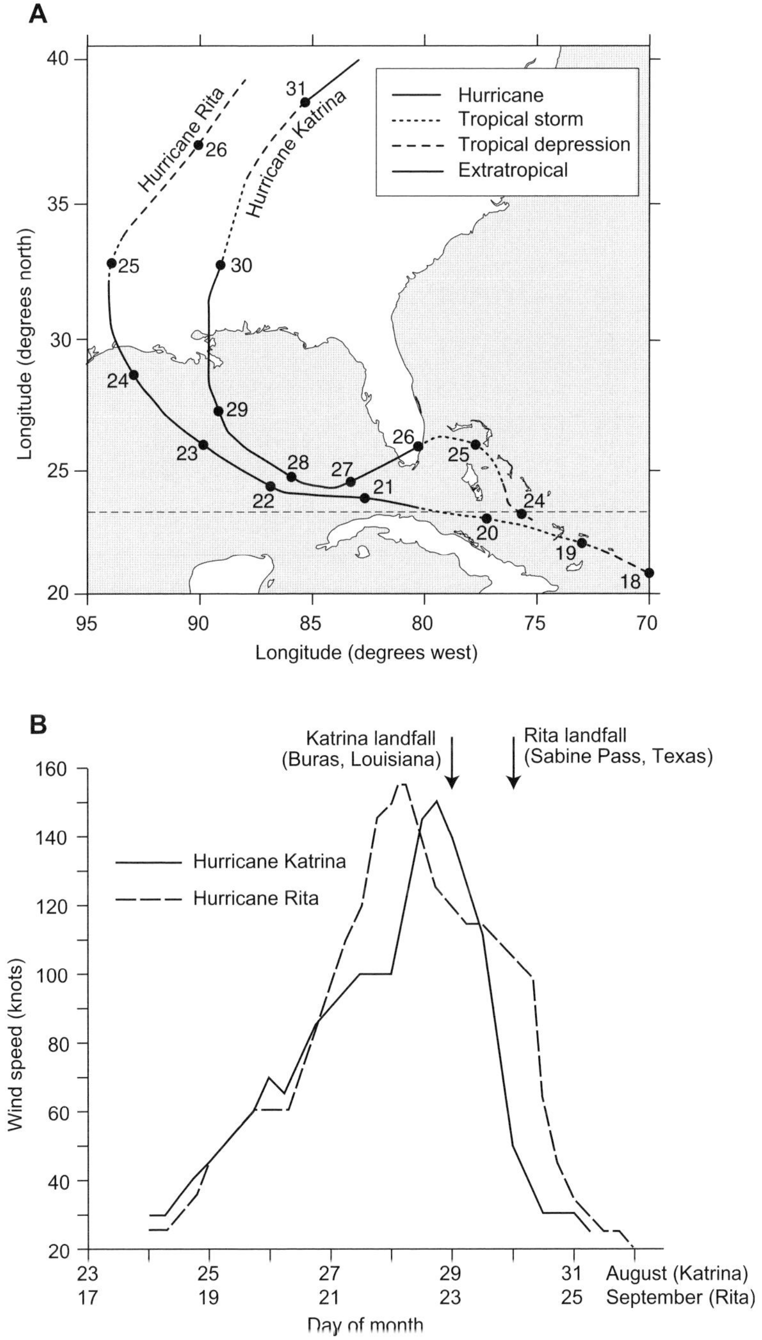

Fig. 7.25. Hurricane Katrina (23–31 August 2005) and Hurricane Rita (18–26 September 2005)
(A) Best track daily positions (circles), with day of month for Katrina (Aug.) and Rita (Sept.) indicated. (B) Best track maximum sustained surface winds.
Sources: Redrawn from Knabb *et al.* (2006*a*, figs 1, 2, pp. 37–8; 2006*b*, figs 1, 2, pp. 30–1).

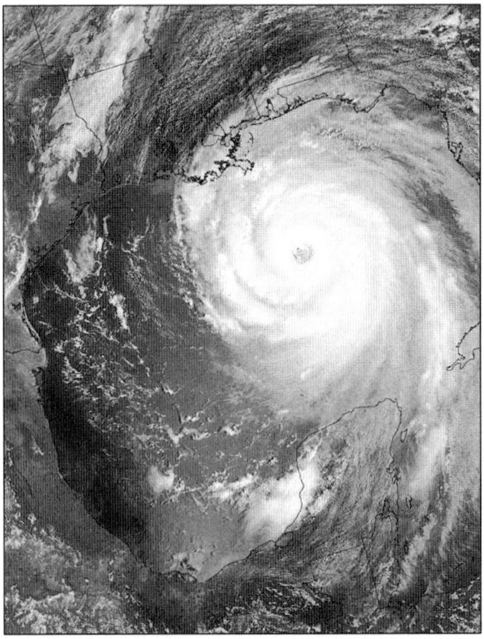

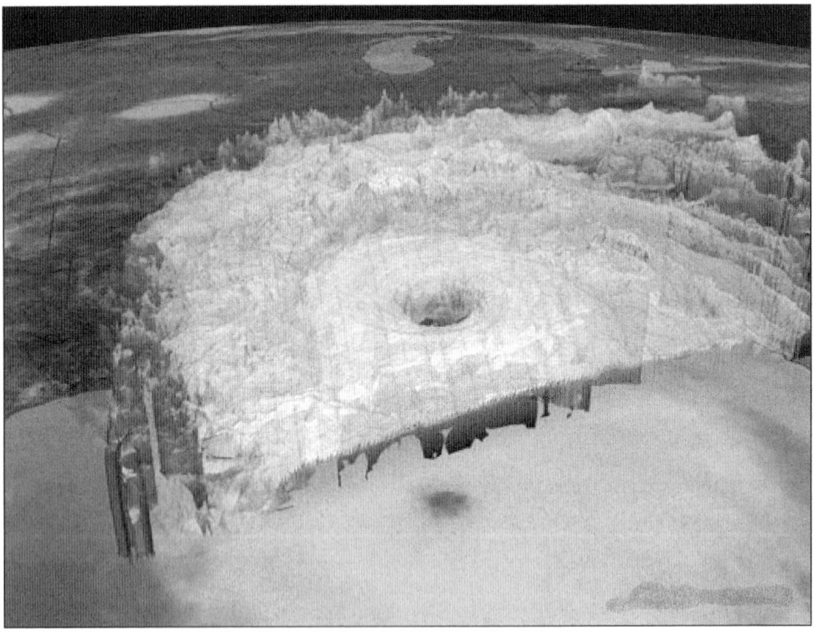

Pl. 7.6. Hurricane Katrina, 28–29 August 2005

Hurricane Katrina made landfall near Buras, Louisiana, as a category 3 hurricane on 29 Aug. 2005. It was one of the deadliest hurricanes to strike the coastal United States in 100 years. Around 1,500 deaths have been directly attributed to the storm, and millions were displaced. Among the consequential diseases reported were methicillin-resistant *Staphylococcus aureus* (MRSA) infection, wound infections due to *Vibrio vulnificus* and *V. parahaemolyticus*, and numerous cases of diarrhoeal disease. The upper image was taken at 08.42 EDT on 28 Aug. and shows the swirl of cloud around the eye of the storm. The lower image was taken at 17.30 EDT on the same day by NASA's Tropical Measuring Mission satellite to reveal the storm's rain structure. Rain ranged from 0.5 inches per hour in the lightest-coloured areas through to at least 2 inches in the darkest.

Sources: Upper image: NASA/Jeff Schmaltz, MODIS Land Rapid Response Team. Lower image: NASA/JAXA.

Table 7.16. Hurricane Katrina: selected diseases and conditions among evacuees in the three weeks following landfall, August–September 2005

Disease/condition[1]	Number of cases	Reporting states
Dermatologic conditions (infectious)		
Methicillin-resistant *Staphylococcus aureus* infections	30[2]	Texas
Vibrio vulnificus and *V. parahaemolyticus* wound infections	24[3]	Arizona, Arkansas, Georgia, Louisiana, Mississippi, Oklahoma, Texas
Diarrhoeal disease		
Acute gastroenteritis (some attributed to norovirus)	~1,000	Louisiana, Mississippi, Tennessee, Texas
Non-toxigenic *V. cholerae* O1	6	Arizona, Georgia, Mississippi, Oklahoma, Tennessee
Non-typhoical *Salmonella*	1	Mississippi
Respiratory disease		
Pertussis	1	Tennessee
Respiratory syncytial virus	1	Texas
Streptococcal pharyngitis	1	Texas
Tuberculosis	1	Pennsylvania
Other conditions		
Presumed viral conjunctivitis	~200	Louisiana

Notes: [1] Other diseases and conditions, variously reported among evacuees and rescue workers, included: scabies; circumferential lesions at waist; contact dermatitis; erythematous immersion foot; prickly heat; influenza-like illness and upper respiratory tract infections; tinea corporis; arthropod bites; and head lice. [2] Three confirmed cases. [3] Six deaths.
Source: Centers for Disease Control and Prevention (2005*b*: 962).

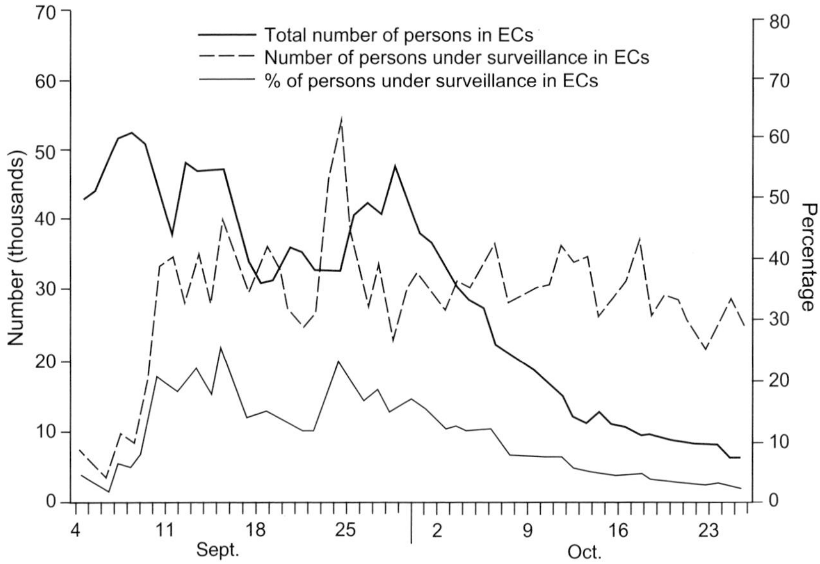

Fig. 7.26. Daily count of persons in hurricane evacuation centres, Louisiana, September–October 2005

Line traces plot the total number of persons in evacuation centres (ECs), and the number and percentage of persons under medical surveillance.

Table 7.17. Signs and syndromes of communicable disease among persons in hurricane evacuation centres, Louisiana, September–October 2005

Condition	Average daily incidence rate[1,2]	Number of cases (largest cluster)
Fever only[3]	0.5 (0–1.9)	10
Bloody diarrhoea	0.1 (0–0.7)	6
Watery diarrhoea[4]	1.8 (0–4.0)	22
Vomiting only[5]	1.3 (0–6.0)	13
Influenza-like illness	4.7 (0–8.8)	47
Rash	2.7 (0–13.8)	35
Scabies, lice, or other infestation	0.6 (0–3.8)	60
Wound infection	1.6 (0–8.5)	34
Conjunctivitis	0.4 (0–1.8)	10

Notes: [1] Incidence rate per 1,000 persons. [2] Range of incidence rates in parentheses. [3] >38°C. [4] With or without vomiting. [5] One episode or more.

Source: Centers for Disease Control and Prevention (2006*d*).

syndromic surveillance for communicable diseases by the Louisiana Department of Health and Hospitals, 4 September–26 October 2005. Summary details of the diseases detected are given in Table 7.17. As the table shows, influenza-like illnesses and rashes were the most commonly recorded conditions, with the largest case clusters due to skin infestation (60 cases), influenza-like illnesses (47 cases), rashes (35 cases), and wound infections (34 cases). It is recognized, however, that some clusters were associated with the significant over-reporting of cases (Centers for Disease Control and Prevention 2006*d*).

Other Communicable Diseases: Toxigenic Vibrio Cholerae

Among the other diseases of note identified in the aftermath of Hurricanes Katrina and Rita, two cases of infection with the El Tor biotype of *Vibrio cholerae* O1 (see Section 9.2.2) were documented in a couple from south-eastern Louisiana in mid-October 2005. Their residence had been severely damaged by the hurricanes, and both had eaten locally caught seafood (crabs and shrimp) in the days before onset of illness. Infection was attributed to the improper handling and/or preparation of the contaminated seafood under difficult living conditions (Centers for Disease Control and Prevention 2006*c*).

7.7 Conclusion

Using a series of case studies, this chapter has illustrated the ways in which planned and unplanned changes to the environment can foster the emergence and re-emergence of infectious diseases. Changes in water management, land use, forest clearance and regeneration, and modifications to local agricultural practices can all create new ecological niches which may be occupied by disease agents and their vectors. At the macro scale, climate change and natural disasters can create their own disease opportunities by bringing humans into contact with unfamiliar epidemiological environments. This unfamiliarity frequently amplifies the consequences of infections. Sometimes this amplification occurs as a result of environmental change in war zones. It is the amplification effect of wars and local conflicts upon disease emergence which we consider in the next chapter.

8

Disease Amplifiers: Wars and Conflicts in the Post-1945 Era

8.1 Introduction

The history of war is replete with examples of novel diseases that have suddenly and unexpectedly erupted into human consciousness. As we noted in Section 2.2, ancient Greek historians such as Herodotus, Thucydides, and Diodorus Siculus provide classical accounts of the devastation wrought by mysterious war pestilences—diseases which, in many instances, elude classification in modern disease systems, and to which the appellation 'antique plague' is occasionally given (Smallman-Raynor and Cliff 2004*b*: 66–73). In more recent times, we saw in Table 1.7 how maladies such as the idiopathic English sweating sickness, along with venereal syphilis, typhus fever, and yellow fever, appeared—ostensibly for the first time—in association with wars of the late medieval and early modern periods. In the twentieth century, trench fever (World War I, 1914–18), scrub typhus (World War II, 1939–45), and Korean haemorrhagic fever (Korean War, 1950–3) provide further instances of the emergence phenomenon (Macpherson *et al.* 1922–3; Philip 1948; Gajdusek 1956).

In addition to sponsoring apparently wholly new conditions, military conflict has also promoted the re-emergence of many infectious and parasitic diseases. Recent examples include African trypanosomiasis (Ugandan Civil War, 1979–86; Berrang Ford 2007), diphtheria and tuberculosis (Tajikistan Civil War, 1992–7; Keshavjee and Becerra 2000; Usmanov *et al.* 2000) and epidemic louse-borne typhus fever (Burundian Civil War, 1993–2005; Raoult, Ndihokubwayo, *et al.* 1998).

8.1.1 Wars as Disease Amplifiers

Figure 8.1 illustrates schematically the sample factors that underpin the war-related emergence and re-emergence of infectious diseases. As Price-Smith (2002: 129) observes, military conflict acts 'as a direct disease "amplifier," creating those physical conditions (poverty, famine, destruction of vital infrastructure, and large population movements) that are particularly conducive to the spread and mutation of disease'. High-level population mobility and mixing, differential patterns of disease exposure and susceptibility, the breakdown of public health infrastructure, and insanitary living conditions are all pertinent to an understanding of the (re-)emergence complex (Lederberg *et al.* 1992: 110–12). Additional factors also attain prominence. Within the schema of Figure 8.1, heightened exposure to the zoonotic pool has played a particularly important role in the war-related precipitation of disease emergence and re-emergence. Historically, ecological changes resulting from warfare, including the burning and firing of forests, the forced abandonment and destruction of agricultural land, and the consequent disruption and alteration of zootic habitats, have served to bring soldiers and civilians into close proximity with disease-bearing wildlife and insects (Gajdusek 1956; Velimirovic 1972), enhancing the possibilities for cross-species disease spread. For combat troops, the risk is magnified by inadvertent deployment in isolated ecological niches to which humans are ill-adapted (Philip 1948), while, in the era of military air transport, the rapid de-deployment and/or evacuation of overseas troops poses an obvious epidemiological threat to the reception country (Neel 1973).

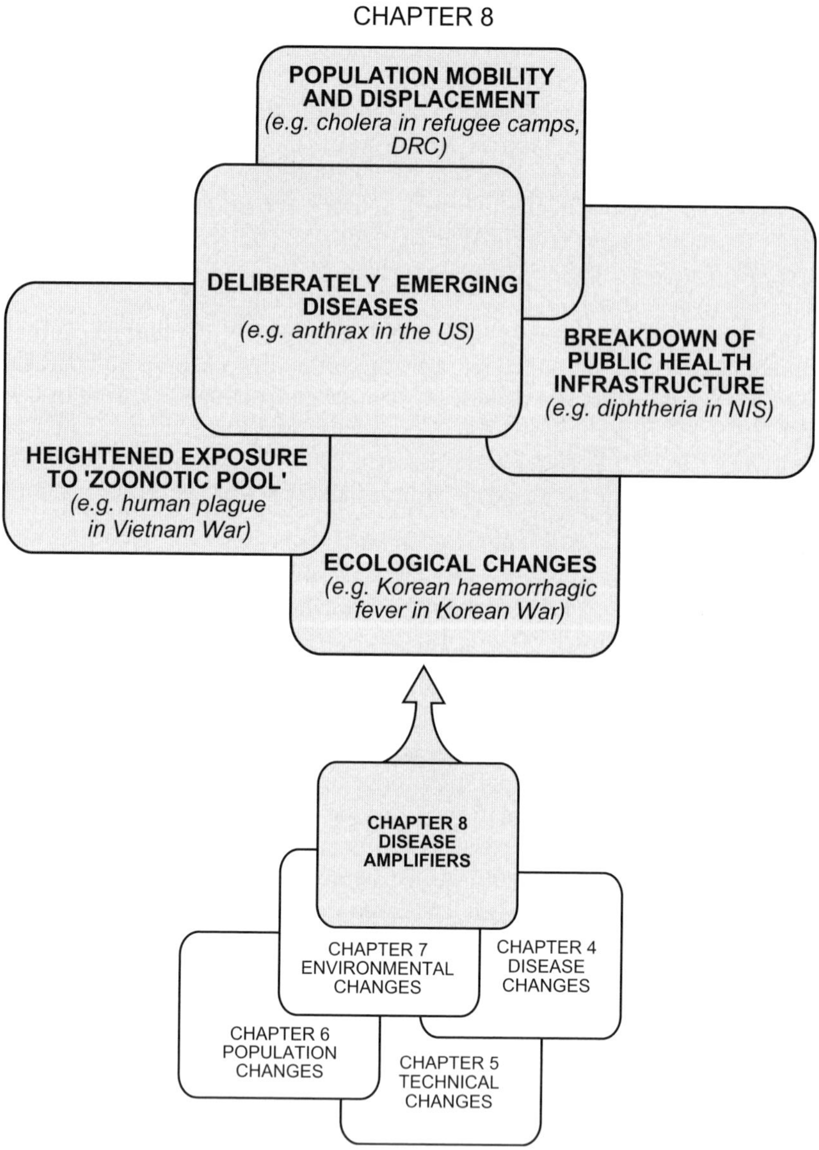

Fig. 8.1. (Upper) Venn diagram showing the facilitating factors for disease emergence and re-emergence associated with wars and conflicts
The lower diagram is redrawn from Fig. II.1 and shows the position of wars and conflicts (shaded box) within the suite of facilitating factors associated with the processes of disease and emergence and re-emergence. DRC = Democratic Republic of the Congo. NIS = newly independent states of the former Soviet Union.

8.1.2 Layout of Chapter and Selection of Examples

Historical perspectives on the intersection of war and disease emergence are provided by Smallman-Raynor and Cliff (2004*b*: 480–526). In the present chapter, we develop the theme in relation to conflicts and diseases in the post-1945 period. We begin by drawing on specific examples of disease emergence and re-emergence in relation to different categories of war in two geographical divisions: international conflicts in East Asia (Section 8.2) and ethnic conflicts and genocide in Central Africa (Section 8.3). In the remainder of the chapter, we summarize evidence for the emergence and re-emergence of diseases in other theatres of war during the late twentieth and early twenty-first centuries (Section 8.4), before turning to the issue of deliberately emerging diseases in the context of biological warfare and bioterrorism (Section 8.5). The chapter is concluded in Section 8.6.

The diseases selected for close examination in Sections 8.2 and 8.3 are listed in Table 8.1, along with summary information on the associated wars, afflicted populations, and emergence factors. Although a rigid classification into *emergent* and *re-emergent* diseases is complicated by the length of time for which most of the sample diseases are known to have been circulating,[1] we follow Smallman-Raynor and Cliff (2004*b*: 489) by drawing a simple distinction between those diseases that, prior to the twentieth century, were essentially unknown to the West (Japanese encephalitis and Korean haemorrhagic fever), and classical diseases that have been known to the West for many centuries (cholera, epidemic louse-borne typhus fever, malaria, and plague). Within this simple division, our selection of diseases, wars, and populations in Table 8.1 has been chosen to span a range of disease agents, populations, and emergence factors.

8.2 International Conflicts in the Far East: Korea and Vietnam

In this section, we use post-1945 conflicts in the Far East to illustrate the war-related processes of virus emergence (Korean War, 1950–3) and parasite and bacterium re-emergence (Vietnam War, 1964–73). Our discussion draws on the studies of Smallman-Raynor and Cliff (2004*b*: 498–524).

8.2.1 Emergent Viruses in the Korean War

The Korean War (1950–3) presented the multinational United Nations (UN) Command with a series of medical challenges that were 'without comparison'

[1] The earliest accounts of the most recently described disease in Table 8.1 (Korean haemorrhagic fever) date to the 1930s.

Table 8.1. Conflicts and diseases selected for examination in Sections 8.2 and 8.3

War/conflict	Disease (aetiological agent)	Population	Geographical location	Emergence factor(s)
East Asia (Section 8.2)				
Korean War (1950–3)	Japanese encephalitis (Japanese encephalitis virus)	UN Command	Korea	Entry of unprotected overseas forces into area of newly recognized clinical infection (Lincoln and Sivertson 1952)
	Korean haemorrhagic fever (Hantaan virus)	UN Command	Korea	Ecological change associated with abandonment of agricultural land; human invasion of ecological niche of rodent reservoir of Hantaan virus (*Apodemus agrarius*) (Paul and McClure 1958)
Vietnam War (1964–73)	Malaria (*Plasmodium* spp.)	US forces	Vietnam/US	Exposure of troops to chloroquine-resistant strains of *P. falciparum*; importation to US by Vietnam returnees (Neel 1973)
	Plague (*Yesinia pestis*)	Vietnamese civilians	Vietnam	War-induced disruption of human and zootic habitats; emergence of resistance to insecticides in principal flea vector (*Xenopsylla cheopis*) (Marshall *et al.* 1967; Velimirovic 1972)
Central Africa (Section 8.3)				
Burundian Civil War (1993–2005)	Epidemic louse-borne typhus fever (*Rickettsia prowazekii*)	Internally displaced populations (IDPs)	Burundi	Internal population displacement; unsanitary conditions in relief camps (Raoult *et al.* 1998)
Rwandan genocide (1994)	Cholera (*Vibrio cholerae* O1 biotype El Tor)	Rwandan refugees	Zaire	International population displacement; residence in relief camps, with exposure to contaminated water supplies (Goma Epidemiology Group 1995)

in the countries from which the bulk of the troops originated (Hunter 1953: 1408). While frostbite, along with other non-battle injuries due to exposure and extreme cold, ranked among the most severe medical problems in the early stages of the war (Anonymous 1953), infectious conditions were widespread. Gonorrhoea and other sexually transmitted infections occurred in epidemic form, while malaria, dysentery, and diarrhoeal diseases, respiratory tract infections (including scattered cases of influenza A), intestinal parasites, and infectious hepatitis were also encountered at various stages of the conflict (Hunter 1953; Ingham 1953). However, two emergent viral diseases that, prior to the mid-twentieth century, were largely unknown in Western medicine achieved particular prominence among UN troops: Japanese encephalitis and Korean haemorrhagic fever (Lincoln and Sivertson 1952; McNinch 1953).

JAPANESE ENCEPHALITIS

Japanese encephalitis (*ICD*-10 A83.0) is a severe, often fatal, disease of the central nervous system due to infection with Japanese encephalitis virus (JEV). The disease is widespread in South-East Asia (including China, Japan, and Korea), having extended westwards into India and Pakistan and eastwards into New Guinea and northern Australia in recent decades (Endy and Nisalak 2002; Mackenzie, Gubler, *et al.* 2004). The virus is transmitted by a mosquito vector from its reservoir (probably wild birds) to humans and other mammals, which, in turn, serve as incidental hosts (Figure 8.2). The fatality rate is 20–50 per cent among cases, with permanent mental impairment, severe emotional instability, and paralysis being the most common sequelae in survivors (Tsai 2000; Heymann 2004: 37–41).

Descriptions of a disease believed to have been Japanese encephalitis can be traced back to 1871. But the importance of the condition was not recognized in Korea until the 1940s. In 1946, JEV was isolated from a US soldier who was stationed in South Korea (Sabin *et al.* 1947), while a serologic survey by Deuel and colleagues (1950) confirmed the widespread nature of inapparent JEV infection in that country. In 1949, a major outbreak, associated with some 5,616 documented cases and 2,729 deaths (attack rate 27.8 per 100,000), resulted in the addition of Japanese encephalitis to the list of notifiable communicable diseases in South Korea (Thongcharoen 1989; Sohn 2000). In terms of Figure 8.1, the infection of UN Command in Korea probably reflected the heightened exposure of soldiers to the zoonotic pool.

The 1950 Epidemic in US Troops

As described by Lincoln and Sivertson (1952), the start of the epidemic can be traced to the second week of August 1950, when a US soldier died after a short illness characterized by fever and coma. Autopsy revealed evidence of encephalitis, and a virus, identified as JEV, was successfully isolated from the

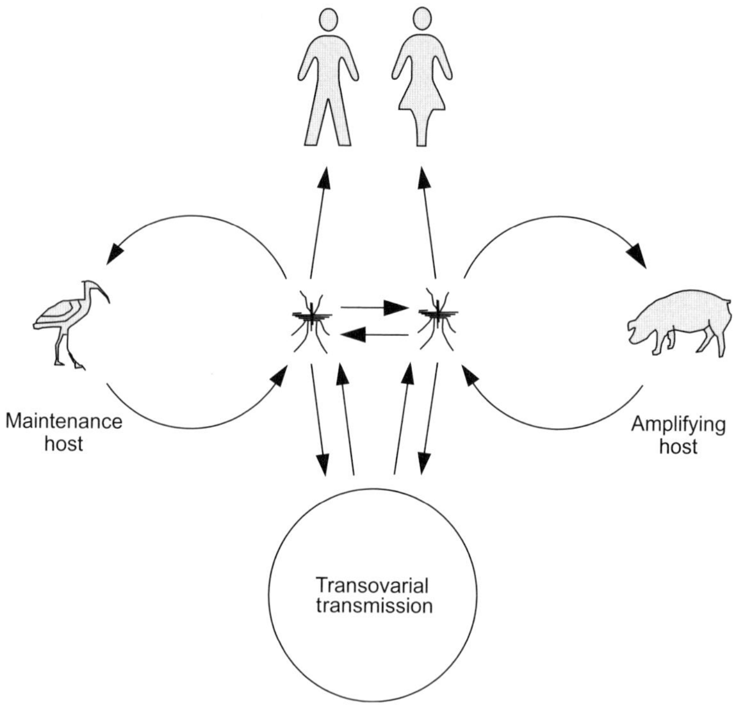

Fig. 8.2. Presumptive natural cycle of Japanese encephalitis virus (JEV)
Japanese encephalitis virus is maintained in nature by a cycle that includes certain species of mosquito (*Anopheles*, *Culex*, and *Mansonia*) and bird (family *Ardeidae*). Mosquitoes may also serve to maintain the virus by transovarial transmission, while domestic pigs are the main amplifying host for the virus. Transmission to man occurs via the bite of an infected mosquito.

Sources: Redrawn from Smallman-Raynor and Cliff (2004*b*, fig. 9.5, p. 499), originally from Thongcharoen (1989, fig. 6, p. 30).

deceased. During the next two months, approximately 300 further cases of Japanese encephalitis were diagnosed in the US contingent of UN Command. Geographically, the epidemic was confined to the 50–100 km radius of the defensive 'perimeter' area (Pusan Perimeter) of south-eastern Korea (Figure 8.3A), with cases occurring both at the front of the perimeter and in the vicinity of the port of Pusan. As judged by a sample of 201 cases admitted to the evacuation hospital at Pusan, the epidemic peaked in the week beginning 17 September, with the last admission on 15 October (Figure 8.3B). Thereafter, Japanese encephalitis declined in importance in UN Command. All US troops in Korea were vaccinated against the disease, and, although the efficacy of the vaccine then remained unproven, subsequent years were to witness little or no disease activity (Hunter 1953).

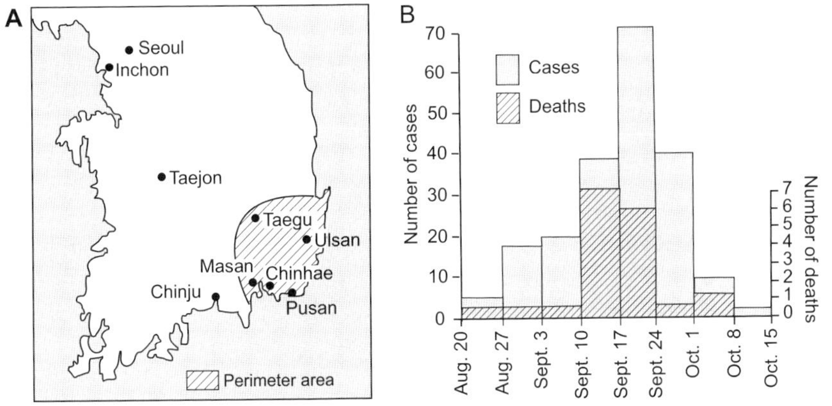

Fig. 8.3. Japanese encephalitis among US troops in the Korean War, August–October 1950

(A) Location of the 50–100 km radius 'perimeter' area (Pusan Perimeter) of south-eastern Korea, within which all cases of Japanese encephalitis among US troops occurred. (B) Weekly count of admissions and deaths for a sample of 201 Japanese encephalitis patients admitted to the evacuation hospital at Pusan.

Sources: Redrawn from Smallman-Raynor and Cliff (2004*b*, fig. 9.6, p. 500), originally from Lincoln and Sivertson (1952, figs 1 and 2, p. 269).

KOREAN HAEMORRHAGIC FEVER

The second year of hostilities presented the UN forces with fresh epidemiological challenges. In the spring and early summer of 1951, troops stationed in the vicinity of the 38th parallel—close to the front line with North Korea—began to present with a severe, frequently fatal, disease characterized by fever lasting 7–14 days, prostration, intense headache behind the eyes, vomiting, and haemorrhages. At first, medical officers suspected the disease to be leptospirosis, acute nephritis, or some other form of renal condition. It soon became apparent, however, that the men of UN Command were suffering from a malady that was previously unknown to Western medicine. Variously termed *Korean haemorrhagic fever* (KHF) or *epidemic haemorrhagic fever* (EHF), the disease had, in fact, already been encountered by Russian and Japanese military physicians in the 1930s (Gajdusek 1956; Paul and McClure 1958; Trencséni and Keleti 1971). Today, KHF is recognized as one of several similar, but distinct, emergent viral fevers of global distribution and to which the general term *haemorrhagic fever with renal syndrome* (HFRS) is applied (Table 8.2; see also Table 7.10). Its emergence is generally attributed to ecological changes including land clearance, aided and abetted by heightened exposure of humans to the resulting zoonotic pool.

Table 8.2. The haemorrhagic fever with renal syndrome (HFRS) group of diseases

Common appellation	Virus	Principal reservoir	Distribution of virus	Severity of associated disease
KHF[1]	Hantaan	*Apodemus agrarius* (striped field mouse)	China, Korea, Russia	Moderate to severe[2]
Haemorrhagic fever	Dobrava-Belgrade	*Apodemus flavicollis* (yellow-neck mouse), *Apodemus agrarius* (striped field mouse)	Balkans; central and north-eastern Europe	Moderate to severe[2]
Haemorrhagic fever	Seoul	*Rattus norvegicus* (Norway rat)	Global	Moderate to severe[2]
Nephropathia epidemica	Puumala	*Clethrionomys glareolus* (bank vole)	Europe, Russia, Scandinavia	Mild[3]

Notes: [1] Korean haemorrhagic fever. [2] Death rate 1–15%. [3] Death rate <1%.
Sources: Smallman-Raynor and Cliff (2004*b*, table 9.5, p. 502), based on information in Schmaljohn and Hjelle (1997, tables 1 and 2, pp. 96–8).

Nature of KHF

The specific aetiological agent of Korean haemorrhagic fever (*ICD*-10 A98.5) is Hantaan virus, whose natural reservoir is the striped field mouse, *Apodemus agrarius*. Incidental transmission to humans arises from exposure to contaminated rodent excreta—probably aerosolized urine. Typically, 30 per cent of patients show a mild clinical course, 50 per cent a moderate course, and 20 per cent develop severe disease. Death occurs in 1–15 per cent of moderate to severe cases. The incubation period of KHF is of the order of 2–3 weeks (range 1–6 weeks). Geographically, KHF is recognized as a significant public health problem in parts of China, Korea, and Russia (Nathanson and Nichol 1998; Heymann 2004: 240–3) (Table 8.2).

KHF in the Korean War

The known distribution of KHF in Korea at about the time of the war is mapped in Figure 8.4A, while Plates 8.1A and 8.1B provide views of the infective terrain. The wartime zone of recognized KHF activity extended along the 38th parallel of latitude, forming a 160 km (east–west) belt that straddled the border between present-day North and South Korea. According to McNinch (1953), the first UN troops to contract KHF were stationed just north of the 38th parallel and were admitted to US medical installations in May and June 1951. The subsequent course of reported disease activity in UN forces is plotted on a weekly basis to January 1953 in Figure 8.5. As the graph shows, cases were concentrated in three clearly defined waves of

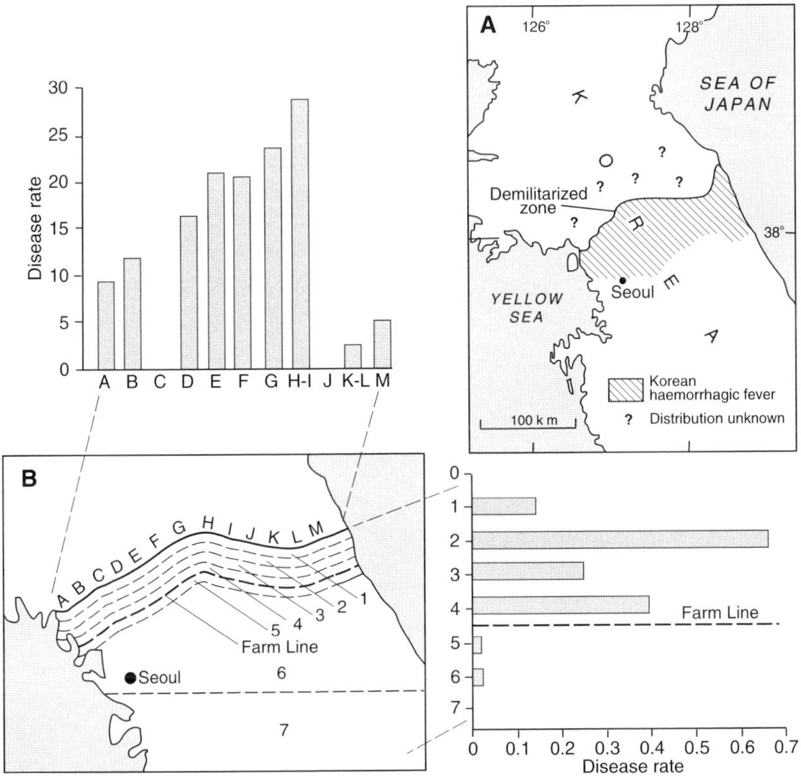

Fig. 8.4. Localized patterns of Korean haemorrhagic fever (KHF) among UN troops fighting on, and near, the front line during the Korean War, April 1952–June 1953 (A) Contemporary map of the known distribution of KHF as defined by Gajdusek (1956). (B) Rates of KHF among UN troops at sample horizontal locations along the front line (coded A–M) and sample vertical locations to the south of the front line (coded 1–7). The position of the 'Farm Line' (dividing vertical locations 4 and 5) marks the northern boundary of continued native agricultural production during the war. Note that disease rates for front-line locations, A–M, are expressed per million man-days of exposure; disease rates for locations south of the front line, 1–7, are expressed per 1,000 estimated population. Disease rates at vertical locations 1–7 relate to the sample period May–June 1953.

Sources: Redrawn from Smallman-Raynor and Cliff (2004*b*, fig. 9.8, p. 505), originally based on Paul and McClure (1958, figs 1, 3, and 4, and table 2, pp. 128–32, 136).

infection, with seasonally based peaks of activity in September–November 1951, and April–July and September–November 1952. As regards mortality, case-fatality rates for KHF declined progressively over the period of the war, falling from 14.6 per cent (April–August 1951) to 5.7 per cent (September 1951–March 1952), 5.1 per cent (April–August 1952), and 2.7 per cent (September 1952–January 1953) for US personnel. The reason for this

A

B

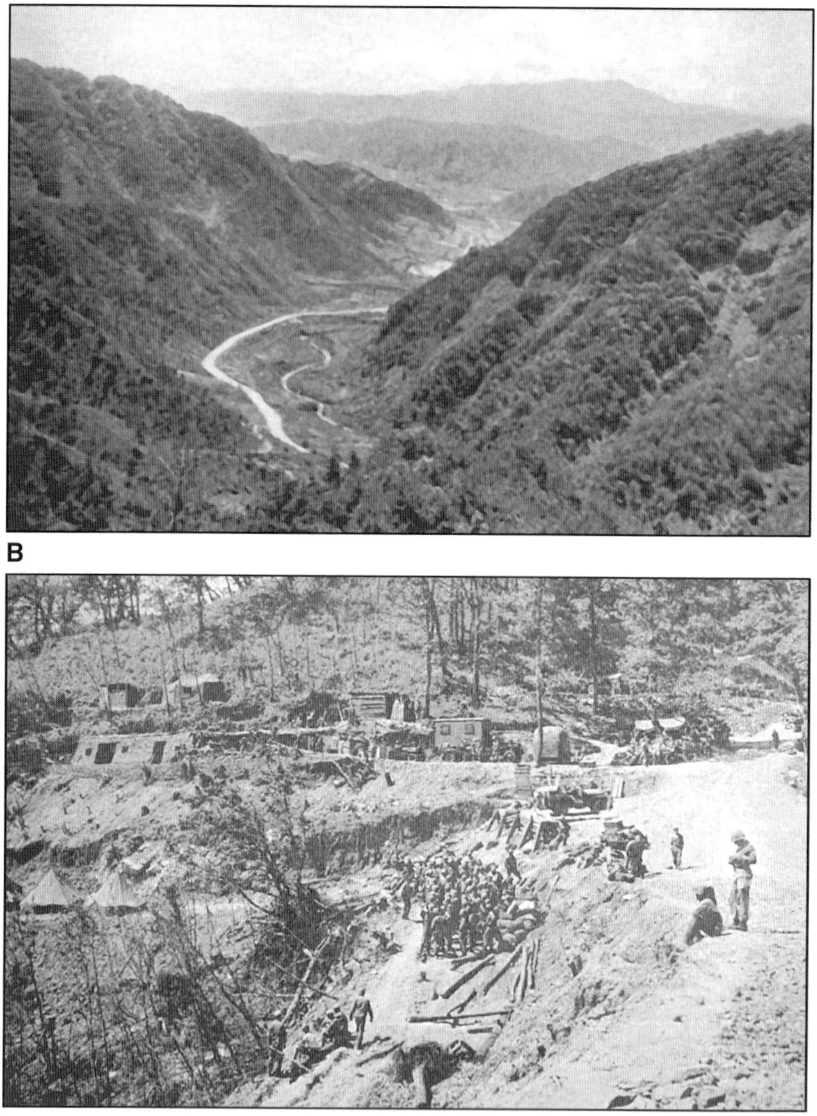

Pl. 8.1. Korean haemorrhagic fever (KHF) in the Korean War, 1950–1953
(A) Characteristic landscape in the endemic region: Hantaan River valley, where the first cases of KHF were identified in UN troops in 1951. (B) Military disruption of natural ecology.

Sources: Smallman-Raynor and Cliff (2004*b*, pls 9.3A,B, p. 507), repr. from Gajdusek (1956, figs 5, 7, pp. 34, 36).

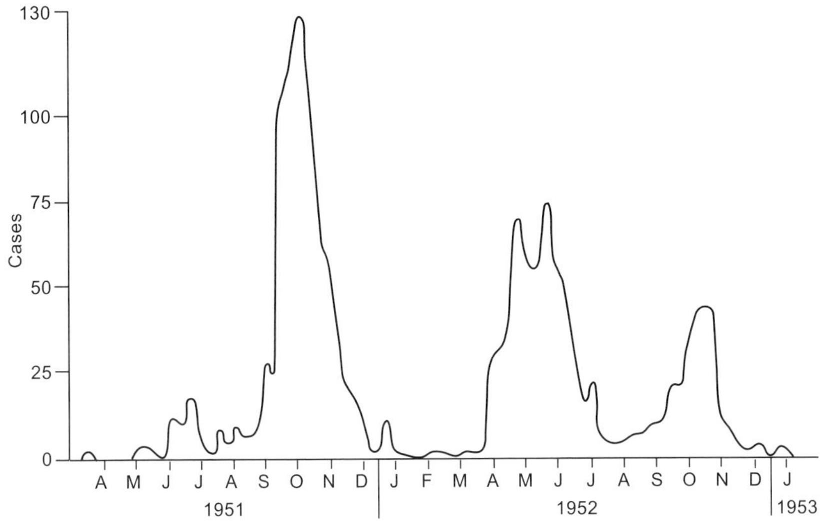

Fig. 8.5. Weekly incidence of Korean haemorrhagic fever (KHF) in UN troops during the Korean War, April 1951–January 1953

Sources: Redrawn from Smallman-Raynor and Cliff (2004*b*, fig. 9.9, p. 506), originally from Trencséni and Keleti (1971, fig. 34, p. 114), after Marshall (1954).

documented decline is uncertain, although Pruitt and Cleve (1953) suggest that the under-reporting of mild cases may account for the apparently high case-fatality rate in the spring and summer of 1951.

Spatial Patterns. The actual locale and circumstances under which UN troops contracted KHF during the period April 1952–July 1953 are examined by Paul and McClure (1958). The study area, along the line of combat to the north of Seoul and the focal point of KHF among UN troops, is mapped in Figure 8.4B; this area forms part of the endemic zone of KHF in Figure 8.4A. The letter codes (A–M) in Figure 8.4B indicate the horizontal positions of 13 UN combat forces during the study period, while the bounded areas running east to west (number-coded 1–5) indicate the vertical positions of troops away from the front line. The disease rates associated with the horizontal (A–M) and vertical (1–5) positions are plotted on the graphs that accompany Figure 8.4B.

From the very first appearance of KHF in UN troops, epidemiological activity had appeared to be most intense in the forward combat area in Figure 8.4B. All land to the north of the front line was under the control of North Korean forces. Away from the front line, vertical cross-sections in Figure 8.4B demarcate the Forward Division (coded 1), the Mid-Division (2), the Rear Division (3), and the Forward Corps Area (4) of UN Command. The latter zone was bordered to the south by the so-called

'Farm Line' (heavy broken line in Figure 8.4B). Between the Farm Line and the Forward Division, all agricultural activity had come to a standstill. The native population had been displaced, villages had been destroyed, secondary invasion of underbrush and weeds had commenced, and the area was studded with military installations of all kinds. Field mice and foxes were in abundance, while rodents found sustenance in the buried food supplies left by the fleeing Koreans. South of the Farm Line, in the Rear Corps Area (coded 5 in Figure 8.4B), the native population continued to live and farm.

The KHF rates for troops in vertical zones 1–5 are given in the right-hand graph of Figure 8.4B, along with rates for those positioned to the south of the Rear Corps Area (areas coded 6–7). Owing to insufficient information on man-days of exposure, rates are expressed per 1,000 estimated population. As the graph shows, disease activity was concentrated in the zone north of the Farm Line, reaching 0.67 cases per 1,000 estimated population in the Mid-Division (area 2). South of the Farm Line, rates fell off dramatically (Paul and McClure 1958).

Interpretation. The evidence highlights the combined role of war-associated population displacement, ecological change, and patterns of combat exposure in the emergence of an apparently 'new' viral disease. The spatially focused nature of the KHF outbreaks, along and just to the south of the front line, corresponds with the ecological changes that accompanied the abandonment of intensive farming activities and which provided an environment conducive to the rodent reservoir of Hantaan virus, *A. agrarius* (Paul and McClure 1958). Some 95 per cent of all KHF cases originated from the area between the front line and the line which demarcated the area of civilian evacuation, with the heightened exposure of troops to rodent excreta in trenches, bunkers, and tents. To the south of this zone, native farming practices continued, ecological changes associated with the war were less marked, and the occurrence of KHF was correspondingly low (Trencséni and Keleti 1971).

Post-War Patterns of KHF, 1950–1986

Although an armistice was agreed in July 1953, UN soldiers continued to contract KHF throughout the autumn of 1953 and the spring of 1954. Only in 1955, with the civilian resettlement of the endemic zone and a reversion of the local ecology to its pre-war form, did levels of disease activity begin to reduce among the military population (Trencséni and Keleti 1971). To illustrate the post-war pattern of KHF activity, the heavy line trace in Figure 8.6 plots the annual count of hospital admissions for KHF in US military personnel stationed in the Republic of Korea, 1950–86; the remaining line traces plot the equivalent information for Korean soldiers (full line) and civilians (broken line). As the graph shows, the post-war annual incidence remained very low among US troops, although occasional outbreaks associated with joint US–Korea military training exercises have been described

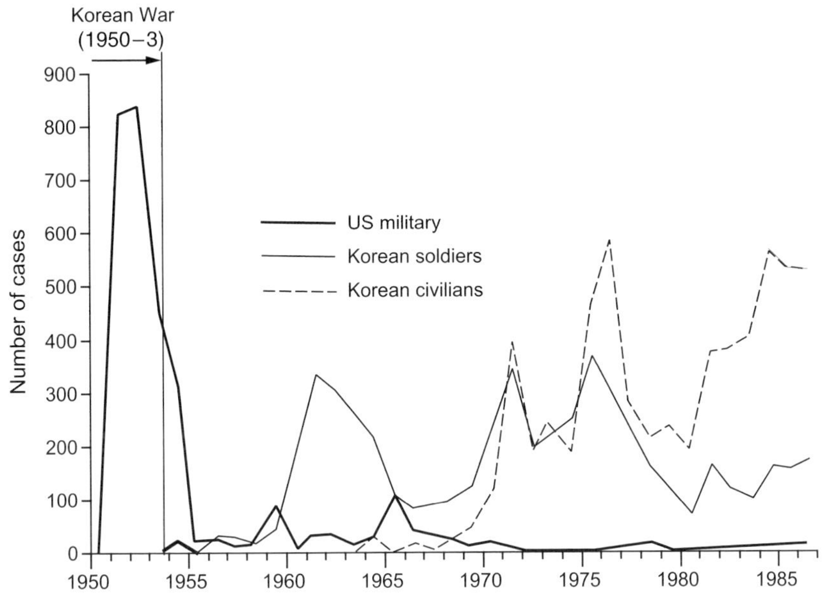

Fig. 8.6. Annual incidence of Korean haemorrhagic fever (KHF) in the Republic of Korea, 1950–1986
Incidence is based on hospital admissions among US military personnel stationed in Korea, Korean soldiers, and civilians.

Sources: Redrawn from Smallman-Raynor and Cliff (2004*b*, fig. 9.10, p. 510), originally drawn from data in Lee (1989, table 1, p. S865).

(Pon *et al.* 1990). However, the disease continued to be of military significance for the Korean army, emerging as a more general problem in the civil population as the virus began a rapid extension southwards—away from its recognized focus in the vicinity of the 38th parallel—in the early 1970s (Lee 1994) (Figure 8.7).

8.2.2 Re-emergent Parasites and Bacteria in the Vietnam War

The health impacts of the Vietnam War (1964–73)[2] are reviewed by Allukian and Atwood (1997). Global estimates of 3 million war dead, 800,000 orphans, 83,000 amputees, 10 million evacuees and refugees, and 600,000 tons of unexploded munitions serve to emphasize the gravity of the conflict. Large-scale population dislocation, the decimation of civil health infrastructure, and overcrowding in relief camps all contributed to the epidemic incidence of tuberculosis and intestinal parasites, while haemorrhagic fevers, leprosy, malaria, plague, and rabies—among a raft of diseases—threatened military

[2] As part of a longer-running civil war between North and South Vietnam (1956–75), the Vietnam War is defined here as the period of hostilities that commenced with large-scale US military involvement after the Gulf of Tonking incident (Aug. 1964) and ended with the withdrawal of US troops under the Paris Peace Accords (Jan. 1973).

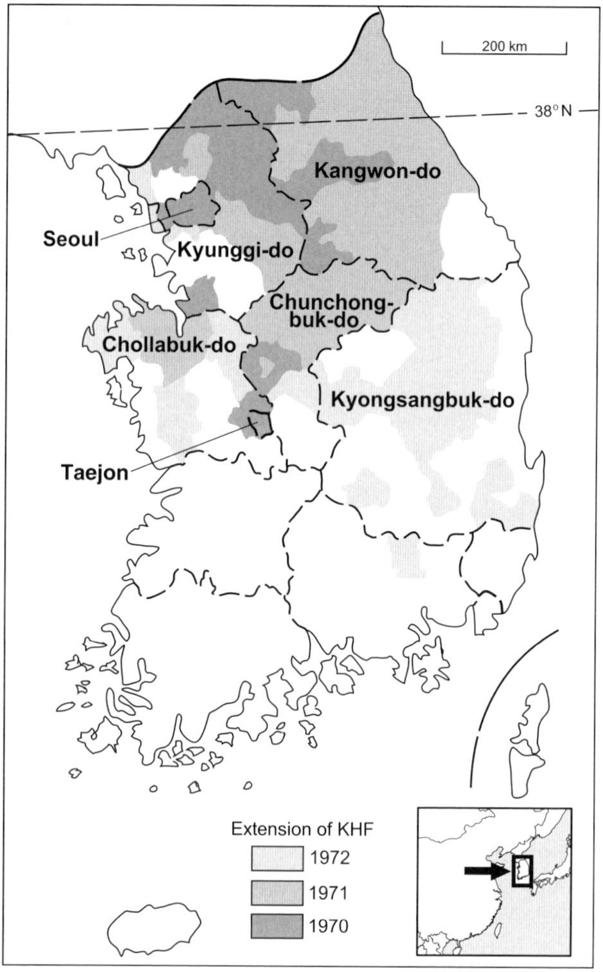

Fig. 8.7. Geographical extension of reported cases of Korean haemorrhagic fever (KHF) in the Republic of Korea, 1970–1972
In the aftermath of the Korean War, KHF remained largely restricted to the demilitarized zone in the vicinity of the 38th parallel. Beginning in the early 1970s, however, the map depicts a rapid southwards extension of the disease into central and southern parts of the country. This development was associated with the upsurge in civilian cases depicted in Fig. 8.6. For further details, see Lee (1994).
Source: Drawn from Lee (1994, figs 3–5, pp. 154–6).

and civil populations alike. Ecological changes wrought by the military use of Agent Orange and other herbicides, war-induced shifts in the ecosystems of rodents and insects, and the circulation of drug-resistant strains of *Plasmodium falciparum* and *Mycobacterium tuberculosis* further contributed to the disease problems of the Vietnam War (Cowley 1970; Neel 1973).

Vietnam and the Theme of Disease Re-emergence

The Vietnam War illustrates the wartime re-emergence of two 'classical' infectious diseases: malaria (US forces) and human plague (Vietnamese civilians). Framed by the more general theme of microbial resistance and change (Chapter 4), our selection of malaria in US forces is founded on the early recognition of chloroquine-resistant strains of the malaria parasite, *P. falciparum*, acquired by combat units in close promixity to the Viet Cong. On the other hand, our selection of plague in Vietnamese civilians reflects the manner in which war-induced alterations to economies and ecosystems may promote the epidemic transmission of previously low-level, endemic, infections such as *Yersinia pestis* (Figure 8.1).

US FORCES AND MALARIA

Malaria represented the single most important medical problem for US forces stationed in Vietnam. As Neel (1973) and Beadle and Hoffman (1993) note, several factors contributed to the particular severity of the disease in the Vietnam War: (i) the relative inexperience of line officers with regard to malaria and malaria discipline in high-risk locations; (ii) the circulation of malignant *P. falciparum* as the predominant species of the malaria parasite; and (iii) the existence of chloroquine-resistant species of *P. falciparum*. During the course of the conflict, malaria accounted for no less than 65,000 admissions and 124 deaths in the combined US army and naval forces (Beadle and Hoffman 1993), while, as an annual average in the sample period 1967–70, the disease ranked second only to the non-specific 'fever of undetermined origin' as a cause of man-days lost from duty in the US army (Table 8.3).

Table 8.3. Average annual admissions rate and average annual number of man-days lost from duty, US army in Vietnam, 1967–1970

Disease/condition	Admissions rate[1]	Man-days lost from duty
Malaria	24.6	198,625
Acute respiratory infections	34.3	71,078
Skin diseases[2]	25.8	65,541
Neuropsychiatric conditions	16.2	119,408
Viral hepatitis	7.3	92,495
Venereal disease[3]	1.8	5,293
Fever of undetermined origin	60.7	225,600

Notes: [1] Rate expressed per 1,000 mean strength. [2] Including dermatophytosis. [3] Excluding cases 'carded for record only'.
Sources: Smallman-Raynor and Cliff (2004*b*, table 9.7, p. 515), based on information in Neel (1973, tables 2 and 3, pp. 34, 36).

Combat Troops, Malaria, and Drug-Resistant P. falciparum

A prominent feature of malaria among US forces in Vietnam was the focus of the disease among combat troops. Some 80 per cent of all malaria cases in the US army were reported from combat units, with tactical missions in the Central Highlands of South Vietnam forming a primary source of exposure to drug-resistant strains of *P. falciparum* in the early stages of the conflict (Neel 1973: 109, 170). By way of illustration, Figure 8.8 is based on Nowosiwsky's (1967) study of drug-refractory *P. falciparum* malaria among US combat units in the northern sector of the Central Highlands area. For each of three military units (coded 'A', 'B', and 'C'), the graphs plot the daily incidence of malaria in relation to tactical missions undertaken between

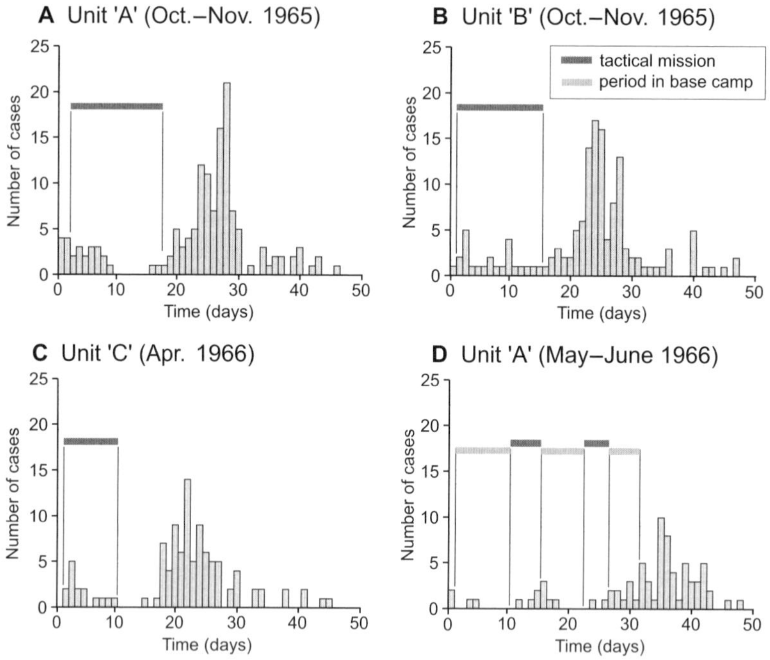

Fig. 8.8. Daily incidence of *Plasmodium falciparum* malaria in sample US military units, Republic of Vietnam, 1965–1966

Graphs plot the daily number of malaria cases in relation to the timing of tactical missions undertaken by units in the north central highlands of South Vietnam. Tactical missions are marked by the black horizontal bars. (A) Unit 'A', Oct.–Nov. 1965 (16-day tactical mission). (B) Unit 'B', Oct.–Nov. 1965 (14-day tactical mission). (C) Unit 'C', Apr. 1966 (9-day tactical mission). (D) Unit 'A', May–June 1966 (5-day and 4-day tactical missions). Graphs A and B are based on the day of onset of symptoms; graphs C and D are based on the day of admission to hospital.

Sources: Redrawn from Smallman-Raynor and Cliff (2004*b*, fig. 9.11, p. 515), originally from Nowosiwsky (1967, figs 1–3, pp. 464–5).

October 1965 and June 1966. The periods associated with the missions are identified on the graphs by black horizontal bars, while the bar charts plot the daily occurrence of malaria in the corresponding unit.[3]

While cases of malaria identified during the tactical missions can be attributed to prior disease exposure, all four graphs in Figure 8.8 are characterized by a marked increase in malaria incidence some 13–19 days after the termination of operations. With a median incubation period of *c*.16 days, estimates of mission-based attack rates range from 8.3 cases per 1,000 man-days of exposure (8.8D) to approximately 12.0 cases per 1,000 man-days of exposure (8.8C). At these levels, and notwithstanding the maintenance of all members of the units on chloroquine–primaquine prophylaxis, a three-month deployment in an endemic area during peak periods of disease transmission would be expected to yield a 90 per cent infection rate among the men.

Changing Levels of Enemy Contact and Malaria. In a subsequent epidemiological investigation of US Marine regiments operative in the Que Son Mountains of north-central Vietnam in 1969–70, Bridges (1973) correlated the level of malaria activity with the estimated size of the local Viet Cong/North Vietnamese (VC/NVA) forces. Between the malaria seasons (September–December) of 1969 and 1970, the disease rate in the Marine regiments fell from 81 per 1,000 strength to 33 per 1,000 strength (Table 8.4). Such a marked decrease, Bridges argues, could not be attributed to changes in vector density or improved malaria discipline alone. Rather, given that the only persons in the foothills and mountain areas were US Marines and VC/NVA soldiers, and that Marines were evacuated on presentation with symptoms of malaria, enemy troops served as the principal reservoir of the disease in

Table 8.4. Malaria rates (per 1,000 strength) in the 5th and 7th US Marine Regiments, Que Son Mountains, Vietnam, during the malaria seasons of 1969 and 1970

	Malaria rate (per 1,000 strength)	
Month	1969	1970
Sept.	136	58
Oct.	72	39
Nov.	87	21
Dec.	28	15
AVERAGE	81	33

Sources. Smallman-Raynor and Cliff (2004*b*, table 9.8, p. 516), originally from Bridges (1973, table III, p. 414).

[3] Precise details of dates and locations were withheld from the original study for operational reasons.

the Que Son Mountains. During the study period, the estimated strength of the VC/NVA force reduced from a high of 16,800 (May 1969) to 8,560 (December 1970), with a corresponding reduction in the reported level of *P. falciparum* malaria in US troops.

VIETNAMESE CIVILIANS AND THE RE-EMERGENCE OF PLAGUE

Vietnam has been regarded as a permanent reservoir of the aetiological agent of plague, *Y. pestis*, since the introduction of the disease to Saigon in 1906 (Cavanaugh *et al.* 1968; Velimirovic 1972). Figure 8.9 is based on information included in Velimirovic (1972) and traces the reported pattern of human plague in the Republic of Vietnam over the seven decades to 1970. The vertical axis has been plotted on a logarithmic scale to allow for widely varying case totals. Although the available evidence is fragmentary, and under-reporting of cases must be suspected, the relative success of French colonial efforts at plague control (including quarantine, vaccination, disinfection, and general measures of rodent and flea control) is clearly reflected in the progressive reduction of disease activity to near-zero levels by the mid-1930s. Thereafter, Japanese occupation (1940–5) was associated with a modest resurgence in human plague, to a peak (335 cases) in the early years of the French Indo-China War (1946–54). However, with the onset of civil war in 1956 and, more particularly, with the escalation of hostilities

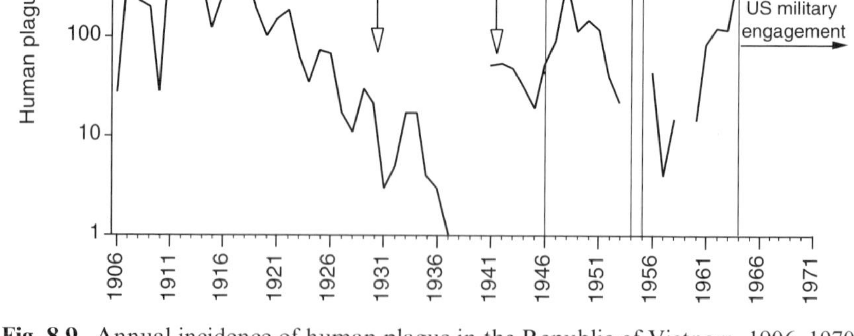

Fig. 8.9. Annual incidence of human plague in the Republic of Vietnam, 1906–1970. Note that the vertical axis is drawn on a logarithmic scale

Sources: Redrawn from Smallman-Raynor and Cliff (2004*b*, fig. 9.12, p. 517), based on Velimirovic (1972, table X, p. 496).

from 1964, Figure 8.9 shows that the reported number of cases spiralled from an annual average of <60 (1956–63) to >3,600 (1964–70).

Factors in Re-emergence

The capacity of plague to re-emerge in the manner depicted in Figure 8.9 serves to underscore the profound epidemiological dangers associated with war-induced disturbances to both human and zootic habitats (Velmirovic 1972). In particular, the upsurge in plague activity during the 1960s was intimately associated with factors that increased the level of contact between human beings, plague-carrying rodents (preliminary studies implicated *Rattus norvegicus*, *R. rattus*, and the house shrew, *Suncus murinus*, in the spread of the epidemic), and their associated fleas. From late 1964, large-scale US bombing and firing resulted in the destruction of an estimated 50 per cent of forest cover and 20 per cent of agricultural land, thereby forcing rodents and humans into close proximity in towns, cities, and relief camps (Velimirovic 1973). The disruption of Vietnam's agricultural economy resulted in a reversal of the regular lines of food shipment and the associated patterns of human–rodent contact. Neel (1973: 171) explains:

> Plague in the Vietnamese civilian population pointed up... the shifting of disease patterns when the normal way of life of any peoples whose structure, economically or environmentally, is altered. Vietnam is a rice-producing and rice-exporting country. Normally, the grain flowed from the rice bowls of the interior to the few major ports of the country. The rodents which infest the areas followed the path of the rice to the ports. There they were controlled; thus, the danger of a serious outbreak of plague was averted. During the war when, for economic reasons, the South Vietnamese began to import grain, a reverse situation was created. The rice was shipped from the ports into the countryside; the rodents followed the flow of the grain inland and created havoc in the form of increased incidence of plague among the native population in areas which had hithertofore been relatively free of the disease.

However, changes in human and rodent habitats formed only part of the re-emergence complex. High resistance to DDT, probably arising from prolonged exposure under the local mosquito–malaria eradication programme, was recognized in the principal flea vector, *Xenopsylla cheopis*, from 1965. Vector resistance to a further insecticide (dieldrin) emerged in some localities from about 1970. With efforts at plague control hindered by the development of vector resistance and with any possibility of the implementation of a comprehensive programme of plague eradication stultified by the ongoing hostilities, the epidemic continued to spread apace in the late 1960s and early 1970s (Marshall *et al.* 1967; Velimirovic 1972).

Spatial Diffusion

Figure 8.10 traces the spatial extension of human plague in Vietnam during the decade to 1970. The annual map sequence shades those provinces in

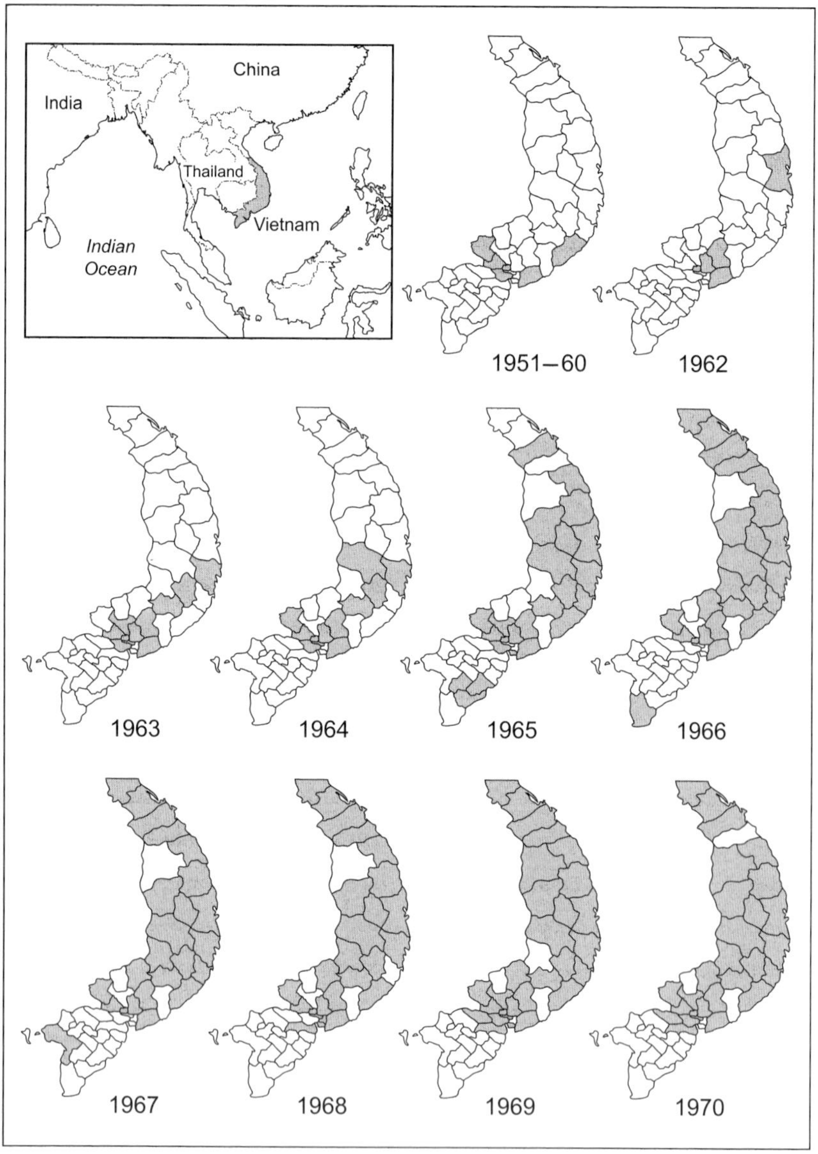

Fig. 8.10. War and the spread of human plague in the Republic of Vietnam, 1951–1970

Provinces in which cases of human plague were reported in a given time period have been shaded.

Sources: Redrawn from Smallman-Raynor and Cliff (2004*b*, fig. 9.13, p. 520), originally from Velimirovic (1972, fig. 9, p. 500).

which cases of plague were reported in the period 1962–70, while aggregate evidence for a 10-year period prior to epidemic onset (1951–60) is shown for reference. From a primary focus of plague activity in south-central Vietnam in 1962, Figure 8.10 depicts a progressive north-eastwards extension of the disease in 1963–4. Coincidental with the escalation of hostilities, rapid colonization of more northerly provinces occurred in 1965–6. As described by Smallman-Raynor and Cliff (2004*b*: 519), this phase of rapid northwards transmission approximated a wave-like (contagious) diffusion process, with the disease pushing out of the central settlements with the associated movement of foodstuffs.

Following the period of rapid geographical expansion in 1965–6, inspection of Figure 8.10 reveals that the overall spatial distribution of plague remained relatively static in the years 1967–70. Plague continued to be reported from virtually all the provinces of central and northern Vietnam at this time, but with an apparent absence from many of the more southerly localities. Spatial contraction of the epidemic followed the US military withdrawal from Vietnam in the early 1970s (Kohn 1998: 353).

VIETNAM RETURNEES: DISEASE THREATS IN THE CONTINENTAL US

As described in Chapter 6, the risk of disease importation as a consequence of international travel represents one of the principal factors in the modern-day emergence and re-emergence of infectious diseases. The particular risk is magnified when many tens of thousands of deployed troops, potentially exposed to one or more of a long list of infectious diseases, begin to return to their homeland (Lederberg *et al.* 1992: 111–12). In this context, the Vietnam War heralded a new era in the mass transfer of US soldiers: for the first time ever, air transport (rather than sea transport) formed the principal means for the return of overseas forces to the continental United States, resulting in travel times shorter than the incubation period of many infectious diseases. Despite the fears, however, Table 8.5 shows that relatively few cases of the anticipated disease threats were identified among Vietnam returnees (Gilbert, Moore, *et al.* 1968; Greenberg 1969). Of the diseases that were generally regarded as potential threats to US forces in Vietnam (Group 1 in Table 8.5), vaccination and other methods of disease prevention and control ensured that very few (or no) cases of cholera, plague, or Japanese encephalitis were identified in returnees. Likewise, many of the actual disease problems among US forces in Vietnam (Group 2 in Table 8.5) yielded few cases on return to the United States.

Malaria. One disease listed in Table 8.5 did, however, gain particular prominence in contemporary discussions of disease re-emergence in the

Table 8.5. Health problems associated with US military personnel stationed in Vietnam and among Vietnam returnees (status: late 1960s)

Disease	Documented occurrence	
	US personnel in Vietnam	US returnees
Group 1: Potential threats		
Tuberculosis	Few cases	Few cases
Plague	5 cases	1 case
Cholera	No cases	No cases
Japanese encephalitis	Few cases	No cases
Filariasis	No clinical cases	—
Helminthiasis	Localized outbreaks	—
Leptospirosis	Few cases	No cases
Melioidosis	72 cases	10 cases
Group 2: Actual disease problems		
Respiratory tract disease	Significant	—
Diarrhoeal disease[1]	Severe local outbreaks	Some cases
Skin disease	Serious problem	—
STDs	Moderate incidence	Few cases
Dengue	Few cases	—
Scrub typhus	Few cases	3 cases
Malaria	Serious problem	2,700 cases (1967)

Note: [1] Dysentery, infectious hepatitis, paratyphoid, and typhoid fevers.
Source: Smallman-Raynor and Cliff (2004*b*, table 9.9, p. 532), based on information in Greenberg (1969).

United States: malaria. Malaria had been the subject of an intensive elimination programme in the US prior to the war, with a correspondingly low incidence in its civil population. Under these circumstances, the danger of increased transmission as a result of importation with military returnees was widely recognized (Gilbert, Moore, *et al.* 1968; Greenberg 1969; Cowley 1970). The concern was well founded. Between 1965 and 1970, the annual count of malaria cases treated in domestic US army medical facilities grew from 62 to 2,222, with a corresponding surge in the national malaria curve (Figure 8.11). In contrast to Vietnam, where the majority of malaria cases in US troops (>90 per cent) were attributable to *P. falciparum*, most cases in returnees (>80 per cent) were due to *P. vivax*—probably arising from partial failure of the army's terminal prophylaxis programme (Barrett *et al.* 1969; Neel 1973). Notwithstanding sporadic reports of mosquito-transmitted *P. vivax* malaria as a consequence of exposure to returnees (Luby *et al.* 1967), lack of evidence for the general re-establishment of malaria in the United States is signalled in Figure 8.11 by the precipitous fall in disease activity at the end of the Vietnam War (Gibson *et al.* 1974).

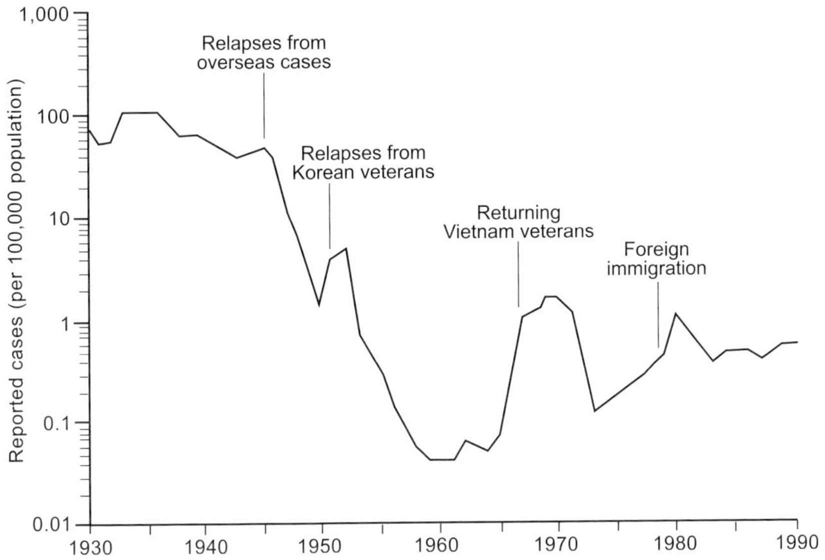

Fig. 8.11. Annual incidence (per 100,000 population) of malaria in the continental United States, 1930–1990

Sources: Redrawn from Smallman-Raynor and Cliff (2004*b*, fig. 9.16, p. 525), originally from Lederberg *et al.* (1992, fig. 2.5, p. 80).

8.3 Ethnic Conflict: Genocide, Displacement, and Disease in Central Africa

Mass population displacement arising in consequence of war has potentially severe epidemiological ramifications for all those involved (Smallman-Raynor and Cliff 2004*b*: 231–99). Large-scale population upheavals—and the circumstances that fuel them—often result in a profound disruption of livelihoods, social support mechanisms, and health delivery systems. Dislocation of food production systems may lead to chronic malnutrition and an increased susceptibility to infectious diseases, while settlement in relief camps may give rise to increased levels of disease transmission. Sexual violence and exploitation raise the threat of HIV/AIDS and other sexually transmitted infections, while environmental changes and/or exposure to new environments may promote the processes of disease emergence and re-emergence (Prothero 1994; Kalipeni and Oppong 1998).

In this subsection, we illustrate the role of wartime population displacement as a facilitating factor in disease emergence and re-emergence with special reference to the ethnic conflicts that erupted in the neighbouring states of Burundi and Rwanda, Central Africa, in 1993 and 1994 (Figure 8.1). The two conflicts yielded well over 2.0 million international refugees, while the number of internally displaced persons (IDPs) still stood at 1.4 million in late 1999. The movements spawned outbreaks of dysentery, malaria, acute respiratory infections, and meningitis. Most prominent among the epidemiological events, however, were explosive camp-based epidemics of louse-borne typhus fever among IDPs in Burundi and cholera among Rwandan refugees in eastern Zaire.

8.3.1 Epidemic Louse-Borne Typhus Fever: Burundian IDPs

The assassination of President Melchior Ndadaye of Burundi on 21 October 1993 precipitated a fierce civil war between the country's Hutu and Tutsi tribal groups. By the end of the year, hostilities had resulted in the internal displacement of an estimated 130,000 persons, with the number growing to 800,000—representing some 13 per cent of the entire population of Burundi—during the events of the next several years. Many hundreds of thousands of others, either unwilling or unable to find sanctuary in Burundi, fled across international borders into neighbouring Rwanda, Tanzania, and Zaire.

The population movements were, from the outset, accompanied by the spread of infectious diseases. As early as December 1993, the sentinel surveillance system of Burundi had detected a substantial increase in the occurrence of dysentery and malaria, while, over the border in Rwanda, non-bloody diarrhoea and respiratory tract infections added to the health problems of the Burundian refugees (Centers for Disease Control and Prevention 1994*b*). The most marked epidemic event, however, occurred in 1996–7 with the spread of epidemic louse-borne typhus fever in the camps of the displaced in Burundi.

The 1996–1997 Epidemic

Clinical and epidemiological details of louse-borne typhus fever are given in Heymann (2004: 583–6). The disease occurs sporadically in the highlands of sub-Saharan Africa, with countries of Central Africa (Burundi and Rwanda), East Africa (Ethiopia), and West Africa (Nigeria) serving as the main endemic foci. As regards the occurrence of the disease in Burundi, an outbreak, associated with some 9,000 reported cases, occurred in 1974–5. Thereafter, the annual incidence of the disease fell to low levels, with no documented cases between 1990 and 1994 (World Health Organization 1997). From November 1995, however, a fever of unknown origin, in association with a proliferation of body lice, began to spread in an overcrowded prison camp in the northern province of N'Gozi (Figure 8.12). The prison outbreak escalated to a peak in January 1996, and, from thereon, an epidemic of louse-borne typhus fever (known locally as *sutama*) began to take hold in the country's internally displaced population (Bise and Coninx 1997; Raoult, Ndihokubwayo, *et al.* 1998). While several thousand cases were

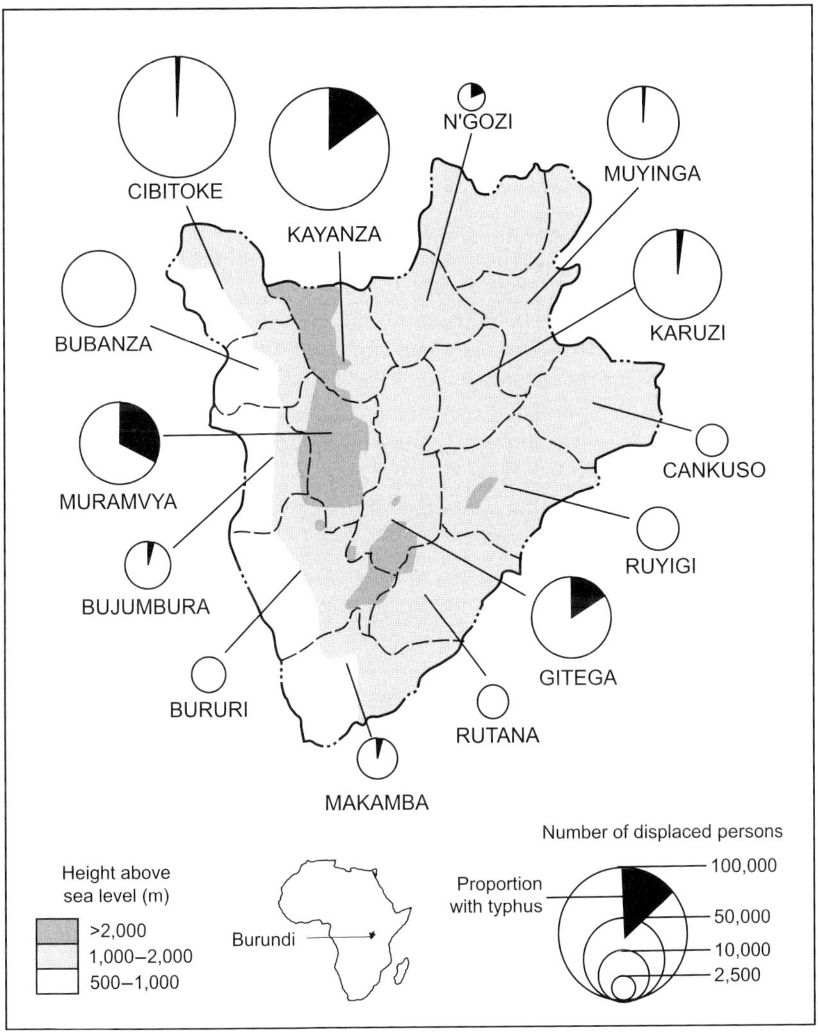

Fig. 8.12. Epidemic louse-borne typhus among residents of camps for the internally displaced in Burundi, Central Africa, January–September 1997
Proportional circles plot the number of internally displaced persons (IDPs) by province, while the black segments mark the percentage proportion of IDPs diagnosed with typhus. Shaded areas of the map mark land above 1,000 metres and 2,000 metres.
Sources: Redrawn from Smallman-Raynor and Cliff (2004*b*, fig. 5.18, p. 291), originally drawn from Raoult, Ndihokubwayo, *et al.* (1998, fig. 1, p. 354, and table 3, p. 356).

reported in 1996, the major period of epidemic transmission occurred in 1997 (World Health Organization 1997).

The proportional circles in Figure 8.12 are based on information included in Raoult, Ndihokubwayo, *et al.* (1998) and plot, by province, the distribution of some 700,000 internally displaced persons in Burundi during 1997. At this time, most of the displaced were resident in 28 large camps. Most camps were located away from towns and cities. Many lacked any form of health care. Based on information for these constituent camps, the shaded sectors in Figure 8.12 indicate the proportion of the displaced population in which louse-borne typhus fever was diagnosed between January and September 1997. All told, 43,971 cases were recorded in the camps, with the highest levels of disease activity in the central highland provinces of Gitega, Kayanza, and Muramvya and in the small refugee population of N'Gozi. While the disease remained largely restricted to the central and northern highland provinces, cases of typhus fever in the lower-lying capital province, Bujumbura, are believed to have resulted from the migration of people from the highlands. Whether the epidemic ultimately developed from a single source or resulted from a series of localized independent outbreaks remains unknown (Raoult, Ndihokubwayo, *et al.* 1998).

While the highland provinces of Burundi are recognized as a focus of the causative agent of louse-borne typhus fever, *Rickettsia prowazekii*, certain predisposing factors appear to have resulted in particularly high levels of disease activity among the displaced in those provinces. Such factors included poor sanitation, a cold climate, and the consequent need for several layers of clothing, thereby promoting conditions favourable to body louse infestation.

Epidemic Control

Although disease activity in the principal foci of the epidemic (Gitega, Kayanza, and Muramvya provinces) began to decline in April–May 1997 (Figure 8.13), substantial difficulties were encountered in the control of the epidemic. Owing to the ongoing hostilities, supplies of insecticides did not become widely available until July. Even then, delousing operations were complicated by the transient nature of the camp populations.

8.3.2 Cholera: Rwandan Refugees in Eastern Zaire

In early April 1994, long-standing ethnic tensions in Rwanda erupted into genocide. Within three months, an estimated 800,000 people—mainly ethnic Tutsis—had perished at the hands of Hutu extremists and other *génocidaires*. By mid-July, however, resurgent Tutsi forces had begun to reassert control in Rwanda, precipitating the flight of 2 million or more ethnic Hutus. While some fled to western Tanzania (580,000 refugees), northern Burundi (270,000), and Uganda (10,000), the majority (1.2 million) moved to Goma

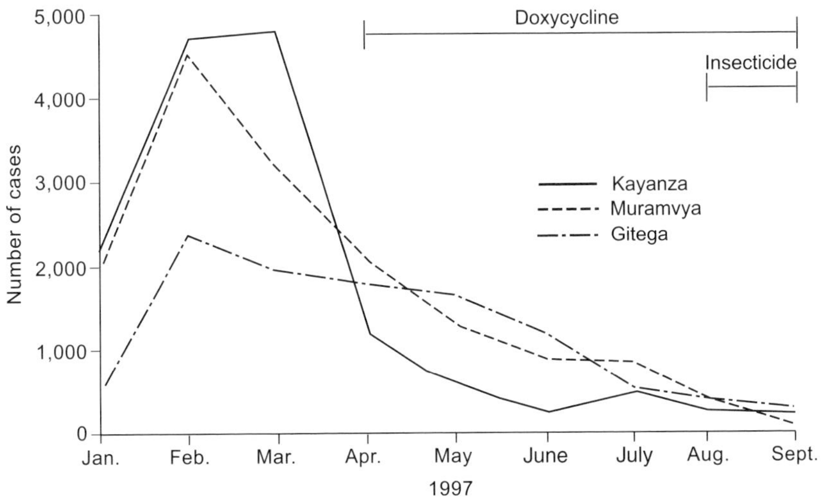

Fig. 8.13. Monthly count of louse-borne typhus fever in the camps of internally displaced persons in three central highland provinces of Burundi, January–September 1997
The period associated with the administration of antibiotic (doxycycline) treatment and insecticides is indicated. The locations of the three provinces (Gitega, Kayanza, and Muramvya) are indicated in Fig. 8.12.
Sources: Redrawn from Smallman-Raynor and Cliff (2004*b*, fig. 5.19, p. 293), originally from Raoult, Ndihokubwayo, *et al.* (1998, fig. 2, p. 355).

and proximal locations in eastern Zaire (United Nations High Commission for Refugees 2000); see Figure 8.14. For the latter contingent, the mortality rates that accompanied the displacement were, in the words of the Goma Epidemiology Group (1995: 343), 'almost unprecedented in refugee populations'. 'The world', the same source adds, 'was simply not prepared for an emergency of this magnitude.'

DEATH RATES AMONG REFUGEES IN ZAIRE

Some impression of the level of mortality sustained by Rwandan refugees in eastern Zaire can be gained from Table 8.6. For a month-long period from the beginning of the displacement (14 July), the lower row of the table is based on a body count of refugees and gives the crude mortality rate (per 10,000 per day) associated with an estimated refugee population of between 0.5 and 0.8 million.[4] The total body count of 48,347 yields a mortality rate of 19.5–31.2 per 10,000 per day, consistent with the death of up to 10 per cent of refugees during the first month of the crisis. The results of population

[4] As described by the Goma Epidemiology Group (1995: 340), the estimate of 0.5–0.8 million is based on water and food ration distribution figures and on agency-based mapping exercises.

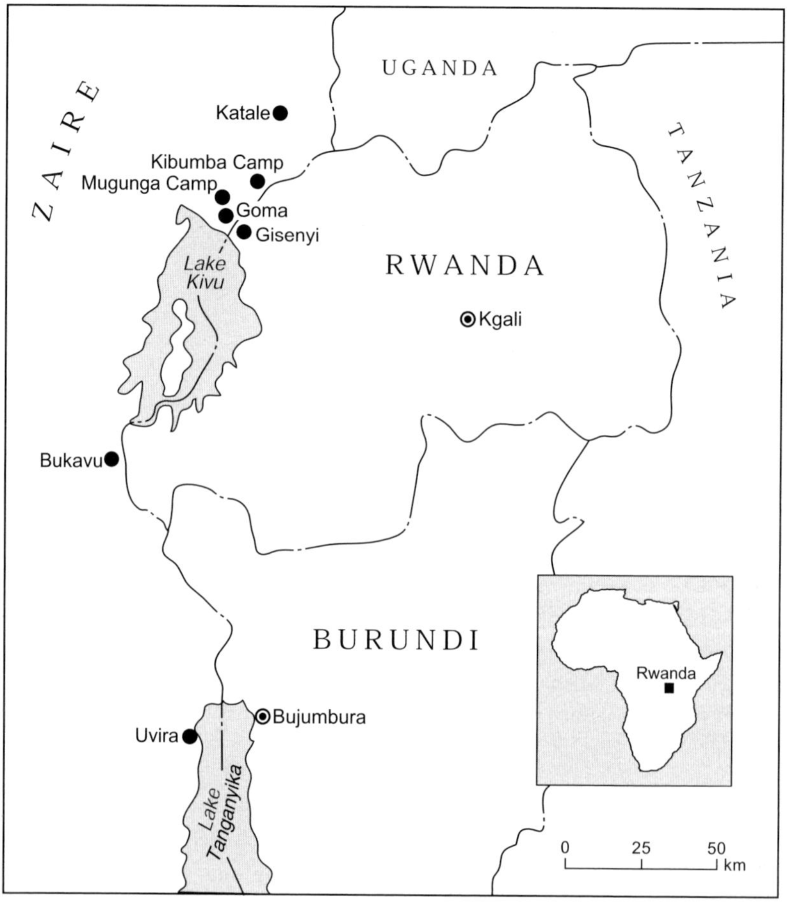

Fig. 8.14. Map showing the location of Rwandan refugee camps in eastern Zaire, 1994

Sources: Redrawn from Smallman-Raynor and Cliff (2004*b*, fig. 5.20, p. 294), originally from Goma Epidemiology Group (1995, fig. 1, p. 339).

surveys in the camps at Katale, Kibumba, and Mugunga, in which many of the refugees were eventually settled (Figure 8.14), provide similarly high estimates of crude mortality (Table 8.6) (Goma Epidemiology Group 1995).

Epidemic Cholera, July–August 1994

Surveys indicate that an overwhelming proportion of all deaths (85–90 per cent) were associated with cholera and other diarrhoeal diseases. The first case of cholera was diagnosed in the refugee population on 20 July, to be followed by an explosive outbreak of the disease associated with *Vibrio cholerae* O1 (biotype El Tor) in the days that followed. Details are sketchy,

Table 8.6. Estimated crude mortality rate for Rwandan refugees in Zaire, 1994

Survey location	Survey period	Estimated population (000)	Estimated crude mortality rate[1]	Estimated percentage mortality
Katale survey	14 July–4 Aug.	80	41.3	8.3
Kibumba survey	14 July–9 Aug.	180	28.1	7.3
Mugunga survey	14 July–13 Aug.	150	29.4	9.1
Body count (all areas)	14 July–14 Aug.	500–800	19.5–31.2	6.0–9.7

Note: [1] Expressed per 10,000 per day.
Source: Goma Epidemiology Group (1995, table 1, p. 340).

but, between 14 July and 12 August, some 62,000 cases of diarrhoeal disease were reported from the refugee health facilities in eastern Zaire, of which an estimated 35,000 were attributable to cholera. Allowing for those cholera cases that did not present to health facilities, the Goma Epidemiology Group (1995) place the actual cholera caseload at 58,000–80,000—equivalent to an attack rate of up to 16 per cent (Goma Epidemiology Group 1995; Van Damme 1995).

Detailed information on the geographical distribution of cholera is unavailable (Goma Epidemiology Group 1995). However, some 57 per cent of all reports of diarrhoeal disease in the seven days to Wednesday 27 July (marking the epidemic peak) originated from health facilities in and around the town of Goma. Untreated water from Lake Kivu, near which the Goma refugees were originally located, is suspected to have operated as a principal source of infection. With the transmission of the disease further fuelled by overcrowding, poor personal hygiene, and lack of adequate sanitation, it seems that cholera spread so rapidly that vaccination would have had no tangible effect on the course of the epidemic (Goma Epidemiology Group 1995).

Subsequent Cholera Outbreaks

The cholera outbreak of July–August 1994 was followed in subsequent years by further outbreaks of the disease among the Rwandan refugees.

Returnees (November 1996). Between 16 and 24 November 1996, some 350,000 refugees from five camps in eastern Zaire re-entered Rwanda through Gisenyi (Figure 8.14). Health personnel of Médecins sans Frontières (MSF) undertook 15,675 consultations along the route of the returnees, of which 8,916 were for watery diarrhoea. Sample tests indicated that an unknown, but probably substantial, proportion of diarrhoeal disease was attributable to infection with *Vibrio cholerae* O1 (Brown, Reilley, *et al.* 1997).

Refugees in Zaire (April 1997). In April 1997, a cholera outbreak was reported among 90,000 Rwandan refugees located between Kisangani and

Ubundu, some 450 km north-east of Goma. During a 16-day period, 4–19 April, a total of 545 cholera patients were admitted to the treatment centre (attack rate 0.9%), of which 67 (12.3%) died. Several factors contributed to the inflated mortality during the outbreak, including (i) lack of adequate food, shelter, or access to health care in the months prior to the appearance of cholera and (ii) logistic difficulties associated with accessing isolated camps by relief personnel. Although intervention strategies (surveillance, health education, provision of potable water, aggressive oral rehydration therapy, and the construction of latrines) may have been effective in preventing the further spread of the disease, such activities ceased on 21 April 1997, when the refugees were dispersed by unidentified militias (Centers for Disease Control and Prevention 1998*a*).

8.4 Other Late Twentieth- and Early Twenty-First-Century Conflicts

In recent years, an undercurrent of academic thought has posited that nuclear weaponry and the end of the Cold War have rendered war obsolete (Black 2000). Yet wars of varying intensity have continued to escalate over the last few decades (Stewart 2002). This escalation has been focused in some of the poorest regions of the world (Figure 8.15), with the increasing participation of non-state organizations, the growing operation of 'low-intensity' conflicts, and the burgeoning involvement of civil populations surfacing as prominent features in these modern conflagrations (van Creveld 1991; United Nations High Commission for Refugees 2000). Emerging and re-emerging diseases feature prominently among the correlates of these developments (see, for example, Hukic *et al.* 1996; Usmanov *et al.* 2007; Berrang Ford 2007), with recent and ongoing conflicts in sub-Saharan Africa, Central and South-West Asia, and elsewhere serving to highlight the contemporary relevance of the problem.

8.4.1 Civil War and Ethnic Rebellion in Sudan

THE SUDANESE CIVIL WAR (1983–2005): VISCERAL LEISHMANIASIS IN SOUTHERN SUDAN

Visceral leishmaniasis (kala-azar) (*ICD*-10 B55.0) is a zoonotic disease of tropical Africa and Asia caused by protozoa of the *Leishmania donovani* complex. The protozoa are transmitted from animals to man by species of sandfly (predominantly *Phlebotomus*). In visceral leishmaniasis, unlike cutaneous and mucocutaneous forms of the disease, cells are infected beyond the subcutaneous and mucosal tissue. Symptoms include fever, diarrhoea,

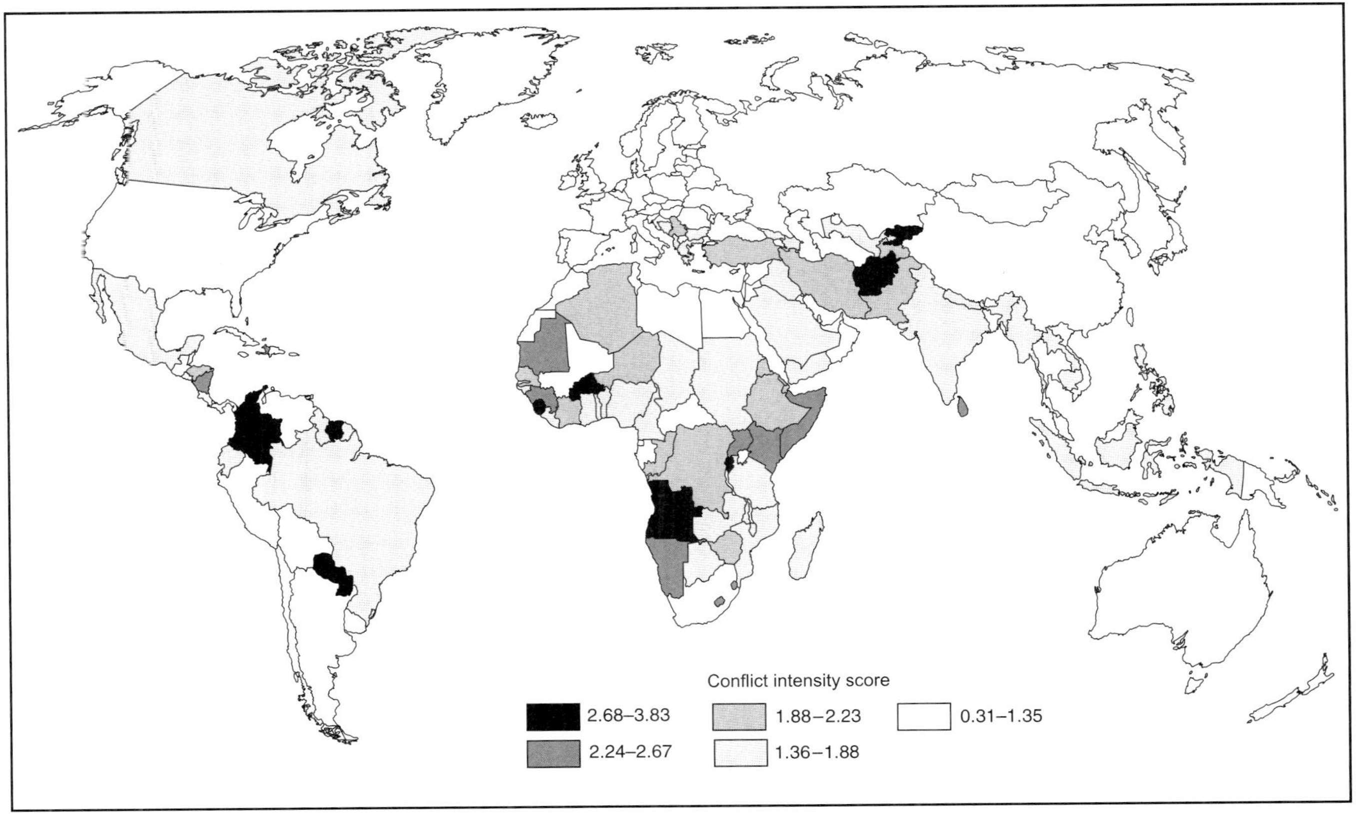

Fig. 8.15. Intensity of military conflict by country, 2000
Conflict intensity is measured according to the number of media reports of external and internal military conflict targeted at each country.
Sources: Redrawn from Smallman-Raynor and Cliff (2004*b*, fig. 13.2, p. 692), originally from Murray, King, *et al.* (2002, fig. 2, p. 347).

wasting, and enlargement of the abdomen, liver, and spleen. For untreated cases of the disease, two-year mortality rates of up to 95 per cent have been reported (Allison 1993; Heymann 2004: 299–301).

Emergence in Southern Sudan

Prior to the mid-1980s, visceral leishmaniasis in the African state of Sudan appeared to be largely restricted to the eastern sector of the country, close to the border with Ethiopia; see Figure 8.16A. Beginning in October 1988, however, medical teams in the Sudanese capital, Khartoum, began to notice an increase in the incidence of visceral leishmaniasis among war-displaced people originating from the purportedly disease-free southern province of Western Upper Nile. Subsequent investigations in the province revealed an epidemic of devastating proportions. By the mid-1990s, an estimated 100,000 people—representing probably one-third of the resident population of Western Upper Nile—had died of the disease (Seaman *et al.* 1996). The source of the infection in the province is unknown, although Perea *et al.* (1991) have postulated importation with soldiers recruited and/or trained in the endemic east of Sudan. These soldiers were subsequently deployed as a consequence of the south's long-running civil war.

Diffusion Patterns. Whatever the source of the epidemic in Western Upper Nile, intra-provincial population movements in response to war and food shortages appear to have played an integral role in the local spread of the disease (Perea *et al.* 1991; Seaman *et al.* 1996). The diffusion pattern, based on the timing of intense disease activity in the various districts of the province, is plotted by the vectors in Figure 8.16B. As the map indicates, the epidemic first peaked in the southern sector of Jikany district in 1988–9, spreading onwards to western, northern, and southern districts in the years that followed.

Mortality Rates. The proportional circles in Figure 8.16B plot the estimated population of sample districts at the time of appearance of visceral

Fig. 8.16. Emergence of visceral leishmaniasis in Western Upper Nile, southern Sudan, 1984–1994

(A) Areas of endemic visceral leishmaniasis in Sudan. The location of Western Upper Nile, situated to the south-west of the main endemic area, is indicated by the heavy border. (B) Epidemic spread of visceral leishmaniasis in Western Upper Nile during the 1980s and 1990s. Vectors trace the routes of disease diffusion while dates mark periods of intense disease activity in various areas of the province. Proportional circles provide estimates of district populations at the time of arrival of visceral leishmaniasis. Shaded sectors give the estimated percentage proportion of the population that subsequently died of the disease. The southernmost districts of the province were unaffected by the epidemic during the time interval under consideration.

Sources: Redrawn from Smallman-Raynor and Cliff (2004*b*, fig. 13.8, p. 722), originally based on Seaman *et al.* (1996, fig. 1, p. 863, and table 4, p. 870).

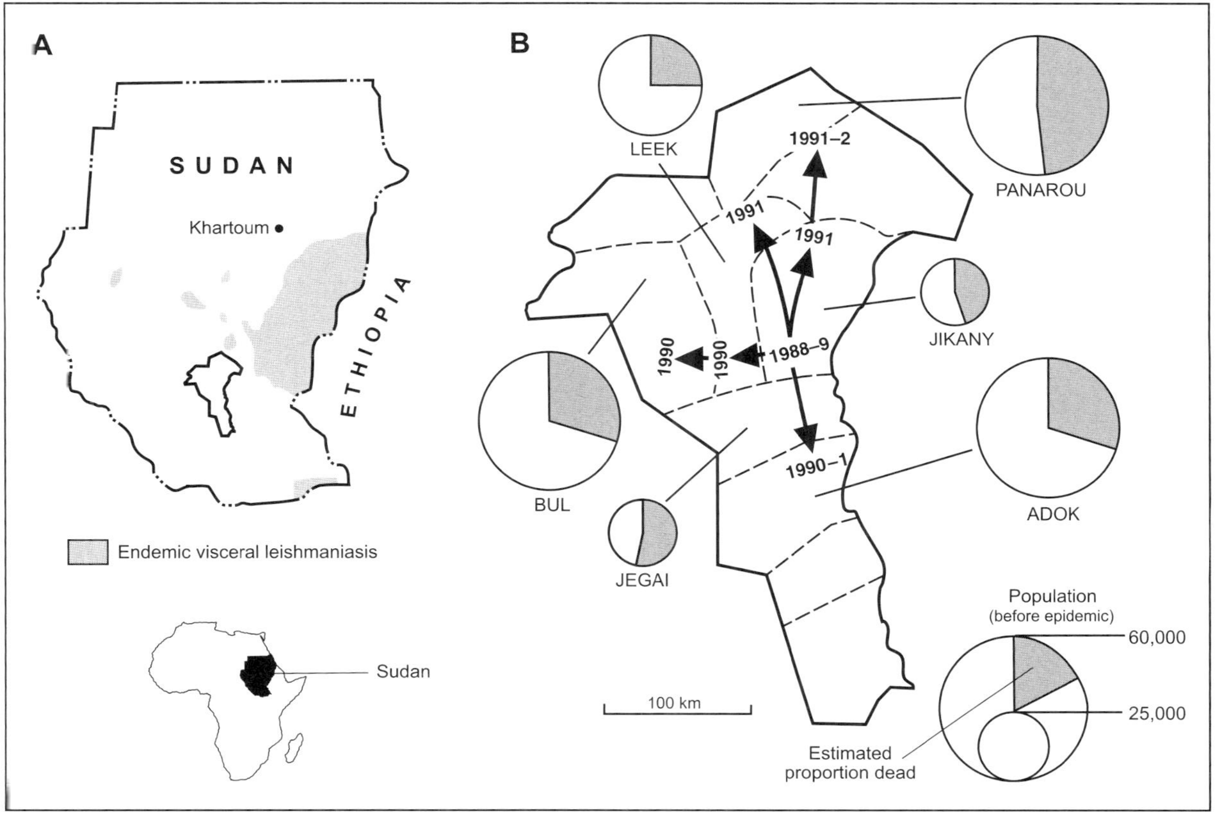
A
SUDAN
Khartoum
ETHIOPIA
Endemic visceral leishmaniasis
Sudan
B
LEEK
PANAROU
JIKANY
BUL
ADOK
JEGAI
1991–2
1991
1991
1988–9
1990
1990
1990–1
100 km
Population
(before epidemic)
60,000
25,000
Estimated
proportion dead

leishmaniasis. The shaded sectors provide percentage estimates of associated mortality in the years that followed. As the map shows, mortality from visceral leishmaniasis is believed to have exceeded 25 per cent in all the sample districts, reaching highs of 48 per cent (Panarou) and 56 per cent (Jegai).

Outlook. A separate epidemic of visceral leishmaniasis was observed in the province of Eastern Upper Nile in 1994. Hundreds are known to have died before the outbreak was identified. As Seaman *et al.* (1996: 871) note, the war-associated disruption of agriculture, relief, and disease-control programmes has ensured that the 'age-old cycle of war, famine and infectious disease is still part of the way of life among the threatened cultures of southern Sudan'. The epidemic has been a human tragedy of major proportions, with conditions of war and famine continuing to favour the establishment of new endemic foci in the region.

DARFUR CONFLICT (2003–PRESENT): HEPATITIS E IN WESTERN SUDAN

In early 2003, just as the Sudanese Civil War finally appeared to be approaching a resolution, a fresh conflict erupted in the region of Darfur, western Sudan (Figure 8.17). Formed along ethnic lines, and with local rebel forces, the Sudanese military, and the Janjaweed militias as the principal combatants, mass violence against civilians (including alleged acts of genocide) had resulted in the internal and international displacement of 1.5–2.0 million people (~25 per cent of the population of Darfur) by September 2004. With limited assistance from charities and other humanitarian organizations, an epidemiological survey of relief camps in South Darfur identified violence, diarrhoeal diseases, and acute malnutrition as the major health problems of the internally displaced (Grandesso *et al.* 2005).

The 2004 Outbreak of Hepatitis E

Hepatitis E (*ICD*-10 B17.2) was identified as a distinct clinical entity in 1980, with hepatitis E virus (HEV) now recognized as the principal cause of enterically transmitted non-A, non-B hepatitis worldwide (Heymann 2004: 266–8). Consumption of faecally contaminated water is the principal route of HEV transmission, with the disease recognized as a potential health problem for refugees and other displaced persons in East Africa since the late 1980s (Toole 1997). Against this background, Guthmann *et al.* (2006) describe the largest outbreak of HEV to be documented in a displaced population: the epidemic in Mornay relief camp, West Darfur, July–December 2004; see Figure 8.17 for location. The camp-based epidemic was associated with 2,621 recorded cases in a total population of 78,800 (attack rate 3.3 per cent); 45 patients died, with a specific case-fatality rate of 31.1 per cent for pregnant women. Risk factors for infection were

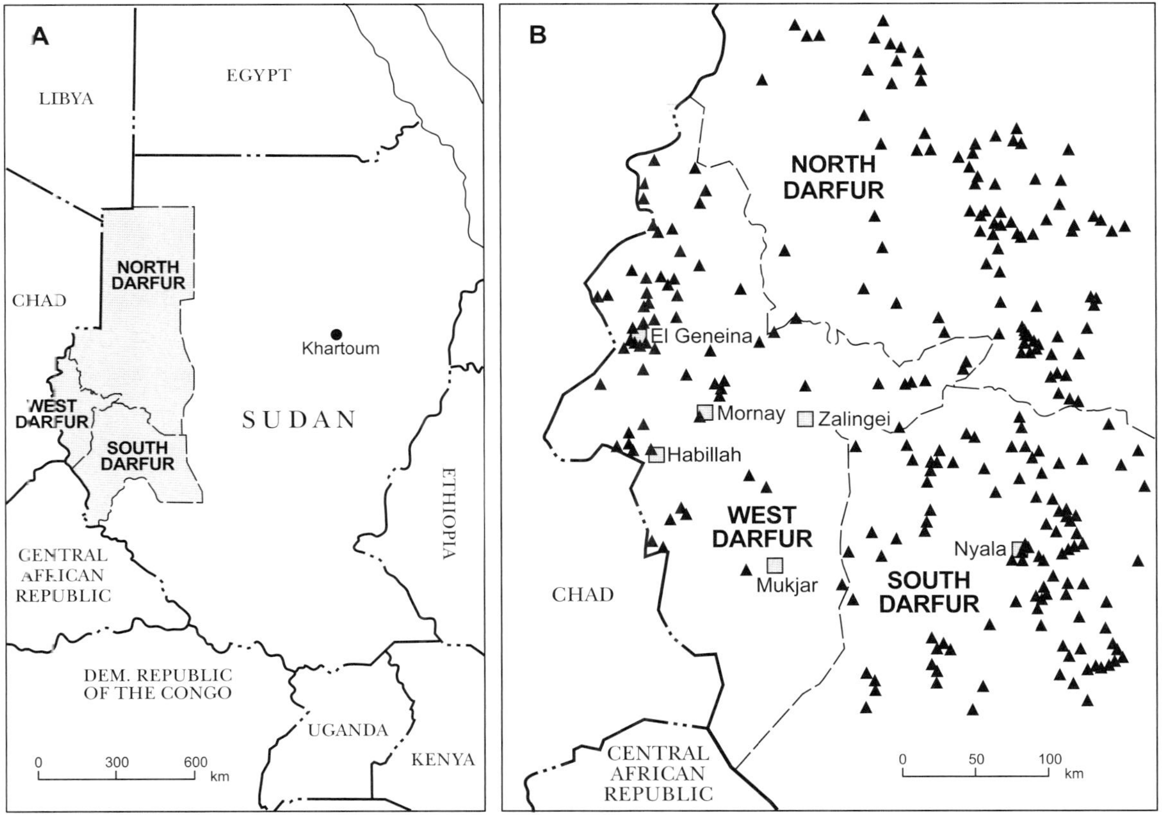

Fig. 8.17. Population displacement in Darfur, western Sudan

(A) Location map of the states of North, South, and West Darfur. (B) Location of relief camps for internally displaced persons (IDPs) in Darfur region (status: Apr. 2007). The location of Mornay Camp, West Darfur, is indicated.

Source: Map B drawn from United Nations High Commission for Refugees (2007).

identified as age (15–45 years) and consumption of chlorinated water, the latter highlighting the potential problems of HEV inactivation in water sources during complex emergencies (Boccia *et al.* 2006; Guthmann *et al.* 2006).

8.4.2 The Middle East and Afghanistan

THE PERSIAN GULF WAR (1991)

Not all modern conflicts have acted as emerging disease amplifiers. A good example is provided by the Persian Gulf War of 1991. In contrast to the estimated 100,000 plus Iraqi civilians believed to have died from the health impacts of the war and associated UN economic sanctions imposed after Iraqi forces overran Kuwait, the impact of infections upon a coalition of US, British, Canadian, and other forces who responded in Operation Desert Shield was minimal. Table 8.7 gives cause-specific counts of non-battle mortality among all US military personnel deployed during the preparatory (Operation Desert Shield) and combat (Operation Desert Storm) phases of the Gulf War, 1 August 1990–31 July 1991.[5] Compared with previous US military campaigns, the remarkable feature of Table 8.7 is the solitary confirmed death from infectious disease—and this in over 0.26 million person-years of deployment. High levels of protection against major infectious diseases were afforded by the administration of vaccines for adenovirus types 4 and 7, hepatitis B, influenza, measles, mumps and rubella, meningococcal disease, poliomyelitis, tetanus, diphtheria, typhoid, yellow fever, and, depending on the situational context, anthrax, botulinum, and rabies (Grabenstein *et al.* 2006). Non-fatal outbreaks of diarrhoeal diseases, including gastroenteritis due to enterotoxigenic *Escherichia coli* and drug-resistant *Shigella sonnei*, did, however, gain prominence in some deployed units (Hyams, Bourgeois, *et al.* 1991).

THE GLOBAL WAR ON TERROR SINCE 2001

In this subsection, we examine the US-led coalition wars in Iraq (Operation Iraqi Freedom, 2003–present) and Afghanistan (Operation Enduring Freedom, 2001–present) that formed part of the Bush administration's ongoing 'Global War on Terror'. Perspectives on the health impacts of the military operations on local civilian populations are provided by Sharp, Burkle, *et al.* (2002), Roberts *et al.* (2004), and Burnham *et al.* (2006), while, as an indicator of trends among deployed Coalition forces, Table 8.8 provides an overview

[5] In addition to the 225 non-battle-related deaths recorded for US forces deployed to the Persian Gulf in Table 8.7, 147 US troops died as a direct result of trauma sustained during Operation Desert Storm (Writer *et al.* 1996).

Table 8.7. Mortality from non-battle causes in US military personnel deployed to the Persian Gulf, 1 August 1990–31 July 1991

Cause	Deaths (rate per 100,000 person-years)
All non-battle-related deaths	225 (84.95)
Unintentional injury	183 (69.09)
Motor vehicle	62 (23.41)
Motorcycle	0 (0.00)
Aircraft	47 (17.74)
Explosions	18 (6.80)
Other	56 (21.14)
Illness	30 (11.33)
Cardiovascular	2 (0.76)
Unexpected/undefined[1]	21 (7.93)
Cancer	0 (0.00)
Infectious disease	1 (0.38)
Other	6 (2.27)
Self-inflicted	10 (3.78)
Gunshot	10 (3.78)
Hanging/asphyxiation	0 (0.00)
Other	0 (0.00)
Homicide	1 (0.38)
Gunshot	1 (0.38)
Other	0 (0.00)
Unknown	1 (0.38)

Note: [1] Includes deaths for which there was no apparent preceding illness or injury and deaths attributed to cardiac or respiratory failure and other causes on casualty reports.
Source: Writer *et al.* (1996, table 1, p. 119).

of the principal infections so far documented in US military personnel in Iraq and Afghanistan.

Iraq: Operation Iraqi Freedom

Severe outbreaks of gastroenteritis were recorded in US and British forces in the opening phases of Operation Iraqi Freedom (Bailey *et al.* 2005; Thornton *et al.* 2005), while diarrhoea and respiratory tract infections gained a more general prevalence in the deployed forces (Sanders *et al.* 2005). Cases of infection and disease associated with the agent of Q fever, *Coxiella burnetii*, have been associated with the deployment of US personnel to northern and western Iraq (Leung-Shea and Danahar 2006; Hartzell *et al.* 2007), while sporadic cases of brucellosis have also been documented (Aronson *et al.* 2006). Among the other conditions in Table 8.8, cutaneous leishmaniasis, severe (acute eosinophilic) pneumonia,[6] and hospital-acquired drug-resistant *Acinetobacter* wound infections have been identified as emergent health issues for the Coalition forces. For cutaneous leishmaniasis, Figure 8.18

[6] The aetiology of the documented cases of severe (acute eosinophilic) pneumonia is unknown and may be non-infectious.

Table 8.8. Infections documented in deployed US forces in Operation Iraqi Freedom and Operation Enduring Freedom

Disease	Iraq (Operation Iraqi Freedom, 2003–)	Sources	Afghanistan (Operation Enduring Freedom, 2001–)	Sources
Acinetobacter infection in war wounds	Antibiotic-resistant *Acinetobacter baumannii* infections in medical evacuees	Centers for Disease Control and Prevention (2004*c*); Jones, Morgan, *et al.* (2006)	Antibiotic-resistant *Acinetobacter baumannii* infections in medical evacuees	Centers for Disease Control and Prevention (2004*c*)
Brucellosis	Few sporadic cases (2003–5)	Aronson *et al.* (2006)		
Gastroenteritis	Severe outbreaks secondary to norovirus and *Shigella* infections in initial phases of the conflict	Aronson *et al.* (2006)	Severe outbreaks secondary to norovirus and *Shigella* infections in initial phases of the conflict	Ahmad (2002); Centers for Disease Control and Prevention (2002); Putnam *et al.* (2006)
Leishmaniasis	Estimated 0.23 per cent of deployed ground forces diagnosed with cutaneous leishmaniasis (Mar. 2003–June 2005)	Aronson *et al.* (2006); Centers for Disease Control and Prevention (2003*b*, 2004*a*)	Sporadic reports of cutaneous and visceral disease	Centers for Disease Control and Prevention (2003*b*, 2004*a*,*b*)
Malaria			Malaria due to *Plasmodium vivax* in military returnees from eastern Afghanistan	Kotwal *et al.* (2006)
Q fever	Sporadic cases and small outbreaks	Leung-Shea and Danahar (2006); Hartzell *et al.* (2007)		
Respiratory illness	Self-reported respiratory illness common; 18 documented cases (9.1 cases per 100,000 person-years of deployment) of acute aeosinophilic pneumonia (AEP), Mar. 2003–Mar. 2004	Gottlieb (2003); Shorr *et al.* (2004); Aronson *et al.* (2006)	Self-reported respiratory illness common	Aronson *et al.* (2006)

Source: Based on Aronson *et al.* (2006).

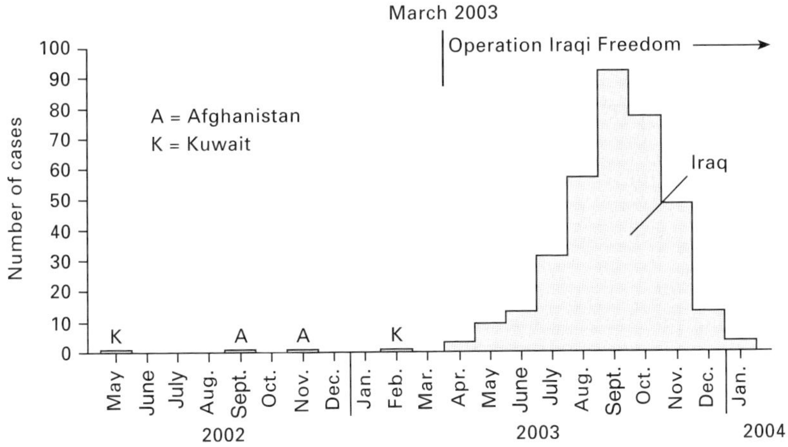

Fig. 8.18. Cutaneous leishmaniasis in US military personnel deployed in Operation Enduring Freedom and Operation Iraqi Freedom, May 2002–January 2004
The graph plots the month of onset of disease in patients deployed to Afghanistan (two cases), Iraq (346 cases), and Kuwait (two cases).
Source: Redrawn from Centers for Disease Control and Prevention (2004*a*: 265).

plots the month of onset of the disease in a sample of 346 parasitologically confirmed cases in US personnel deployed to Iraq, with additional cases in US personnel deployed to Kuwait (two cases) and Afghanistan (two cases) also indicated. As the graph shows, the first cases of cutaneous leishmaniasis were recorded in April 2003, with the number rising to a peak of >90 in September 2003, and declining thereafter. The majority of the cases were members of the Active Force component of the army, with many having been positioned near the Iraq–Syria and Iraq–Iran borders.

Afghanistan: Operation Enduring Freedom
Among Coalition forces in Iraq, Table 8.8 indicates that outbreaks of severe gastrointestinal diseases secondary to noroviruses and other infectious agents were documented in personnel deployed in the early stages of Operation Enduring Freedom. Sporadic cases of cutaneous and visceral leishmaniasis have also been recorded in US personnel, while the identification of malaria due to *P. vivax* in US military returnees from eastern Afghanistan has been attributed to suboptimal compliance with preventive measures.

8.4.3 Other Wars and Deployments: UN Peacekeeping Forces

One major development in global military activity over the past half-century has been the international deployment of armed forces to oversee, to maintain, and increasingly to create the conditions of peace in ceasefires and armistices (Renner 1997). Under the auspices of the UN Peacekeeping Operations, over 61 peacekeeping missions had been authorized by the United Nations in the six decades to the end of 2006. These missions are plotted, by year of operation, as the bar chart in Figure 8.19. In the period prior to 1990, the UN undertook only 18 different peacekeeping missions. But, with the end of the Cold War, the number of missions spiralled so that 43 new missions in well over 30 countries of Africa, the Americas, Asia, Europe, and Oceania were authorized by the United Nations in the period 1990–2006.

Fatality Trends

As the fine line trace in Figure 8.19 shows, late twentieth-century developments in peacekeeping duties were associated with an upsurge in the number of deaths among UN personnel (Seet and Burnham 2000). Of these, 24.5 per cent were classified in the category 'illness'; the annual series is plotted as the heavy line trace in Figure 8.19.

Infectious Diseases

Table 8.9 lists the occurrence of infectious diseases and disease agents in sample UN and NATO peacekeeping operations since 1956. Among the

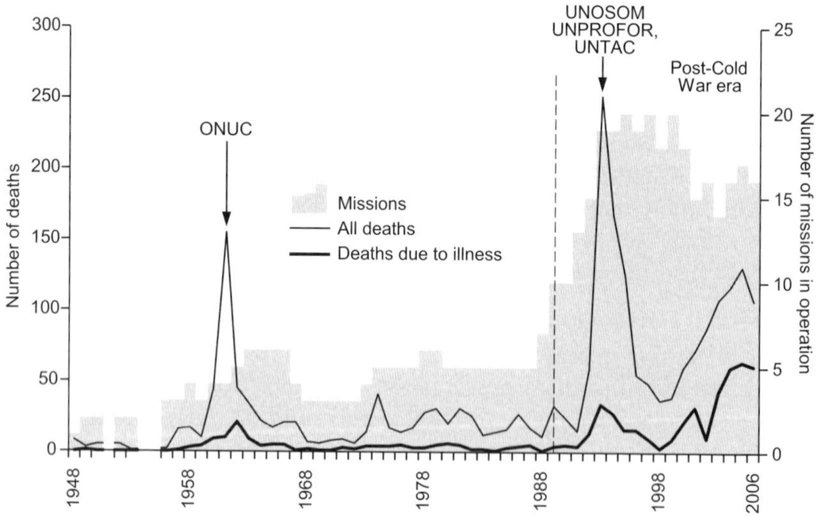

Fig. 8.19. United Nations peacekeeping missions, 1948–2006
The bar chart plots the number of peacekeeping missions in operation during a given year. The line traces plot the annual number of deaths in UN peacekeeping forces from all causes (fine line trace) and illness (heavy line trace). For reference, the end of the Cold War has been set at 1990. Periods of peak mortality associated with operations in the Congo (ONUC) in 1961, and Cambodia (UNTAC), Somalia (UNOSOM), and the former Yugoslavia (UNPROFOR) in 1993, are indicated.
Source: Data from United Nations Peacekeeping (2008).

Table 8.9. Some infectious diseases and disease agents documented in a sample of UN and NATO peacekeeping operations

Year	Peacekeeping operation	Nationality of troops	Disease/infection	Cases	Reference
1956–62	UN Emergency Force in Gaza	Multinational	Hepatitis A	207	Hesla (1992)
1978	UN Interim Force in Lebanon	Multinational	Hepatitis A	83	Hesla (1992)
1983–4	Multinational Force and Observers, Sinai Desert (Egypt)	Fijian	Cutaneous leishmaniasis	63[1]	Norton *et al.* (1992); Fryauff *et al.* (1993)
1985	UN Peacekeeping Force in Cyprus	Swedish	Sandfly fever	8[2]	Eitrem *et al.* (1990)
1989–90	UN Transition Assistance Group, Namibia	Multinational	Respiratory tract infection	2,593[3]	Steffen *et al.* (1992)
1992–3	UN Transition Authority, Cambodia	Multinational	HIV	7[4]	Soeprapto *et al.* (1995)
	Operation Restore Hope, Somalia	US	Dengue fever	14	Kanesa-thasan *et al.* (1994)
1994 (19 Sept.–4 Nov.)	Operation Uphold Democracy, Haiti	US	Dengue fever & other febrile diseases	106	Centers for Disease Control and Prevention (1994*d*)
1995	UN Mission in Haiti	Bangladeshi	Hepatitis E[5]	4	Drabick *et al.* (1997)
1995–6 (19 weeks)	Operation Resolute, Bosnia-Hercegovina	British	Enteric disease	1,139[6]	Croft and Creamer (1997)
1996	Operation Resolute, Bosnia-Hercegovina	British	Rubella	4	Adams *et al.* (1997)
1997	UN Stabilization Force, Bosnia-Hercegovina	Czech	Q fever	26	Splino *et al.* (2003)

Notes: [1] Fifteen further cases were recorded in Australian/New Zealander (1 case), British (1), Colombian (6), Dutch (1), Italian (1), US (2), and Uruguayan (3) peacekeepers. [2] Cohort study. [3] Outpatient consultations, Apr. 1989–Mar. 1990. [4] Results from prevalence study sample. [5] Infection imported from Bangladesh to Haiti. [6] Data for entire 19-week period; an 'explosive' outbreak of gastrointestinal disease was recorded during week 2 of operations.
Source: Based on Smallman-Raynor and Cliff (2004*b*, table 13.7, p. 720).

more noteworthy events were outbreaks of hepatitis A among multinational forces in Gaza and the Lebanon in the 1950s–1970s, cutaneous leishmaniasis among Fijian and other troops in Egypt during 1983–4, and dengue fever among US troops stationed in Somalia and Haiti in the early and mid-1990s. Although the outbreaks documented in Table 8.9 were generally small and deaths were few in number, Adams *et al.* (1997) note that the spread of infectious diseases represents a potentially serious drain on peacekeeping personnel.

8.4.4 Diseases of Undetermined Aetiology: Post-Combat Syndromes

One marked feature of many past wars has been the development among the veteran populations of debilitating syndromes characterized by a complex of signs and symptoms. In a review of these post-combat syndromes, Hyams, Wignall, *et al.* (1996) have identified a series of examples—from the American Civil War (Da Costa syndrome) to the Gulf War (Gulf War syndrome)—that have variously manifested as fatigue or exhaustion, shortness of breath, headache, diarrhoea, dizziness, disturbed sleep, and forgetfulness (Table 8.10).[7] As Jones, Hodgins-Vermaas, *et al.* (2002: 323) conclude of the historical evidence: 'Post-combat syndromes have arisen from all major wars over the past century, and we can predict that they will continue to appear after future conflicts. What cannot be accurately forecast is their form, as they are moulded by the changing nature of health fears and warfare . . . '

GULF WAR SYNDROME

Gulf War syndrome, manifesting as a spectrum of unexplained illnesses in US, British, and other veterans of the Persian Gulf War of 1991 (Section 8.4.2), is the most intensively studied of the post-combat syndromes in Table 8.10. Although no new or unique medical condition has yet been formally identified among Gulf War veterans (Shapiro *et al.* 2002), considerable speculation has surrounded possible factors, over and above the psychological dimensions of active combat, that may have adversely affected the symptomatic health of many tens of thousands of servicemen. Particular attention has focused on the side-effects of measures undertaken to protect the combatants from the threat of chemical and biological warfare, including multiple vaccinations against such biological agents as plague and anthrax (UK troops) and anthrax and botulism (US troops). Various other factors, including troop exposures to depleted uranium, organophosphate pesticides, nerve agents (sarin), and the toxins released by oil fires, have all been mooted in the aetiology of Gulf War-related illnesses (Wessely *et al.* 2001).

[7] Earlier evidence for the possible occurrence of a post-combat syndrome following deployment in the Crimean War (1853–6) and the First War of Indian Independence (1857–8) is provided by Jones and Wessely (1999).

Table 8.10. Symptoms commonly associated with war-related medical and psychological illnesses

Symptom	War and illness[1] US Civil War: Da Costa syndrome	World War I: Effort syndrome	World War II: Combat stress reaction	Vietnam War: Agent Orange exposure	Vietnam & other wars: Post-traumatic stress disorder (PTSD)	Gulf War: Gulf War syndrome
Fatigue/exhaustion	+	+	+	+	+	+
Shortness of breath	+	+	+		+	+
Palpitations/tachycardia	+	+	+		+	
Pre-cordial pain	+	+			+	+
Headache	+	+	+	+	+	+
Muscle and joint pain				+	+	+
Diarrhoea	+		+	+	+	+
Excessive sweating	+	+	+			
Dizziness	+	+	+	+	+	
Fainting	+	+				
Disturbed sleep	+	+	+	+	+	+
Forgetfulness		+	+	+	+	+
Difficulty concentrating		+	+	+	+	+

Notes: [1] '+' indicates a commonly reported symptom.
Sources: Smallman-Raynor and Cliff (2004*b*, table 13.9, p. 727), from Hyams, Wignall, *et al.* (1996, table 1, p. 399).

8.5 Deliberately Emerging Diseases: Biological Warfare and Bioterrorism

Biological weapons are generally regarded as representing one of the foremost threats to global security in the twenty-first century. Biological weapons are relatively inexpensive to produce and transport, and have the capacity for immense destruction over wide areas. In addition, the capability has been developed for pathogen delivery via a number of weapons systems including long-range missiles, dispersers on manned and drone aircraft, bombs, and bomblets. Once the secret preserve of a handful of leading states, bioweapons technology is increasingly finding its way to lesser state powers, non-state organizations, and others who have been attracted by the potential destructiveness of such weapons (Dando 1994; Henderson 2000). 'The history of weapons development', Henderson (2000: 64) remarks, 'tells us that weapons that have been produced, for whatever reason, will eventually be used. One would hope that the history of biological weapons might be the exception to the rule, but it would be hazardous to believe that.'

THE CONCEPT OF DELIBERATELY EMERGING DISEASES

Following the categorization of Morens *et al.* (2004) in Section 1.2, the term 'deliberately emerging diseases' refers to diseases and disease agents that have been developed by man 'usually for nefarious use'. The microbial agents of deliberately emerging diseases may be naturally occurring, and may or may not have been genetically engineered to facilitate delivery or to enhance virulence. The 2005 revision of the *International Health Regulations* has strengthened WHO's role in global surveillance for deliberately emerging diseases. Under the revised regulations, member states are required to notify WHO of *all events which may constitute a public health emergency of international concern* (Article 6.1)—whether naturally occurring, intentionally created, or unintentionally caused. In the event of notification of the intentional release of a biological agent, international response and containment is coordinated through the WHO's Global Outbreak Alert and Response Network (GOARN) (Heymann 2004, pp. xxxii–xxxiv).

8.5.1 Biological Weapons: Definitions and Disease Agents

The World Health Organization (2004*f*: 5) defines biological weapons as 'those that achieve their intended target effects through the infectivity of disease causing microorganisms and other such entities, including viruses, infectious nucleic acids and prions'. Although a large number of disease agents have been posited as possible agents in biological weapons (Table 8.11), a series of factors (including cultivation and effective dispersal, transmission dynamics,

Table 8.11. Sample biological entities identified by the World Health Organization (WHO) for possible development in weapons

Disease (*disease agent*)[1]	Mortality (%)
Bacteria	
Anthrax (*Bacillus anthracis*) [A22]	*c*.100 (inhalational)
Brucellosis (*Brucella* spp.) [A23]	<2
Glanders (*Burkholderia mallei*) [A24.0]	*c*.95
Tularaemia (*Franciscella tularensis*) [A21]	≤5
Cholera (*Vibrio cholerae*) [A00]	≤80
Plague (*Yersinia pestis*) [A20]	*c*.100 (pneumonic)
Fungi	
Coccidioidomycosis (*Coccidioides immitis*) [B38]	low
Rickettsiae	
Q fever (*Coxiella burnetii*) [A78]	low
Rocky Mountain spotted fever (*Rickettsia rickettsii*) [A77.0]	
Typhus fever (*Rickettsia prowazekii*) [A75]	≤70
Viruses	
Chikungunya [A92.0]	very low
Crimean–Congo haemorrhagic fever [A98.0]	≤50
Dengue [A90/91]	very low (non-haemorrhagic cases)
Eastern equine encephalitis [A83.2]	≤80
Influenza [J10, J11]	usually low
Japanese encephalitis [A83.0]	≤50 (encephalitis cases)
Marburg vival disease [A98.4]	25
Tick-borne encephalitis [A84.0]	≤40
Smallpox [B03]	≤30
Venezuelan equine encephalitis [A92.2]	low
Western equine encephalitis [A83.1]	3–15
Yellow fever [A95]	≤40

Note: [1] *ICD*-10 code for each disease given in square brackets.
Sources: Smallman-Raynor and Cliff (2004*b*, table 13.4, p. 707), based on World Health Organization (1970*a*, 2004*f*) and Dando (1994, table 2.2, p. 31).

environmental stability, infectious dose size, and availability of prophylactic and therapeutic measures) suggest that relatively few agents have strategic potential. As far as present-day developments are concerned, comparative biological advantage—including ease of agent production, resistance to destruction, and the potential for aerosol dispersal—appears to favour the anthrax bacillus (*Bacillus anthracis*) over many other candidates (Henderson 1999, 2000).

8.5.2 Historical Dimensions of Biological Warfare

The history of biological warfare is reviewed by Christopher *et al.* (1997), Gould and Connell (1997), Henderson (2000), Metcalfe (2002), and Balmer (2002), among others. While the deployment of diseased cadavers, animals and animal carcasses, and other infective materials as weapons of war can be traced to classical times,[8] the strategic planning and scientific development of biological weapons—contingent on advances in microbiology—is a phenomenon of the last 100 years. During World War I, the Germans are alleged to have developed a biological warfare programme with the specific intent of contaminating Allied livestock and animal feed with the agents of anthrax and glanders. Notwithstanding efforts to control the use of biological weapons under the 1925 Geneva Protocol, the first viable programme of biological warfare emerged with the establishment of Japan's notorious germ warfare unit, Detachment 731, in the 1930s. By the end of World War II, Japanese forces are alleged to have deployed a range of biological entities (including the agents of plague, typhoid, cholera, and dysentery) in the war against China (Christopher *et al.* 1997; Gould and Connell 1997).

POST-WORLD WAR II DEVELOPMENTS

In the aftermath of World War II, a number of countries—including Belgium, Britain, Canada, the United States, and the Soviet Union—pursued offensive biological weapons programmes. By the late 1960s, the United States alone had stockpiled a large biological arsenal of lethal agents (including *B. anthracis* and botulinum toxin), incapacitating agents (including *Brucella suis* and Venezuelan equine encephalitis virus), and anti-crop agents (including rice blast and rye stem rust). Under the Nixon administration, however, the US programme was terminated in 1969–70, with the reputed destruction of the entire biological arsenal by February 1973 (Christopher *et al.* 1997).

USSR: Sverdlovsk Anthrax Outbreak

While the 1972 Biological and Toxic Weapons Convention prohibited the possession, development, and stockpiling of pathogens or toxins in excess of

---

Pl. 8.2. Geographical spread of anthrax associated with the airborne escape of spores from the military microbiology facility at Sverdlovsk, former USSR, April–May 1979 Sverdlovsk is a city of about 1.2 million, situated 1,400 km to the east of Moscow. During Apr. and May 1979, an outbreak of anthrax occurred among humans and livestock in a zone extending downwind from the city's military facility. The outbreak among humans was associated with a documented 66 deaths from inhalational anthrax—the largest recorded epidemic in history. (A) Satellite photograph showing the probable location of patients at time of exposure to anthrax in early Apr. 1979 (numbers), along with calculated contours of constant anthrax dosage (black lines). (B) Villages (letter-coded) where livestock died of anthrax in Apr. 1979, with calculated contours of constant anthrax dosage (black lines).

Sources: Smallman-Raynor and Cliff (2004*b*, pl. 13.1, pp. 710–11), repr. from Meselson *et al.* (1994, figs 2 and 3, pp. 1204–5).

[8] Trevisanato (2007*b*), for example, hypothesizes that the 'Hittite plague' of the late 14th century BC may have been an epidemic of tularaemia whose spread was promoted, at least in part, by the deployment of contaminated animals in the ranks of the enemy during the Neshite–Arzawan War of 1320–1318 BC.

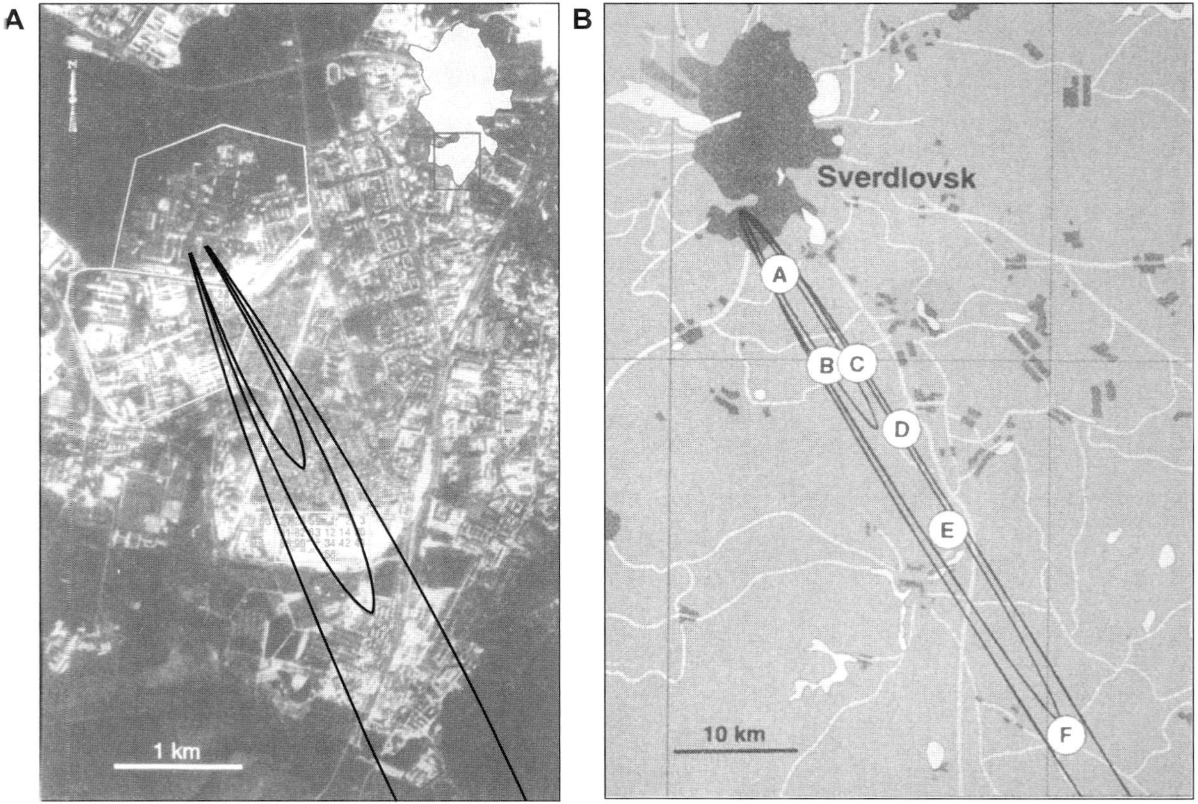
A
1 km
B
Sverdlovsk
A
B
C
D
E
F
10 km

the quantities required for 'peaceful purposes', several signatories to the Convention continued to participate in outlawed activities. For example, during the 1970s and 1980s, the former USSR is reputed to have solved many technical problems in bioweapons development including the production of antibiotic-resistant microbes, the preparation of microbes for aerosol dissemination, and pathogen delivery in missiles and warheads. The developments were not without incident. In April and May 1979, an inhalation anthrax outbreak occurred among people who lived and worked up to 4 km downwind of a military establishment in the Soviet city of Sverdlovsk; an outbreak was also recorded in livestock along an extended axis of the human epidemic zone for a distance of some 50 km (Meselson *et al.* 1994) (Plate 8.2). The outbreak was associated with 77 human cases and 66 deaths—the largest epidemic of inhalational anthrax ever documented. In 1992, after years of international dispute over the matter, President Boris Yeltsin conceded that the epidemic was the result of an unintentional release of anthrax spores from the Sverdlovsk biological facility (Christopher *et al.* 1997; Gould and Connell 1997).

Developments in the 1990s: Evidence from Iraq

Although a number of countries (including China, Cuba, India, Iran, Israel, Libya, North Korea, Russia, and Syria) are either known, or suspected, to have contributed to the international proliferation of biological weapons in the late twentieth century, the Iraqi programme has been subject to the closest scrutiny by the international community in recent years. In the aftermath of the Persian Gulf War (Section 8.4.2), UN weapons inspectors in Iraq uncovered evidence of offensive biological programmes involving *B. anthracis*, rotavirus, and camel pox virus, among other disease agents. Pathogen production and storage included 20,000 litres of botulinum toxin and 8,000 litres of anthrax spore suspension, with the capability for long-range delivery in the warheads of SCUD missiles (Gould and Connell 1997; Henderson 1999).

8.5.3 Bioterrorism in the United States

Recent years have been marked by an escalating concern over the threat of bioterrorism in the United States (Hughes 1999; Tucker 1999). Prior to the late 1990s, the FBI typically investigated a dozen cases each year involving the acquisition or use of biological, chemical, and nuclear materials. The number of investigations grew to 74 in 1997 and 181 in 1998. While some 80 per cent of the investigations were associated with hoaxes, a number were concerned with failed attacks (Tucker 1999). As regards the nature of the perpetrators, religious fundamentalism emerged as a motivating factor from the mid-1990s, while general civil populations and symbolic buildings and/or organizations were the most common (threatened or intended) targets of attack (Tucker 1999). As Tucker (1999: 503) warns:

> the historical record suggests that future incidents of bioterrorism will probably involve hoaxes and relatively small-scale attacks, such as food contamination. Nevertheless, the diffusion of dual-based technologies relevant to the production of biological and toxin agents, and the potential availability of scientists and engineers formerly employed in sophisticated biological warfare programs such as those of the Soviet Union and South Africa, suggest that the technical barriers to mass-casualty terrorism are eroding.

BIOTERRORIST-RELATED ANTHRAX IN THE UNITED STATES, 2001

In the days and weeks that followed the atrocities of 11 September 2001, the civil population of the United States became the target for terrorist attacks with *B. anthracis*, the causative agent of anthrax. While the nature of anthrax (*ICD*-10 A22) is summarized in Heymann (2004: 20–5), we note here that human infection with *B. anthracis* manifests in three clinical forms: cutaneous, gastrointestinal, and inhalational. All three human forms are potentially lethal, although, as in the case of the Sverdlovsk incident in Section 8.5.2, discussions of anthrax bioweapons have centred on the particular lethality of inhalational anthrax.

The 2001 Attacks

Prior to 2001, documented cases of the inhalational form of anthrax—nationally and worldwide—were largely associated with occupational exposure to contaminated animals and animal products (Figure 8.20). On 2 October 2001, however, the Florida Department of Health was notified of a possible case of inhalational anthrax in an office worker from Palm Beach County. The case history of the patient—a photographic editor with a Florida newspaper—revealed exposure to a suspicious (powder-containing) letter on 19 September; the patient succumbed on 5 October (Bush *et al.* 2001). By 7 November, a further 21 cases of confirmed or suspected bioterrorist-related anthrax had been identified in the United States (Centers for Disease Control and Prevention 2001*b*). The distribution of cases by form of disease (cutaneous or inhalational anthrax), status of infection (confirmed or suspected), and geographical location (city or state) is given in Table 8.12; for reference, Figure 8.21 plots the cases by day of symptom onset.

As Figure 8.21 shows, the case distribution was characterized by two temporally discrete periods of activity: (i) late September–early October (9 cases), which, with the exception of two cases of inhalational anthrax in Florida, was centred on the north-eastern states of New York and New Jersey; and (ii) mid-to-late October (13 cases), dominated by cases of inhalational anthrax in the District of Columbia and New Jersey (Cliff, Haggett, and Smallman-Raynor 2004: 191–2). As regards exposure to *B. anthracis*,

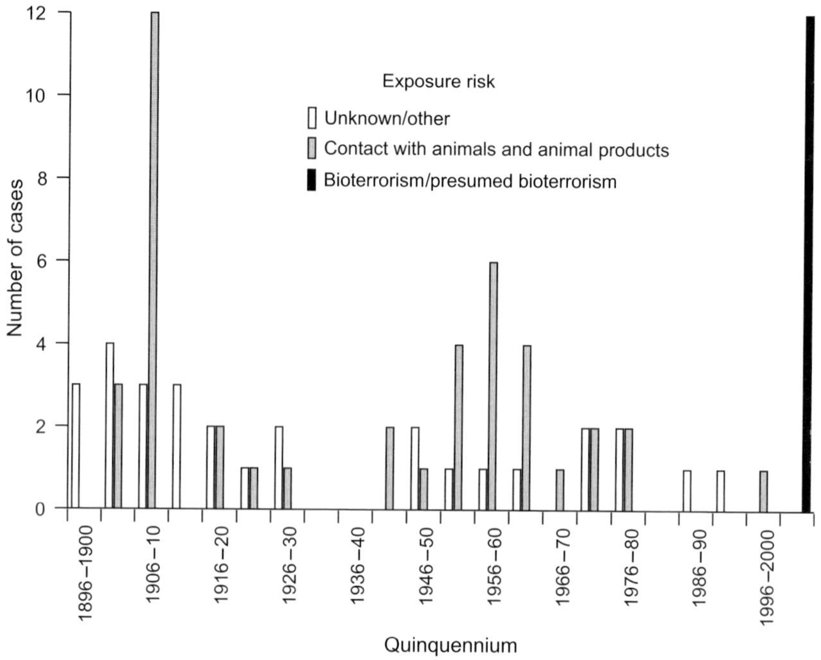

Fig. 8.20. Inhalational anthrax: global series of documented cases by exposure risk, 1900–2005

Cases of inhalational anthrax associated with the Sverdlovsk episode of 1979 (Sect. 8.5.2) have been omitted from the series.

Source: Drawn from data in Holty *et al.* (2006, app. table 2, pp. W-46–W-50).

Table 8.12. Cases of bioterrorism-related anthrax in the United States (status: 7 November 2001)

Category of case	Florida	New York City	District of Columbia	New Jersey	Total
Inhalational					
Confirmed	2	1	5	2	10
Suspected	0	0	0	0	0
Cutaneous					
Confirmed	0	4	0	3	7
Suspected	0	3	0	2	5
TOTAL	2	8	5	7	22

Sources: Smallman-Raynor and Cliff (2004*b*, table 13.6, p. 713), from Centers for Disease Control and Prevention (2001*b*, table 1, p. 973).

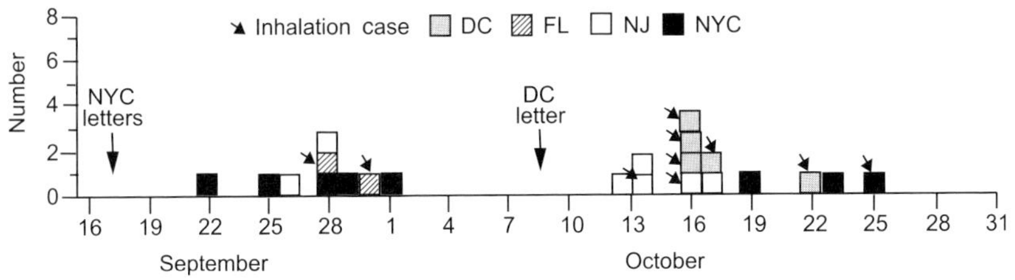

Fig. 8.21. Cases of bioterrorism-related anthrax by day of onset, United States, September–October 2001

Cases are geo-coded according to the place of work of patients. The postmarked dates of *B. anthracis*-contaminated letters sent to New York City (NYC) and the District of Columbia (DC) are indicated for reference. FL = Florida. NJ = New Jersey.

Sources: Redrawn from Smallman-Raynor and Cliff (2004*b*, fig. 13.6, p. 713), originally based on Centers for Disease Control and Prevention (2001*a*, fig. 1, p. 941).

one or more cases in each of the geographical clusters had direct or indirect contact with contaminated letters and/or postal facilities. The strain of *B. anthracis* used in the various attacks was subsequently identified as one commonly found in laboratories and, although processed for the purposes of aerosolization, the bacillus had not been engineered to enhance virulence.

8.5.4 Prospects: Future Threats

PRIORITY THREATS

The Bioterrorism Preparedness and Response Program of the US Centers for Disease Control and Prevention (CDC) provides a categorization of microbial agents on the basis of the probability that their use would result in an overwhelming adverse impact on public health; see Rotz *et al.* (2002). The three-category division, from Category A (*high-priority agents that pose a risk to national security*) to Category C (*emerging pathogens that could be engineered for mass dissemination*), is summarized in Table 8.13. In addition to classical agents—such as *B. anthracis*, *Variola major*, and *Y. pestis*—whose potential for use in biological weapons is well established, Table 8.13 identifies a number of newly recognized disease agents as current and/or future threats. Prominent among the latter are the filoviruses that cause Ebola–Marburg viral diseases (Category A), enterohaemorrhagic strains of *E. coli* (Category B), and the encephalitogenic Nipah virus (Category C).

OTHER POTENTIAL THREATS: POLIOMYELITIS

Poliovirus is not generally viewed as representing an immediate bioterrorist threat because of the currently high levels of immunity to the virus that have been achieved through the WHO's Global Polio Eradication Initiative

Table 8.13. Potential bioterrorism diseases/agents by CDC-defined category

CATEGORY A. *High-priority agents that pose a risk to national security because they: can be easily disseminated or transmitted from person to person; result in high mortality rates and have the potential for major public health impact; might cause public panic and social disruption; and require special action for public health preparedness*

- Anthrax (*Bacillus anthracis*)
- Botulism (*Clostridium botulinum* toxin)
- Plague (*Yersinia pestis*)
- Smallpox (*Variola major*)
- Tularaemia (*Francisella tularensis*)
- Viral haemorrhagic fevers
  - filoviruses (including Ebola, Marburg)
  - arenaviruses (including Lassa, Machupo)

CATEGORY B. *Agents that: are moderately easy to disseminate; result in moderate morbidity rates and low mortality rates; and require specific enhancements of existing diagnostic capacity and enhanced disease surveillance*

- Brucellosis (*Brucella* spp.)
- Epsilon toxin of *Clostridium perfringens*
- Food safety threats (e.g. *Salmonella* spp., *E. coli* O157:H7)
- Glanders (*Burkholderia mallei*)
- Melioidosis (*Burkholderia pseudomallei*)
- Psittacosis (*Chlamydia psittaci*)
- Q fever (*Coxiella burnetii*)
- Ricin toxin from *Ricinus communis*
- Staphylococcal enterotoxin B
- Typhus fever (*Rickettsia prowazekii*)
- Viral encephalitis
  - alphaviruses (including Venezuelan, eastern and western encephalitis)
- Water safety threats (e.g. *Vibrio cholerae* and *Cryptosporidium parvum*)

CATEGORY C. *Emerging pathogens that could be engineered for mass dissemination in the future because of: availability, ease of production and dissemination; and potential for high morbidity and mortality rates and major health impact*

- Hantaviruses
- Nipah virus

Source: Centers for Disease Control and Prevention (2008*b*).

(Smallman-Raynor, Cliff, Trevelyan, *et al.* 2006). This situation could change, however, with the cessation of vaccination in the post-eradication era. While the containment of poliovirus stocks, with a view to limiting both the unintentional and intentional release of the virus, forms a central component of the Global Polio Eradication Initiative's (2003) Strategic Plan 2004–2008, the laboratory synthesis of poliovirus has raised fresh concerns over the bioterrorist threat (Nomoto and Arita 2002). In 2002, researchers at the State University of New York reported the successful assembly of poliovirus from stretches of mail-order DNA on the basis of a genetic blueprint from the Internet (Cello *et al.* 2002). As Cello and colleagues (2002: 1018) observe, 'Any threat from bioterrorism will arise only if mass vaccination stops and herd immunity against poliomyelitis is lost. There is no doubt that technical advances will permit the rapid synthesis of the poliovirus genome, given access to sophisticated resources.'

8.6 Conclusion

In this chapter, we have examined the role of war as a mechanism in the emergence and re-emergence of infectious diseases. Foremost among the factors examined, heightened exposure to the 'zoonotic pool' has regularly promoted the wartime transmission of animal- and insect-borne diseases for which human beings are incidental and potentially highly susceptible hosts. The military invasion of isolated ecological niches, the disruption of human and zootic habitats, and the promotion of local conditions favourable to the wildlife reservoirs of disease agents, all add to the wartime risk of disease emergence and re-emergence. The evolution of drug-resistant pathogens and insecticide-resistant vectors has further contributed to the (re-)emergence complex, while, in the era of mass air transport, the rapid de-deployment of troops has threatened the reintroduction of pathogens into disease-free areas.

For military populations, a prominent feature of the present chapter has been the role of front-line combat troops in both the emergence of apparently 'new' diseases and the re-emergence of old plagues. In the Korean War, for example, outbreaks of KHF were focused on UN combat troops who were bivouacked in the environs of the 38th parallel. Likewise, during the Vietnam War, the occurrence of chloroquine-resistant *P. falciparum* malaria was associated with tactical missions that brought US troops into contact with Viet Cong forces. Such examples underscore the importance of active military operations and enemy engagement as factors in the wartime emergence and re-emergence of infectious diseases.

Whatever the conflict and whatever the geographical setting, war-displaced populations in the modern era have fallen victim to a common set of ailments: diarrhoeal diseases, measles, acute respiratory tract infections, and malnourishment. Cholera, malaria, hepatitis, and meningococcal disease have occasionally appeared, and, on rare occasions, diseases such as epidemic louse-borne typhus fever have been recorded. As the examples of Burundian IDPs and Rwandan refugees in this chapter have shown, the age-old vulnerability of war-displaced populations to the spread of infectious diseases reflects the profound disruption of livelihoods, social support mechanisms and health delivery systems, insanitary living conditions, and intensive population mixing in relief camps. The epidemiological risks are magnified when the displacements occur in remote locations, rapidly and at a scale that is beyond the immediate response capacity of humanitarian organizations.

Deliberately emerging diseases, resulting from the intentional dispersal of biological agents, pose an immediate and direct threat to global security in the twenty-first century. While events in the United States have highlighted the potential importance of the phenomenon, the future risk of such events is neither predictable nor quantifiable. Under such circumstances, strengthened national and global surveillance and outbreak preparedness form a front line of response to the threat (Heymann 2004, pp. xxxii–xxxiv).

9

Temporal Trends in Disease Emergence and Re-emergence: World Regions, 1850–2006

9.1 Introduction

In Chapters 4–8, we have examined a series of processes that, often working in combination, have served to precipitate the emergence and re-emergence of infectious and parasitic disease agents in the human population. In this chapter, we conclude our survey with an analysis of temporal trends in disease emergence and re-emergence since 1850. The discussion is informed by long-term shifts in the underlying causes of mortality encapsulated in Omran's model of epidemiological transition (Section 1.4.1), paying particular attention to the manner in which sample infectious and parasitic diseases have waxed and waned at a variety of geographical scales from the global to the local over the last ~150 years.

LAYOUT OF CHAPTER

Our choice of examples strikes a balance between coverage of geographical regions and epidemiological environments, and coverage of important diseases that we have not so far examined in detail. Our consideration is structured by geographical scale:

(1) At the global level, we discuss three major human diseases that have undergone phases of rapid global expansion since 1850—plague, cholera, and HIV/AIDS (Section 9.2).
(2) At the regional level, we examine twentieth-century trends in general infectious disease mortality in the advanced economies of Europe, North America, and the South Pacific, 1901–75, before looking at time sequences for sample emerging (Ebola–Marburg) and cyclically re-emerging (meningococcal) diseases in sub-Saharan Africa (Section 9.3).
(3) At the national level, we use Hall's (1993) data to establish the main trends in morbidity due to infectious diseases in Australia, 1917–91 (Section 9.4).
(4) At the local level, we extend our examination of long-term disease trends in London, described for the pre-1850 period in Section 2.4, into the late twentieth century (Section 9.5).

The chapter is concluded in Section 9.6.

9.2 Global Pandemic Surges

In this section, we examine long-term trends in three major human infectious diseases that have undergone phases of global expansion in the last 150 years: plague (Section 9.2.1); cholera (Section 9.2.2); and HIV/AIDS (Section 9.2.3). Set within historical context, the pandemic events are identified by the shaded bars in Figure 9.1 and include the Third Plague Pandemic (1850s–1950s), the Third to Seventh (and the putative Eighth) Cholera Pandemics (1852–present), and the currently recognized HIV/AIDS Pandemic (1981–present). The cyclical surges witnessed for plague and cholera have been driven primarily by the exponential increases in inter-location connectivity resulting from the transport changes described in Sections 6.3–6.5. In the case of cholera, the process has been enhanced by microbial changes (Chapter 4). For HIV/AIDS, previously unrecognized pathogens have entered the human

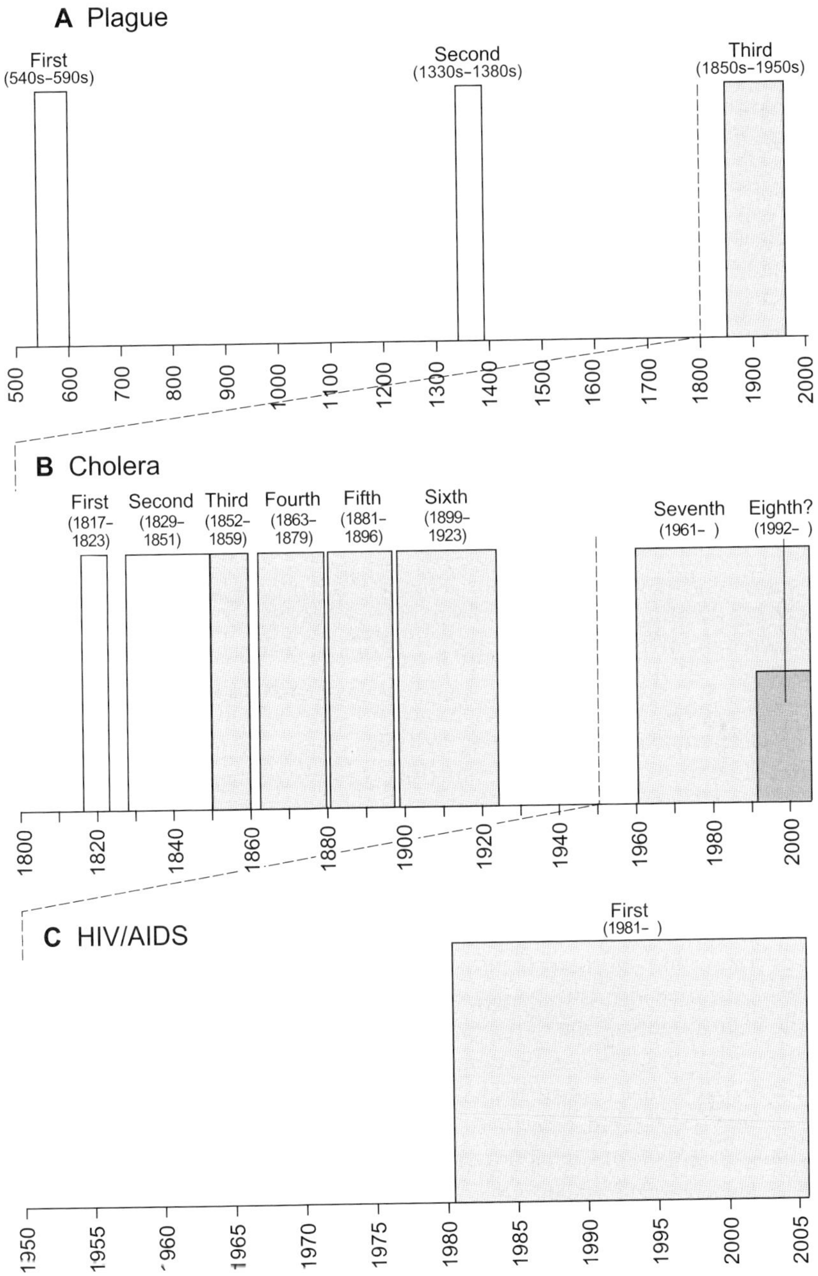

Fig. 9.1. Historical sequence of plague, cholera, and HIV/AIDS pandemics
The time periods encompassed by the three plague pandemics (graph A), seven cholera pandemics (graph B), and the recognized HIV/AIDS pandemic (graph C) are indicated. Pandemics encompassed by our survey period (post-1850) are shaded. The timings of 19th-century cholera pandemics follow the evidence of Pollitzer (1959) and Barua and Greenough (1992) in Table 2.6.

population by zoonotic transmission (Sections 1.5.1, 4.2, and 7.2–7.5) to start the pandemic.

9.2.1 Plague

An overview of the nature and history of plague to 1850 is given in Section 2.3.2. The several centuries of heightened outbreak activity that followed the Second Plague Pandemic (1330s–1380s) were superseded, from the mid-eighteenth century, by an apparent geographical retreat of *Yersinia pestis* to permanent enzootic foci in Central Asia and East Africa. The period of epidemiological quiescence, however, came to an end in the latter half of the nineteenth century as the disease re-emerged in the form of the Third Plague Pandemic (Figure 9.1A).

THE THIRD PANDEMIC (1850s–1950s)

The global diffusion of the Third Plague Pandemic is reconstructed in Figure 9.2. The ultimate origin of the pandemic can be traced to west Yunnan, China—part of the vast enzootic focus of the disease in the Central Asia Highland—in the mid-1850s.[1] From here, plague spread slowly at first, through China, eventually to reach the port cities and international shipping hubs of Canton and Hong Kong in 1894. Details of the subsequent rapid global spread of the disease from these centres are provided by Pollitzer (1954) and Rodenwaldt and Jusatz (1954–61), but Figure 9.2 shows that, fuelled by late nineteenth-century developments in the size, speed, and efficiency of steamships (Section 6.3.1), plague had circumnavigated the world by 1910. As Raettig (1954–61: III/33) observes of this period, 'New foci of sylvan plague arose everywhere . . . lying between 20°C summer isotherms of the northern and southern hemispheres and in which it was possible for the plague causative agents to be transmitted from the rats of the harbour towns to the wild rodents in the vast steppes and semi-desert regions.'

The global time series of reported plague cases associated with the main phase of pandemic transmission, 1899–1953, is plotted in Figure 9.3. The curve displays a rapid growth to a sharp peak in 1911, with pronounced fluctuations superimposed on a steady and progressive decline in reported disease incidence over the next several decades. By the 1950s, Raettig (1954–61: III/33) could report that the pandemic was finally drawing to a close: 'Statistics of the infection show that the prognosis is a favourable one, as plague is receding in all the foci which are still active. The vast pandemia . . . is dying out.' A final assessment of the overall mortality due to the pandemic is

[1] Pollitzer (1954: 15) attributes the disruption of the epidemiological equilibrium of plague, resulting in the initial spread of the disease from a focus in west Yunnan, to the population flux that resulted from the suppression of the Mohammedan Rebellion of 1855.

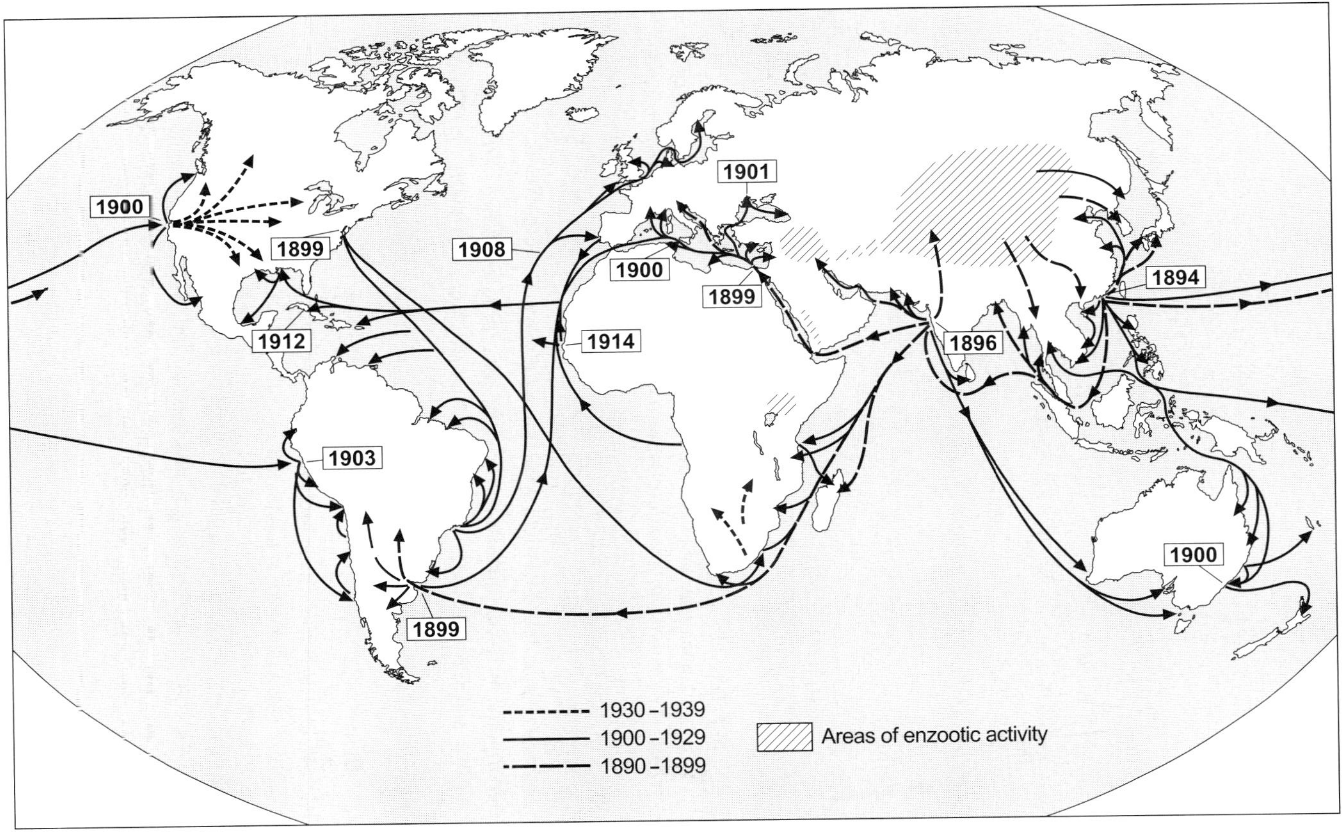

Fig. 9.2. Global spread of the Third Plague Pandemic, 1850s–1950s
Vectors show the diffusion of plague from permanent enzootic foci (diagonally shaded) in Central Asia and East Africa.
Source: Drawn from Rodenwaldt and Jusatz (1954–61, map III/87).

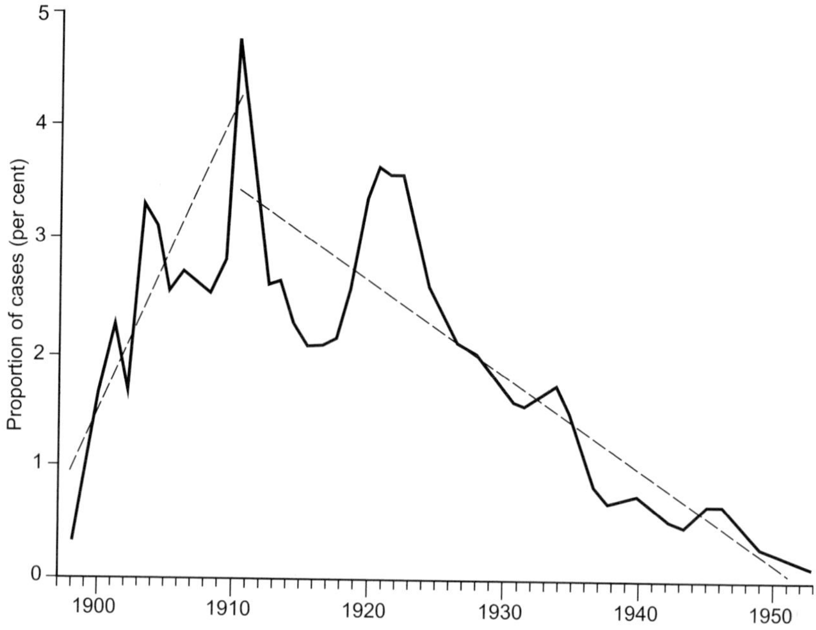

Fig. 9.3. Global curve of annual plague incidence, 1899–1953
Annual counts of plague cases are expressed as a percentage proportion of all cases in the 55-year observation period. Underpinning trends are indicated for the periods 1899–1911 and 1911–53 by the broken lines.
Source: Redrawn from Raettig (1954–61, fig. 1, p. III/33).

precluded by the fragmentary nature of the available evidence, although a global figure of >10 million deaths—mainly in Asia—is cited by Khan (2004).[2]

GLOBAL TRENDS AND EARLY TWENTY-FIRST CENTURY OUTBREAKS

A broad—albeit incomplete—impression of the global trend in plague can be gained from Figure 9.4, which plots, as a histogram, the annual count of recorded human cases in the principal regional centres of disease activity (Africa, the Americas, and Asia), 1935–2003. Following the termination of the period of heightened disease activity associated with the tail-end of the Third Plague Pandemic in the 1940s and 1950s, Figure 9.4 identifies two phases of modestly raised plague incidence:

[2] Pollitzer (1954: 16–70) provides a detailed review of documented plague mortality in individual countries and regions. See also the regional overviews by Raettig *et al.* (1954–61*a,b,c*).

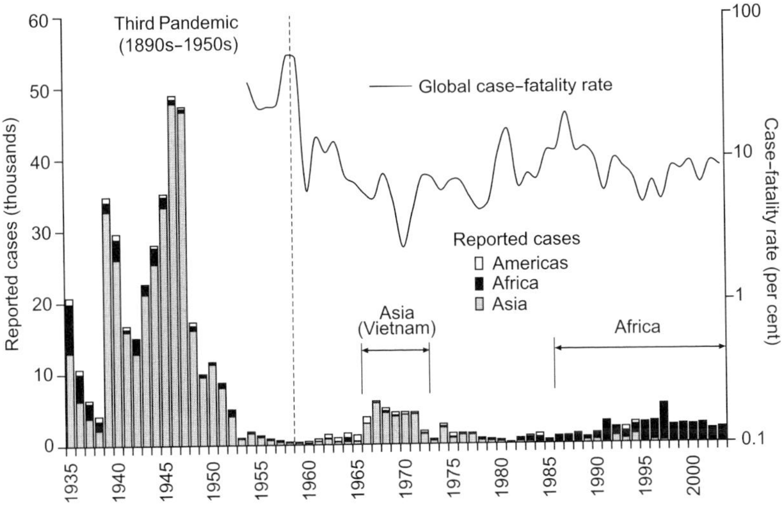

Fig. 9.4. Global trends in plague, 1935–2003

The bar chart plots the annual count of reported plague cases by continent. The line trace is based on plague cases and deaths reported to the WHO and plots the estimated global case-fatality rate, 1954–2003. Locations associated with heightened plague activity in the late twentieth and early twenty-first centuries are indicated.

Sources: Drawn from data assembled from World Health Organization (1949, table 1, pp. 144–5; 2000*b*, table 3.1; 2004*b*, table 1, pp. 304–6), Pollitzer (1954, table II, p. 27), Raettig *et al.* (1954–61*a*, table C, p. III/27; 1954–61*c*, table C, p. II/48), and Velimirovic (1972, tables III, VI, VII, VIII, X, pp. 484, 489, 491, 492, 496).

(i) *late 1960s/early 1970s*, centred on Asia and associated with the re-emergence of plague in consequence of the ecological and economic disruptions engendered by the Vietnam War (Velimirovic 1972);

(ii) *mid-1980s onwards*, centred on East and Central Africa, notably the Democratic Republic of the Congo, Madagascar, and Tanzania (see, for example, Kilonzo *et al.* 1992; World Health Organization 1992*b*; Chanteau *et al.* 1998), and marking a shift in the epicentre of reported disease activity away from the Asian continent.

Factors associated with the evolution of phase (i) are described in Section 8.2.2, while the events surrounding the dramatic reappearance of human plague in India in 1994—after almost 30 years of silence in the subcontinent—are reviewed in Section 11.2.4.

Early Twenty-First-Century Outbreaks

Figure 9.5 plots the location of human plague outbreaks as documented in the WHO Epidemic and Pandemic Alert and Response's (EPR) *Disease Outbreak News*, 2001–6, against a backdrop of known and probable foci of

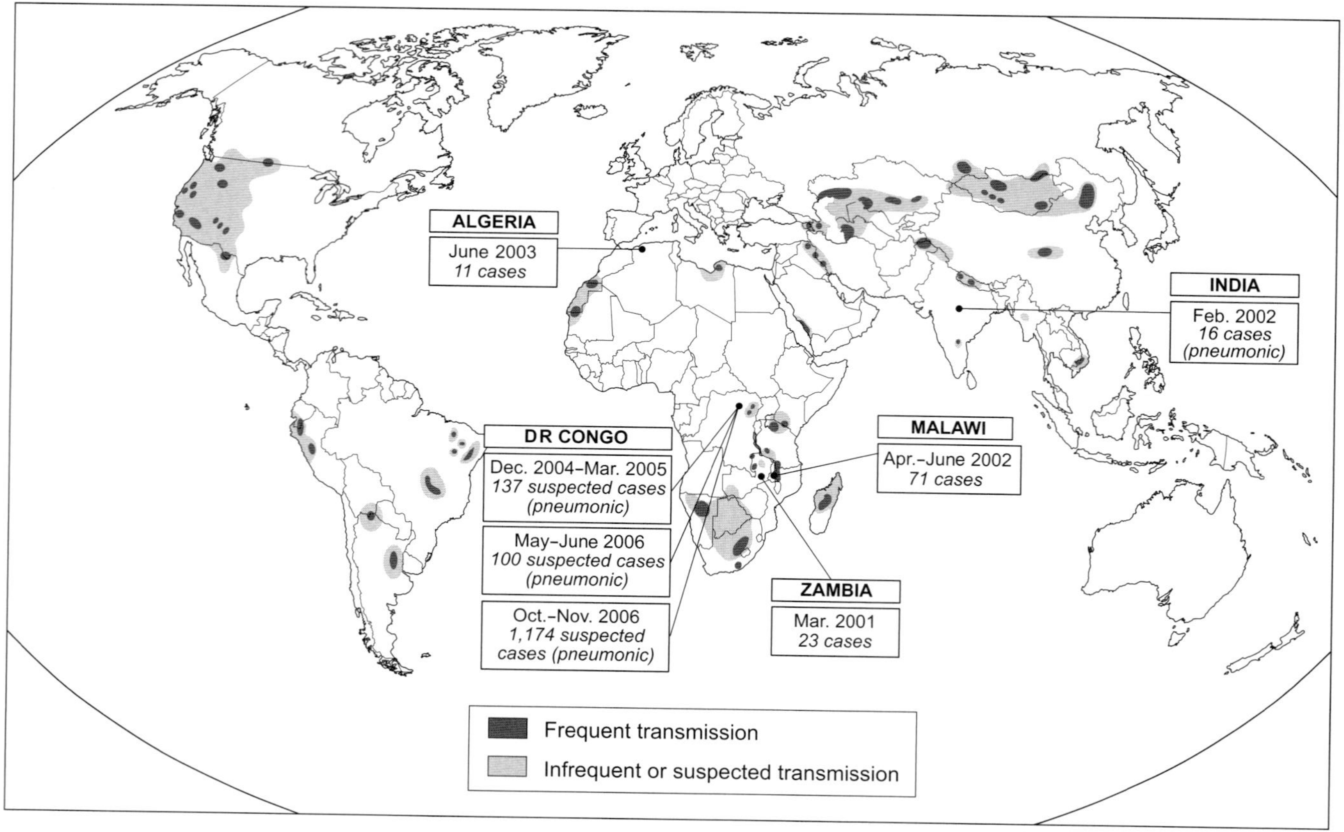

Fig. 9.5. Early twenty-first-century outbreaks of plague
The locations of outbreaks of human plague as documented in the WHO Epidemic and Pandemic Alert and Response's (EPR) *Disease Outbreak News*, 2001–6, are set against a backdrop of known and probable foci of plague transmission.
Sources: Redrawn from Cliff, Haggett, and Smallman-Raynor (2004, fig. 2.12, p. 24), with additional information from World Health Organization Epidemic and Pandemic Alert and Response (2008).

plague transmission. As the map shows, plague foci are present on all continents (except Australia) within a broad belt of tropical, subtropical, and warmer temperate climates between parallels 55° N and 40° S. Within this distribution, Figure 9.5 identifies a series of documented outbreaks of bubonic and suspected pneumonic plague in the Central African states of Zambia (2001), Malawi (2002), and the Democratic Republic of the Congo (2004–5, 2006). To the north, the re-emergence of plague in Algeria (2003) after a 50-year absence may have been associated with a previously unrecognized natural focus of the disease, while, in Asia, a small outbreak (16 cases) of pneumonic plague was recorded in India during 2002 (World Health Organization 2004*b*).

PROSPECTS FOR THE FUTURE

Concerns over the future re-emergence of plague arise from anthropogenic changes associated with the increasing human invasion of natural plague foci, the special challenges posed by war-related population displacements, and the deteriorating sanitary conditions in the urban centres of developing countries. As Dennis (1998: 180) explains of the latter:

> Throughout the developing world, massive urbanization has outstripped sanitary and hygienic measures needed to control rats at acceptable levels. Socioeconomic deprivation of recent immigrants, slums, unprotected food stores, uncollected garbage, lack of sewage facilities, and tolerance of rat infestations characterize these rapidly growing urban centers. It is surprising that large epidemics of urban bubonic plague have not happened in the second half of the 20th century, since the environmental conditions appear to be ripe for such occurrences.

The issues of antimicrobial resistance discussed in Section 4.3 also gain prominence. The recent recovery of multidrug-resistant (MDR) strains of *Y. pestis* from patients in Madagascar has raised concerns over the treatment and prevention of the disease. Although antimicrobial resistance in the plague bacterium is still considered rare, the potential for the rapid natural evolution of high levels of drug resistance warrants the need for systematic global surveillance of the phenomenon (Galimand *et al.* 2006; Welch *et al.* 2007).

9.2.2 *Cholera*

An overview of the nature and history of Asiatic cholera to 1850 is given in Section 2.3.4. As described there, the cholera pandemics of 1817–23 (First Cholera Pandemic) and 1829–51 (Second Cholera Pandemic) signalled the onset of a cycle of global pandemic events, of greater or lesser intensity and duration, that has continued through to the present day (Figure 9.1B).

PANDEMIC EVENTS, 1850–1925

Following the timings of Pollitzer (1959) in Table 2.6, four pandemics (referred to in the historical sequence of Figure 9.1B as the Third to Sixth Cholera Pandemics) followed hard on the heels of each other in the period 1850–1925. The specific strains of *V. cholerae* associated with the early events are unknown, although the Sixth Pandemic has been ascribed to the classical biotype of *V. cholerae* O1 (Barua 1992; Kaper *et al.* 1995). As illustrated for major phases of the Fourth (1863–79) and Fifth (1881–96) Pandemics in Figure 9.6, cholera travelled on each occasion from the Indian subcontinent into Asia and Europe via the great trade routes, spreading eventually to Africa and—with the exception of the Sixth Pandemic—the Americas. On each occasion, certain common factors conspired to accelerate the progression of the pandemics. The annual pilgrimages to Mecca (haj) were one such factor, as described by Rodenwaldt (1952: I/13) for the early stages of the Fourth Cholera Pandemic (Figure 9.6A):

> The disastrous spread of this epidemic [in May 1865] was due to the fact that it coincided with the Hadj Festival [*sic*]...Tens of thousands of people gathered in Jidda and Mecca under primitive conditions...
>
> Among the pilgrims gathered in Mecca panic broke out in the first days of May. They fled in all directions. By 19th of May cholera had broken out in Suez. Early in June all parts of Lower Egypt including Alexandria were infected. From there, during June and July, almost all important Mediterranean ports were infected via the sea route. The disease reached Malta on 20th June. In August cholera appeared in the ports of the Black Sea...
>
> Meanwhile, fleeing pilgrims had carried the disease through the interior of Arabia to the Shatt-al-Arab, and in August the ports on the Persian Gulf were infected.

Major wars (Chapter 8) also regularly fuelled pandemic transmission, as illustrated by the events of the Crimean War (1853–6) in the Third Pandemic, the Austro-Prussian War (1866) in the Fourth, and the Philippine–American War (1899–1902) in the Sixth (Smallman-Raynor and Cliff 1998*a*,*b*, 2004*a*,*b*).

TIME TRENDS

Figure 9.7 has been drawn from reports assembled by the WHO and plots the annual incidence of cholera by world region, 1935–2006. As the graph shows, cholera was confined largely to Asia in the decades that followed on from the 1899–1923 pandemic.[3] Beginning in the early 1960s, however, the disease re-emerged in the form of the Seventh Cholera Pandemic (Figure 9.1B).

[3] The 1947 epidemic of cholera in Egypt, associated with some 20,500 deaths, represents a noteworthy exception to this apparent geographical confinement (Barua 1992: 15–16).

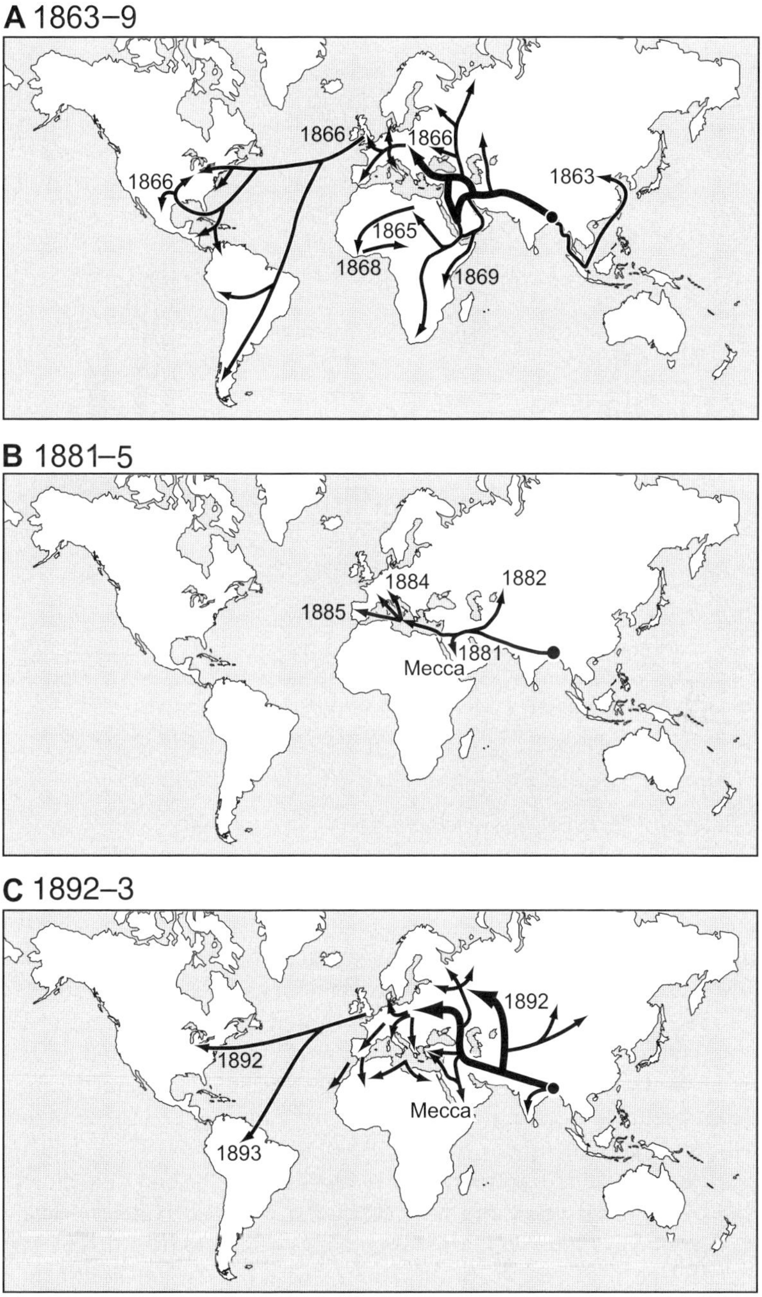

Fig. 9.6. Global diffusion routes of two late nineteenth-century cholera pandemics Vectors show the diffusion of cholera associated with major phases of the Fourth (1863–9; map A) and Fifth (1881–5, 1892–3; maps B, C) Cholera Pandemics.

Source: Redrawn from Cliff and Haggett (1988, fig. 1.1D, p. 5).

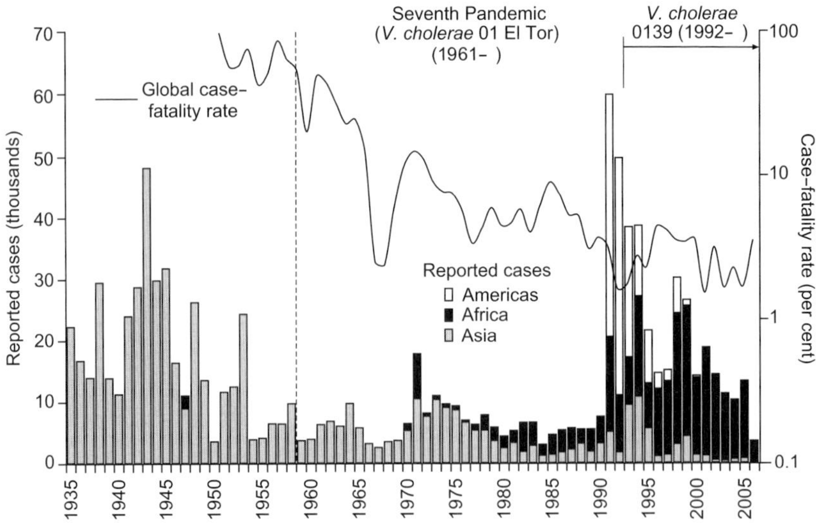

Fig. 9.7. Global trends in cholera, 1935–2006
The bar chart plots the annual count of reported cholera cases by continent, 1935–2006. The line trace is based on cholera cases and deaths reported to the WHO and plots the estimated global case-fatality rate, 1954–2006.
Sources: Drawn from data in World Health Organization (1947, table 1, p. 140; 2008*b*).

The Seventh (El Tor) Cholera Pandemic (1961–present)

The year 1961 marked the spread, apparently for the first time, of the El Tor biotype of *V. cholerae* serogroup O1 as a pandemic infection.[4] While each of the preceding six pandemics had originated in the Indian subcontinent, the source of the El Tor pandemic can be traced to the Indonesian island of Sulawesi. Epidemics of El Tor cholera were first observed in southern Sulawesi in 1937–8 and, again, in 1939–40, 1944, and 1957–8. Beginning in 1960–1, outbreak activity began to extend to the north of the island and on to other parts of the Indonesian archipelago (Mukerjee 1963; Hermann 1973). From thereon, Figure 9.8 shows that the El Tor pandemic spread to mainland Asia (1960s) and subsequently to Africa (1970s) and Europe (1970s). The appearance of the disease in the Americas (1990s) marked the end of a cholera-free period of over 100 years and was associated with the explosive upsurge in cases depicted in Figure 9.7. Major epidemics were also recorded in Africa in the 1990s (see, for example, Section 8.3.2), with the African continent emerging as the primary regional focus of reported cholera activity by the early

[4] *V. cholerae* O1 (biotype El Tor) was first identified in Indonesian pilgrims at the El Tor quarantine station, Egypt, in 1905.

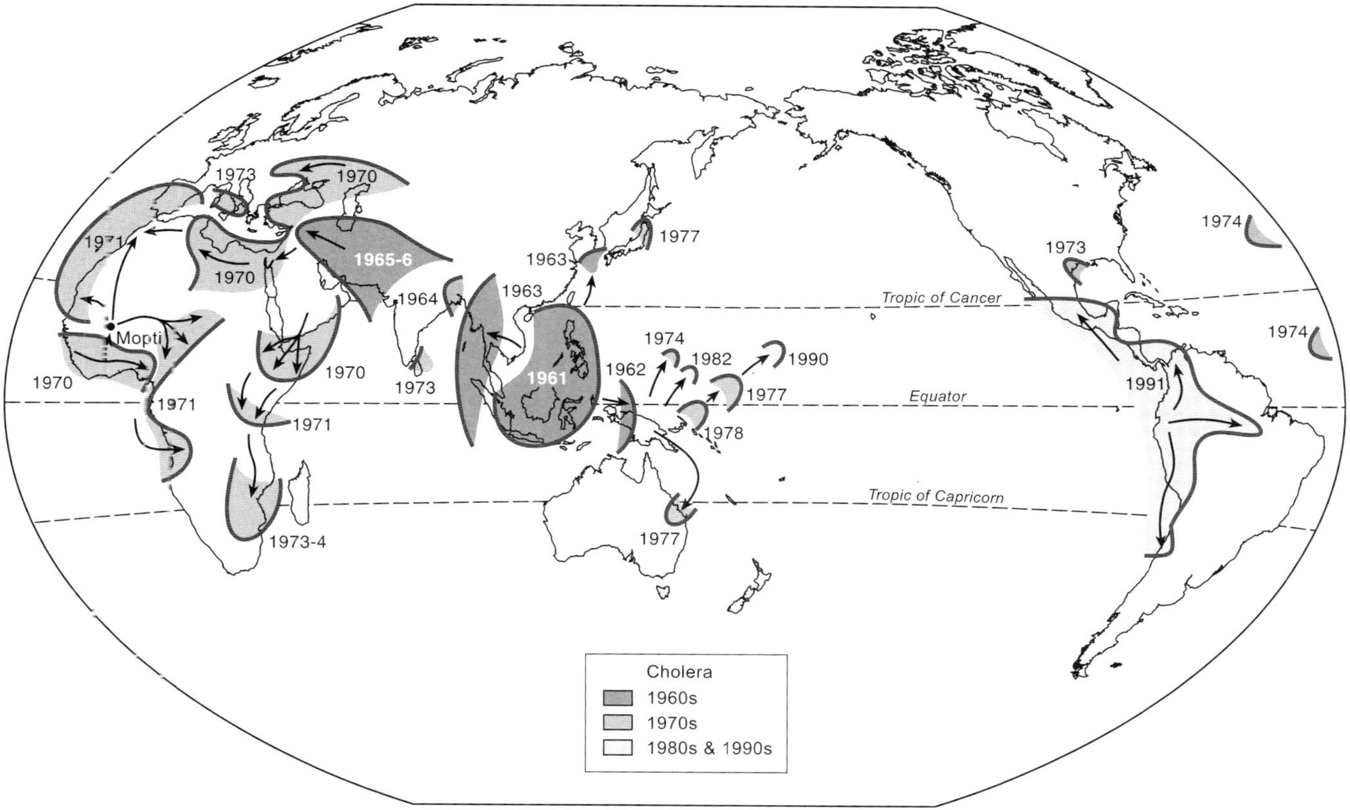

Fig. 9.8. The Seventh Cholera Pandemic (El Tor biotype), 1961–present
Global spread of the seventh pandemic of cholera from an Indonesian source.

Sources: Redrawn from Cliff, Haggett, and Smallman-Raynor (2004, fig. 2.27, p. 31), originally from Barua and Greenhough (1992, fig. 1, p. 132).

twenty-first century (Figure 9.7). Kaper *et al.* (1995) cite the following factors that contributed to the extensive spread of El Tor cholera after 1961: (i) the enhanced capacity for El Tor vibrios to survive in environmental niches; (ii) the relatively mild nature of El Tor cholera and the high frequency of asymptomatic excretors; and, as described in Chapter 6, (iii) the heightened opportunities for disease dispersal with air passenger traffic.

The Emergence of V. cholerae *O139*

While the Seventh Pandemic continues, recent developments have pointed to the possible emergence of a putative Eighth Cholera Pandemic associated with a novel epidemic strain, *V. cholerae* O139 (Swerdlow and Ries 1993; Kaper *et al.* 1995) (Figure 9.1B). Cholera due to *V. cholerae* O139 was first observed during major epidemics in Bangladesh and India in 1992 and, soon thereafter, in Afghanistan, China, Kazakhstan, Malaysia, Nepal, Pakistan, and Thailand (Kaper *et al.* 1995). Since that time, *V. cholerae* O139 has demonstrated a propensity to pulse-retreat and re-emerge within its original foci of infection (Mukhopadhyay *et al.* 1998; Faruque *et al.* 2003). Although the bacterium has been carried to other continents by travellers, epidemic activity still remains confined to South-East Asia (Heymann 2004: 106).

Trends in Cholera Mortality

The line trace in Figure 9.7 plots, on a logarithmic scale, annual estimates of the global case-fatality rate for cholera, 1951–2006. Beginning with very high estimates (>50.0 per cent) in the 1950s, the early years of the El Tor pandemic were coincident with a pronounced reduction of case-fatality rates to low levels (<5.0 per cent) from the mid-1970s. This reduction reflects (i) the milder nature of El Tor cholera vis-à-vis classical cholera and, since the 1970s and 1980s, (ii) the wider availability of oral rehydration therapy and other improved treatments. Marked regional variations in case-fatality rates persist, however, with early twenty-first-century estimates ranging from <0.3 per cent (Asia) to >3.0 per cent (Africa).

TWENTY-FIRST-CENTURY OUTBREAKS

Cholera remains a major and growing disease threat in the early twenty-first century. The Seventh Pandemic shows some signs of intensifying rather than abating, while the appearance of *V. cholerae* O139 has prompted close international surveillance by the WHO. Figure 9.9 is based on information included in the WHO Epidemic and Pandemic Alert and Response's (EPR) *Disease Outbreak News*, and plots, by geographical region, the number of countries in which outbreaks of cholera were documented each year, 2001–6. Geographical locations which reported especially large outbreaks (>10,000 cases) in each annual period are indicated. Consistent with the geographical trend in Figure 9.7, countries of Africa accounted for the majority (91 per

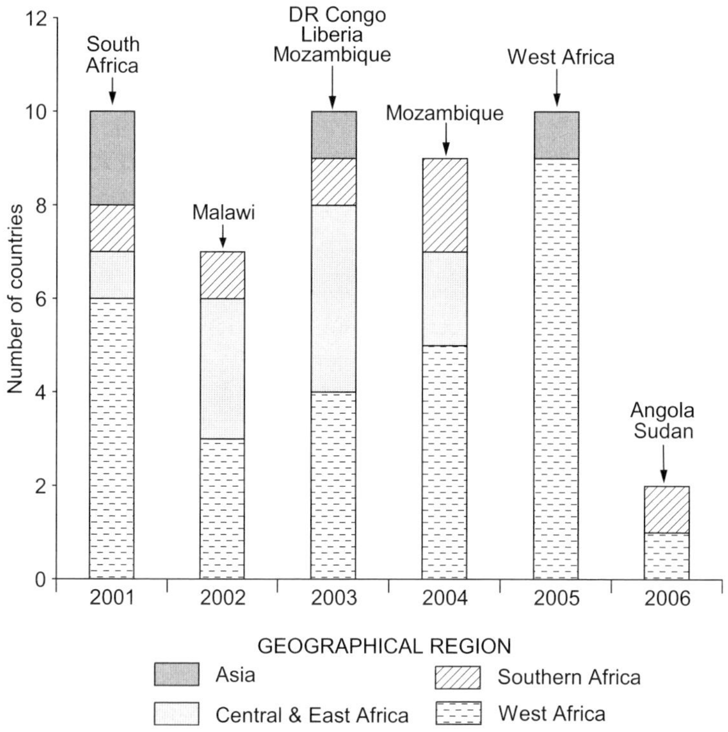

Fig. 9.9. Geographical distribution of cholera outbreaks reported in the WHO Epidemic and Pandemic Alert and Response's (EPR) *Disease Outbreak News*, 2001–2006 Bars show the annual count of countries in which outbreaks were documented, 17 April 2001–21 June 2006. Countries reporting large outbreaks (>10,000 cases) in a given year are named.

Source: Based on World Health Organization Epidemic and Pandemic Alert and Response (2008).

cent) of documented outbreaks in Figure 9.9, with events in South Africa in 2001 (>86,000 cases), Malawi in 2002 (>22,000 cases), the Democratic Republic of the Congo in 2003 (>13,000 cases), Mozambique in 2003–4 (>27,000 cases), West Africa in 2005 (>77,000 cases), and Angola in 2006 (>46,000 cases) being of particular magnitude.

9.2.3 HIV/AIDS

The acquired immunodeficiency syndrome (AIDS) is a severe, life-threatening, disease which was first recognized as a distinct clinical syndrome in 1981. The syndrome is a manifestation of advanced infection with the human immunodeficiency virus (HIV). The general term 'HIV/AIDS' is used by the Joint United Nations Programme on HIV/AIDS (UNAIDS) and other official bodies to refer to the pandemic of infection and disease associated with HIV, and we adopt that term in the present discussion.

NATURE OF AIDS

The immune system usually serves to safeguard the body against the invasion of disease-causing micro-organisms such as bacteria, protozoa, and viruses. In AIDS, however, the immune system collapses and leaves the body open to potentially life-threatening opportunistic infections, the development of rare and unusually aggressive cancers, dementia, wasting, and other severe conditions. The immune dysfunction that eventually gives rise to AIDS is a continuous process over a variable, but usually protracted, period of several years or more. During this time, an HIV-infected person will typically pass through a series of stages ranging from an acute retroviral syndrome (a short-lived glandular-fever-type disease) in the very early stages of infection with HIV, through a prolonged period of asymptomatic infection associated with a progressive subclinical immune dysfunction, an early symptomatic stage (sometimes referred to as AIDS-related complex, or ARC), eventually progressing to advanced or late-stage disease (AIDS). During the long course of infection, the disease manifestations range from none, through non-specific illnesses and opportunistic infections, to autoimmune and neurological disorders and several types of malignancy, especially Kaposi's sarcoma. For further details, see Heymann (2004: 1–9).

The Human Immunodeficiency Virus (HIV)

The human immunodeficiency virus is classified as a member of the lentivirus sub-family of the virus family *Retroviridae*. Two serologically distinct types of HIV are currently recognized, HIV-1 and HIV-2. While HIV-1 is the virus associated with the global AIDS pandemic, HIV-2 appears to be less aggressive and more geographically limited in distribution (largely restricted to West Africa). Human beings are the reservoir of HIV, and three primary routes of virus transfer can be identified: sexual, parenteral, and perinatal. Susceptibility to HIV infection and associated immune deficiency appears to be general. The incubation period for AIDS is highly variable, with the observed time from primary infection with HIV to the diagnosis of AIDS ranging from <1 year to >15 years. In more developed countries, at least, the increasing availability of effective antiretroviral therapies has served to reduce the development of clinical AIDS since the mid-1990s (Heymann 2004: 1–9).

ORIGINS AND GLOBAL DISPERSALS

The geographical origins of the global HIV/AIDS pandemic have been the subject of intense speculation over the last quarter-century. Early hypotheses pointed to the Caribbean island of Hispaniola in general, and the country of Haiti in particular, as the possible source of the disease (see Smallman-Raynor, Cliff, and Haggett 1992: 129–31). By the mid-1980s, however, scientific debate about the geographical origins of the then newly identified HIV-1 and HIV-2 had switched to the African continent. A number of virologists now consider that the origins of HIV lie with the cross-species transmission of related viruses of non-human primates (simian immunodeficiency viruses, or SIVs) in sub-Saharan Africa (Van Heuverswyn and Peeters 2007).[5] Recent research has pointed to the emergence of pandemic strains of HIV-1 as a result of cross-species transmission of an SIV from chimpanzees (*Pan troglodytes troglodytes*) in Central Africa (Gao, Bailes, *et al.* 1999; Keele *et al.* 2006). Similar studies have attributed the emergence of HIV-2 to the cross-species transmission of an SIV from the sooty mangabey (*Cercocebus atys*) in West Africa (Gao, Yue, White, *et al.* 1992; Gao, Yue, Robertson, *et al.* 1994). As for the timings of these events, HIVs are known to have been infecting humans in the 1950s and 1960s (Smallman-Raynor, Cliff, and Haggett 1992: 120–8), with current evidence pointing to human infection with the common ancestral virus of the pandemic HIV-1 group M prior to the 1940s (Sharp, Bailes, *et al.* 2001).

Global Diffusion Patterns I: HIV-1

A number of models have attempted to reconstruct the geographical corridors by which HIV-1 has spread from its postulated origin in central Africa to establish itself as a global pandemic infection (Shannon *et al.* 1991: 40–50; Smallman-Raynor, Cliff, and Haggett 1992: 143–6). Foremost among the models proposed is that of Robert C. Gallo, co-discoverer of the virus. Figure 9.10A is underpinned by the Gallo model and shows one possible scenario for the time-sequenced global spread of HIV-1. Gallo hypothesized that, from a hearth in sub-Saharan Africa, HIV-1 was carried to Haiti by Haitian technicians and professionals who had been working in the erstwhile Zaire (now the Democratic Republic of the Congo) under the auspices of the United Nations during the 1960s and 1970s. These workers, who had replaced the expelled Belgian administrators following Zairean independence in 1960, began to return at a time when Haiti was becoming a vacation destination for North American homosexuals. Haiti was then seen as a stepping stone for HIV spread into North America, from whence the virus diffused to the rest of the world (Gallo 1987; Smallman-Raynor, Cliff, and Haggett 1992: 144–6). Although the estimated timings of events vary, the initial spread sequence invoked by the model (Central Africa → Haiti → United States) is consistent with the early phylogenetic analysis of Li, Tanimura, *et al.* (1988) and, more recently, Gilbert, Rambaut, *et al.* (2007).

[5] For an alternative perspective, see Hooper (1999).

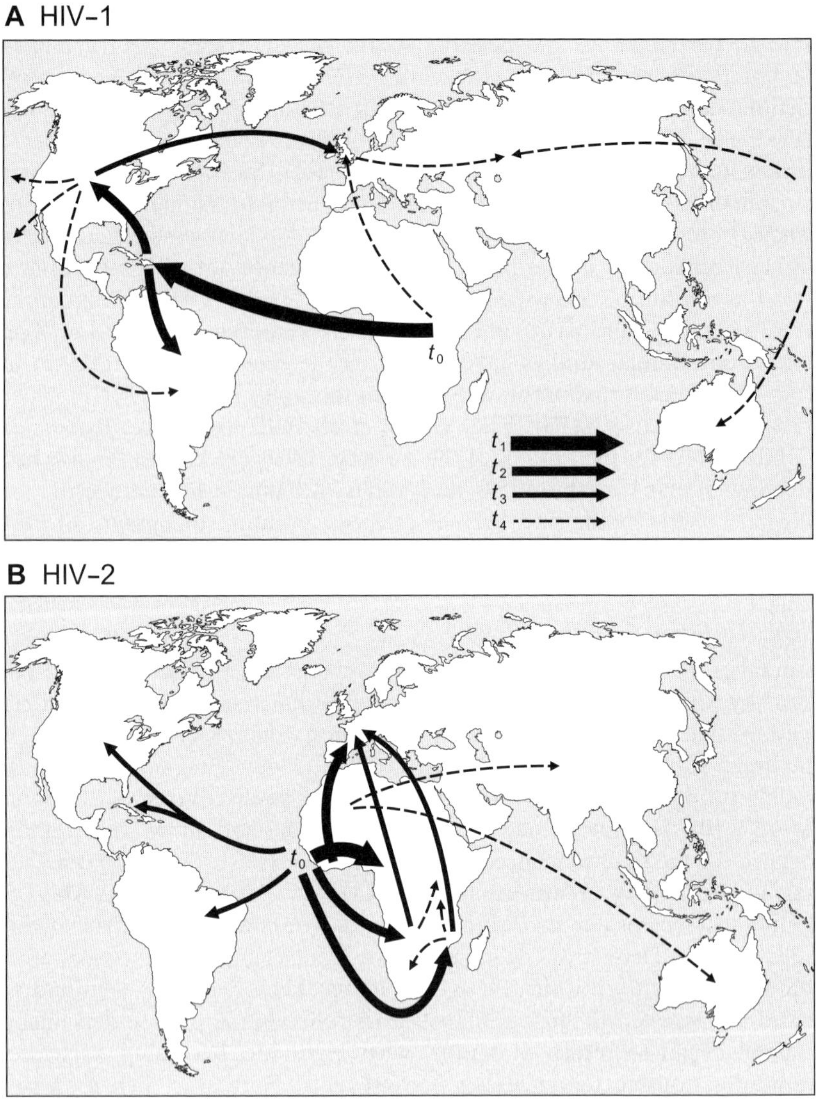

Fig. 9.10. Global diffusion routes of HIV-1 and HIV-2
(A) Global spread of HIV-1, illustrating the Gallo hypothesis of an initial series of linkages between Central Africa, the Caribbean, and North America. (B) Global spread of HIV-2, based on the case histories of patients reported in the 1980s and the early 1990s. Vector weights indicate the inferred time sequences (t_1, ..., t_4) of virus transmission.

Source: Adapted from Smallman-Raynor, Cliff, and Haggett (1992, figs 4.1A and 4.9C, pp. 144, 181).

Global Diffusion Patterns II: HIV-2

The global extent of HIV-2 differs fundamentally from that of HIV-1. At the time of its first isolation in 1983–4, HIV-1 was already firmly established in much of the Americas, Europe, and Central Africa. In contrast, HIV-2, originally isolated from West African patients in 1986, is still primarily concentrated in sub-Saharan Africa. Although there has been limited spread to other regions, and this evidence has been used by Smallman-Raynor, Cliff, and Haggett (1992: 174–82) to construct the general model of global transmission in Figure 9.10B, HIV-2 has not established itself as a pandemic infection of HIV-1 proportions. Indeed, since the available evidence points to West Africa as the source of the virus, it appears that HIV-2 has remained largely concentrated in its original heartland.

GLOBAL PANDEMIC TRENDS

The current size of the HIV/AIDS pandemic can be judged from Table 9.1. As global estimates for the year 2007, UNAIDS reported that 33.2 million people were living with HIV, 2.5 million people were newly infected with HIV, and 2.1 million people had died of AIDS. Whether viewed in terms of mortality or overall disease burden, HIV/AIDS ranks as one of the most important infectious health threats in the early twenty-first century (Cliff, Haggett, and Smallman-Raynor 2004: 157–8).

Table 9.1. Estimated HIV/AIDS statistics for 2007

Geographical area	Adults and children living with HIV[1] (000)	Adults and children newly infected with HIV[1] (000)	Adult (15–49 years) HIV prevalence (%)	Adult and child deaths due to AIDS[1] (000)
Sub-Saharan Africa	22,500	1,700	5.0	1,600.0
North Africa & Middle East	380	35	0.3	25.0
South & South-East Asia	4,000	340	0.3	270.0
East Asia	800	92	0.1	32.0
Oceania	75	14	0.4	1.2
Latin America	1,600	100	0.5	58.0
Caribbean	230	17	1.0	11.0
Eastern Europe & Central Asia	1,600	150	0.9	55.0
Western & Central Europe	760	31	0.3	12.0
North America	1,300	46	0.6	21.0
TOTAL	33,200	2,500	0.8	2,100.0

Note: [1] Adults defined as individuals aged ≥15 years.
Source: UNAIDS (2007, table 1, p. 7).

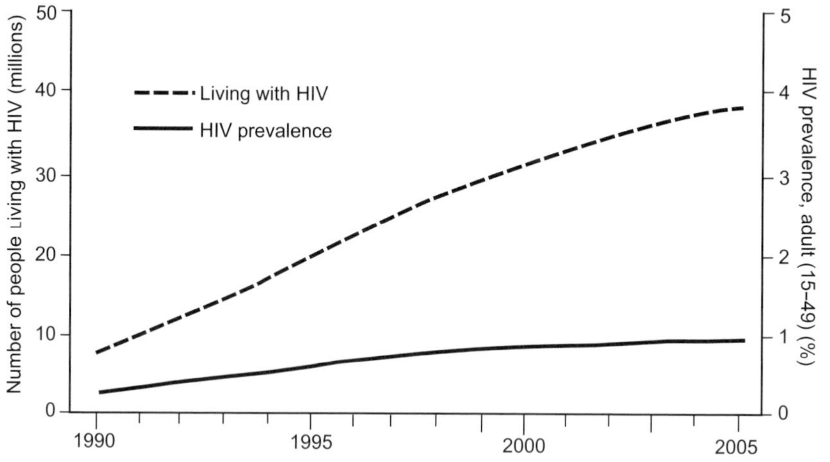

Fig. 9.11. Global trends in HIV/AIDS
The graph plots, by year, UNAIDS estimates of the number of people living with HIV (upper line trace) and the prevalence of HIV infection for adults aged 15–49 years (lower line trace), 1990–2007.
Source: Redrawn from UNAIDS (2007, figs 1, 2, pp. 4, 5).

Time Series

Some impression of the growth of the HIV/AIDS pandemic to its 2005 level can be gained from Figure 9.11. The growth curves plot, on an annual basis, UNAIDS global estimates of the number of people living with HIV infection (upper line trace) and the prevalence of HIV infection in adults aged 15–49 years (lower line trace), 1990–2005. Two prominent features of the global pandemic emerge from the growth curves. First, the rapid and sustained increase in the number of people living with HIV, from <10 million (1990) to >33.2 million (2005), reflects the effects of both natural population growth and, from the mid-1990s, the availability of life-prolonging antiretroviral treatments. Second, consistent with evidence for changes in HIV incidence,[6] the latter years of the observation period were associated with an apparent stabilization of the overall prevalence of HIV in adults at a little under 1.0 per cent.

Map Sequences

The spatial evolution of the HIV/AIDS pandemic is traced in Figure 9.12. The maps plot UNAIDS estimates of the prevalence of HIV in adults aged 15–49 years for 1985 (map A), 1995 (map B), and 2007 (map C); summary

[6] We use the term 'incidence' to refer to newly reported HIV diagnoses as distinct from recent HIV infections. Estimates of the latter have been facilitated by recent advances in HIV testing technologies and are increasingly being reported in US HIV publications. See Centers for Disease Control and Prevention (2008*c*) for further details.

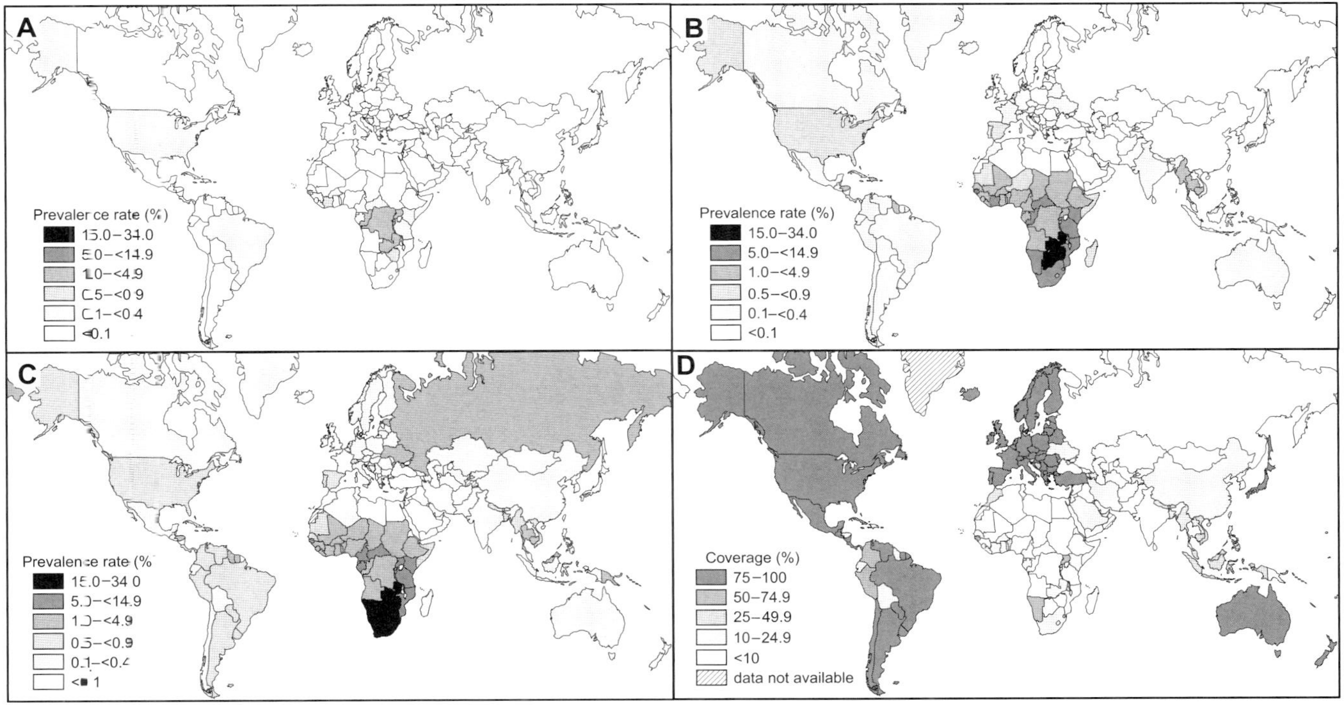

Fig. 9.12. The global HIV/AIDS pandemic
UNAIDS estimates of HIV prevalence rates (per cent) for adults aged 15–49 years in (A) 1985, (B) 1995, and (C) 2007. Map D shows, for a sample point in time (June 2005), national estimates of the percentage proportion of people on antiretroviral therapy among those in need.

Sources: Redrawn from UNAIDS (maps A–C) and WHO/UNAIDS (map D), accessed via World Health Organization (2007*f*).

regional statistics for the 2007 map are given in Table 9.1. Maps 9.12A–C show generally high and intensifying levels of HIV infection in sub-Saharan Africa, with a pronounced geographical shift in the principal focus of activity from Central and East Africa (1985, map A) to southern Africa (2007, map C) over the observation period. By 2007, an estimated 5.0 per cent of adults aged 15–49 years were infected with HIV in sub-Saharan Africa (Table 9.1), with levels of 15.0–28.0 per cent in the southern sector of the region (Figure 9.12C). Elsewhere, the maps identify certain sharp increases in HIV prevalence in some countries of the Americas, Asia, and eastern Europe, although, as regional aggregates, the majority tendency is for levels of infection to lie below the global estimate of 0.8 per cent (Table 9.1).

PROSPECTS

With distant prospect of a marketable HIV vaccine (Steinbrook 2007), the prevention of HIV/AIDS continues to depend on education, condom promotion, and the treatment and control of other sexually transmitted diseases. Once HIV infection has been acquired, antiretroviral drugs have the potential to lengthen life, as well as to reduce the risk of interpersonal HIV transmission and HIV transmission from mother to child. But antiretroviral therapy is expensive, and, despite general use in the industrialized countries of North America, western Europe, and the Pacific, it is largely unavailable to the needy in much of Africa, Asia, and parts of eastern Europe (Figure 9.12D). Unless unforeseen changes occur, the ravages of the HIV/AIDS pandemic are likely to persist well into the present century and beyond.

9.3 Regional Epidemics: Trends and Time Sequences

In this section, we turn to a consideration of infectious diseases in major regional divisions of the world. We begin by establishing general trends in disease mortality for the advanced regional economies of Europe, North America, and the South Pacific, 1901–75 (Section 9.3.1). Moving from temperate to tropical latitudes, we then examine in Section 9.3.2 sample time sequences of disease emergence (Ebola–Marburg viral diseases) and cyclical re-emergence (meningococcal disease) in sub-Saharan Africa.

9.3.1 Twentieth-Century Trends in Mortality: Advanced Regional Economies

THE DATABASE

This subsection makes use of the monumental collection of mortality data assembled by Alderson (1981) in his *International Mortality Statistics.*

Details of the data set are provided by Smallman-Raynor and Cliff (2004*b*: 130–43). For the purposes of the present analysis, we draw on Alderson's estimates of age- and sex-standardized mortality ratios (SMRs) for 24 infectious causes of death and pneumonia (Table 9.2) in 29 economically advanced countries (Table 9.3) over 15 quinquennial periods, 1901–5 to 1971–5. Here, our designation of the sample countries as 'economically advanced' is based on their classification by the World Bank (2008) as upper-middle- and high-income economies in terms of gross national income (GNI).

Construction of Regional Mortality Series

While European countries dominate the geographical sample in Table 9.3, we note that there are representatives from North America (Canada, US) and the South Pacific (Australia, New Zealand) on which to undertake a world regional comparison of trends in advanced economies. For each of the 25 causes of death in Table 9.2, the average SMR in a given quinquennium was calculated across the constituent countries of each of the designated regions in Table 9.3 to yield 25 (disease) $\times$ 15 (quinquennia) matrices of average SMRs for Europe, North America, and the South Pacific. The regional matrices of average SMRs form the basis of all analysis in this subsection.

A Note on the Sample Diseases

In making the selection of diseases in Table 9.2, the overlapping categories of 'typhoid and paratyphoid fever', 'typhoid fever', and 'paratyphoid fever and other salmonella infections' have been included. Following Alderson (1981), the decision to include all three reflects the distinction, contingent on diagnostic developments, which was drawn between the different forms of salmonellosis in the mortality statistics of some countries from the early twentieth century. We also note here that Alderson's category 'pneumonia' is formed to include mortality from pneumonias of infectious and non-infectious aetiologies and the results should be interpreted accordingly.

Table 9.2. International mortality trends, 1901–1975: list of 25 causes of mortality selected from Alderson (1981)

Anthrax	Plague
Brucellosis	Pneumonia
Cholera	Poliomyelitis
Diphtheria	Respiratory infections
Dysentery	Tuberculosis (all forms)
Gonococcal infection	Tuberculosis (non-respiratory)
Hepatitis (infectious)	Tuberculosis (respiratory)
Influenza	Typhoid and paratyphoid fever
Leprosy	Typhoid fever
Malaria	Typhus and other rickettsial diseases
Measles	Whooping cough
Meningococcal infections	Yellow fever
Paratyphoid fever and other salmonella infections	

Table 9.3. International mortality trends, 1901–1975: list of countries selected from Alderson's (1981) data set for analysis in Section 9.3.1

Country	Designated region	Country	Designated region
Australia	South Pacific	New Zealand	South Pacific
Austria	Europe	Norway	Europe
Belgium	Europe	Poland	Europe
Bulgaria	Europe	Portugal	Europe
Canada	North America	Romania	Europe
Czechoslovakia	Europe	Spain	Europe
Denmark	Europe	Sweden	Europe
Eire	Europe	Switzerland	Europe
Finland	Europe	Turkey	Europe
France	Europe	UK: England and Wales	Europe
Greece	Europe	UK: Northern Ireland	Europe
Hungary	Europe	UK: Scotland	Europe
Iceland	Europe	US	North America
Italy	Europe	Yugoslavia	Europe
Netherlands	Europe		

EUROPEAN TRENDS

We begin with a consideration of disease trends in Europe. For each of the 25 causes of death in Table 9.2, Figure 9.13A plots the time series of average SMRs in a standardized format by setting the values in the first quinquennium (1901–5) equal to 100, and indexing later values with respect to first values. For reference, the series of average SMRs for all infections, abstracted as an additional cause-of-death category from Alderson's *International Mortality Statistics*, is plotted as the heavy line trace in Figure 9.13A. Finally, to pick out the aggregate trends, the maximum and minimum values and the three quartiles (Q1, median, and Q3) recorded across the 25 diseases in a given quinquennium are plotted as index numbers (1901–5 = 100) in Figure 9.13B.

The broad trends in Figure 9.13 are clear. Bearing in mind that the vertical axes of both graphs are plotted on a logarithmic scale, mortality rates generally declined exponentially over the observation period. For the majority of diseases studied, average SMRs at the end of the period were <10.0 per cent of their 1901–5 values (Figure 9.13A). However, within this general decline the envelope of maximum and minimum values expanded (Figure 19.3B), indicative of an increasing divergence of mortality trends for the sample diseases over the 75 years.

Relative Trends: Cluster Analysis

A fundamental question that can be asked of Figure 9.13A is whether a given disease category (fine line traces) became more or less important as a cause of mortality, relative to the aggregate pattern for all infections (heavy line

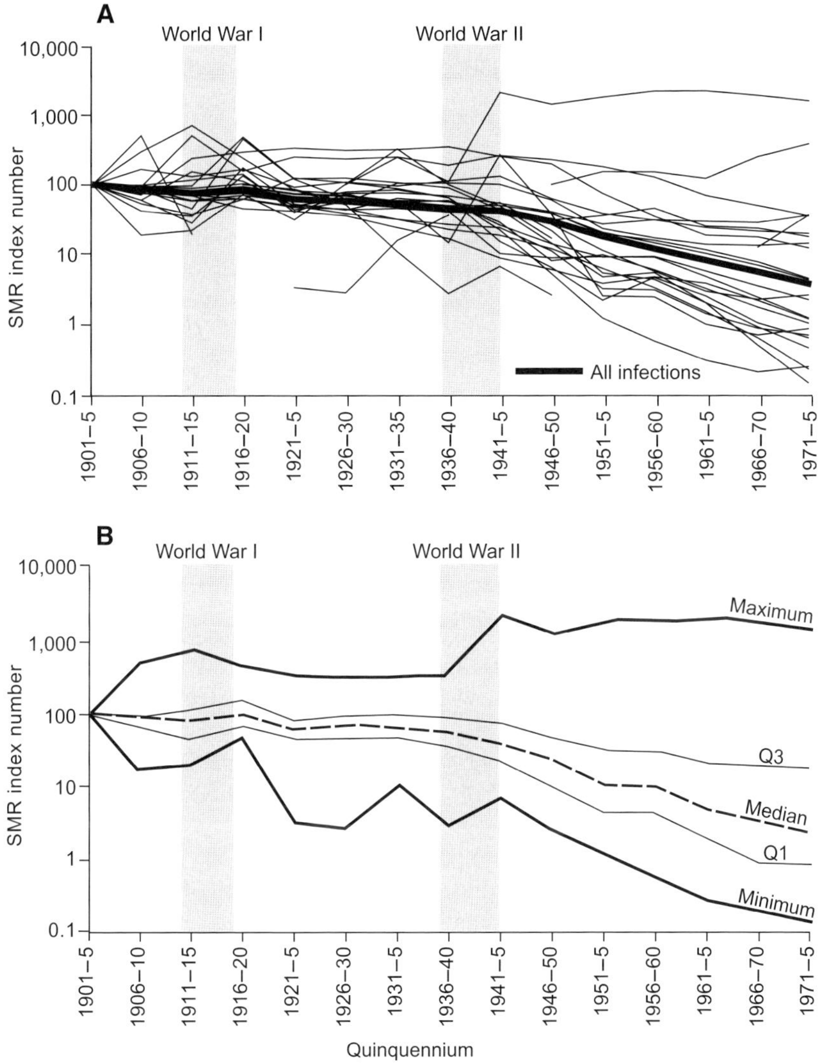

Fig. 9.13. Average trends in 25 causes of death, Europe, 1901–1975
The line traces in graph A plot the values of sex-standardized mortality ratios (SMRs) averaged across the 25 European countries listed in Table 9.3. For reference, the average SMR for all infections is plotted as the heavy line trace. Graph B plots the maximum and minimum values and the three quartiles (Q1, median, and Q3) of the times series in graph A. All series are plotted as index numbers (1901–5 = 100).
Source: Alderson (1981).

trace), over the eight-decade observation period. To assess this, let SMR'_{it} denote the SMR index number (as plotted in Figure 9.13A) for a given infectious cause of death *i* in quinquennium *t*. We then define the ratio

$$SMR'_{it}/SMR'_{t}, \tag{9.1}$$

where SMR'_{t} is the corresponding SMR index number for all infections. Application of equation 9.1 to each of the causes of death in Table 9.2 yielded 25 (diseases) × 15 (quinquennia) time series of ratios, which, in turn, were classified in terms of their temporal activity by complete linkage cluster analysis (Everitt *et al.* 2001). The dendrogram in Figure 9.14 identifies three well-defined groups of diseases, labelled groups 1–3. The median time series for the causes which comprise each group are plotted as the index numbers (1901–5 = 100) in Figure 9.15. Taken relative to all infections, values >100 mark an increase in mortality associated with the group and values <100 mark a decrease in mortality.

Viewed in terms of their relative trends, Figure 9.15 allows us to classify the three groups of diseases in Figure 9.14 as 'emerging' (group 1), 'retreating' (group 2), and 'emerging/retreating' (group 3) as causes of mortality in twentieth-century Europe. We consider each group in turn.

(1) *Group 1: Emerging diseases.* This group comprises a spectrum of diseases of viral, bacterial, and mixed aetiologies, with a predominance of conditions associated with the upper and lower respiratory tract (influenza, pneumonia, respiratory infections, and respiratory tuberculosis) and the central nervous system (meningococcal infections and poliomyelitis[7]) (Figure 9.14). The median mortality curve is characterized by a steady and progressive increase to very high index values (>300) in the later years of the observation period (Figure 9.15).

(2) *Group 2: Retreating diseases.* This group comprises a series of classical viral, bacterial, and rickettsial diseases, including several of the great quarantine diseases (cholera, typhus fever and other rickettsial diseases, and yellow fever) and some vaccine-preventable childhood infections (diphtheria, measles, and whooping cough) (Figure 9.14). The median mortality curve is characterized by a steady and progressive fall to very low index values (<30) in the latter years of the observation period (Figure 9.15).

(3) *Group 3: Emerging/retreating diseases.* This small group comprises diseases that, with the exception of one protozoal disease (malaria),

[7] Smallman-Raynor, Cliff, Trevelyan, *et al.* (2006) provide a monograph-length treatment of the rise of poliomyelitis as one of the important emerging diseases of the early and mid-20th century. As described there, the introduction of safe and effective poliovirus vaccines in the 1950s served to curb disease activity in many developed countries of the world, while, since 1988, the WHO Global Polio Eradication Initiative has pushed wild poliovirus back to a handful of endemic areas in Africa, Eastern Mediterranean, and South-East Asia.

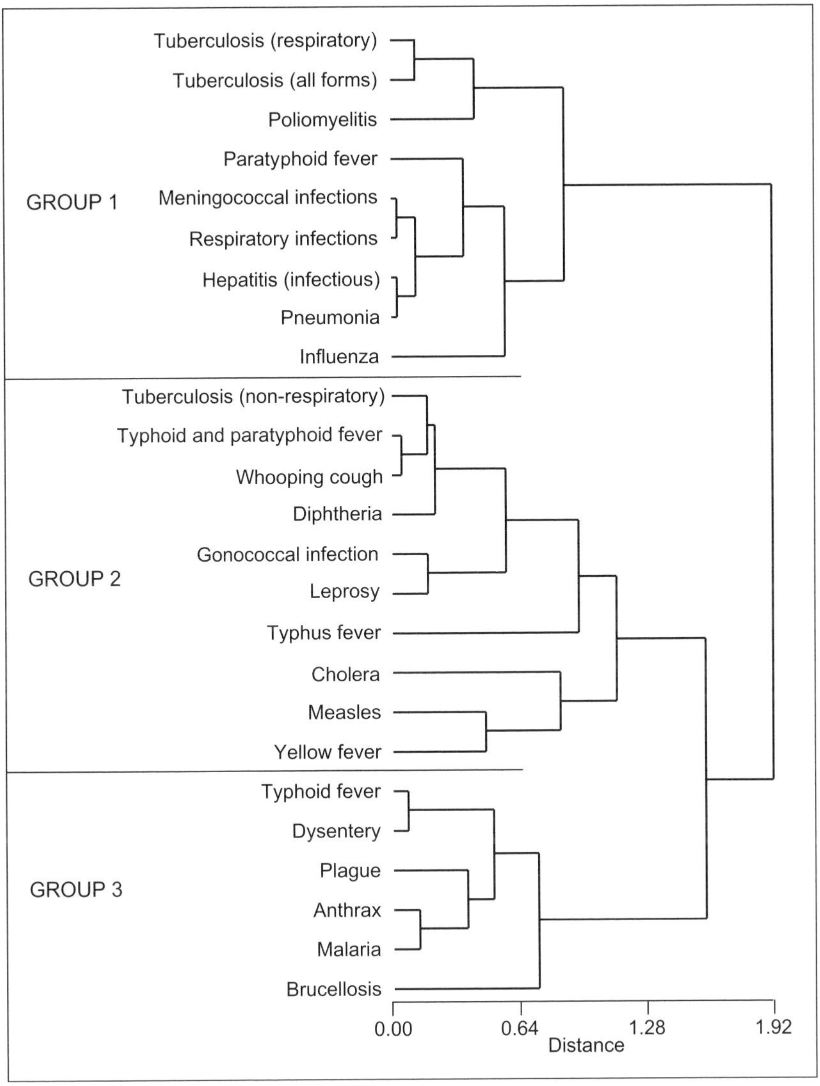

Fig. 9.14. Classification of 25 causes of death in terms of their relative time series behaviour, Europe, 1901–1975
Three principal disease groups (labelled groups 1–3), defined by complete linkage cluster analysis, are indicated. Note that the titles of some disease categories are given in abbreviated form; see Table 9.2 for full titles.
Source: Alderson (1981).

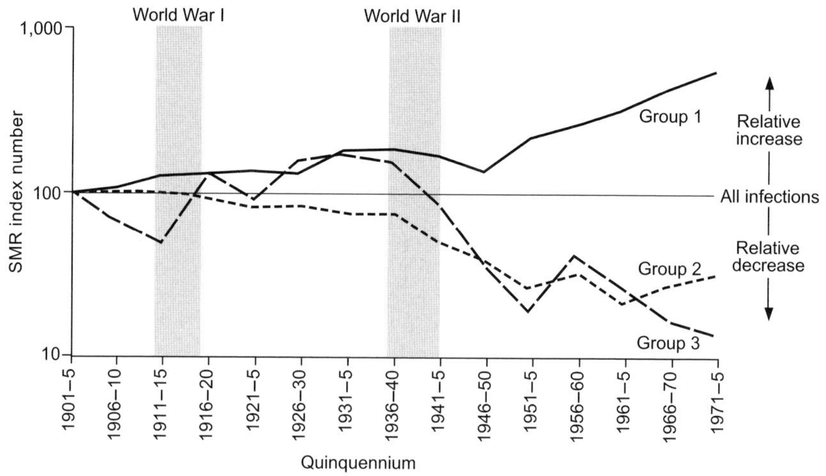

Fig. 9.15. Relative trends in mortality for the three groups of diseases in Fig. 9.14 Line traces plot the median series for the causes of death which comprise groups 1–3 in Fig. 9.14. The time series have been standardized on an initial value of 100 in the first quinquennium (1901–5), and subsequent values have been indexed with respect to this initial value. Index numbers >100 mark a relative increase in cause-specific mortality, while index numbers <100 mark a relative decrease in cause-specific mortality. SMR = sex-standardized mortality ratio.

are of bacterial aetiology (anthrax, brucellosis, dysentery, plague, and typhoid fever) (Figure 9.14). The median mortality curve shares characteristics of the curves for groups 1 and 2, with (i) an initial increase to relatively high index values (>150) in the inter-war years, followed by (ii) a steep fall to very low index values (<30) in the post-1945 period (Figure 9.15).

INTER-REGIONAL ANALYSIS

To broaden the regional analysis of relative mortality trends, the complete linkage cluster analysis for Europe in Figure 9.14 was extended to include the entire set of 75 series (25 diseases × 3 regions) of average SMRs for Europe, North America, and the South Pacific. As before, equation 9.1 was used to scale the input series by (region-specific) average SMRs for all infections. The results of the cluster analysis mimicked those for Europe, with three well-defined groups of 'emerging' (group 1), 'retreating' (group 2), and 'emerging/retreating' (group 3) diseases. For each of the three regions, the Venn diagrams in Figure 9.16 identify those diseases classified in (A) group 1, (B) group 2, and (C) group 3.

Figures 9.16A and B isolate 11 diseases which, relative to regional trends in mortality for all infections, display a common pattern of emergence

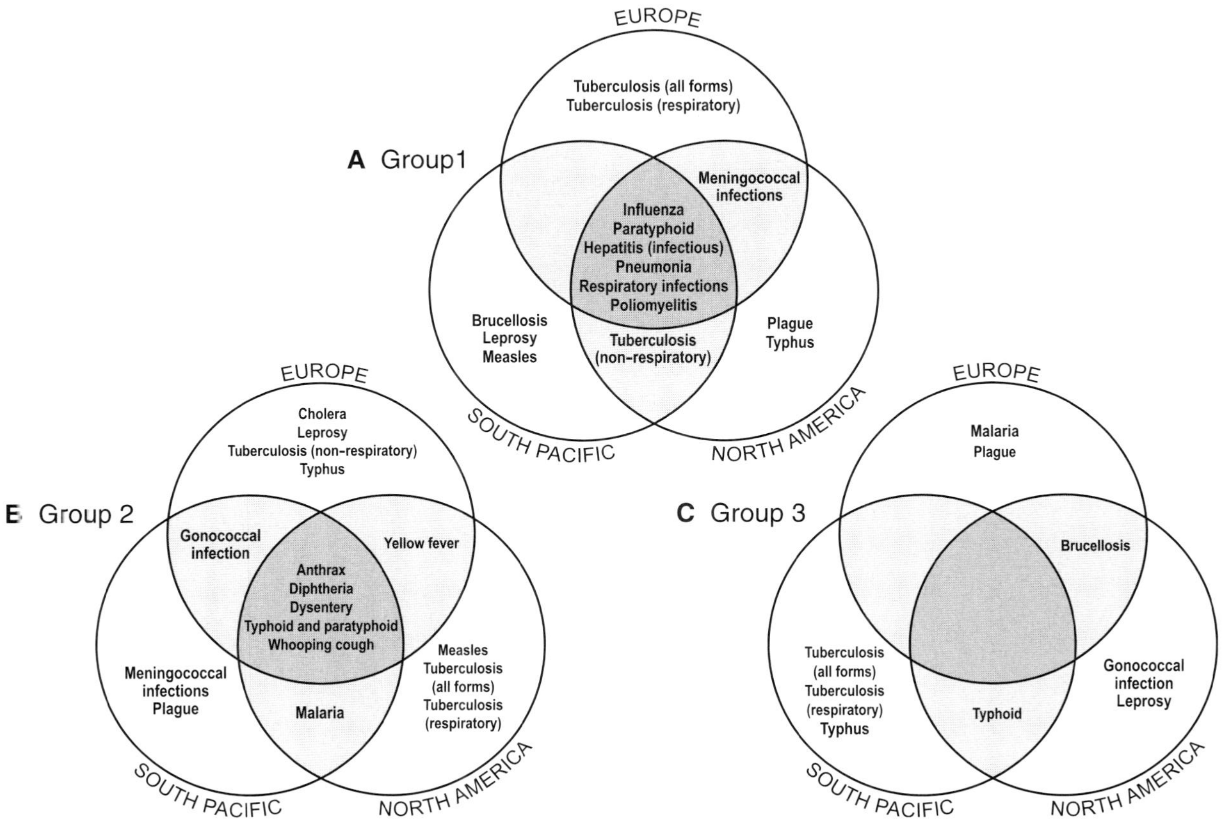

Fig. 9.16. Venn diagrams showing the regional distribution of diseases by relative mortality trend, 1901–1975
Diseases are classified by group as emerging (group 1, diagram A), retreating (group 2, diagram B), and emerging/retreating (group 3, diagram C) as a cause of mortality, relative to all infections, in the regions of Europe, North America, and the South Pacific. Trends associated with each group mimic those depicted in Fig. 9.15. Note that the titles of some disease categories are given in abbreviated form; see Table 9.2 for full titles.

(infectious hepatitis,[8] influenza, paratyphoid fever and other salmonella infections, pneumonia, poliomyelitis, and respiratory infections; Figure 9.16A) or retreat (anthrax, diphtheria, dysentery, typhoid and paratyphoid fever, and whooping cough; Figure 9.16B) across the regions of Europe, North America, and the South Pacific. Other diseases in Figure 9.16 display more complex patterns, with multiple regional pairings and, for some diseases, regionally distinctive trends. Illustrating the latter, the South Pacific is singled out by the emergence of brucellosis, leprosy, and measles[9] (Figure 9.16A), the retreat of meningococcal infections and plague (9.16B), and the emergence/retreat of tuberculosis and typhus (9.16C). Similarly distinct patterns of disease emergence, retreat, and emergence/retreat are observed in Figure 9.16 for Europe and North America.

SUMMARY

In the advanced regional economies of Europe, North America, and the South Pacific, the twentieth century was characterized by a stark decline in mortality caused by many of the diseases included in Table 9.2. A disease-specific review of the complex of factors that have contributed to this decline, including improvements in sanitation and hygiene, nutrition, immunization, antimicrobial therapy, and vector control, is provided by Lancaster (1990: 497–502). Our analysis has demonstrated that the mortality decline was not uniform for all the diseases studied, and, when examined relative to mortality from all infections, patterns of emergence and retreat—akin to Thomson's (1955, 1976) description of the ebb and flow of infectious diseases (Section 1.1)—can be deciphered. Some of the developments were specific to the epidemiological environments of the individual regions. Others, however, were common to all regions and include the relative rise (infectious hepatitis, influenza, paratyphoid fever and other salmonella infections, and poliomyelitis) and fall (anthrax, diphtheria, dysentery, typhoid and paratyphoid fever, and whooping cough) of mortality from some of the major human viral and bacterial diseases.

9.3.2 Time Sequences of Emergence and Cyclical Re-Emergence in Sub-Saharan Africa

Insufficient data of the type and quality included in Alderson's (1981) *International Mortality Statistics* exist to establish overall trends in infectious

[8] For the time period under consideration (1901–75), the data presented by Alderson (1981) do not distinguish between the different types of viral hepatitis (A, B, C, D, and E). We note here, however, that trends in viral hepatitis vary substantially by type and by geographical area, and that there have been marked reductions in hepatitis A and B incidence where vaccination programmes have been implemented.

[9] For a consideration of the emergence and eventual retreat of measles in the South Pacific in the period, 1850–1990, see Cliff, Haggett, and Smallman-Raynor (1993: 119–41, 184–8, 212–14, 268–9).

disease activity for the economically less advanced regions of the world. Frequently, however, sufficient data are available to piece together long time sequences for individual diseases of regional importance. In this subsection, we examine the time sequences associated with two categories of disease that, during the twentieth century and beyond, have risen to prominence in sub-Saharan Africa: (i) cyclically re-emerging meningococcal disease and (ii) the recently emerging Ebola–Marburg viral diseases.

CYCLICAL RE-EMERGENCE: MENINGOCOCCAL DISEASE

Meningococcal disease (*ICD*-10 A39) is the broad term for clinical illnesses due to infection with the bacterium *Neisseria meningitidis*. Invasive disease may present as meningitis (inflammation of the meninges) and, less commonly, septicaemia (with or without meningitis). Meningococcal meningitis is also known as 'cerebrospinal meningitis' or 'cerebrospinal fever' and is the cause of many thousands of deaths each year. The disease has a worldwide distribution, but, as we describe below, it displays a special spatial concentration with cyclic epidemics in the African continent.

Nature of Meningococcal Disease

Overall, the clinical pattern of meningococcal disease is similar in all epidemiological situations (Stephens *et al.* 2007). A typical incubation period of 3–4 days (range: 2–10 days) gives way to the sudden onset of fever, intense headache, photophobia, nausea and, frequently, vomiting, a stiff neck, and a characteristic petechial rash with pink macules. Delirium and coma often appear, with sudden prostration and ecchymoses. Historically, case-fatality rates of >50 per cent have been recorded during epidemics. But, with early diagnosis, antibiotic therapy, and supportive measures, the fatality rate has fallen to 8–15 per cent. For survivors, long-term sequelae may include neurological deficit, deafness, and loss of limbs (Heymann 2004: 359).

Six serogroups of *N. meningitidis* (serogroups A, B, C, Y, W-135, and X) are known to be associated with outbreaks of life-threatening disease. Serogroups A, B, and C account for the majority of cases worldwide, with serogroups B and C predominating in Europe and North America and serogroups A and C predominating in Africa and Asia. Some regions have reported an increase in cases due to serogroups Y and W-135 in recent years. The reservoir of *N. meningitidis* is humans. The mode of transmission is by direct contact, including respiratory droplets from the nose and throat of infected people. Carriage of *N. meningitidis* in the nose and throat is common and at any time may be seen in up to 10 per cent of the population; invasion causing systemic disease is comparatively rare. Communicability persists until meningococci are no longer present in discharges from the nose and mouth. Susceptibility to the clinical disease is low and decreases with age. For further details, see Heymann (2004: 359–66).

Meningococcal Disease and the African 'Meningitis Belt'

'Epidemic convulsions' are mentioned in tenth-century China, and a possible description by Willis in England in 1684 suggests that meningococcal disease has been present in the human population for some centuries (Patterson 1993). Epidemic cerebrospinal meningitis (CSM) is described in detail in the early months of 1805 in Geneva, and, from then on, CSM outbreaks were reported from both sides of the Atlantic (Table 2.2) (Hirsch 1883–6: iii. 547–94). The record for Africa, however, is more fragmentary and begins later. The initial pattern of intermittent outbreaks, as illustrated by the records of meningococcal disease in the mining communities of South Africa in the 1880s, was very similar to the record for Western countries. However, the start of the twentieth century marked the onset of the first of a series of recognized epidemic cycles which have repeatedly spread across a vast swath of the African continent to form the so-called 'meningitis belt' (Jusatz 1954–61; Lapeyssonnie 1963).

Delimitation of the meningitis belt. The African meningitis belt is delimited in Figure 9.17. It stretches across the savannah zone south of the Sahara, extending over states that comprise both the WHO Africa region and, to the east of the zone, the WHO Eastern Mediterranean region.[10] The reasons for the focus of disease activity in this belt, with a strong concentration of outbreak activity in the dry season (December–May), are not fully understood. Suggestions include a possible physiological link with dry and dusty environmental conditions that may impair the nasopharyngeal mucosa,

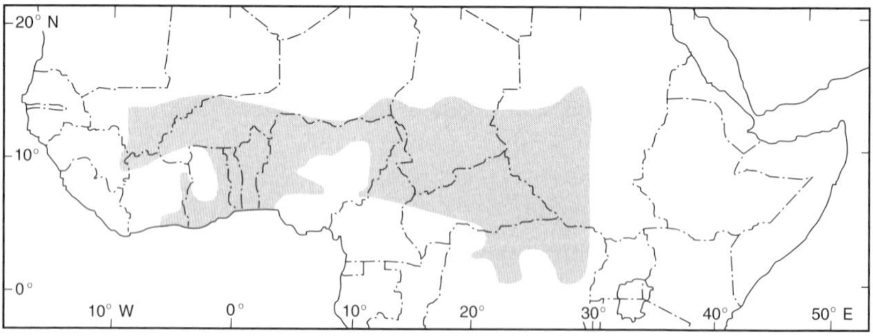

Fig. 9.17. The African meningitis belt in the late twentieth century
The belt across tropical Africa lies in a zone between 5° and 15° N of the Equator. It is characterized by an annual rainfall between 30 cm and 110 cm.

Sources: Redrawn from Cliff, Haggett, and Smallman-Raynor (2004, fig. 7.39, p. 111), originally based on Peters and Gilles (1989, fig. 778, p. 192) and World Health Organization (1998*b*, fig. 2, p. 6).

[10] See Figure 3.1 for a delimitation of the world regions used by the WHO.

thereby increasing the risks of invasive disease in the host. A number of environmental variables (including absolute humidity, dust and rainfall profiles, and land cover type) have been shown to correlate with the historical and contemporary distribution of outbreaks in Africa, although their exact role in disease activity remains undefined (Molesworth, Cuevas, *et al.* 2002; Molesworth, Thomson, *et al.* 2003). Additional contributory factors may include the presence of other respiratory pathogens, crowding, and poor hygiene (Moore *et al.* 1989).

Epidemic cycles, 1900–1999. Jusatz (1954–61) identifies four major cycles in the African meningitis belt in the period 1900–60: First Cycle (1900–8); Second Cycle (1914–26); Third Cycle (1927–41); Fourth Cycle (1942–58). Figure 9.18 is drawn from information provided by Jusatz and identifies, for each of the four cycles, years of epidemic activity in sample countries of the region. Although the evidence is fragmentary and unavailable for some countries in earlier periods, sufficient information exists to infer an extension of each cycle along the greater part of the belt's east–west axis. By way of illustration, the course of the Third Cycle (1927–41)—diffusing as a contagious transmission wave east → west from a suspected origin in the province of Mongalla in southern Sudan—is mapped in Figure 9.19.

Evidence for the strong cyclicity of meningococcal disease in more recent decades is illustrated for five sample countries of the meningitis belt in Figure 9.20.[11] The length of epidemic cycles in these countries varies between 8–9 years (Niger) and 10–15 years (Burkina Faso). More generally, Moore *et al.* (1989) observe that epidemics typically occur every 8–12 years and affect up to 1 per cent of the population. Between epidemics, the disease is hyperendemic.

Time–Space Sequences: Recent Emergence Events in the Meningitis Belt

Recent events have highlighted the introduction of new strains of *N. meningitidis* rather than the resurgence of established strains as a driver of the epidemic cycles in the meningitis belt (Moore 1992; Nicolas *et al.* 2005). By way of illustration, Figure 9.21 is based on the study of Nicolas *et al.* (2005) and charts the time–space sequence of detection of three different sequence types of *N. meningitidis* in 13 sample countries of the belt, 1988–2003. Available evidence indicates that the sequence type mapped in Figure 9.21A (serogroup A ST-5) was first introduced into the belt in 1987 via the series of inter-regional linkages plotted in Figure 9.22. As the diffusion map shows, the source of ST-5 can be traced to South Asia, where it was circulating in epidemic form in the mid-1980s. Westwards spread into the Eastern Mediterranean region occurred in association with the annual haj to Mecca in

[11] It is important to recognize that the major epidemics depicted in Figure 9.20 are superimposed on annual cycles of disease activity, with the latter accounting for a considerable burden of meningococcal disease in the region.

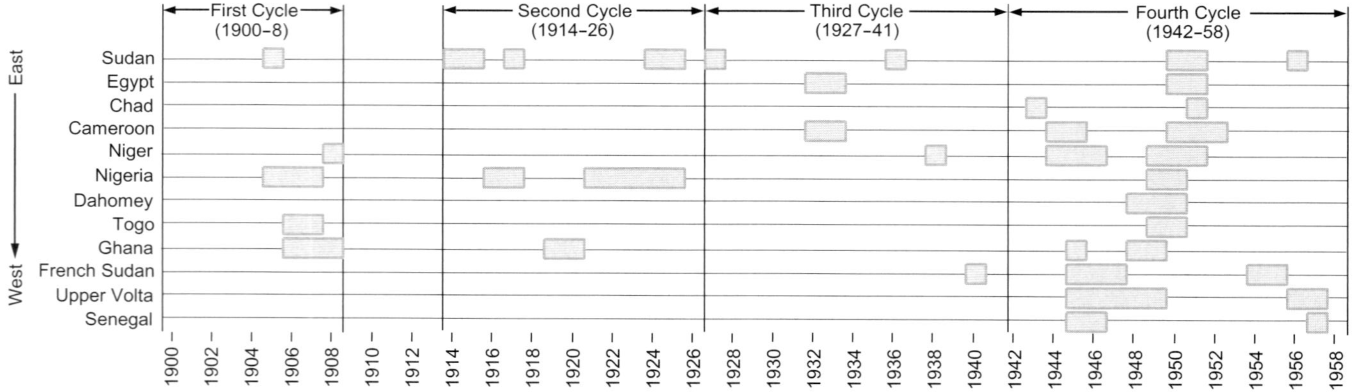

Fig. 9.18. Major cycles of meningococcal disease in the African meningitis belt, 1900–1958
The diagram is drawn from Jusatz (1954–61) and highlights years of epidemic activity in sample countries. The counties have been arranged according to their approximate position on the dominant east (upper)–west (lower) axis of the belt. Country names follow the usage of Jusatz: Dahomey (Benin); French Sudan (Mali); and Upper Volta (Burkina Faso, including Côte d'Ivoire until 1947). The period encompassed by each disease cycle is indicated. Note that the diagram is indicative only; information is missing for some countries and time periods.

Source: Based on Jusatz (1954–61: III/44–44*b*).

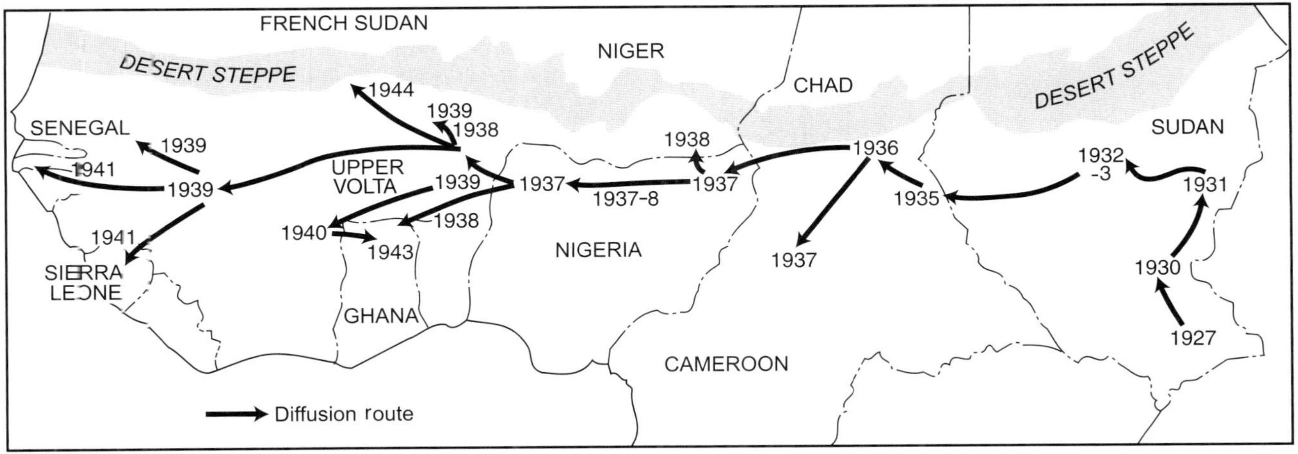

Fig. 9.19. Epidemic spread of the third recognized cycle of meningococcal disease in the African meningitis belt, 1927–1941 Vectors show the inferred diffusion corridors of the disease. The area of desert steppe (semi-desert) that borders the southern Sahara is indicated for reference.

Source: Based on Rodenwaldt and Jusatz (1954–61, special map 1, reverse of map III/89).

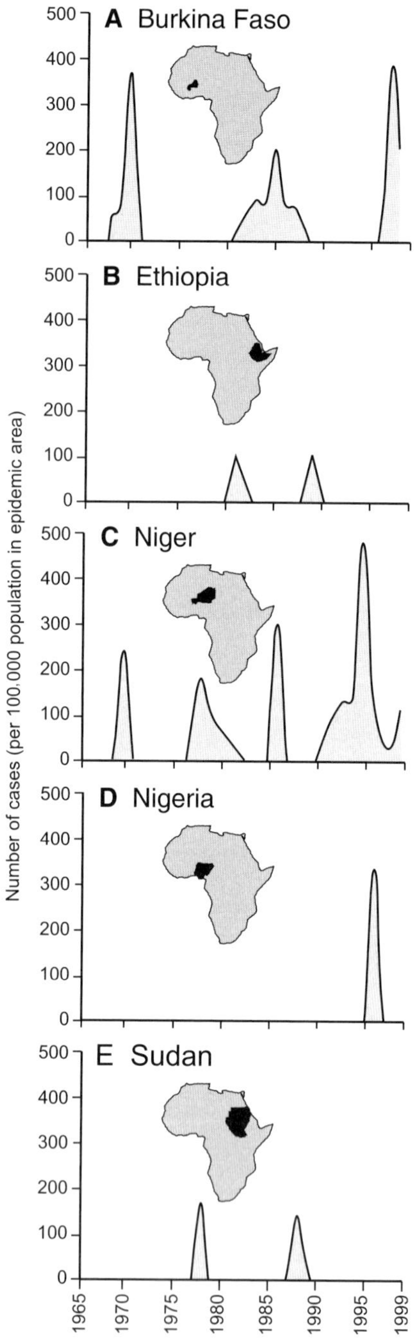

Fig. 9.20. Meningitis cycles in Central Africa

Epidemic cycles of meningococcal disease for five African countries, 1966–99. Data for less than 50 cases per 100,000 are not available.

Sources: Redrawn from Cliff, Haggett, and Smallman-Raynor (2004, fig. 7.40, p. 111), originally from World Health Organization (2000*c*, fig. 5.1, p. 58).

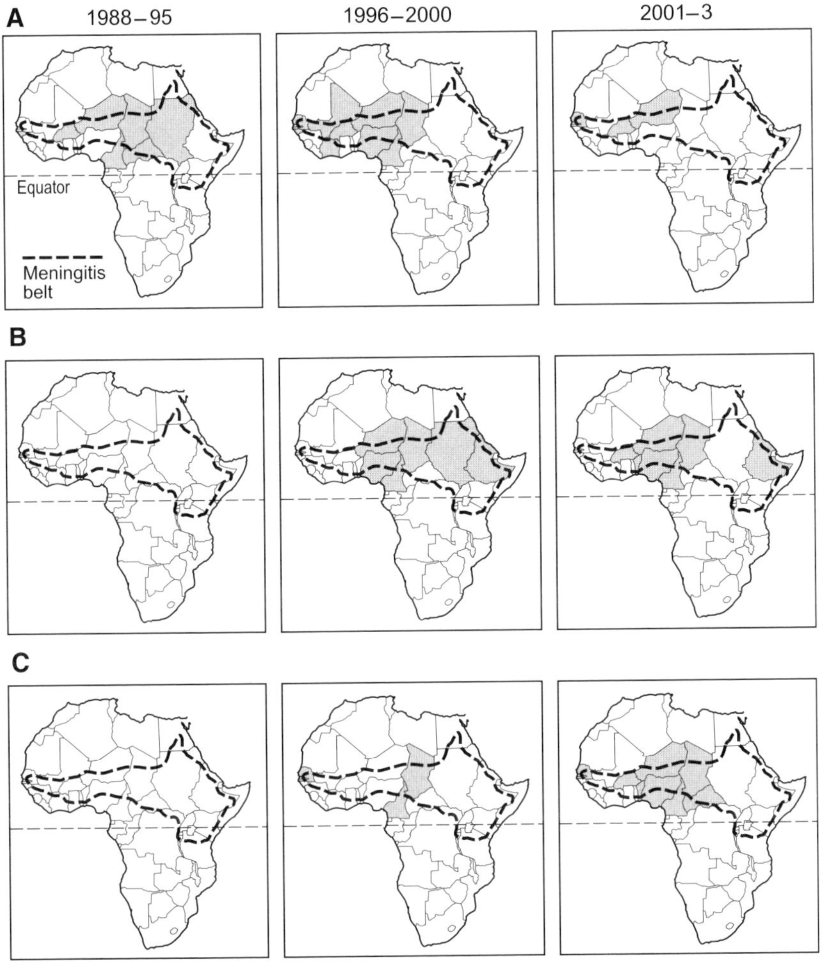

Fig. 9.21. Emergence and expansion of different serogroups of *N. meningitidis* in the African meningitis belt, 1988–2003

The maps are based on sample evidence and shade those countries in which different serogroups of *N. meningitidis* were recovered in the years 1988–95, 1996–2000, and 2001–3. (A) Serogroup A ST-5. (B) Serogroup A ST-7. (C) Serogroup W135 ST-11. The extent of the currently recognized meningitis belt is indicated for reference.

Source: Based on Nicolas *et al.* (2005, table 1, pp. 5131–2).

1987. From there, pilgrims returning to Africa carried the bacterium into the meningitis belt. Beginning with major epidemics in N'Djamena (Chad) and Khartoum (Sudan) in the spring of 1988, the new strain spread throughout the zone (Figure 9.21A) to emerge as the cause of most documented epidemics in the decade to 1997 (Moore *et al.* 1989; Nicolas *et al.* 2005).

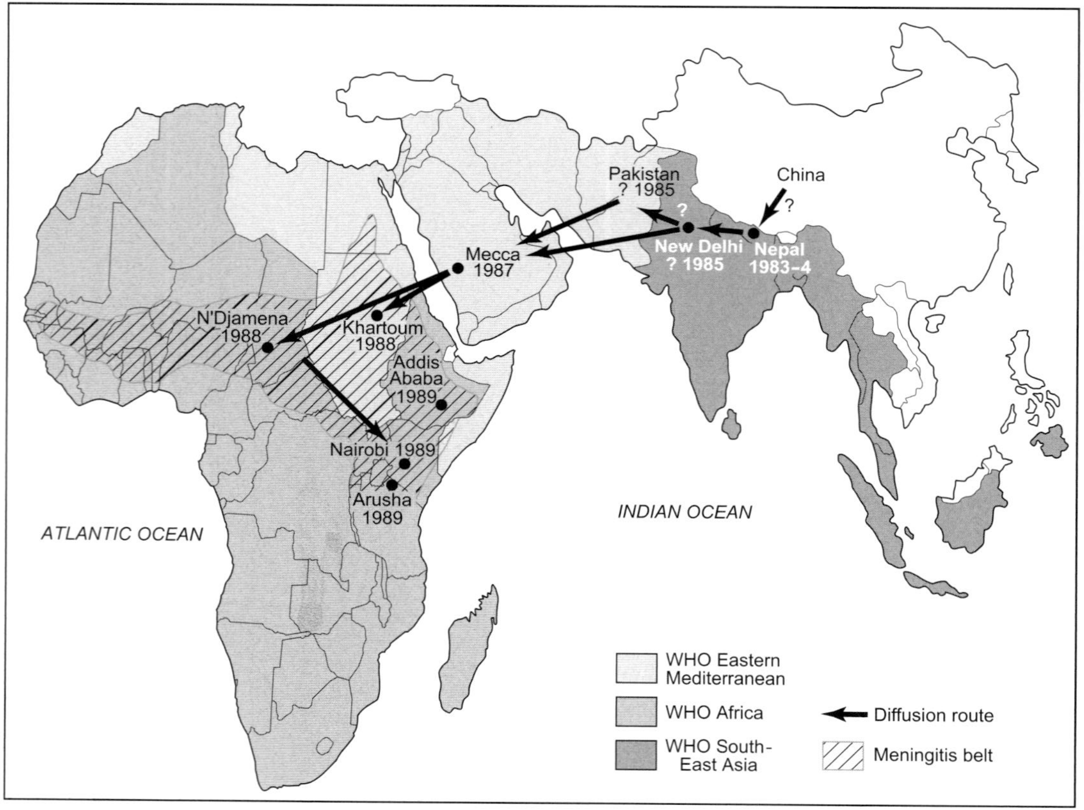

Fig. 9.22. Inter-regional transmission corridors of serogroup A ST-5 *N. meningitidis*, 1983–1989
Vectors depict the diffusion of the bacterium implicated in severe epidemics of meningococcal meningitis in the WHO regions of South-East Asia, Eastern Mediterranean, and Africa in the 1980s. The extent of the currently recognized meningitis belt is shaded for reference.

Sources: Based on Moore *et al*. (1989, fig. 2, p. 261), Moore (1992, fig. 4, p. 519), and Centers for Disease Control (1990*a*).

Figures 9.21B and C show that two further sequence types of *N. meningitidis* began to expand in the meningitis belt in the period 1996–2003:

(i) serogroup A ST-7 (maps 9.21B). This serogroup first emerged in the belt in the mid-1990s and totally replaced the previously circulating serogroup A ST-5 by 2002;

(ii) serogroup W135 ST-11 (maps 9.21C). The history of amplification of this serogroup in the belt was coincidental with the worldwide outbreak of W135 meningococcal disease that occurred among haj pilgrims and their contacts in 2000 (Section 6.5.2) (Lingappa *et al.* 2003; Nicolas *et al.* 2005). Although W135 strains were detected towards the end of epidemics in Central and West Africa in 2001 (World Health Organization 2001*a*), the first major epidemic attributed to the strain was recorded in Burkina Faso in 2002 (Koumaré *et al.* 2007). Koumaré and colleagues (2007) hypothesize that the extensive prior use of serogroup A + C vaccines provided a niche for the new bacterium which contributed to the rapid spatial expansion mapped in Figure 9.21C.

Future Prospects

There has been some suggestion that epidemics of meningococcal disease have become more frequent in Africa in recent years, although the evidence is equivocal. While the geographical core of the classical meningitis belt, first defined by Lapeyssonnie (1963), has generally held, the last decade has seen increased outbreaks of meningococcal disease in areas adjacent to the belt, as well as in several countries to the east and south of the African continent. The evidence suggests that the belt may be expanding, possibly in association with a reduction in rainfall and absolute humidity in sub-humid areas adjacent to the belt (Greenwood 2006);[12] see Chapter 7 for a full discussion of environmental changes as an emerging disease driver.

EMERGENCE: EBOLA–MARBURG VIRAL DISEASES

Ebola–Marburg viral diseases (*ICD*-10 A98.3, A98.4) are severe viral illnesses that were first recognized in the course of virulent outbreaks during the 1960s and 1970s. The disease complex is also known as 'African haemorrhagic fever', and the constituent diseases are sometimes referred to as 'Marburg virus haemorrhagic fever' and 'Ebola virus haemorrhagic fever'. The diseases share high fatality rates (20–90 per cent) linked to excessive bleeding (hence the term 'haemorrhagic'), but each has distinctive viral characteristics. To date, documented outbreaks under natural conditions have been limited to certain countries of the WHO Africa region and the

[12] While the data show that countries outside the meningitis belt do have outbreaks of meningococcal disease, none of these has been documented as having the particular pattern of meningococcal disease, with annual cycles and superimposed epidemics every 8–12 years, characteristic of the meningitis belt itself.

adjacent country of Sudan in the WHO Eastern Mediterranean region (Figure 3.1).

Nature of Ebola–Marburg Viral Diseases

The causative agents of Ebola–Marburg viral diseases (Ebola virus and Marburg virus) are distinct members of the *Filoviridae* family. The mode of transmission is through person-to-person contact with infected blood, secretions, organs, or semen; healthcare workers are at high risk of infection, while nosocomial transmission (due to exposure to contaminated needles and syringes) has been recognized as a frequent source of infection in outbreaks. The period of communicability for both fevers is as long as blood and secretions contain virus. Susceptibility appears to be general (Heymann 2004: 182).

Ebola and Marburg viral diseases are virtually indistinguishable on clinical grounds. An incubation period of 2–21 days gives way to the sudden onset of high fever, headache, and malaise. Other symptoms include pharyngitis, vomiting, diarrhoea, and maculopapular rash. The haemorrhagic diathesis is often accompanied by hepatic damage, renal failure, and central nervous system involvement. This may lead to terminal shock with multi-organ collapse. Observed case-fatality rates range between 50–90 per cent (Ebola) and 25–80 per cent (Marburg) (Heymann 2004: 180).

The natural reservoirs of Ebola and Marburg viruses remain unknown despite extensive studies. In the case of epidemics, it has usually been possible to trace the source back to a human or non-human primate index case, but no further. Suspected reservoirs have included spiders, ticks, and bats, but there is as yet no field evidence to incriminate any of these. Human and non-human primates are the only disease targets involved to date, but they are not thought to serve as reservoirs (Peterson, Bauer, *et al.* 2004; Peterson, Carroll, *et al.* 2004).

Time Sequences of Outbreak Activity

Figure 9.23 plots, by WHO region, the annual count of countries in which outbreaks of Marburg (graph A) and Ebola (graph B) viral diseases have been documented in the four decades to 2005. Summary details of the individual outbreaks are given in Tables 9.4 and 9.5, while a geographical overview of the first recognized Marburg epidemic (1967) is provided in Section 6.4.3. In general terms, the pattern of Ebola–Marburg viral diseases is sporadic. Three principal elements are involved: (i) individual cases and occasional outbreaks in countries of the WHO Africa region (from Liberia to Kenya) and neighbouring Sudan; (ii) hospital cases (Europe) and non-clinical infections (United States) associated with monkeys imported from Africa (Uganda) and the Western Pacific (Philippines) respectively; and (iii) sporadic cases among travellers in sub-Saharan Africa. Available evidence indicates that the viruses are endemic in parts of East, Central, and possibly West Africa, while the Philippines may be a source area for Ebola virus in the Asia–Pacific region.

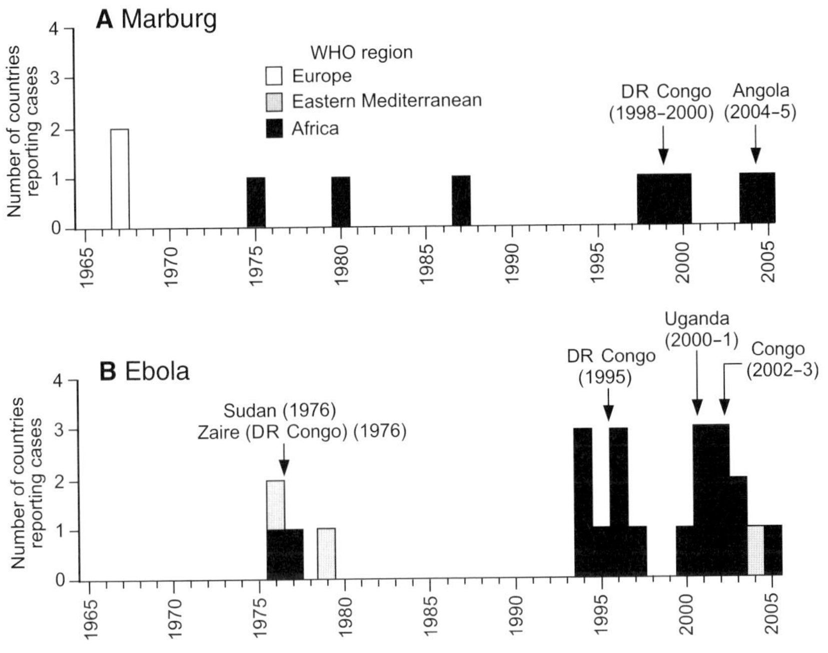

Fig. 9.23. Trends in outbreaks of Ebola–Marburg viral diseases, 1965–2005 Graphs plot, by WHO region, the number of countries in which documented outbreaks of Ebola–Marburg viral diseases were in process during a given year. (A) Marburg viral disease. (B) Ebola viral disease. Details of the outbreaks are provided in Tables 9.4 and 9.5. Outbreaks associated with >100 reported cases are indicated.

Sources: Based primarily on World Health Organization (2004*c*, table 1, p. 438; 2005*a*).

Ebola outbreaks in Africa. As described in the classic reports by the WHO/International Study Team (1978) and the International Commission (1978), Ebola viral disease was first recognized in 1976, when it caused near-simultaneous outbreaks associated with >600 documented cases in two districts 150 km apart: (i) the Maridi region of southern Sudan and (ii) the Bumba zone of Equateur region in northern Zaire (Table 9.5). With the exception of further limited occurrences in Zaire and Sudan in the late 1970s, Ebola virus largely retreated as the cause of documented human disease,[13] to re-emerge in the form of a series of outbreaks of varying magnitude from the mid-1990s (Figure 9.23B and Table 9.5). Some impression of the spread of outbreak

[13] Jezek *et al.* (1999) record evidence of sporadic human infections with Ebola virus, with low levels of secondary transmission, in Zaire in the period 1981–5. In addition, a subtype of Ebola virus (Ebola-Reston) was responsible for several outbreaks of Ebola viral disease among cynomolgus monkeys (*Macaca fascicularis*) imported from the Philippines to the US and Italy between 1989 and 1996; several human infections were identified in association with these events, although no Ebola-related illnesses were reported (Centers for Disease Control 1990*b*; World Health Organization 1992*a*; Miranda *et al.* 1999; Rollin *et al.* 1999).

Table 9.4. Documented outbreaks of Marburg viral disease, 1967–2005

Year	Location	Number of cases	Number of deaths	Notes
1967	Germany and the former Yugoslavia	31	7	Handlers of monkeys and monkey tissue, medical attendants, and a sexual contact
1975	South Africa (via Zimbabwe?)	3	1	Two travellers and a medical attendant
1980	Kenya	2	1	A European who had visited Kitum Cave, Mount Elgon National Park, and a Kenyan medical attendant
1987	Kenya	1	1	A European who had visited Kitum Cave, Mount Elgon National Park
1998–2000	Democratic Republic of the Congo	154	128	Majority of cases were male workers at a gold mine in Durba
2004–5	Angola	374	329	Largest outbreak on record, believed to have originated in Uige province in October 2004

Source: Based primarily on World Health Organization (2005*a*).

Table 9.5. Documented outbreaks of Ebola viral disease, 1976–2005

Year	Country	Number of cases	Number of deaths	Virus subtype[1]
1976	Sudan	284	151	Ebola-Sudan
	Zaire (DR Congo)	318	280	Ebola-Zaire
1977	Zaire (DR Congo)	1	1	Ebola-Zaire
1979	Sudan	34	22	Ebola-Sudan
1994	Gabon	52	31	Ebola-Zaire
	Côte d'Ivoire	1	0	Ebola-Côte d'Ivoire
	Liberia	1	0	Ebola-Côte d'Ivoire
1995	DR Congo	315	250	Ebola-Zaire
1996	Gabon	31	21	Ebola-Zaire
	South Africa	1[2]	1	Ebola-Zaire
1996–7	Gabon	59	44	Ebola-Zaire
2000–1	Uganda	425	224	Ebola-Sudan
2001–2	Gabon	65	53	Ebola-Zaire
	Republic of Congo	59	44	Ebola-Zaire
2002–3	Republic of Congo	143	128	Ebola-Zaire
2003	Republic of Congo	35	29	Ebola-Zaire
2004	Sudan	17	7	Ebola-Sudan
2005	Republic of Congo	12	9	Ebola-Zaire

Notes: [1] A fourth virus subtype, Ebola-Reston, was detected in Oct. 1989 in Reston, Virginia (US), in a colony of cynomolgus monkeys (*Macacus fascicularis*) imported from the Philippines. [2] Nurse involved in the treatment of an Ebola patient transferred from Gabon to South Africa. DR Congo = Democratic Republic of the Congo.
Source: Based primarily on World Health Organization (2004*c*, table 1, p. 438).

activity can be gained from Figure 9.24, which maps, as proportional circles, the time-sequenced occurrence of Ebola outbreaks in the period 1976–2005. Summary details are provided in Table 9.5. Inspection of the main map in Figure 9.24 reveals an extension of Ebola outbreak activity in Central Africa, beyond the initial foci in southern Sudan and northern Zaire in the mid-1970s, to Gabon (1990s) and the Republic of the Congo and Uganda (2000s). Elsewhere, sporadic cases of Ebola viral disease were recorded in West Africa (Côte d'Ivoire and Liberia) and southern Africa (South Africa) in the mid-1990s.

The strain of Ebola virus associated with the majority of the recent human outbreaks recorded in Table 9.5 (Ebola-Zaire subtype) has been implicated in massive die-offs of wild apes (gorillas and chimpanzees) in parts of western equatorial Africa since the mid-1990s (Leroy *et al.* 2004). These die-offs have tended to lead and appear to be epidemiologically linked to human outbreaks, thereby implying an underpinning spatial expansion of the virus in wildlife. Against this background, the vectors in Figure 9.24 are based on the analysis of Walsh, Biek, *et al.* (2005) and show the hypothesized route of epizootic diffusion of the Ebola-Zaire virus subtype from a best-fit origin in northern Democratic Republic of the Congo. The evidence is consistent with

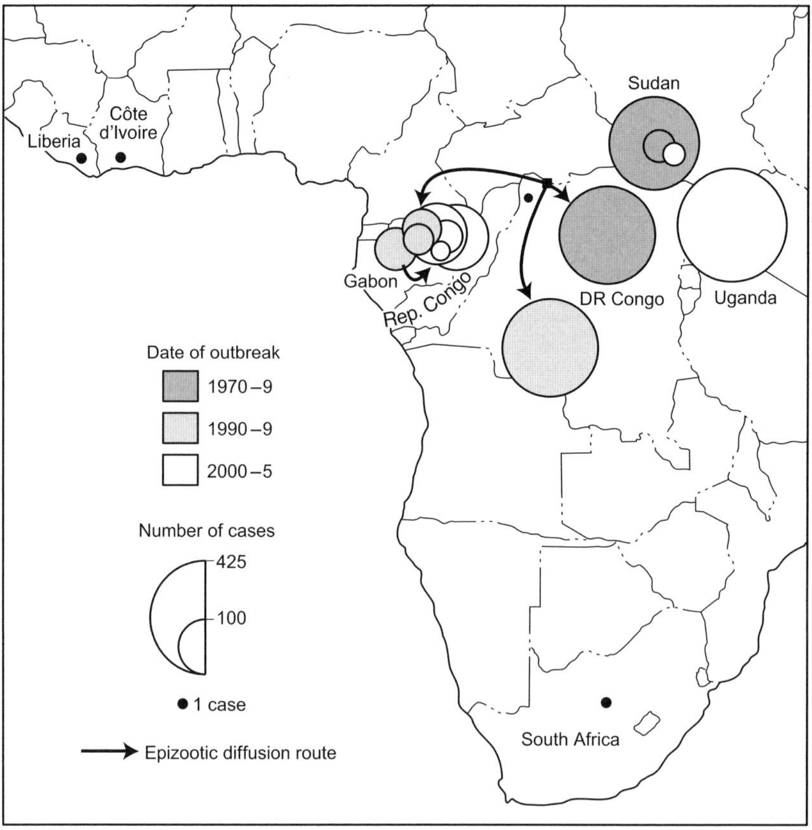

Fig. 9.24. Recorded outbreaks of Ebola viral disease, 1976–2005
The maps are based on the evidence in Table 9.5 and plot, as proportional circles, the locations of Ebola viral disease outbreaks in Africa. Circles are shaded according to the dates of outbreaks, with relatively early outbreaks represented by the relatively darker shading categories. Note that no outbreaks were recorded in the 1980s. Vectors are based on the analysis of Walsh, Abernethy, *et al.* (2005, fig. 1, p. 1947) and depict the hypothesized route of epizootic diffusion of Ebola virus (Ebola-Zaire subtype) from a best-fit origin in northern Democratic Republic of the Congo.
Source: Outbreak data based primarily on World Health Organization (2004*c*, table 1, p. 438).

a wave-like advance of the epizootic southwards and westwards through western equatorial Africa at an estimated rate of approximately 50 km per year (Walsh, Biek, *et al.* 2005). The advance of the wave would account for the catastrophic decline of great apes in some parts of the region (Walsh, Abernethy, *et al.* 2003; Leroy *et al.* 2004; Rouquet *et al.* 2005) and, through the handling of animal carcasses, the corresponding increase in human outbreaks in the Democratic Republic of the Congo, Gabon, and the Republic of the Congo since the mid-1990s (Walsh, Biek, *et al.* 2005).

Future Threats

While the cumulative total number of recorded human cases of Ebola–Marburg viral diseases is small to date, the potential threat from the diseases is high. Outbreaks of Ebola viral disease (Democratic Republic of the Congo and Uganda, 2007) and Marburg viral disease (Uganda, 2007) have continued to be reported beyond the time-frame of Tables 9.4 and 9.5 (World Health Organization 2007*a*,*b*), while importations of the viruses into Europe and North America with shipments of non-human primates have underscored the potential threat of the disease beyond the assumed endemic areas. There are no vaccines, no specific treatments, and current therapy consists of maintaining fluid and electrolyte balance and the administration of blood and plasma to control bleeding. Safe handling of these viruses is limited to a very few laboratories around the world, and, at the moment, rapid recognition of the diseases, advice on protective measures, strict isolation of patients, and barrier nursing are the first lines of defence.

9.4 National Examples: Australia

Our regional examination of twentieth-century mortality trends in Section 9.3.1 included two countries (Australia and New Zealand) that comprised the region of the South Pacific. In the present section, we undertake a closer examination of developments in disease activity for Australia. We begin, in Section 9.4.1, by supplementing the original analysis of mortality trends for 25 diseases in the South Pacific with a parallel examination of morbidity trends for 89 diseases in Australia. Our Australian morbidity series, 1917–91, terminates in the early years of a decade when several novel viruses of bats were identified for the first time as causes of human disease in the Australia continent. We therefore conclude our review, in Section 9.4.2, with a brief consideration of the sequence of events associated with these 'virus spill-overs'.

9.4.1 Morbidity Trends

This subsection draws on the analysis of Smallman-Raynor and Cliff (2004*b*: 124–6). Notifiable disease data have been routinely collected by the states and territories of Australia since 1917. The task of pulling the data into a consistent body of statistics covering the time-span to the late twentieth century has been undertaken by Robert Hall of the Australian Department of Health, Housing, Local Government, and Community Services, and it is his annual data on reported cases and case rates for 89 communicable diseases and other conditions, 1917–91, that are analysed in this section.

The diseases are listed in Hall (1993) and cover a wide spectrum of infections, ranging from quarantine diseases (for example, plague and yellow fever) to common respiratory infections (influenza and measles), parasitic diseases, and haemorrhagic fevers. Although Hall attaches the usual 'health warnings' to the published statistics, and data points are entirely missing for some years (1941, 1943, and 1951), we note here that the data represent the best available estimates of long-term trends in notifiable disease activity for Australia.

TREND ANALYSIS

Over the 75 years to 1991, 2,200,194 notifications were received by Australia's routine disease notification system. The peak number in any one year was 120,023 in 1919, when 89,941 cases of influenza were reported. Figure 9.25A plots as line traces the annual notified case rate per 100,000 population for each of the 89 diseases in Hall's data set. A logarithmic scale has been used. The heavy lines mark the maximum case rate and the three quartiles (Q1, median, and Q3) recorded each year across the 89 diseases. No attempt has been made to pick out individual diseases. The broad trends follow those of the European mortality curves in Figure 9.13, with case rates in Figure 9.25 declining exponentially over the 75-year period. Up to the beginning of World War II, the band of rates is effectively horizontal, with a slight hint of an increasing range to the encompassing envelope through the 1930s. After 1945, the steady fall in case rates that has persisted through to the present day set in, although there is some evidence for a levelling out in the speed of fall after *c*.1970. From *c*.1950, the range of rates also declined as compared with 1917–39.

To aid comparison between the rates for different diseases over time, Figure 9.25B replots from Figure 9.25A the line traces for the maximum case rate and the three quartiles as index numbers (1917 = 100). Again, a logarithmic scale has been used for the vertical axis. In contrast to Figure 9.25A, the use of index numbers enables the time series for the minimum annual rates to be illustrated avoiding a plotting problem that arises when showing the raw data on a log scale—namely, many years with zero or near-zero rates. Like graph A, graph B shows the sharp fall in rates after 1945. The time series for minimum rates emphasizes this decline by reflecting the very low rates for many infectious diseases at the end of the twentieth century.

Figure 9.26 emphasizes the morbidity trends shown in Figure 9.25 by plotting, on an annual basis, the mean, standard deviation, and the coefficient of variation of the notified rates as index numbers. In each year of the time series, these summary statistics have been calculated across the rates for the 89 diseases. We define CV as

$$CV = 100(s/\bar{x}), \tag{9.2}$$

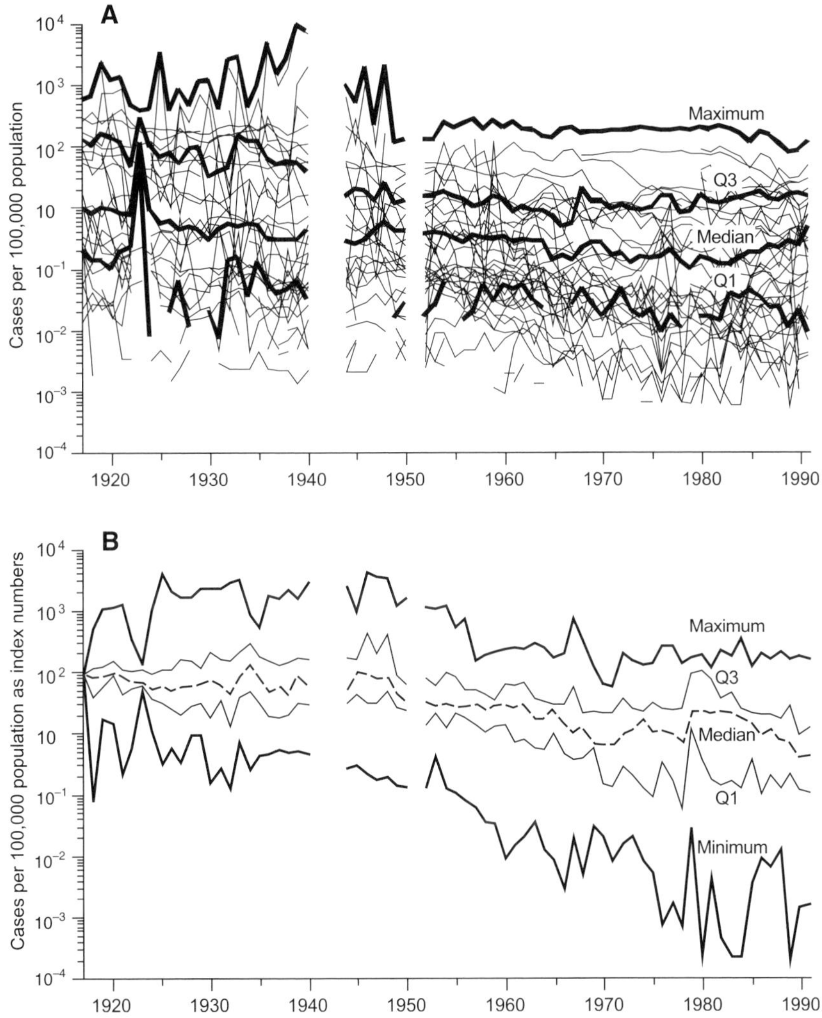

Fig. 9.25. Australia, 1917–1991: annual morbidity rates from 89 infectious diseases (A) The line traces plot the notified number of cases per 100,000 population at the national level. The heavy lines give the maximum rate and the three quartiles (Q1, median, and Q3) calculated on an annual basis across the 89 diseases. A logarithmic scale has been used for the vertical axis. (B) Maximum and minimum rates and three quartiles replotted as index numbers (1917 = 100).

Sources: Redrawn from Smallman-Raynor and Cliff (2004*b*, fig. 3.1, p. 127), based on Hall (1993)

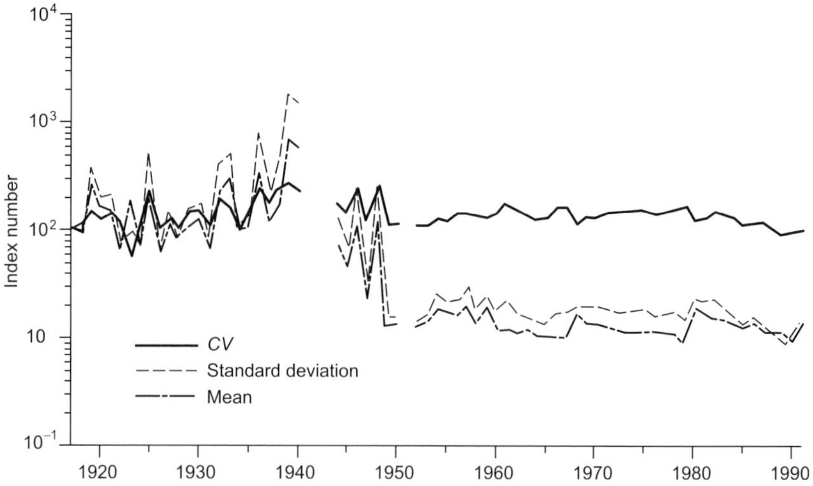

Fig. 9.26. Australia, 1917–1991: summary statistics for annual morbidity rates from 89 infectious diseases

Mean, standard deviation, and coefficient of variation (*CV*) of rates plotted as index numbers (1917 = 100). The statistics have been calculated annually across the notified rates for the 89 diseases.

Sources: Redrawn from Smallman-Raynor and Cliff (2004*b*, fig. 3.2, p. 128), originally based on Hall (1993).

where $\bar{x}$ and s are the arithmetic mean and standard deviation respectively of the 89 rates in each year. The coefficient is large where there is great variation in relation to the mean, and small when the variation is relatively low. Because the three time series are in different units, they have been converted to index numbers (1917 = 100) to aid comparisons; a logarithmic scale has been used for the vertical axis.

While the coefficient of variation remained effectively constant over the entire period, Figure 9.26 makes clear (i) the roughly constant or slightly rising level (mean) and variation (standard deviation) of rates between 1917 and 1940; (ii) the shift to a lower level and degree of variability after 1945; and (iii) the sharpest decline in rates and variability in the immediate post-World War II period from 1946 to 1951.

9.4.2 Recent Emergence Events: 'Virus Spillovers' from Bats

Recent disease emergence events in Australia are summarized by Beaman (1997), Mackenzie (1999), and Mackenzie, Chua, *et al.* (2001). While the general pattern has mimicked developments in other industrialized countries, with food- and water-borne infections and antimicrobial resistance high on the public health agenda, special interest has attached to a number of emerging vector-borne and zoonotic viral diseases in the Australian continent; see Figure 9.27. Among the vector-borne diseases, the indigenous Barmah Forest virus, along with importations of Japanese encephalitis and dengue viruses, have been associated with multiple disease outbreaks in the Australian continent since the early 1990s (see, for example, Lindsay, Johansen, *et al.* 1995; Mackenzie, Chua, *et al.* 2001; Hanna *et al.* 2006). To these developments can be added the emergence of three zoonotic viral agents (Hendra, Menangle, and Australian bat lyssavirus) whose recognition as the cause of human disease can be traced to virus spillovers from bats.

THE GEOGRAPHICAL PATTERN OF VIRUS SPILLOVERS

Figure 9.28 charts the location of recorded sporadic cases and outbreaks of disease associated with Hendra virus (HeV), Menangle virus (MenV), and Australian bat lyssavirus (ABLV) in humans and other animal species by 2005. The distribution of sample species of fruit bat (*Pteropus* spp.), identified as reservoirs for one or more of the viruses, is delimited by the shaded area. As the map shows, outbreaks of the three viruses have been concentrated along the east coast of Australia, within the known range of the bat reservoirs. Factors that underpin the virus spillovers are unclear, although man-induced changes in bat ecology—including the possible effects of habitat loss and roost disturbance on viral dynamics and levels of inter-species contact—may be facilitating the emergence process (Breed *et al.* 2005).

Hendra Virus (HeV)

Hendra virus (*ICD*-10 B33.8) is classified with Nipah virus (Section 7.4.1) as a member of the novel *Henipavirus* genus of the *Paramyxoviridae* (Heymann 2004: 245–7). As summarized in Table 9.6, the first recognized outbreaks of Hendra viral disease occurred among horses and their human contacts in the widely separated locations of Brisbane and Mackay, Queensland, in August–September 1994 (Figure 9.28). The two outbreaks were associated with 23 equine infections (including 16 deaths) and thee human infections (two deaths), with human cases variously presenting with respiratory disease and prolonged fatal meningoencephalitis (Paterson *et al.* 1998). As Figure 9.28 shows, further outbreaks of Hendra viral disease were subsequently recorded in Cairns (1999, 2004) and Townsville (2004), Queensland (Breed *et al.* 2005). Reservoir studies have identified HeV in fruit bats (*Pteropus* spp.) all along the eastern coast of Queensland (Young *et al.* 1996),[14] and a bat → horse → human transmission chain is inferred for the initial outbreaks. The manner in which horses acquired HeV from bats is unknown (Paterson *et al.* 1998).

[14] Evidence of Hendra virus infection has been documented in the spectacled fruit bat (*P. conspicillatus*), the black fruit bat (*P. alecto*), the little red fruit bat (*P. scapulatus*), and the grey-headed fruit bat (*P. poliocephalus*). See Young *et al.* (1996) for further details.

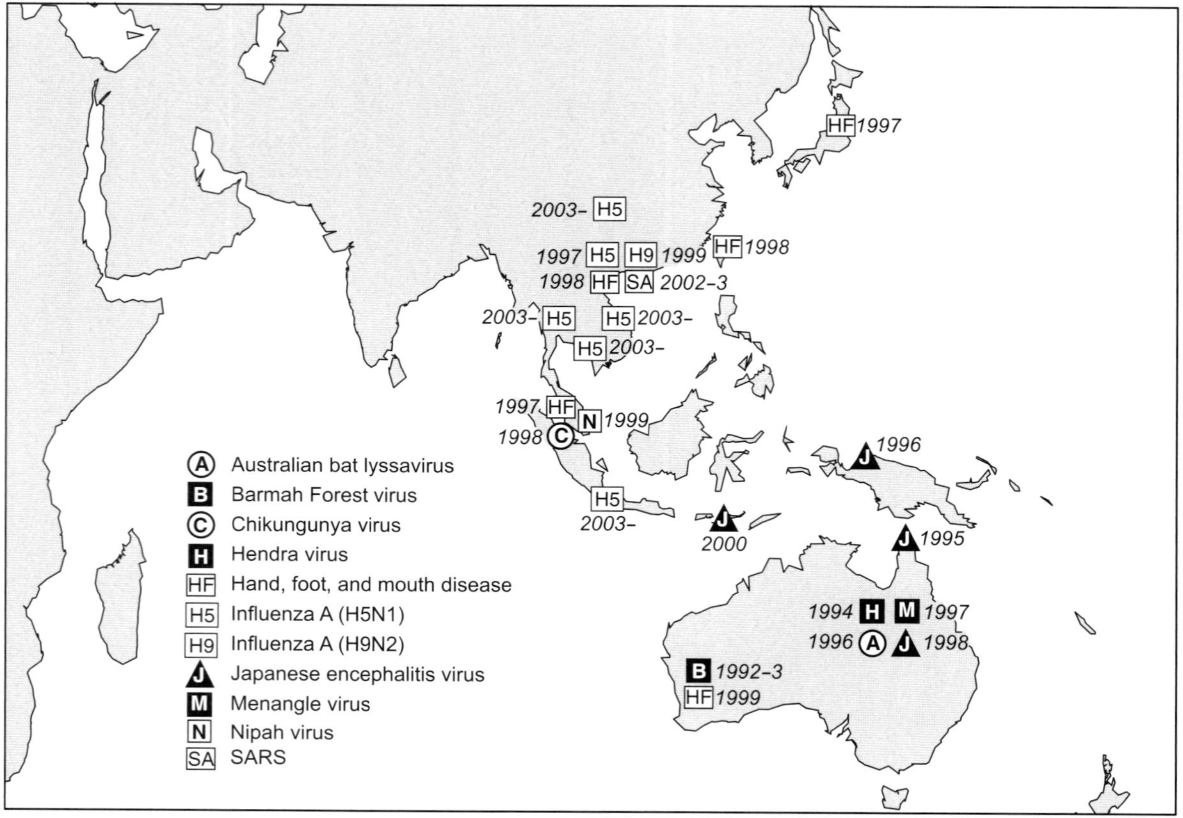

Fig. 9.27. Sample outbreaks of emerging viral diseases in South-East Asia and the western Pacific, 1991–2005
Source: Based in part on Mackenzie, Chua, *et al.* (2001, unnumbered fig., p. 497).

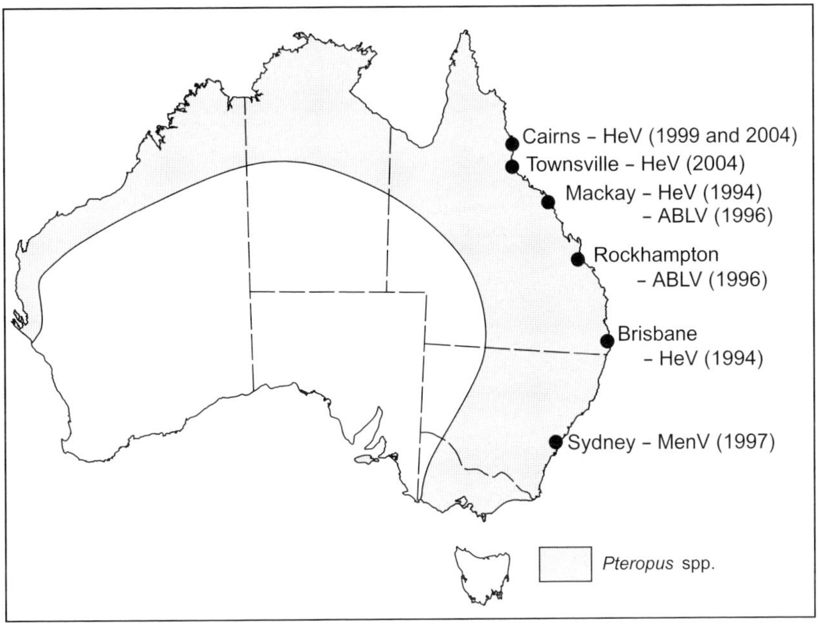

Fig. 9.28. Location of identified virus spillovers from bats to humans and other animal species in Australia, 1994–2005
Dates and places of virus spillovers are indicated for Australian bat lyssavirus (ABLV), Hendra virus (HeV), and Menangle virus (MenV). The aggregate distribution of fruit bat reservoirs of the spillover viruses (*Pteropus alecto*, *P. poliocephalus*, *P. conspicullatus*, and *P. scapulatus*) is indicated by the shaded area.
Source: Adapted from Breed *et al.* (2005, fig. 1, p. 60).

Menangle Virus (MenV)

Menangle virus is a newly recognized member of the *Rubulavirus* genus of the *Paramyxoviridae*. The virus was first isolated from stillborn piglets with abnormalities of the brain, spinal cord, and skeleton at a commercial piggery in New South Wales, Australia, in 1997 (Figure 9.28). Serologic studies indicated that at least two piggery workers were infected with the virus, apparently resulting in a severe febrile illness. Infection with MenV was subsequently identified in grey-headed fruit bats (*P. poliocephalus*) and little red fruit bats (*P. scapulatus*) that were roosting in close proximity to the piggery, and a bat → pig → human transmission chain is presumed (Philbey *et al.* 1998).

Australian Bat Lyssavirus (ABLV)

Prior to the mid-1990s, Australia was considered to be free of rabies and rabies-like viruses. In 1996, however, a new lyssavirus (ABLV) was recovered from a black fruit bat (*P. alecto*). Since that date, fatal human cases of a

Table 9.6. Sequence of events associated with the identification of Hendra viral disease in Australia, 1994–1996

Year	Month	Event
1994	Aug.	Two horses in Mackay, Queensland, die of unidentified illness
	Aug.	Patient 1 develops aseptic meningitis
	Sept.	18 horses in Brisbane, Queensland, fall ill (14 die)
	Sept.	Patient 2 develops an influenza-like illness
	Sept.	Patient 3 develops a fatal respiratory illness
1995	Sept.	Patient 1 develops fatal encephalitis
1996	Sept.	Hendra virus isolated from bats

Source: Paterson *et al.* (1998, table 2, p. 117).

rabies-like disease due to ABLV have been associated with distinct virus strains that circulate in both frugivorous and insectivorous bats in mainland Australia (Warrilow *et al.* 2003; Breed *et al.* 2005) (Figure 9.28).

9.5 Local Patterns: The London Series, 1850–1973

In this subsection, we examine mortality trends for sample infectious diseases in the city of London since 1850. For continuity with our consideration of pre-1850 mortality trends in the city (Section 2.4), we draw upon relevant information contained in two 13 (cause) × 371 (year) data matrices of deaths and death rates per 1,000 population in London, 1603–1973. Full details of the data matrices are provided in Section 2.4.2. Here we note that all mortality data for the 124-year period under review, 1850–1973, are based on information abstracted from the Registrar General's *Annual Report* (1850–1920) and *Statistical Review* (1921–73); our series terminates with the cessation of the *Statistical Review* and the regular reporting of mortality statistics for London. For reference, Table 9.7 gives average annual counts of mortality associated with the 13 causes of death (all causes and 12 diseases), along with the corresponding death rates per 1,000 population, for intervals in the period 1850–1973.

9.5.1 Mortality Curves

Over 9.96 million deaths were registered in London during the period 1850–1973. As the annual curve of death rates in Figure 9.29 shows, the first 70 years of the observation period were marked by a continuation of the long mortality decline that began in the mid-eighteenth century (Section 2.4.2) and which came to an abrupt end at about the time of the Spanish influenza pandemic of 1918–19. Thereafter, death rates fluctuated around a low and approximately stable level of 11–12 per 1,000 population.

Table 9.7. Average annual mortality due to sample infectious diseases, London, 1850–1973

	Average annual count of deaths[1]		
Cause of death	1850–99	1900–49	1950–73
Cholera	451 (0.14)	4 (0.00)	0 (0.00)
Diphtheria	1,018 (0.17)	634 (0.09)	1 (0.00)
Influenza	315 (0.06)	1,900 (0.25)	516 (0.07)
Leprosy	0 (0.00)	0 (0.00)	0 (0.00)
Measles	1,979 (0.47)	1,052 (0.14)	11 (0.00)
Meningococcal disease	3 (0.00)	107 (0.01)	26 (0.00)
Plague	0 (0.00)	0 (0.00)	0 (0.00)
Scarlet fever	2,002 (0.54)	189 (0.03)	2 (0.00)
Smallpox	728 (0.20)	4 (0.00)	2 (0.00)
Syphilis	384 (0.09)	371 (0.05)	211 (0.03)
Tuberculosis (pulmonary)	8,174 (2.04)	6,029 (0.80)	677 (0.08)
Whooping cough	2,541 (0.63)	819 (0.11)	8 (0.00)
All causes	75,184 (18.33)	82,988 (10.84)	89,213 (11.41)

Note: [1] Average annual death rate (per 1,000 population) in parentheses.

As described in Section 2.4.2, two of the sample diseases in Table 9.7 had ceased to be significant causes of recorded mortality in London by the late seventeenth century (plague) and early nineteenth century (leprosy). For the remaining 10 diseases, the main graphs in Figure 9.30 plot the annual series of death rates per 1,000 population, 1850–1973. To set the trends in a longer-term perspective, the inset graphs are replotted from Figure 2.13 and give, by decadal period, the average annual death rates per 1,000 population for 1603–1849 (unshaded bars) and 1850–1973 (shaded bars).

Subject to the limitations of the available data, Figure 9.30 highlights the continued and locally complex pattern of disease succession in the modern period (Thomson 1955, 1976). Set against the decline to very low levels of recorded mortality for cholera (graph A), measles (D), scarlet fever (F), smallpox (G), pulmonary tuberculosis (I), and whooping cough (J), the remaining diseases—diphtheria (B), influenza (C), meningococcal disease (E), and syphilis (H)—emerged to prominence in the recorded statistics after 1850.

Diphtheria (Figure 9.30B). The emergence of diphtheria in London in the late 1850s coincided, in Creighton's (1891–4: ii. 736) words, with a 'sudden uprising of the malady all over the globe'. 'Of its novelty to nearly the whole British [medical] profession in 1858', Creighton adds, 'there can be no question.' The disease was distinguished in the Registrar General's *Reports* for the first time in 1859, having previously been merged with scarlet fever. Diphtheria exerted a significant influence on London's mortality record throughout the latter half of the nineteenth century, to achieve an

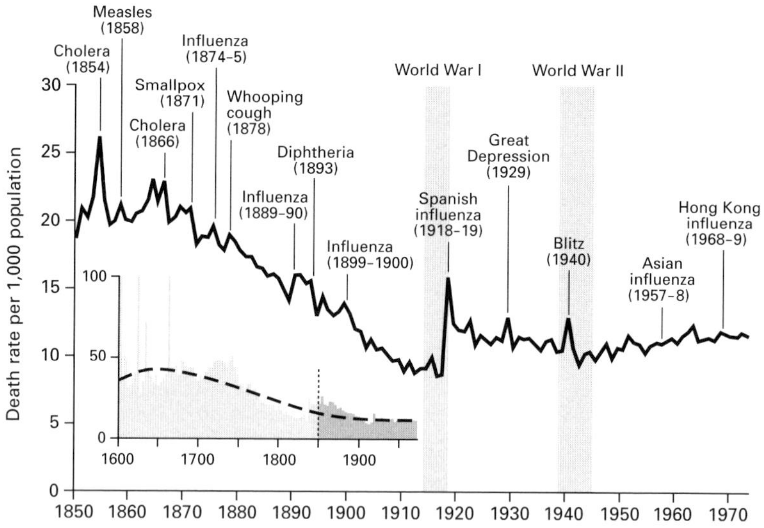

Fig. 9.29. Annual death rates per 1,000 population for all causes, London, 1850–1973 The line trace plots annual death rates for 1850–1973, with sample epidemics and other mortality-related events indicated. The inset graph is redrawn from Fig. 2.12 and plots the estimated annual death rate per 1,000 population for London for 1603–1849 (light bars) and 1850–1973 (dark bars). A polynomial regression line fitted by ordinary least squares (broken line trace) depicts the overall trend in mortality in the inset graph.

'extraordinary severity' in the 1890s (Creighton 1891–4: ii. 741). A secondary peak of mortality occurred in the 1920s, and this was followed by progressive retreat to near-zero death rates by the mid-twentieth century (Table 9.7).

Influenza (Figure 9.30C). Although the epidemic record for influenza and influenza-like illnesses in England and Wales can be traced back to at least 1510 (Thompson 1852; Creighton 1891–4: i. 398–9), the influenza curve for London displays a step-function increase in recorded mortality from the time of the 1889–90 pandemic. While all subsequent events are dwarfed by the towering spike of morality associated with the Spanish influenza pandemic (1918–19), the inter-war period marked the onset of a gradual but perceptible decline in the background level of recorded influenza death rates.

Meningococcal disease (Figure 9.30E). Cerebrospinal fever first appeared as a distinct disease category in the mortality records of London in the early 1880s although, as late as 1894, the disease merited no more than an appended note in Creighton's (1891–4: ii. 863–4) *Epidemics in Britain*. As Figure 9.30E shows, the disease struck its first major blows in London during World War I (1914–18) and continued to yield inflated levels of recorded

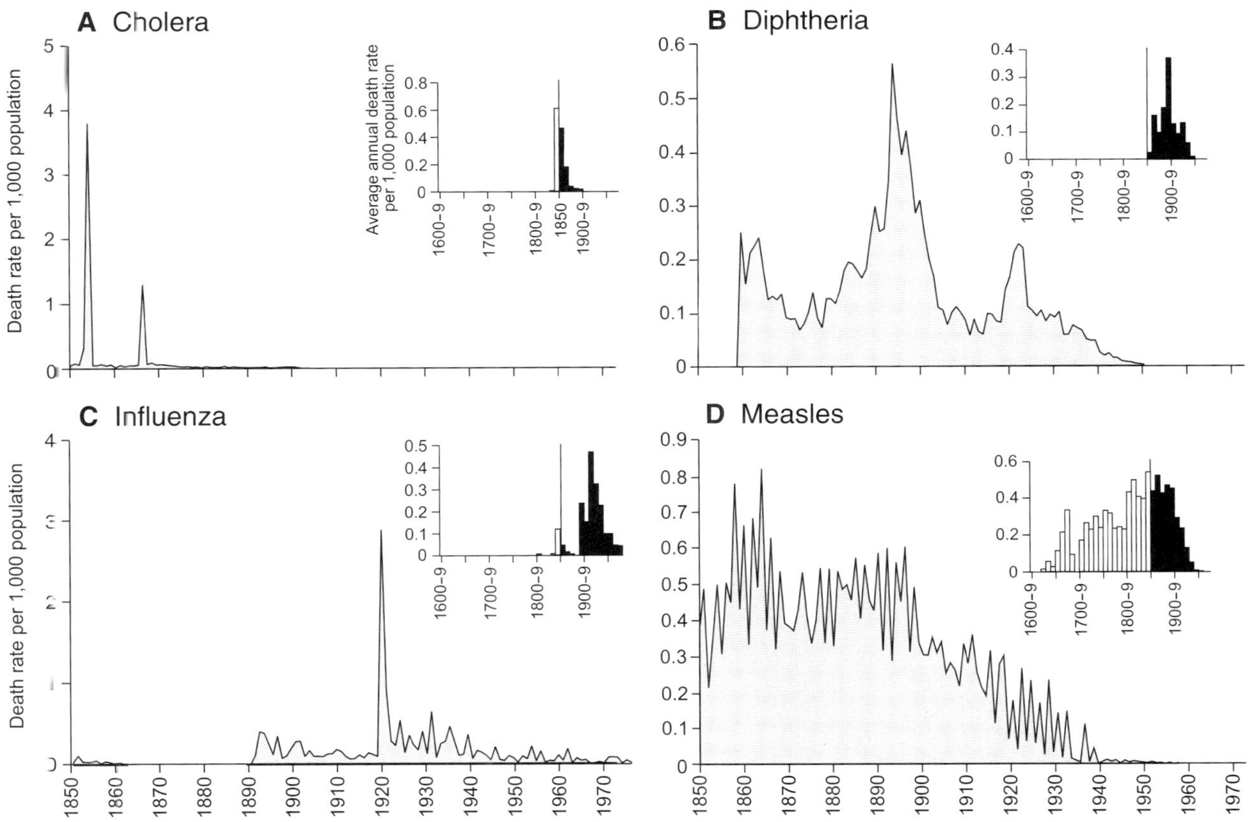

Fig. 9.30. Time series of reported mortality from sample infectious diseases, London, 1850–1973
For each disease, the main graphs plot the annual death rate per 1,000 population for 1850–1973. The inset graphs are redrawn from Fig. 2.13 and plot, by decadal period, the average annual death rate per 1,000 population for 1603–1849 (unshaded bars) and 1850–1973 (shaded bars). (A) Cholera. (B) Diphtheria. (C) Influenza. (D) Measles. (E) Meningococcal disease (cerebrospirial meningitis). (F) Scarlet fever. (G) Smallpox. (H) Syphilis. (I) Tuberculosis (pulmonary). (J) Whooping cough.

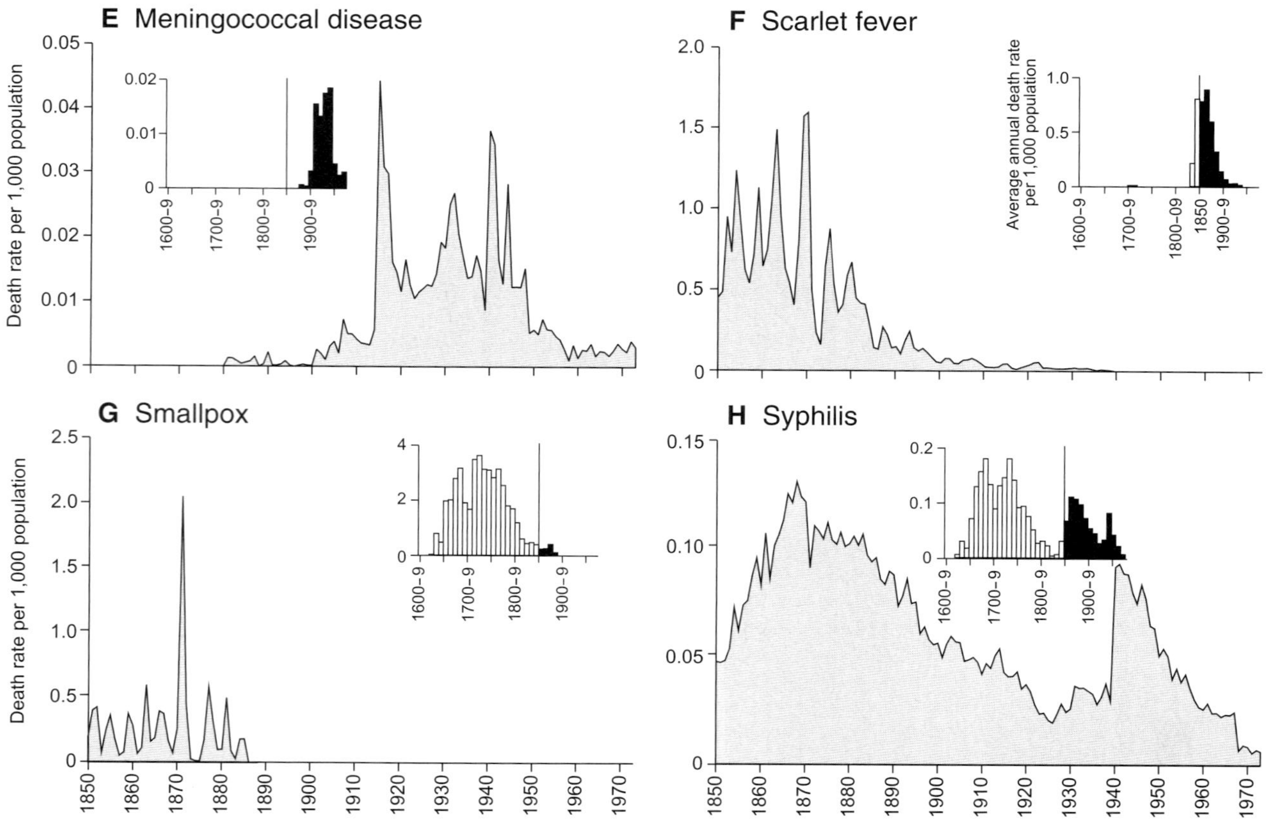

Fig. 9.30. (Continued)

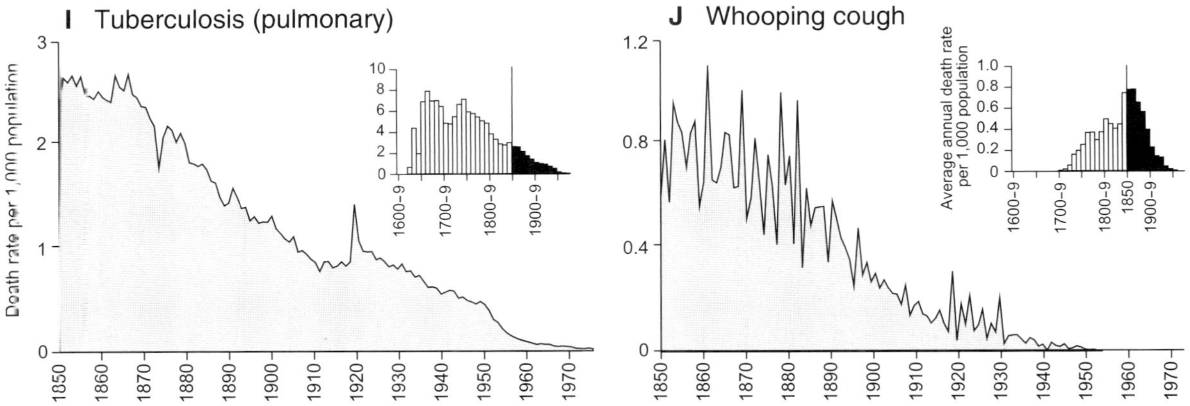

Fig. 9.30. (Continued)

mortality in the decades to the 1950s. Thereafter, death rates subsided to pre-war levels (Table 9.7).

Syphilis (Figure 9.30H). A striking feature of Figure 9.30H is the wave-like resurgence of syphilis, from a 200-year low in recorded death rates in the 1820s and 1830s to a new peak—albeit somewhat below the historic highs of the seventeenth and eighteenth centuries—in the 1860s and 1870s. Thereafter, a long and steady decline in syphilis death rates was temporarily interrupted by the nationwide epidemic that occurred in association with World War II and its immediate aftermath (Green *et al.* 2001).

9.5.2 Epidemic Wavelength

The graphs in Figure 9.31 have been generated as described for Figure 2.15. They plot as circles the dominant wavelength (in years) of epidemics for eight infectious diseases in London.[15] Wavelengths for the sample periods 1850–99, 1900–49, and 1950–73 are represented by the black circles, while, for reference, wavelengths for sample periods prior to 1850 are represented by the white circles. Although the overall pattern is complex, certain prominent features emerge from Figure 9.31: (i) the establishment of steady 2-yearly epidemic cycles for measles from the early nineteenth century (graph C) and for whooping cough from the early twentieth century (graph H); (ii) the progressive reduction from 6- to 2-yearly epidemic cycles for influenza since 1800 (graph B); and (iii) the sharp increase in epidemic wavelength as smallpox retreated as a significant cause of reported mortality from 1850 (graph E). For the remaining diseases, a common pattern of increasing epidemic wavelengths to 6- or 7-yearly cycles in the period 1900–49 is followed, where calculable, by a reduction in wavelength in the truncated period 1950–73.

9.5.3 Epidemic Magnitude

Following the method described for Figure 2.16, the detrended (first differenced) time series of death rates per 1,000 population for each of the eight diseases in Figure 9.31 was examined to determine the largest (maximum) and smallest (minimum) annual rates in (i) each 10-year period from 1850–9 to 1960–9 and (ii) the truncated period 1970–3. The resulting 13-element series of maxima (peaks) and minima (troughs) for each disease are plotted in Figure 9.32. Long-term trends in each series were determined using the linear regression model in equation 2.2; the fitted regression lines are plotted in Figure 9.32, while Table 9.8 gives the slope coefficients, along with the

[15] Of the 10 sample diseases in Figure 9.30, two diseases (cholera and meningococcal disease) were omitted from the wavelength analysis in Figure 9.31 on account of the limited time series available for inter-temporal comparisons in the post-1850 period.

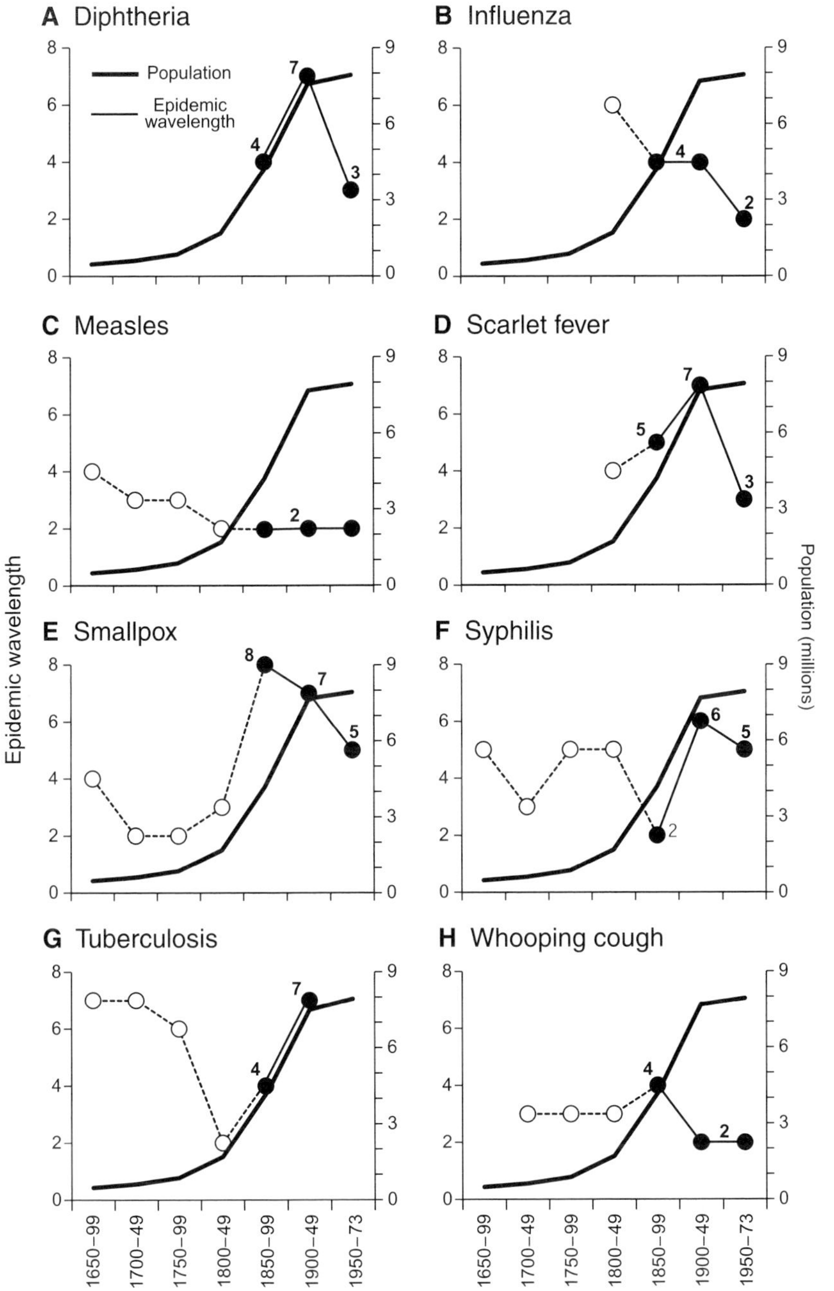

Fig. 9.31. Dominant wavelength (in years) of epidemic cycles for eight sample infectious diseases, London, 1850–1973

Graphs plot the shift in the dominant epidemic wavelength for sample intervals in the period 1850–1973 (black circles), along with the equivalent information for sample intervals in the period 1650–1849 (white circles) where available. Wavelengths (years) are indicated by the numerals attached to the circles. The population of London (heavy line trace) is plotted for reference. (A) Diphtheria. (B) Influenza. (C) Measles. (D) Scarlet fever. (E) Smallpox. (F) Syphilis. (G) Tuberculosis (pulmonary). (H) Whooping cough. Evidence for the period 1650–1849 is considered in Sect. 2.4.2.

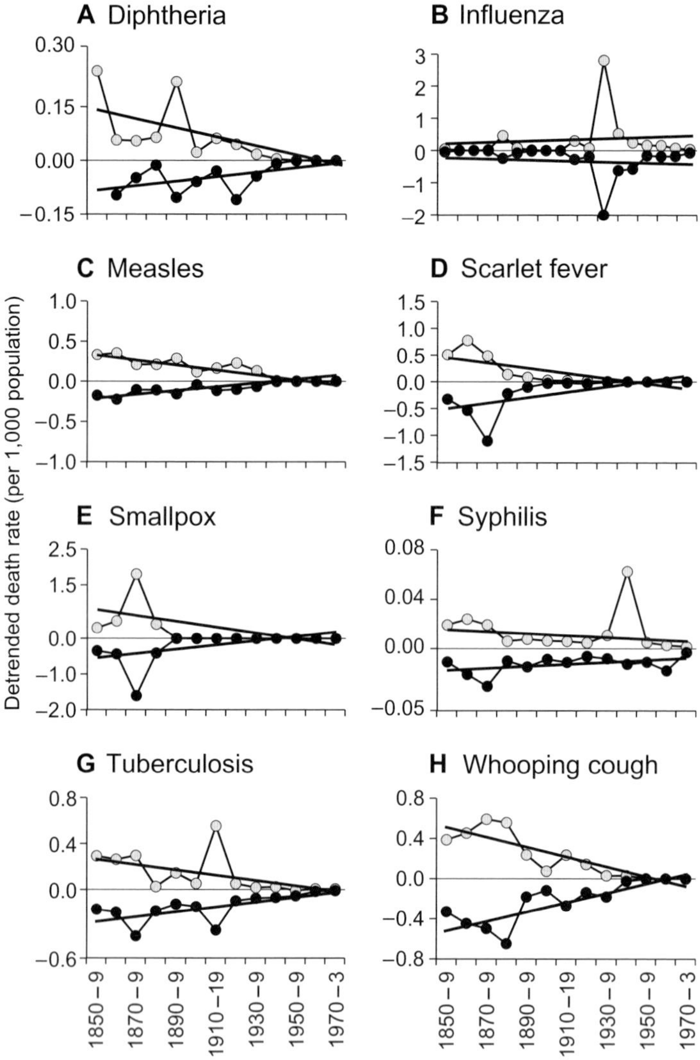

Fig. 9.32. Changing epidemic magnitude, London, 1850–1973
Graphs plot, by 10-year period, the series of maximum (shaded circles) and minimum (solid circles) annual death rates for each of eight diseases. (A) Diphtheria. (B) Influenza. (C) Measles. (D) Scarlet fever. (E) Smallpox. (F) Syphilis. (G) Tuberculosis (pulmonary). (H) Whooping cough. Trends are depicted by the linear regression lines fitted to the series of maxima and minima by ordinary least squares. The slope coefficients of the fitted regression models are given in Table 9.8.

Table 9.8. Regression slope coefficient values for OLS trend lines fitted to maximum (peaks) and minimum (troughs) annual death rates by 10-year period, London, 1850–1973

	Peaks			Troughs		
Disease	Slope coefficient (t-statistic)	R^2 (F-ratio)	Direction of trend	Slope coefficient (t-statistic)	R^2 (F-ratio)	Direction of trend
Diphtheria	−0.01 (−3.04*)	0.46 (9.25*)	Falling	0.01 (2.46*)	0.38 (6.07*)	Rising
Influenza	0.01 (0.14)	0.00 (0.02)	Stable	−0.02 (−0.39)	0.01 (0.16)	Stable
Measles	−0.03 (− 7.14**)	0.82 (51.03**)	Falling	0.03 (6.11**)	0.77 (37.28**)	Rising
Scarlet fever	−0.05 (− 4.18**)	0.61 (17.43**)	Falling	0.05 (2.90*)	0.43 (8.44*)	Rising
Smallpox	−0.07 (− 2.11)	0.29 (4.45)	Stable	0.07 (2.28*)	0.32 (5.18*)	Rising
Syphilis	−0.00 (− 0.42)	0.02 (0.18)	Stable	0.00 (1.66)	0.20 (2.75)	Stable
Tuberculosis	−0.02 (−2.25*)	0.32 (5.08*)	Falling	0.02 (3.06*)	0.46 (9.39*)	Rising
Whooping cough	−0.05 (− 5.74**)	0.75 (32.99**)	Falling	0.04 (4.74**)	0.67 (22.42**)	Rising

Notes: *Significant at the $p = 0.05$ level (one-tailed test). ** Significant at the $p = 0.01$ level (one-tailed test).

associated *t*-statistics, the coefficients of determination (R^2), and the *F*-ratios. As before, statistically significant slope coefficients at the $p = 0.05$ level (one-tailed test) are used to classify the trends as 'rising' (positive slope coefficient) or 'falling' (negative slope coefficient); trends associated with non-significant slope coefficients are classified as 'stable'.

Inspection of Figure 9.32 and Table 9.8 reveals that five of the eight diseases (diphtheria, measles, scarlet fever, pulmonary tuberculosis, and whooping cough) share a common pattern of falling peaks and rising troughs over the period 1850–1973. This pattern implies that the reduction in mortality witnessed for the five diseases in Figure 9.30 was driven by (i) changes in excess mortality associated with epidemic flare-ups rather than (ii) changes in the underpinning pattern of mortality in inter-epidemic periods. Of the remaining diseases, the approximately flat trend lines for two (influenza and syphilis) imply a basic stability in the magnitude of epidemic swings over the time period. Finally, interpretation of the atypical pattern of stable peaks and rising troughs for smallpox is limited by virtue of the retreat of this disease as a significant cause of recorded mortality by 1900.

9.6 Conclusion

In this chapter, we have examined in both advanced and developing countries trends in morbidity and mortality over the 150 years or so since 1850. Continuing the pattern of earlier times (Section 2.3), pandemic cycles of plague and cholera—aided in their speed and direction of diffusion by dramatic improvements in transport and technology—have cast a long shadow over the globe. Towards the end of the twentieth century, they were joined by another pandemic scourge (HIV/AIDS), which, a quarter of a century after its first recognition, still eludes the efforts of medical science to develop an effective vaccine. Within specific epidemiological environments, the same basic patterns of emergence and cyclical re-emergence have been played out by other diseases and at a variety of spatial scales. Meningococcal disease and Ebola–Marburg viral diseases in sub-Saharan Africa (regional level), virus spillovers from bats in Australia (national level), and the recognition of new (diphtheria and cerebrospinal fever) and the resurgence of old (syphilis) disease categories in the mortality statistics for London (local level) are all illustrative of the phenomenon.

In the economically more advanced regions of the world, patterns of disease emergence and re-emergence have been superimposed on an exponential decline in infectious disease morbidity and mortality since 1900. Although infectious diseases are far from eliminated and, in some instances, still cause significant levels of ill health, they have been replaced by cancer, heart, and circulatory disorders as the main causes of death in these countries. In the developing countries, the picture is different. Infectious diseases remain of central importance as causes of death, although the story here is also one of retreat in the face of the WHO's Expanded Programme of Immunization. The use of vaccination to control infectious diseases is discussed further in Section 11.3, while Cliff, Haggett, and Smallman-Raynor (2004: 133–51) discuss the various WHO immunization campaigns to eradicate the vaccine-preventable diseases of smallpox and poliomyelitis.

PART III

The Future for Emergent Disease Control

10

Spatial Detection of (Re-)emerging Diseases

10.1 Introduction

The development of models and surveillance systems to give early warning of a new or re-emerging disease is an important first step in devising control strategies to protect the public health. In this chapter, we discuss and illustrate modelling and surveillance approaches to (re-)emerging disease detection before considering in Chapter 11 what control strategies might be used to mitigate new threats.

We begin by reviewing in Section 10.2.1 the generic SIR (susceptible ⇒ infected ⇒ removed) mass action models commonly used to model the spread of infectious diseases in human and many animal populations, before moving on to present a robust spatial derivative, the so-called *swash–backwash* model (Section 10.2.2). This model is applied in Section 10.3 to data from France, Iceland, and a small English town, Cirencester, to show, for the cyclically re-emerging disease of influenza, how the model readily separates pandemic years from the normal run of influenza seasons. While it is encouraging that the model can spot pandemic years in the train of annual epidemics, influenza is an odd disease in that pandemics occur when a new strain of the causative A virus emerges to afflict the human population. To test the model further, we apply it in Section 10.4 to a set of 14 measles waves for Iceland, 1916–75, waves caused by an unchanging virus in a changing population. Our discussion of the swash–backwash model is concluded in Section 10.5, where it is shown how it can be used as part of a real-time surveillance-based early-warning system for new disease threats.

Any modelling approach to identifying newly emergent or re-emerging diseases can only be as good as the data which are supplied to the models. Accordingly, in Section 10.6, advances in surveillance methodology are outlined which have been facilitated by developments in communications technology, especially the Internet. The chapter is concluded in Section 10.7.

10.2 Wave Analytic Methods

The ways in which diseases are transmitted from person to person have attracted mathematical interest from Bernoulli onwards: the classic accounts are given by Bailey (1975) in his *Mathematical Theory of Infectious Diseases* and by Anderson and May (1991) in their *Infectious Diseases of Humans: Dynamics and Control*. To give a flavour of their approach, a very simplified diagram of the spread of an infectious disease through a human population is illustrated in Figure 10.1. The population is divided into three sub-populations—those at risk (susceptibles, S), those with the disease (infectives, I), and those who have recovered (recovereds, R). Propagation of an epidemic occurs by homogeneous mixing (mass action) between the S and I populations at a rate β. This generates new cases by the transition $S \Rightarrow I$. Infectives recover at a rate μ, while the susceptible population is renewed for future epidemics by births at the rate γ. Population stocks are updated by simple accounting equations. That for I is shown in Figure 10.1—i.e. the number of new infectives at $t+1$ is given by the number at t, plus new infectives generated by the transition $S \Rightarrow I$, minus those infectives at t who recover by $t+1$. If an epidemic is to be sustained, a continuous chain of infectives must be

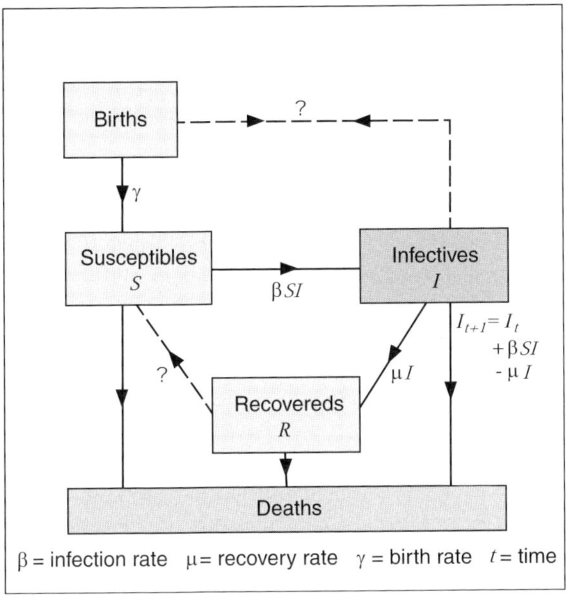

Fig. 10.1. Simplified model of an infection process
The mass action model is based upon person-to-person contact between infectives, *I*, and susceptibles, *S*, at a rate β which generates new cases of the disease. Infected individuals recover at a rate μ and enter the removed population, *R*.
Source: Cliff, Haggett, and Smallman-Raynor (1993, fig. 16.1 upper, p. 414).

maintained. Such a chain will continue as long as transmission of infection from infectives to susceptibles can occur.

10.2.1 Spatial Mass Action Models

A number of early writers, notably Bartlett (1957) and Black (1966) developed the SIR model into a geographical setting by studying the mixing process between susceptibles and infectives in populations distributed in systems of towns of different sizes. Under these conditions, the parameter β cannot be assumed to be constant. The upshot of their work was to establish a direct relationship between the population size of a town and the frequency of epidemic waves. As described in Section 6.2.1, they divided waves into three types found in towns of successively smaller population size: *Type I* waves (large towns), where chains of infection remained continuous and major epidemics flared up at regular intervals; *Type II* waves (medium-sized towns), in which regular epidemics occurred but where the disease disappeared completely between epidemics; and *Type III* waves (small towns) in which epidemics occurred irregularly and infrequently, separated by long inter-epidemic periods of unpredictable duration when no cases of the disease were reported. The population threshold crossed when towns cease to display Type II waves and experience Type I waves is called the *critical community size*; it defines the transition from epidemic to endemic behaviour.

Figure 10.2 shows these ideas schematically. In large towns above the critical community size, like town A, a continuous trickle of cases is reported. These provide the reservoir of infection which sparks a major epidemic when the population at risk (susceptibles, *S*) builds up to a critical mass. For many simple infectious diseases like rubella, measles, and whooping cough on which much of the basic theory was developed, this build-up can only occur as children are born, lose their mother-conferred immunity, and escape either vaccination or the disease (which is assumed to confer lifelong immunity). Eventually the *S* population will become sufficiently large for an epidemic to break out. When this happens, the *S* population is diminished and the stock of infectives, *I*, increases as individuals are transferred by infection from the *S* to the *I* population. This generates the characteristic 'D'-shaped relationship over time between the sizes of the *S* and *I* populations shown on the end plane of the block diagram.

If the total population of a town falls below the critical community size, as in communities B and C of Figure 10.2, epidemics can only arise when the disease agent is introduced into it by the influx (e.g. by migration or journey to work) of infected individuals (so-called *index cases*) from reservoir areas. These movements are shown by the broad arrows. In such smaller towns, the *S* population is insufficient to maintain a continuous record of infection. The disease dies out and the *S* population grows in the absence of infection. Eventually the *S* population will become big enough to sustain an epidemic when an index case arrives. Given that the total population of the community is insufficient to renew by births the *S* population as rapidly as it is diminished by infection, the epidemic will eventually die out.

It is the repetition of this basic process which generates the successive epidemic waves witnessed in most communities. Of special significance is the way in which the continuous infection and characteristically regular Type I epidemic waves of endemic communities break down as population size diminishes into, first, discrete but regular Type II waves in town B and then, second, into discrete and irregularly spaced Type III waves in town C. Since the *S* population continues to grow by births in the absence of infection, very large epidemics can occur in small and isolated communities if build-up takes place over a long period of time in the absence of vaccination and index cases. Note also, in communities below the population size threshold, that the base of the 'D' relationship between the *S* and *I* populations is at zero with respect to *I* between epidemics. This contrasts with towns like A where the non-zero base reflects the continuous trickle of cases in the inter-epidemic phases.

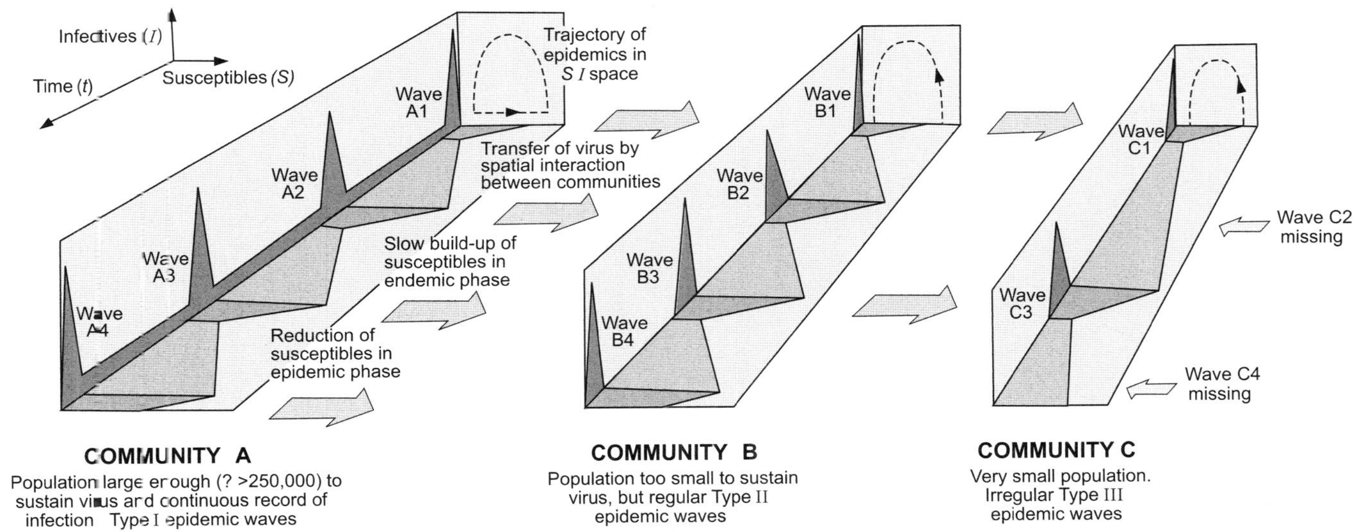

Fig. 10.2. Spatial version of the mass action model
Conceptual view of the spread of a communicable disease in and between towns of different population sizes. Types I–III waves correspond to the Bartlett model described in the text.

Source: Cliff and Haggett (1988, fig. 6.5A, p. 246).

A large literature has developed around the SIR model in which refinements have been added to the model to allow (for example) for: inhomogeneous mixing among the population subgroups, especially spatially; vaccination; the latent period of the disease; carrier states; and population recycling from $R \Rightarrow S$ (see, for example, Keeling and Grenfell 1997). The model has often given profound insights into the spread of epidemics, but it is complex to fit to space–time data without heroic assumptions about the stationarity of model parameters and isotropisms of the underlying processes. The longer the time series and the greater the geographical area being studied, the less likely are such assumptions to be tenable, not least because the sensitivity and specificity of disease reporting is unlikely to have remained constant over time. Over the long term, morbidity/mortality recording is likely to be skewed, with the degree of bias often unknown and non-constant. Even over the short term, it is not clear whether during a period of high disease incidence (for example, the peak of an influenza pandemic), cases and deaths are over-reported because of assumptions about the prevailing cause or under-recorded because reporting physicians are overwhelmed by more pressing clinical demands upon their time. Historical evidence can be adduced to support both points of view.

Epidemiologists are not alone wanting to develop models from data of uncertain accuracy; economists, in particular, have been plagued by trying to establish economic trends from historically variable sources (Morgenstern 1963). Among the many methods proposed to overcome this problem, the work of John Tukey has been particularly important in devising robust methods (what he termed Exploratory Data Analysis, or EDA) to work alongside classical statistical models (Hoaglin *et al.* 1983).

In the next subsection, we develop in the Tukey tradition a robust SIR model for exploring from long-term morbidity and mortality data the speed of epidemic waves, which is particularly helpful in identifying *re-emerging* communicable diseases. The spatial velocity of epidemic waves across human populations has attracted considerable theoretical interest (for example, Abramson *et al.* 2003; Grenfell *et al.* 2001; Zhao and Wang 2004) and is a matter of practical public health concern (Meltzer *et al.* 1999; Fedson 2003). The faster a wave of infection strikes a susceptible population, the less is the time available for implementing protective responses such as isolation and vaccination. Estimating velocity is thus particularly important both with resurgent old diseases with changing characteristics, such as pandemic outbreaks of influenza where genetic shifts in the causative A virus can mean that an infection is introduced into a population with little or no resistance to the new strain (Hay *et al.* 2001; Patterson 1986), and new diseases (e.g. SARS) where, simply because of newness, population resistance and community preparedness is likely to be low. The model is developed in Section 10.2.2. To illustrate its use with cyclically re-emerging diseases, it is applied in Section 10.3 to long time series of influenza epidemics at three diminishing geographical scales—a continental country, France, 1887–1999 (Section 10.3.1), an island community, Iceland, 1916–76 (Section 10.3.2), and a small English market town, Cirencester, 1963–76 (Section 10.3.3).

10.2.2 Swash–Backwash Models

We have demonstrated elsewhere using measles and poliomyelitis data that the spatial extent of infected units within a geographical area, and the time taken from the start of an epidemic for a disease to reach each unit, may be used to measure the spatial velocity of an epidemic wave (Cliff and Haggett 1981; Trevelyan *et al.* 2005; Cliff and Haggett 2006). In this section, we propose a robust *swash–backwash model* for estimating spatial velocity which uses only the binary presence/absence of disease reports rather than the actual number of reported cases/mortality.

THE MODEL

Following Cliff and Haggett (2006), we begin with the observation that a single epidemic wave in any large geographical area is a composite of the waves for each of its constituent sub-areas. That is, the composite wave at the larger geographical scale (say, a country) can in principle be broken down into a series of multiple waves for its constituent sub-areas (say, its regions) at the smaller geographical scale.

Assuming that both the sub-areas and the time periods are discrete, we use the following notation.

A = Area covered by an epidemic wave in terms of the number of sub-areas infected where a_i is a sub-area in the sequence $1, 2, \ldots, a_i, \ldots, A$.

T = Duration of an epidemic wave, defined in terms of a number of discrete time periods, t_j, in the sequence $1, 2, \ldots, t_j, \ldots, T$.

Q = Total cases of a disease recorded in a single epidemic wave measured over all sub-areas and all time periods. Thus, q_{ij} is the number of cases recorded in the cell formed by the i-th sub-area and the j-th time period of the $A \times T$ data matrix.

To illustrate the method, we assume in Figure 10.3 a simple epidemic wave where $A = 12$, $T = 10$, and $Q = 122$. Thus, in Figure 10.3A we begin with a hypothetical map which is converted into a 12×10 space–time data matrix in which 122 recorded cases of a disease are distributed to simulate an array typical of an epidemic wave. Note that, whereas this overall wave is continuous (no time periods with zero cases), for individual sub-areas the record may be discontinuous with one or more time periods with zero cases.

For any one of the rows in the data matrix in Figure 10.3A, two cells can be identified which mark the 'start cell' and the 'end cell' of a recorded outbreak; if the infection only lasts for one time period, the start and end cell are the

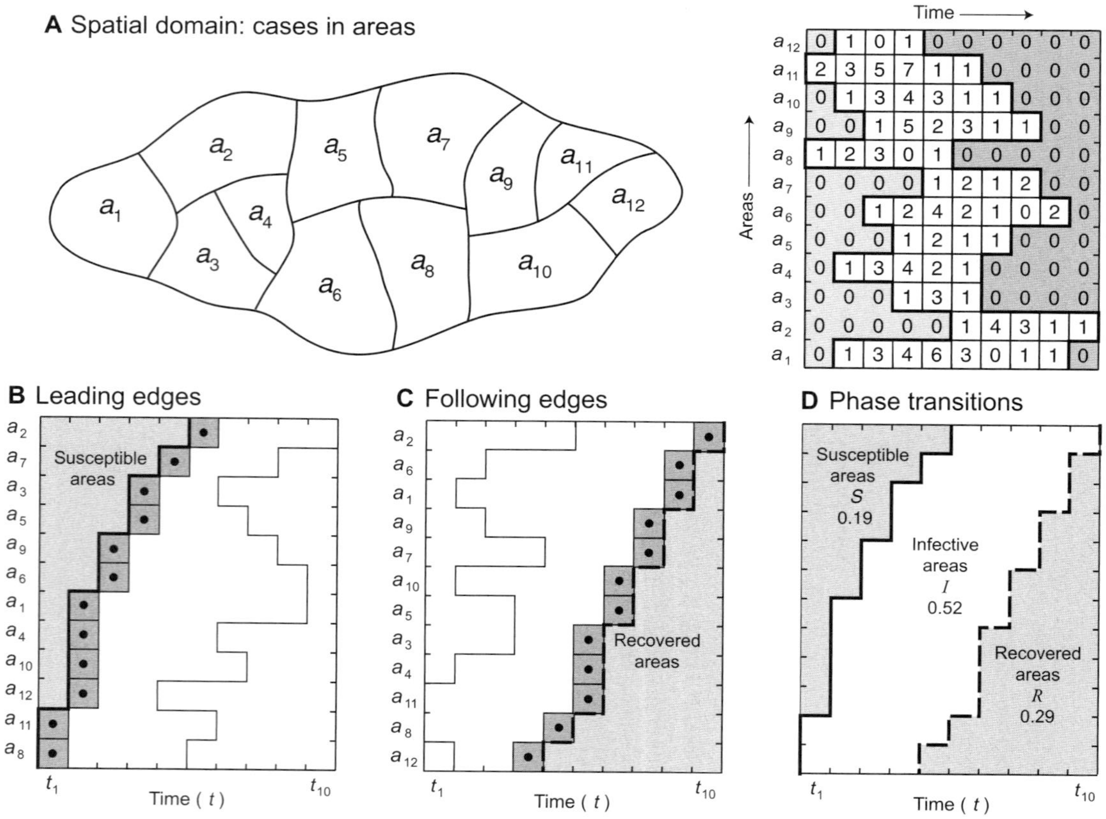

Fig. 10.3. Swash–backwash model: hypothetical 12-area example
(A) Base map with areas reference coded as $a_1 \ldots a_{12}$, and associated space–time data matrix with reported cases for each area given in cells. (B) Matrix rearranged to order leading edges, *LE*, and (C) following or trailing edges, *FE*. (D) Leading and following edges plotted as a phase-transition diagram with susceptible (*S*), infected (*I*), and recovered (*R*) integrals for areas.

same. Figures 10.3B and C analyse these start and end cells. In Figure 10.3B the 12×10 matrix is rearranged so as to position the start cells in an ascending temporal order. This line of cells (dark shading) defines the position of the leading edge (LE) marking the start of the epidemic wave in the different subareas. To the left and above this line lies a zone of cells (light shading) which have yet to be infected and thus may be regarded as areas to which the epidemic has yet to spread.

Equally, the 12×10 matrix can be organized as in Figure 10.3C, so as to arrange the end cells in ascending temporal order. This line of cells (dark shading) defines the position of the trailing edge or following edge (FE), marking the completion of the epidemic waves in each of the different subareas. To the right and below this line lies a zone of cells which have ceased to be infected and which thus may be regarded as areas which have recovered from infection.

Both the edges, LE and FE, can be combined as in Figure 10.3D to identify cells which are in susceptible, S, infected, I, and recovered, R, states. The resulting graph may be regarded as a *phase transition* or *SIR diagram*. It has two roles: first, it defines the boundaries of the two phase shifts from susceptible to infective status ($S \Rightarrow I$) and from infective to recovered status ($I \Rightarrow R$), and second, it integrates the three phases, S, I, and R, as areas within the graph. As discussed in Cliff and Haggett (2006), the phase diagram assumes characteristic configurations depending upon the velocity, duration, and ultimate spatial extent of an epidemic wave as it passes through a region.

Three model parameters relating to the phase diagram are especially useful. We refer to these here as V_{LE} and V_{FE}, the velocities of the leading and following edges of the wave which are functions of the average temporal position of the edges in the phase diagram; and R_{0A}, here defined as the *spatial basic reproduction number*. The relevant equations are summarized in Appendix 10.1.

SPATIAL BASIC REPRODUCTION NUMBER

In conventional SIR models, the *basic reproduction number*, R_0, is one of the most useful parameters used to characterize mathematically infectious disease processes. R_0 is defined as the ratio (in terms of Figure 10.1) between an infection rate (β) and a recovery rate (μ), i.e. $R_0 = \beta/\mu$. In terms of cases, R_0 is interpreted as the average number of secondary infections produced when one infected individual is introduced into a wholly susceptible population. Methods for estimating the basic reproduction number for infectious diseases are considered by Dietz (1993) and Farrington *et al.* (2001); an example of their use is given in Watts *et al.* (2005).

In the spatial domain, as shown in Figure 10.3D, the S, I, and R integrals define the boundaries of the two phase shifts from susceptible to infective status ($S \Rightarrow I$) and from infective to recovered status ($I \Rightarrow R$). This raises the prospect of defining a spatial version of R_0. The spatial basic reproduction number, R_{0A}, is the average number of secondary areas produced from one infected area in a virgin region. The integral S parallels the reciprocal of β in that a small value indicates a very rapid spread, while the integral R parallels the reciprocal of μ in that a small value indicates very rapid recovery. As detailed in Appendix 10.1, we can compute R_{0A} as the ratio of S_A:R_A. Values of R_{0A} calibrate the velocity of spread (the larger the value, the greater the rate of spread).

10.3 Cyclical Re-emergence: Spotting Influenza Pandemics

The nature of the influenza A virus which causes the cyclical appearance of global influenza pandemics is discussed in Section 4.2.2.

10.3.1 France: A Continental Country

DATA SOURCES

Influenza mortality data for France for various geographical units (towns, *départements*, regions, nation) have been either collected or estimated on an annual, monthly, or weekly basis since 1887, making them the longest continuous spatially disaggregated influenza time series available in the world. Inevitably over a time period of this duration, the nature of the data reported changed several times in both geographical and temporal resolution. So we begin by summarizing what is available and the steps taken to produce a consistent data set for analysis.

(1) *1887–1900*. For ~100 towns (depending upon the year) with a population in excess of 20,000 inhabitants.[1] These data give the monthly deaths recorded from pneumonia, bronchopneumonia, and acute and chronic bronchitis. Also given, remarkably, is the output of a model used to estimate from the pneumonia and bronchopneumonia data the number of deaths attributable to influenza determined by the concept of excess mortality. This approach has been routinely used in the United States by the Centers for Disease Control and Prevention to estimate influenza mortality from its weekly returns of pneumonia deaths in 121 cities published in *Morbidity and Mortality Weekly Return* (*MMWR*). In 1900 and 1906, summary volumes of *Statistique*

[1] République Française, Ministère de l'Intérieur. *Statistique sanitaire des villes de France et d'Algérie*. Paris: Imprimerie Nationale/Imprimerie Administrative.

sanitaire des villes de France et d'Algérie (*tableaux récapitulatifs*) were published giving, for France, the monthly time series of deaths from influenza, 1887–1905, estimated by the excess mortality approach from reported deaths from pneumonia and bronchopneumonia.

(2) *1901–5*. For these years, France recorded the monthly number of deaths from influenza for towns down to a population of 30,000[2]—59 towns in 1901, 71 in 1905. The national series of deaths by cause was recorded for towns whose populations exceeded 5,000.

(3) *1906–67*. From 1906, *Statistique sanitaire des villes de France et d'Algérie* was successively retitled *Statistique sanitaire de la France*,[3] *Statistique du mouvement de la population*, and then *Statistique des causes de décès*.[4] France reported the annual number of influenza deaths by *départements*, as well as the French national series throughout (annually through 1942 and monthly thereafter).[5] In many years, summary data are also available for groups of towns and *arrondissements*.

(4) *1968–99*. After 1968, monthly influenza mortality data are available by *départements* from the Institut National de la Santé et de la Recherche Médicale (INSERM).[6]

Thus, for the 113-year window from 1887, it is possible to patch together two matrices giving the time series of monthly influenza mortality for two geographical frameworks: (i) $n = 51$ towns (Figure 10.4) $\times$ 168 months, 1887–1900, and (ii) $n \approx 90$ *départements* $\times$ 1,188 months, 1901–99, by mapping the 51 towns for which data were recorded, 1901–5, to their *départements* and stitching this to the *département* data recorded 1906–99. Details of the patching process are given in Appendix 10.2. These two matrices form the basis for the analysis reported below.

Figure 10.5 illustrates the temporal pattern of recorded deaths from influenza in France over the period.[7] Figure 10.5A shows the seasonal distribution of mortality, with its winter peak characteristic of Northern Hemisphere countries. For this reason, in the analysis which follows, we have used as our temporal unit an *influenza season* running from 1 July to 30 June of the following year, rather

[2] République Française, Ministère de l'Intérieur. *Statistique sanitaire des villes de France et d'Algérie*. Paris: Imprimerie Nationale/Imprimerie Administrative.

[3] République Française, Ministère de l'Intérieur. *Statistique sanitaire de la France*. Melun: Imprimerie Administrative.

[4] République Française, Ministère de l'Économie Nationale/Ministère des Finances et des Affaires Économiques/Ministère des Affaires Économiques/Ministère de l'Économie et des Finances. *Statistique du mouvement de la population, 2^E Partie: Les Causes de décès/Statistique des causes de décès*. Paris: Imprimerie Nationale.

[5] Missing years of data occurred between 1920–4 and 1936–9, when deaths by cause are not known.

[6] The assistance of Professor A. Flahault (Université Pierre et Marie Curie, Paris) in supplying these data electronically and in interpreting them is gratefully acknowledged.

[7] For 1901–5, the national series of deaths by cause was recorded for towns whose populations exceeded 5,000.

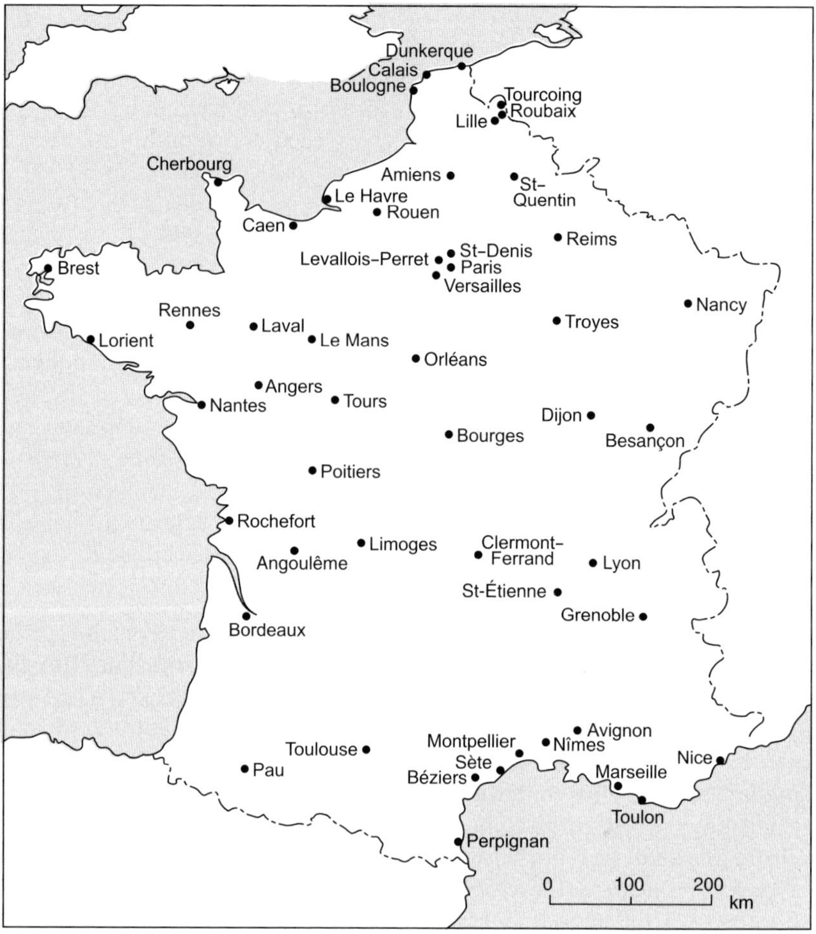

Fig. 10.4. Towns of France, 1887
Geographical distribution of 51 towns with populations in excess of 30,000 used to estimate the spatial velocity of influenza waves in France, 1887–1905.

than calendar years, which split months of high influenza mortality across year boundaries. Figure 10.5B charts the annual time series. In Europe, pandemics (marked) occurred as follows within this 113-year window (Dowdle 1999):

(i) *1889*. First deaths were reported in France in November 1889; the peak month was January 1890. The pandemic occurred in three successive waves in most parts of the world, producing mortality and morbidity greater than had been seen in decades. H2N? was the likely strain.
(ii) *1900*. Dowdle (1999) has queried whether this was truly a pandemic. Excess mortality was reported in North America and in England and Wales but not globally. H3N? was the likely strain.

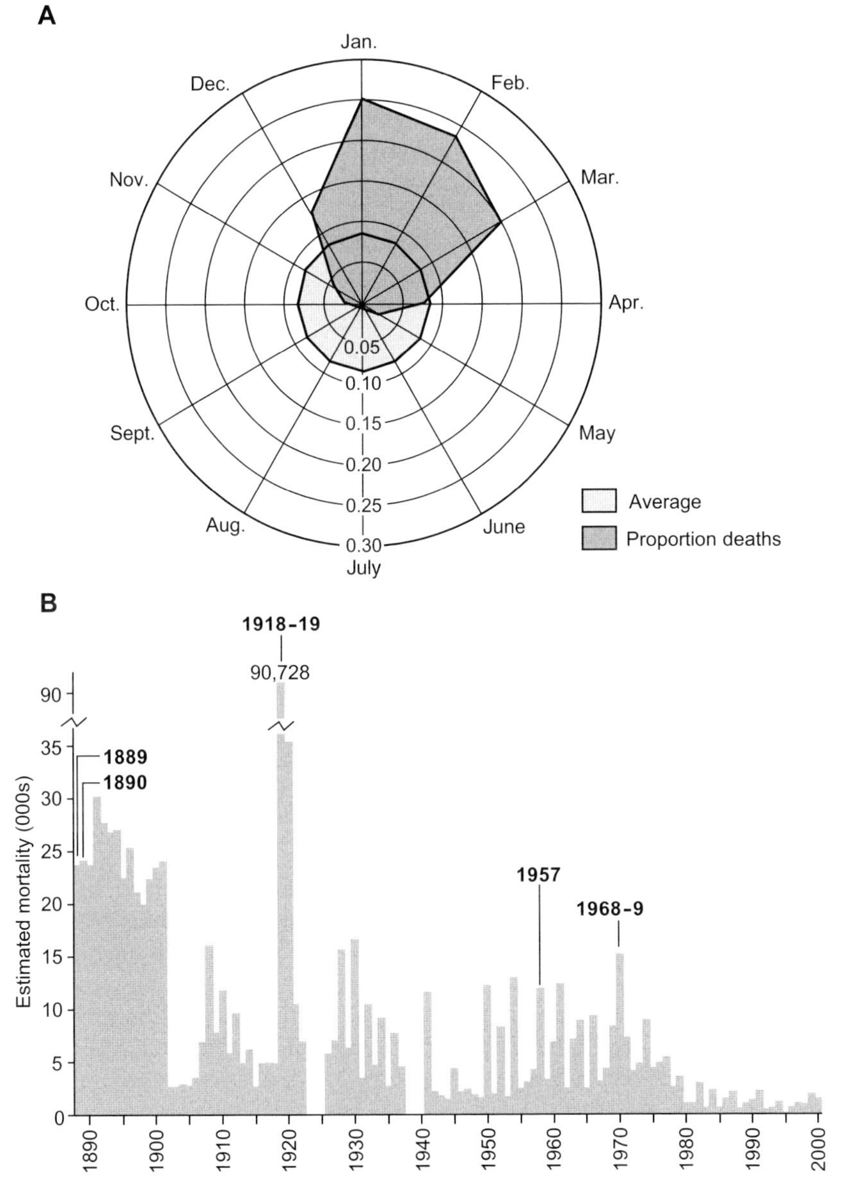

Fig. 10.5. Influenza mortality in France, 1887–1999
(A) Radar chart showing the proportion of deaths reported in each month over the period (dark shading). The average monthly proportion is marked by light shading.
(B) Time series of annual deaths from influenza reported in French records.

(iii) *1918–19*. This occurred in three waves as follows—Wave I: April–July 1918; Wave II: August–November 1918; Wave III: March 1919 (Patterson and Pyle 1991). It produced mortality unequalled in recorded history—up to 50 millions or more worldwide. H1N1 was the likely strain.

(iv) *1957*. This pandemic occurred in two main waves—Wave I: February–December 1957; Wave II: October 1957–January 1958 (Cliff, Haggett, and Smallman-Raynor 2004). H2N2 was the causative virus.

(v) *1968–9*. Wave I: 1968–9 (30 per cent of deaths); Wave II: 1969–70 (70 per cent of deaths). Wave I primarily affected North America and to a lesser extent Europe. In Wave II the situation was reversed and was associated with significant drift in the N surface antigen (Viboud, Grais, *et al.* 2005). H3N2 was the causative strain.

Figure 10.5B shows that, as in most countries of the world, the 1918–19 pandemic stood alone in France in terms of mortality caused. While the long-term trend in mortality is steadily downwards, nevertheless it is the case that pandemic years generally experienced heightened mortality as compared with adjacent years.

The time series illustrated in Figure 10.5B reinforces the need for robust methods of analysis. Apparently influenza mortality ran at a much higher level between 1887 and 1900, when mortality was estimated from excess pneumonia deaths, than in the rest of the time series, when influenza mortality was recorded directly.

Figure 10.6A plots the results for the spatial basic reproduction ratio, R_{0A}, and the two edge parameters, V_{LE} and V_{FE}, along with the linear regression trend lines. It shows that the long-term trend in the spatial basic reproduction ratio was slowly downwards over the last century; i.e. the rate of geographical propagation of influenza epidemics gradually diminished, probably reflecting less intense epidemics arising from (i) improved standards of living and health care, and (ii) no shift of virus strain since 1969. This century-long declining trend in R_{0A} is reflected in a similar decline in the leading edge (*LE*) velocity parameter, and a rising trend in the following edge (*FE*) parameter, implying that epidemics have arrived later and ended sooner in each influenza season; influenza seasons have become of shorter duration.

Within these long-term trends, however, the pandemic seasons of 1900, 1918–19, 1957, and 1968–9 showed a locally raised R_{0A}. In the case of 1889, this is not evident, while the rise to a higher level in 1969 persisted for four seasons. In the latter case, this is consistent with the description by Viboud, Grais, *et al.* (2005) of the 1968–9 pandemic as a 'smouldering pandemic'. From the late 1980s, R_{0A} oscillated wildly, suggestive of locally intense epidemics in each influenza season involving only a few *départements* rather than the entire country. It is tempting to think that the peaks for R_{0A} from the late 1980s might correspond with years in which influenza virus strains

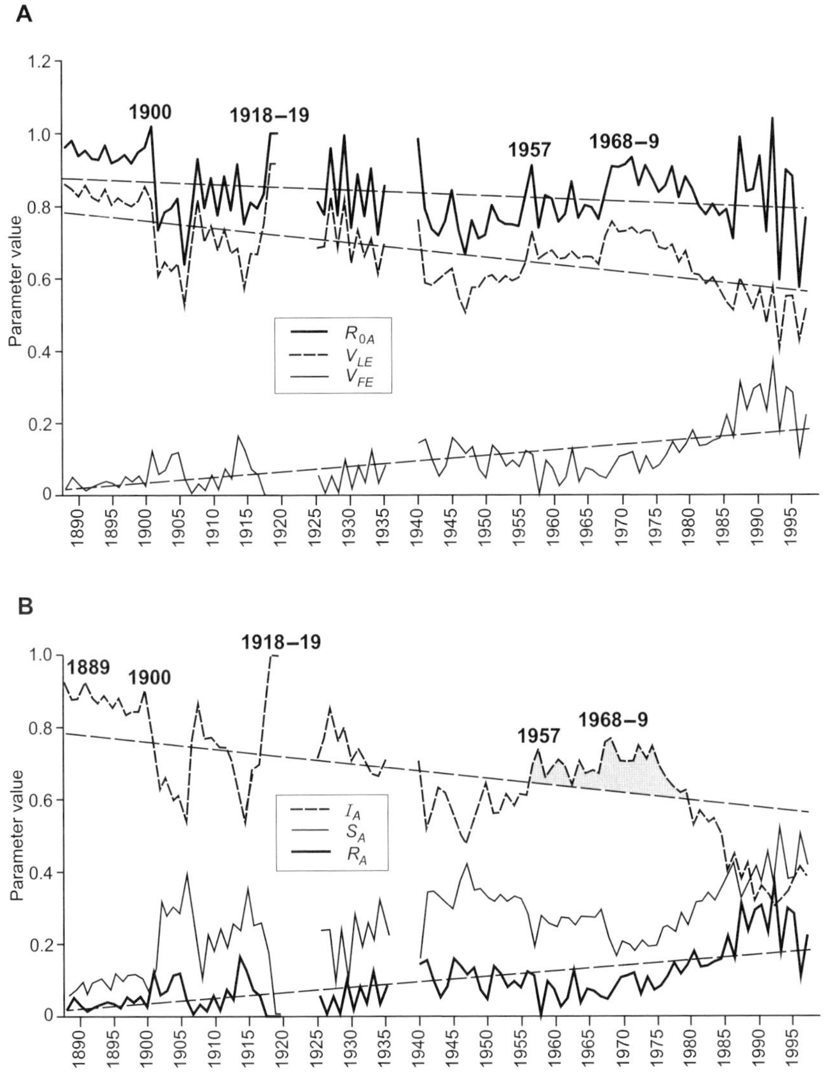

Fig. 10.6. Swash model parameters for influenza in France, 1887–1999
(A) Time series plots of calculated values for the spatial basic reproductive number, R_{0A}, and for the edge velocity parameters, V_{LE} and V_{FE}. (B) Time series of the infected (I), susceptible (S), and recovered (R) integrals. Linear regression trend lines are also shown.

Table 10.1. French influenza strains, 1985–1999, with recorded morbidity

Winter	Cases of recorded morbidity (millions)	Strain circulating
1985–6	3.9	A/H3N2
1986–7	1.4	A/H1N1
1987–8	1.4	A/H3N2
1988–9	*4.9*	*B,A/H1N1*
1989–90	4.9	A/H3N2
1990–1	0.7	B
1991–2	*2.1*	*A/H3N2*
1992–3	1.8	A/H3N2
1993–4	*3.2*	*A/H3N2*
1994–5	1.1	A/H3N2
1995–6	*2.9*	*A/H1N1*
1996–7	*3.1*	*A/H3N2*
1997–8	2.4	A/H3N2
1998–9	*3.1*	*A/H3N2*

Note: Rows in italic correspond with peak values for R_{0A} between 1985 and 1999 on Figure 10.6A.

other than the dominant H3N2 were co-circulating, but Table 10.1 (italicized rows) shows this only to have been the case in two seasons. These seasons were, however, seasons in which recorded morbidity was generally higher than in other years in this time window.

Table 10.2 highlights the difference between pandemic and non-pandemic seasons in France. The 103 seasons for which data were available have been classified into three groups: (*a*) pandemic-affected (11), (*b*) high-intensity interpandemic (54), with death rates greater than the lowest pandemic season, and (*c*) low-intensity interpandemic (38), with death rates lower than the lowest pandemic season. The average velocity of the leading edge ($\bar{t}_{LE}$, equation 10.A1, Appendix 10.1) for the three groups is (*a*) = 2.39 months, (*b*) = 3.59 months, and (*c*) = 4.93 months. The results for V_{LE} in Table 10.2 confirm that pandemic seasons had higher velocities than interpandemic years. This higher velocity was maintained even compared with interpandemic influenza seasons of similar intensity levels as pandemic seasons. Moreover, pandemic seasons appeared to be of greater spatial intensity (larger R_{0A}) and were slower to clear (lower following edge velocities).

The plots of the susceptible and recovered integrals in Figure 10.6B show rising trends over the twentieth century, and this is consistent with the generally declining trend in the infective integral. As noted in Figure 10.6B, these trends imply declining intensity of influenza epidemics over the century-long study period. Again the pandemic years bucked the trend with raised infective integral values. The main other variations in the long-term fall in the infectives integral occurred following the arrival of Asian influenza in 1957,

Table 10.2 Characteristics of 103 influenza waves: France 1887–1888 to 1998–1999

Type of influenza wave	Mortality (mean/100,000 population per season)	Start $\bar{t}_{LE}$ (mean in months)	Velocity (V_{LE})	End $\bar{t}_{FE}$ (mean in months)	Velocity (V_{FE})	R_{0A} (mean)
Pandemic[a] ($n = 11$)	27.29	2.39	0.80	11.45	0.05	0.93
Interpandemic						
High-intensity[b] ($n = 54$)	14.91	3.59	0.70	11.20	0.07	0.84
Low-intensity[c] ($n = 38$)	3.14	4.93	0.59	10.12	0.16	0.80

Notes: [a] Pandemic seasons of 1889–91, 1900, 1918–19, 1957–8, 1968–9. [b] High-intensity = deaths per 100,000 population greater than the least intense pandemic season. [c] Low-intensity = deaths per 100,000 population less than the least intense pandemic season. Data unavailable for seasons 1920–4 and 1936–9.

when the infected integral remained above the trend (shaded in Figure 10.6B) for the next quarter of a century, and then, from the mid-1980s, when the integral remained resolutely below the trend line. The extended period of higher values for the infectives integral post-1957 may be attributed to the combined action of three effects: (i) the long interval since the last major strain shift (40 years since 1918); (ii) the shift from H2N2 to H3N2 in 1968–9; and (iii) the re-emergence in 1976 of Russian influenza (strain H1N1), which has been co-circulating with the Hong Kong strain ever since. Together these effects meant that a greater proportion of the French population was likely to be susceptible to one or other of the mix of circulating strains than if just a single strain had been present over the period. After a generation, with no new major strains emerging, herd immunity appears to have caught up from the mid-1980s, leading to a general collapse of nationwide epidemics.

10.3.2 Iceland: An Island Location

This subsection is based upon Cliff, Haggett, and Smallman-Raynor (2008).

DATA SOURCES

Since 1895, Iceland has required direct notification of influenza cases by physicians (Cliff, Haggett, and Ord 1986). This concern for data collection stems from the island's early history, which was marked by disastrous externally introduced epidemics, including the 1843 influenza outbreak, which, although lasting only two months, doubled the expected death rate for the year (Schleisner 1851). Annual totals and other summary data have been published in that country's annual public health reports (*Heilbrigðisskýrslur*) since that date with, for influenza, national monthly morbidity time series available from 1913 (Figure 10.7A). Of exceptional interest is the 61-year period spanning the middle of the twentieth century from 1915 (Figure 10.7B). For these years, monthly data are broken down to a local level for some 50 medical districts (Figure 10.7C). This allows mapping of ways in which the disease spread around the island, along with calculation of general estimates of its changing spatial and temporal velocity over the period.

RESULTS

Over the whole 61 years studied, Iceland's doctors reported 530,276 cases of influenza, half of them from Reykjavík and immediate surrounding areas (Figure 10.7D). Although reported cases are likely to be underestimates, the broad shape of outbreaks in both space and time is readily discernible. The distribution throughout the year shows clear peaks in March–April with the low periods in August–September, a pattern which, as we have

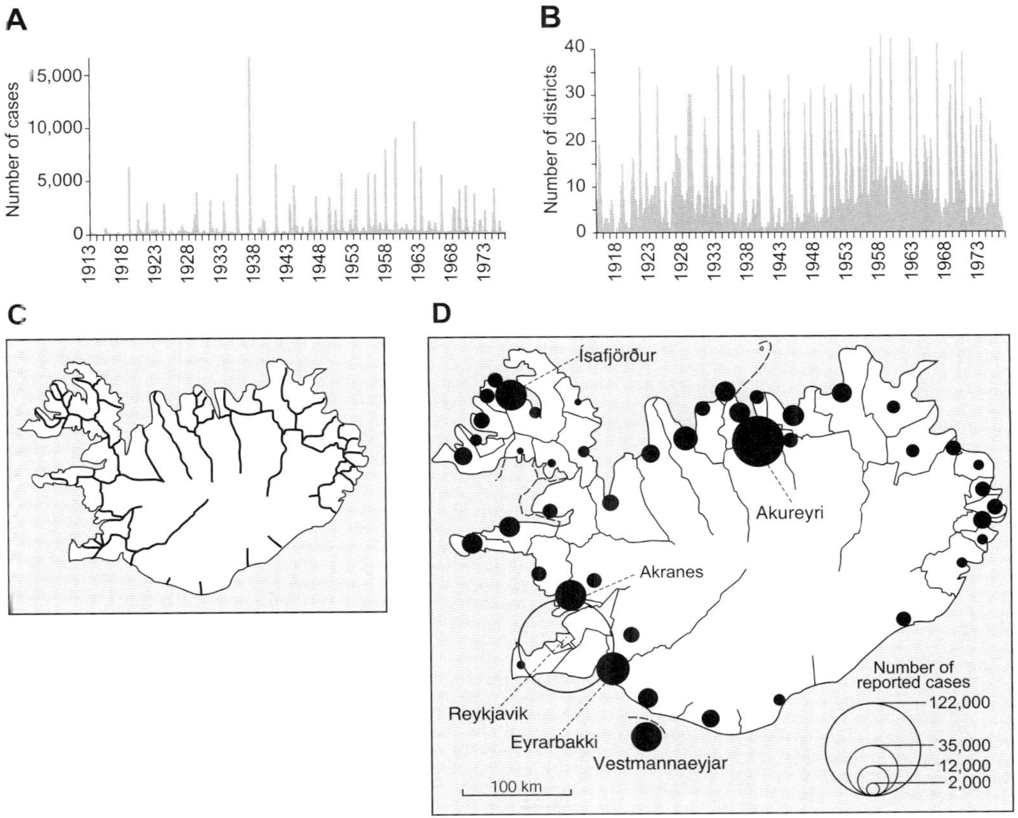

Fig. 10.7. Reported influenza morbidity in Iceland
(A) Monthly records for total reported influenza cases from Jan. 1913 to Dec. 1976. (B) Monthly record of the number of Icelandic medical districts reporting one or more cases of influenza, Jan. 1915–Dec. 1976. (C) Map of boundaries of Icelandic medical districts for the year 1945. Central Iceland is unpopulated icecap and boundaries are undefined. (D) Cumulative total of reported monthly influenza cases for each Icelandic medical district in the period Jan. 1915–Dec. 1976. Circles are drawn proportional to the cumulative number of cases but note the special position of the capital city, Reykjavík. All influenza data based on *Heilbrigðisskýrslur* ('Public Health in Iceland').

seen for France in Figure 10.5A, is typical of many northern latitude countries. However, the sub-Arctic climate of Iceland pushes the peak influenza months slightly later in the influenza season than in France, and so we use for Iceland a slightly different definition of season, running from 1 September to 31 August the following year.

The intricate spatial infrastructure of medical districts allows the local spread of the disease to be monitored across the island. This spatial network is, however, unstable over time as district boundaries have been modified to reflect changes in population and medical provision. Major changes to the 1907 medical district boundaries current at the beginning of our study period occurred in 1932, 1945, and 1955. We have therefore developed a standardized set of districts, based upon the 1945 configuration, which preserves spatial continuity over time (Figure 10.7C).

The swash–backwash model of Section 10.2.2 was applied to Iceland as a whole. The time series of both edges is shown in Figure 10.8A. Despite marked year-to-year variation, the average trend shown by the linear regression line for the leading edge is distinctly upward, implying that waves have speeded up over time, i.e. influenza waves moved around the island faster at the end than at the beginning of the study period. By contrast, the position of the following edge when influenza incidence ceased in any influenza season has remained essentially unchanged. This implies that the duration of reported influenza incidence grew slowly longer, from around 2.5 months in 1915–16 to nearly 4.0 months in 1975–6 (Figure 10.8B), a finding which differs from that for France.

Three of the 61 seasons studied were associated with pandemics of influenza A (the Spanish, Asian, and Hong Kong pandemics). Figure 10.9 uses data on the spatial extent of influenza in each season to plot the position of the pandemic front with reference to the three seasons which immediately preceded or followed it. In the Spanish and Asian pandemics the front stands out clearly, but in the third (Figure 10.9C) the Hong Kong front appears, as in France, to have been spread over two seasons.

Although pandemic years had large numbers of influenza cases, they were not the largest recorded over the period. The 1937–8 season had the largest number of cases (21,977) and the highest monthly rate, and, as Figure 10.7A shows, monthly case numbers in several interpandemic years exceeded those with pandemics. For Iceland in Table 10.3, as for France in Table 10.2, we have divided the 61 seasons into three groups: (*a*) pandemic (3); (*b*) high-intensity interpandemic (24), with case rates greater than the lowest pandemic season; and (*c*) low-intensity interpandemic (34), with case rates lower than the lowest pandemic season. The average velocity of the leading edges (*LE*) for the three groups is (*a*) = 2.83 months, (*b*) = 5.53 months, and (*c*) = 6.03 months. Echoing the results for France, this suggests that pandemic seasons have higher velocities than interpandemic years, and that

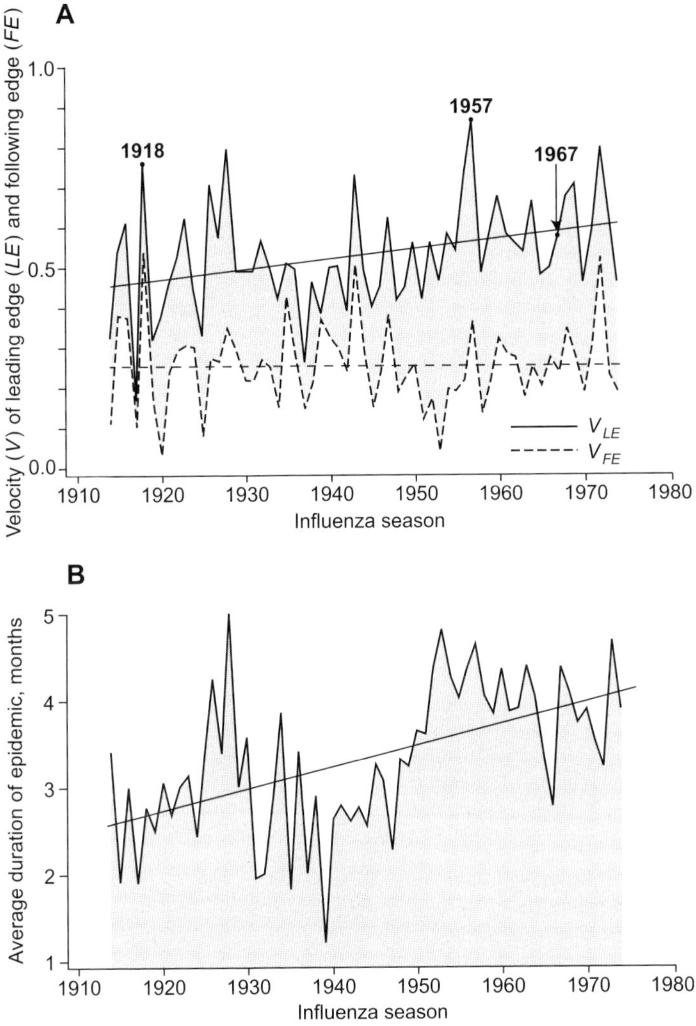

Fig. 10.8. Velocity of epidemic waves in Iceland for the influenza seasons 1915–1916 to 1975–1976
(A) Velocities of the leading edge (*LE*, solid lines) and following edge (*FE*, pecked lines) are shown as the velocity ratios, V_{LE} and V_{FE}, defined in App. 10.1 equation 10.A2. V is in the range $0 \leq V \leq 1$. The larger the value of V, the faster the edge. (B) The widening time gap between the two edges illustrated in A is confirmed in this graph, which plots the average duration of each district's epidemic wave in months. In both A and B the trend lines were determined by OLS linear regression

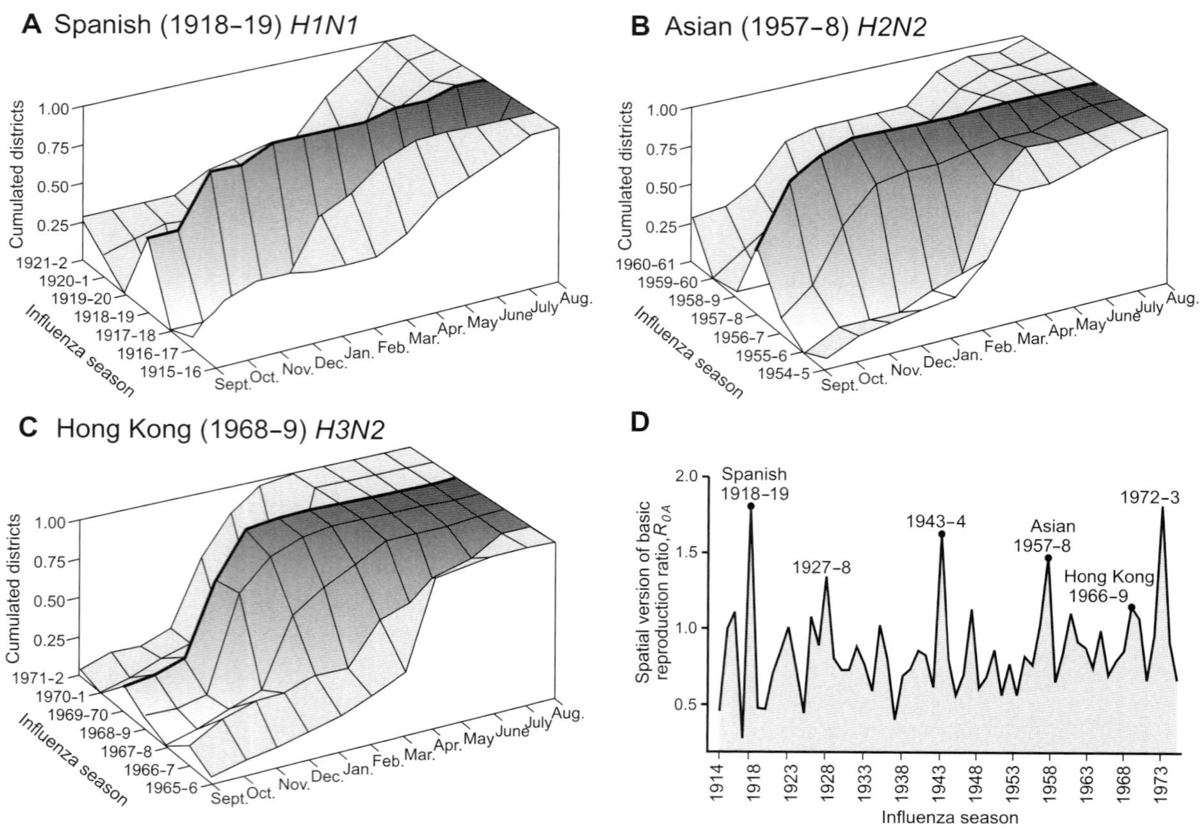

Fig. 10.9. Pandemic seasons in the Icelandic records
(A–C) Profiles showing the cumulative number (scaled to unity) of medical districts reporting influenza cases by month as a measure of the spatial extent of influenza in Iceland for the three shift seasons of 1918–19, 1957–8, and 1968–9. In each case the profile for the shift season is compared with the profiles of the three preceding and three following non-shift seasons. (D) Value of the spatial version of the basic reproduction ratio, R_{0A}, for Iceland for the influenza seasons 1915–16 to 1975–6. Peaks are associated with the three viral shift years for influenza A (1918–19, 1957–8, and 1968–9) and for three other non-shift seasons (1927–8, 1943–4, and 1972–3).

Table 10.3. Characteristics of Iceland's 61 influenza waves, 1915–1916 to 1975–1976

Type of influenza wave	Morbidity (mean cases/season)	Start ($\bar{t}_{LE}$) (mean in months)	Velocity (V_{LE})	End ($\bar{t}_{FE}$) (mean in months)	Velocity (V_{FE})	Duration (mean in months)	R_{0A} (mean index)
Pandemic waves[a] ($n = 3$)	11,027	2.83	0.76	7.03	0.41	3.82	1.48
Interpandemic waves							
High-intensity[b] ($n = 24$)	10,113	5.53	0.54	9.14	0.24	3.56	0.84
Low-intensity[c] ($n = 34$)	2,302	6.03	0.50	9.04	0.25	3.10	0.80

Notes: [a] Three pandemic seasons of 1918–19, 1957–8, and 1968–9. [b] High-intensity = cases per 100,000 population greater than the least intense pandemic wave. [c] Low-intensity = cases per 100,000 population less than the least intense pandemic wave.

this higher velocity is maintained even compared with interpandemic influenza seasons of similar intensity levels as pandemic seasons.

Table 10.3 also shows that values for R_{0A}, when calculated for the three categories of influenza season, (*a*), (*b*), and (*c*), defined above, produced the same differentials as the leading and following edge parameters.

DISCUSSION

Application of the swash–backwash model to Iceland's influenza morbidity records has shown that (i) the onset of waves speeded up over the period 1914 to 1975 and (ii) waves in three viral shift (pandemic) seasons spread significantly faster and were of longer duration than other equally large waves in non-shift (interpandemic) seasons. These are identical to the results reported for France in Section 10.3.2. It suggests that both the swash model and the findings are robust across the transfer of geographical scales from a large country (France) to a small country (Iceland), and from a continental to an island setting.

We now apply the model at the smallest of our spatial scales by looking at influenza waves between 1947–8 and 1975–6 in the English market town of Cirencester.

10.3.3 Cirencester: A Small English Town

Cirencester is a small market town lying between Gloucester and Swindon in the English Cotswolds. It had a population of about 12,000 in 1957 (Figure 10.10B). Based in the town, R. E. Hope-Simpson ran a general practice covering an area of about 210 km^2 from a centrally located surgery. In this practice, individual patients were identified and influenza was diagnosed and studied by a single doctor and his partner over a 30-year period following the end of World War II. The panel consisted of between 3,000 and 4,000 patients, and Hope-Simpson kept very detailed records of the incidence of several infectious diseases, but especially influenza, for each patient. Working with the help of his wife and later with the support of the UK's Medical Research Council and the Public Health Laboratory Service, he set up an Epidemiological Research Unit in Cirencester. By converting cottage rooms at his surgery in Dyer Street, he established a laboratory to permit identification of the viruses isolated from his patients. As a result, this unique practice became internationally known and it provides an unrivalled window into the behaviour of influenza epidemics at the micro scale.

DATA SOURCE

Hope-Simpson recorded every case of influenza identified in the practice, along with the causative strain of the virus and the geo-coordinates of the

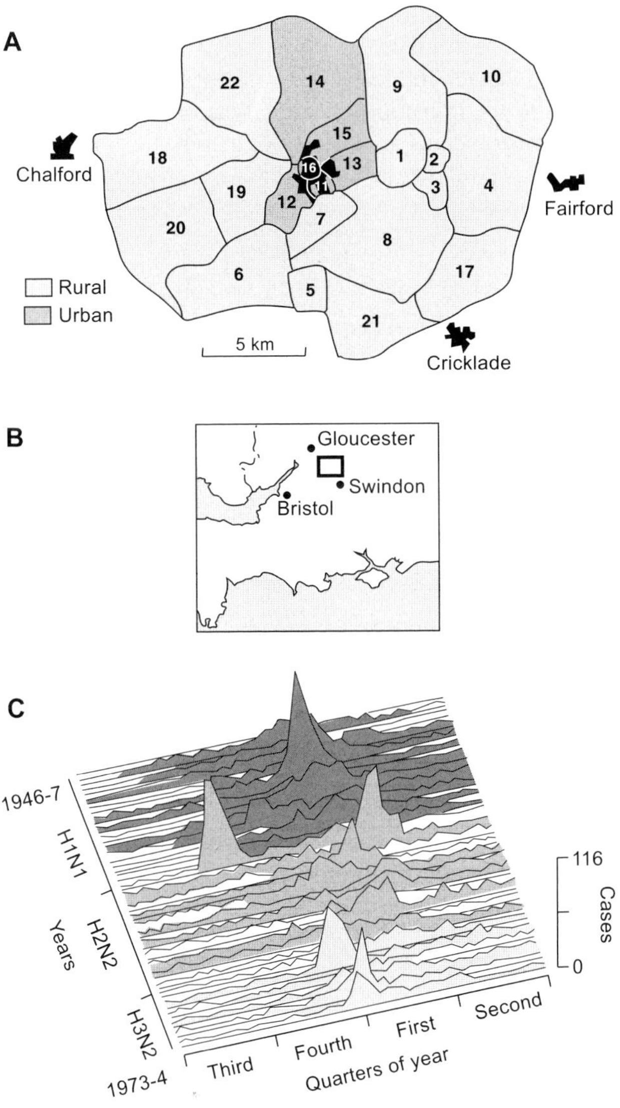

Fig. 10.10. Influenza waves in an English GP practice
The country practice of a local doctor, Edgar Hope-Simpson, near Cirencester. Hope-Simpson made a special study of influenza in the area for some 30 years. (A) Boundaries of the 22 geographical units used by Hope-Simpson for data collection. (B) Location map of Cirencester. (C) Block diagram of cases of clinically diagnosed influenza A weekly, 1946–74. The earlier appearance of influenza in the pandemic seasons of 1957–8 and 1968–9 is striking, as is the greater number of cases reported.
Source: R. E. Hope-Simpson in Cliff, Haggett, and Ord (1986, figs 3.1, 3.12, pp. 48, 65).

patient. Figure 10.10A maps the geographical framework used by Hope-Simpson for data collection, along with a block diagram (Figure 10.10C) of the cases reported in each influenza season, 1946–74. The earlier appearance of influenza in the town in the pandemic seasons of 1957–8 and 1968–9 is striking. This appearance of an early peak at times of antigenic shift in the causative virus can be related to the larger stock of susceptibles available for immediate infection on such occasions.

RESULTS

In Figure 10.11, the results of applying the swash–backwash model to the Hope-Simpson data from 1963–75 are summarized. They echo those already obtained for France and Iceland, with a sharp upturn in R_{0A} and an increase in the leading edge velocity in the second season of Hong Kong influenza (1969). Thereafter R_{0A} fell slowly to reach pre-1968 levels by 1973.

DISCUSSION

In Section 10.3, the swash–backwash model has been applied to records of influenza from France (1887–1999), Iceland (1916–75), and Cirencester (1963–75), locations of vastly different geographical scales and settings. But common threads have been found: pandemic influenza at all three spatial scales appeared (i) earlier than normal in the influenza season and (ii) spread spatially more

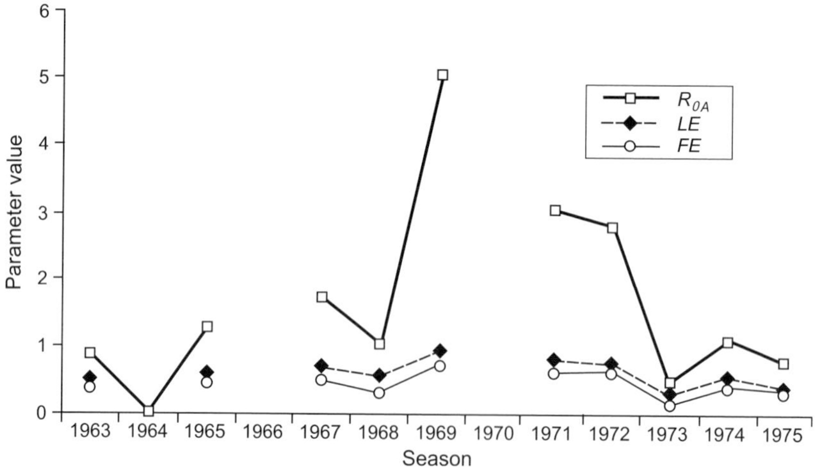

Fig. 10.11. The 1968–1969 pandemic of influenza in the Hope-Simpson GP practice in Cirencester, England
Values of the reproductive ratio, and leading and following edge velocities for the swash–backwash model, 1963–75. As in France and Iceland, influenza moved more rapidly and struck earlier in 1968 than in non-pandemic seasons.

rapidly than normal. If our findings are confirmed elsewhere, this will have wider implications for public health measures. It would suggest that any new influenza pandemic in the twenty-first century, whether emerging from avian influenza or other sources, will give little lead time if the public health is to be protected. This conclusion underscores the role of surveillance and virus watch systems, issues to which we turn later in Section 10.6.

10.4 Measles in Iceland

In the previous section, the swash model was used to show that influenza pandemics have distinctive features in terms of R_{0A} and their velocity of travel. These distinctive features arise from the new virus strain which enters circulation in pandemic years. It is this strain shift which enables pandemics to be picked out from the normal run of annual influenza outbreaks which occur with varying degrees of intensity in the winter season of Northern Hemisphere countries. But what of diseases caused by unchanging agents? Can the swash model yield insights into the characteristics of temporally periodic epidemic waves which may vary in their spatial intensity. We address this issue via an analysis of measles outbreaks on the island of Iceland over a 60-year period, January 1915–December 1974. Our account is based upon Cliff and Haggett (2006).

10.4.1 Periodic Waves: Measles in Iceland

Between 1915 and 1974, 14 measles epidemic waves struck Iceland. The summary characteristics are given in Table 10.4. They show that wave duration was generally less than two years, with the spatial extent tending to be widespread; roughly 90 per cent of the 50 districts shown in Figure 10.7C became infected in each wave. Typically, some 6,000 cases were reported for each wave, with, on average, a rate of around 40 per 1,000 of the Icelandic population becoming infected. The gap between epidemic waves was on average around three years. Whereas the first three characters in Table 10.4 do not show significant trends

Table 10.4. Iceland measles waves, 1915–1974: characteristics

Character	Maximum	Minimum	Mean/Median
Duration (T) (months)	27 (Waves IX, XV)	10 (Wave X)	20.0/21.5
Spatial extent (A) (districts)	49 (Waves VI, VIII)	23 (Wave X)	43.5/45
Numbers infected (Q) (reported cases)	8,408 (Wave VI)	1,872 (Wave X)	5,806/6141
Intensity (cases per 1,000 population)	71.9 (Wave VI)	12.5 (Wave X)	42.0/43.7
Gap between epidemic waves (months)	91 (Wave III)	1 (Wave XV)	36.0/27

over time, the remaining two are highly time-dependent. The five early waves in the period up to 1945 showed much higher attack rates and longer gaps between waves; the nine later waves tended to have lower attack rates and are bunched closer together.

A detailed description of the waves based on original data in the annual volumes of *Heilbrigðisskýrslur* ('Public Health in Iceland') and on doctors' accounts has already been published in monograph form (Cliff, Haggett, Ord, and Versey 1981, account, pp. 59–88; data tables, pp. 201–29) and will not be repeated here. Figure 10.12 shows the time series with the original monthly data aggregated into three-month (quarterly) format on the x-axis of the graph. The y-axis shows not the number of reported cases but the spatial extent of the epidemic waves in each quarter in terms of the number of Icelandic medical districts reporting cases. Waves I and II (in 1904 and in 1907–8, respectively) lack specific spatial detail for analysis. So here we begin our record in 1915 but retain the original wave numbering and look at our first wave (Wave III) in some detail and then at comparative results for the full set of waves.

RESULTS FOR A SINGLE EPIDEMIC WAVE (WAVE III)

The first of the Icelandic measles waves to be analysed was triggered by the arrival in Reykjavík harbour in April 1916 of a ship from Norway with a sailor still infectious with measles. It came nearly eight years after its predecessor. A scatter of measles notifications had been reported over the intervening years (56 cases in all) but preventive measures were swiftly enforced by local doctors, secondary cases were rare, and no major epidemics had occurred. Wave III, when fully developed, was a major epidemiological event with 4,944 reported cases (an attack rate of 55 per 1,000 population) and 118 deaths (a rate of 23.9 deaths per 1,000 measles cases). It lasted for 14 months, peaked in July 1916, only four months after onset, and spread widely over the island, infecting all but seven of Iceland's 50 medical districts.

The form of the epidemic in the time domain is shown in Figure 10.13. We begin with the monthly time series for the number of cases reported and for the number of districts infected: both are shown in Figure 10.13A. In each case the curves are strongly skewed to the left, indicating a rapid build-up of both cases and infected districts. The monthly time series of reported cases per infected district is shown as an inset in Figure 10.13B and confirms both early peaking (based on Reykjavík) and a late but smaller surge (based on Akureyri).

The monthly time series of the number of districts newly infected (i.e. when measles cases were *first* recorded) and of the number of districts where infection terminated (i.e. when measles cases were *last* recorded) are shown in Figure 10.13C. Differences between the two series plotted in (C)

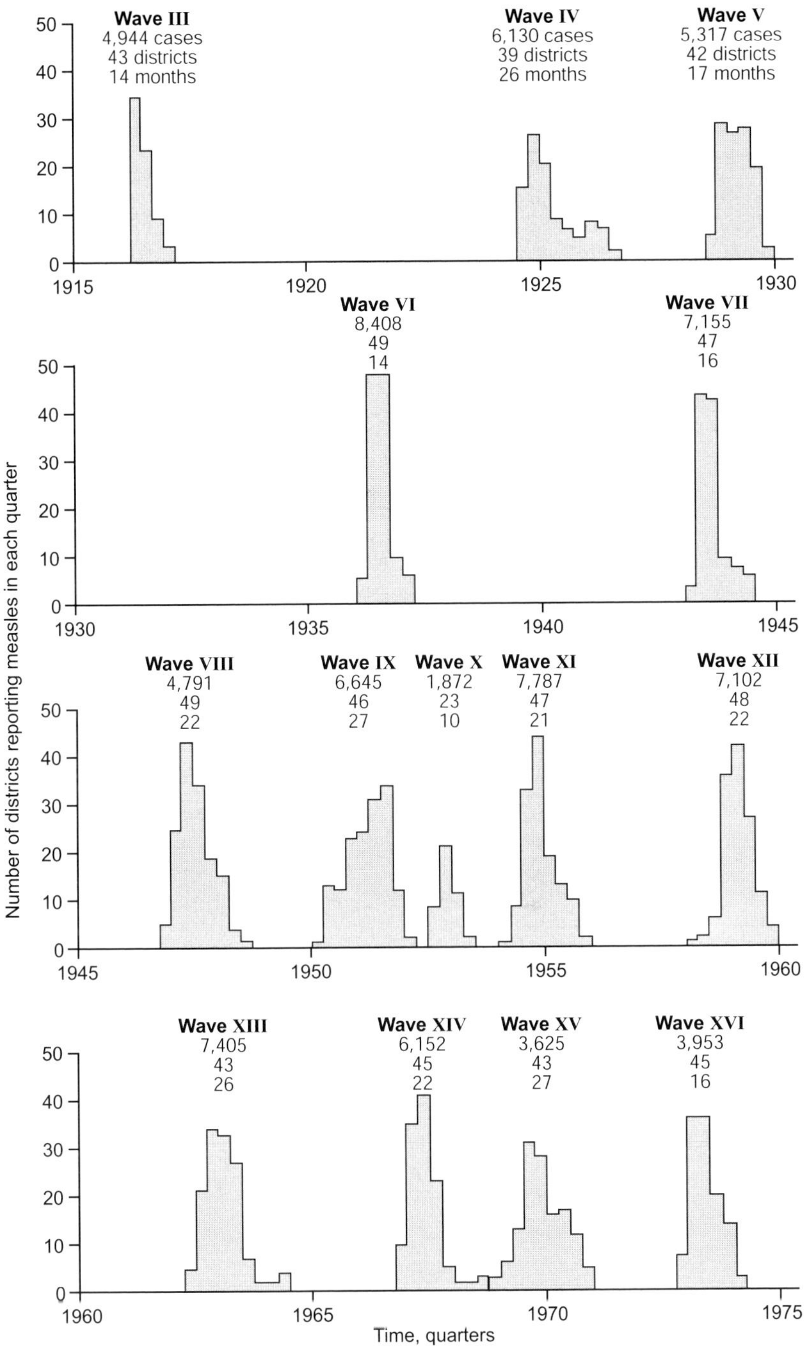

Fig. 10.12. Time series of epidemic measles waves for Iceland over a 60-year period, 1916–1974

Monthly figures have been aggregated to give the number of districts reporting measles cases in each of the four quarters of the year.

Sources: Monthly series in *Heilbrigðisskýslur*, summarized in Cliff, Haggett, Ord, and Versey (1981, data tables, pp. 202–29).

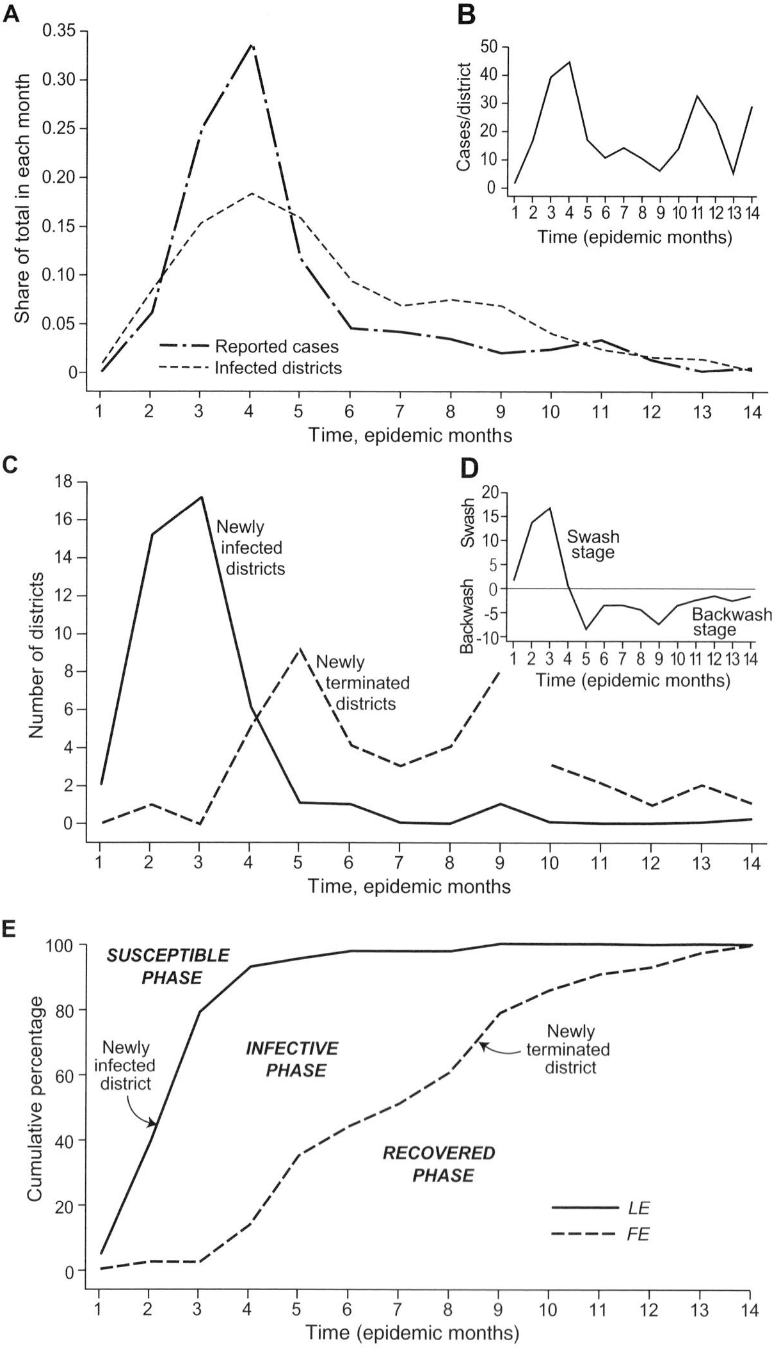

A
Share of total in each month
Reported cases
Infected districts
Time, epidemic months
B
Cases/district
Time (epidemic months)
C
Number of districts
Newly infected districts
Newly terminated districts
Time, epidemic months
D
Swash
Backwash
Swash stage
Backwash stage
Time (epidemic months)
E
Cumulative percentage
SUSCEPTIBLE PHASE
INFECTIVE PHASE
RECOVERED PHASE
Newly infected district
Newly terminated district
LE
FE
Time (epidemic months)

are illustrated in Figure 10.15D. The mean values for the two series are used to define the swash (epidemic wave burgeoning) and backwash (epidemic wave retreating) stages of Wave III in Figure 10.13D. Finally, cumulative curves for the number of newly infected and newly terminated districts used to define susceptible, infective, and recovered districts appear in Figure 10.13E.

RESULTS FOR A TRAIN OF EPIDEMIC EVENTS (WAVES III TO XVI)

How far are the results for the first wave (Wave III) representative of the whole 60-year sequence of waves? To give an overall picture, we summarize in Table 10.5 the range and average characteristics of the wave train in terms of their spatial structure. The average for the leading edges tends to fall in the sixth month of an outbreak, with the following edge about six months later. In terms of the three integrals defined in Appendix 10.1, equations 10.A4–A6, susceptibles make up around one-quarter, infectives around a third, and recovereds the residual space (around 40 per cent) of the phase diagram defined in Figure 10.3D.

Table 10.5. Iceland measles waves, 1915–1974: spatial characteristics in terms of the swash–backwash model

Character	Maximum	Minimum	Mean/Median
Leading edge ($\bar{t}_{LE}$) (months)	10.4 (Wave IX)	2.95 (Wave III)	6.02/5.47
Following edge ($\bar{t}_{FE}$) (months)	19.76 (Wave IX)	7.44 (Wave III)	11.83/11.31
Susceptibles integral (S_A)	0.395 (Wave XII)	0.139 (Wave III)	0.245/0.233
Infectives integral (I_A)	0.415 (Wave XVI)	0.260 (Wave IV)	0.347/0.347
Recovered integral (R_A)	0.541 (Wave XIV)	0.268 (Wave IX)	0.408/0.397
Swash stage[1]	55.8 (Wave IX)	32.2 (Wave XIV)	44.6/44.4
Backwash stage[1]	67.8 (Wave XIV)	44.2 (Wave IX)	55.4/55.6
Basic reproduction ratio, R_{0A}	1.88 (Wave XIV)	0.89 (Wave IX)	1.28/1.29

Notes: [1] The values for swash–backwash stages are given in standardized form as percentages where 100 is the overall duration of the wave, *T* months. Integral values are dimensionless numbers.

Fig. 10.13. Some wave parameters for Icelandic measles Wave III
(A) Monthly time series for the number of cases reported and for the number of districts infected. (B) Monthly time series of density of reported cases per infected district. (C) Monthly time series of the number of districts newly infected (i.e. measles cases *first* recorded) and of the number of districts where infection terminated (i.e. measles cases *last* recorded). (D) Differences between the series plotted in C used to define *swash* and *backwash* stages of the epidemic. (E) Cumulative curves for the number of newly infected and newly terminated districts used to define susceptible, infective, and recovered districts.
Source: Cliff and Haggett (2006, fig. 6, p. 240).

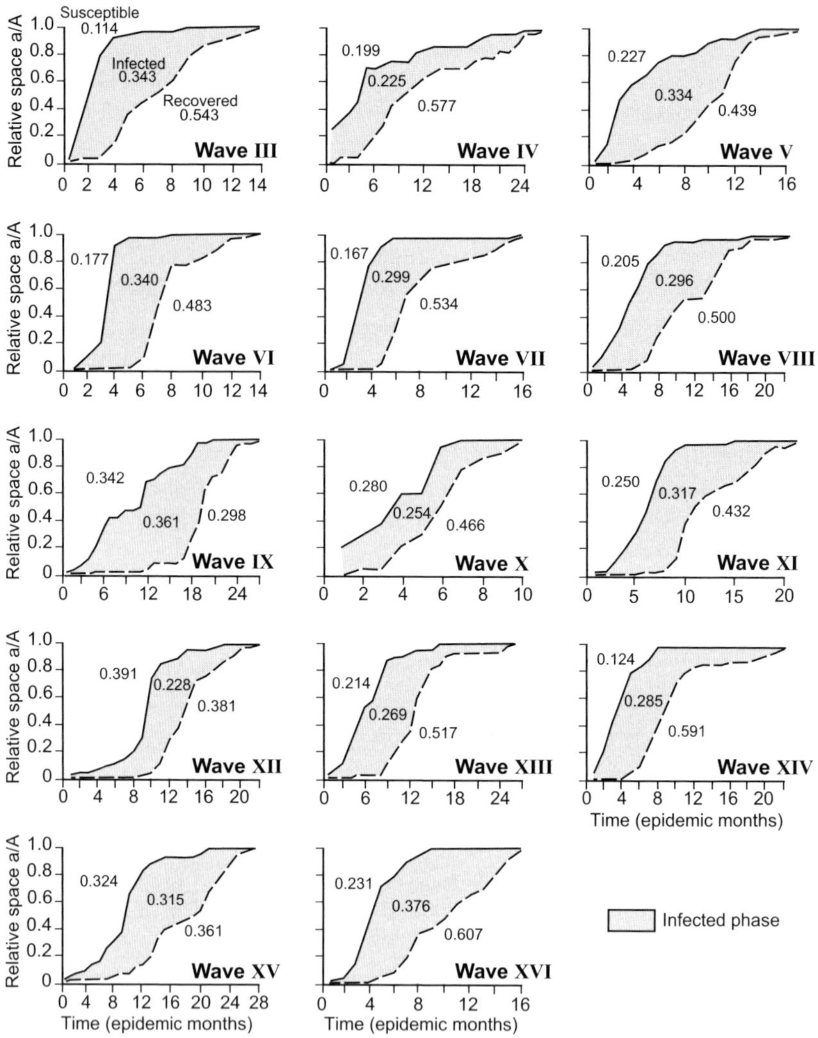

Fig. 10.14. Phase transition diagrams for 14 Icelandic measles waves
The numbers given are integrals which measure the area under each of the three curves as a proportion of the total. As in Fig. 10.17 (later), time and space axes are measured in relative terms.

Source: Cliff and Haggett (2006, fig. 9, p. 244).

Analysis at the individual wave level is given in Figure 10.14, which shows the superimposed cumulative curves from the previous figure to define susceptible, infective, and recovered zones when plotted on a phase transition diagram (cf. Figure 10.3D). Comparative wave data are also

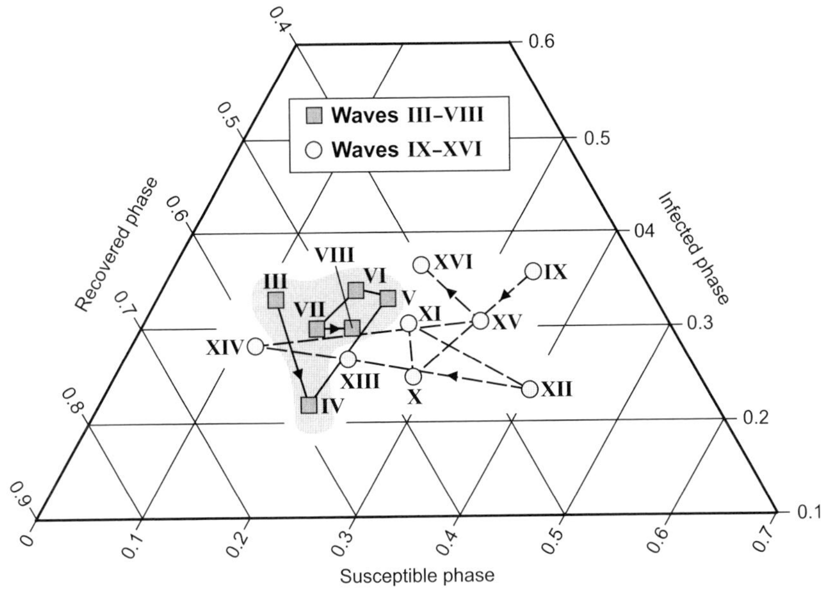

Fig. 10.15. Values for the susceptible, infective, and recovered phases for the 14 epidemic Icelandic measles waves plotted as a ternary diagram
Source: Cliff and Haggett (2006, fig. 10, p. 245).

given in Figure 10.15, which plots the three dimensions of the susceptible, infective, and recovered phases for the 14 waves as a ternary diagram. It is notable that the early waves (shaded) lie broadly to the left of the later, post-World War II, waves on the susceptible phase axis of the ternary diagram. This implies that the early waves showed a more rapid transition from susceptible to infected phases than later waves.

VELOCITY OF THE LEADING AND FOLLOWING STAGES

In Figures 10.13C and D we presented the ideas of swash (newly infected districts) and backwash (newly terminated districts) for the geographical spread of an epidemic wave. But Figure 10.13 and the values in Table 10.5 point to pronounced asymmetry, with the swash stage being shorter and steeper than the backwash stage. This implies in turn that the velocity of the infection phase is faster than that of the recovery phase.

For a fast-moving wave, the average time to infect an area will be relatively small and, for a slow-moving wave, relatively large. Table 10.6 confirms that the leading edge is very significantly faster whether measured in months (nearly three months faster) or when standardized by the overall duration of the epidemic wave (14 per cent faster).

Table 10.6. Iceland measles waves, 1915–74: comparisons between the velocity of leading edges and following edges

Velocity parameters	Measure	Expected relationship	Leading edge (*LE*)	Following edge (*FE*)	Velocity difference confirmed?	Difference[1]
Location	Mean (months)	*LE* < *FE*	8.99	11.82	Yes	2.83 ***
	Mean (%)	*LE* < *FE*	44.82	59.19	Yes	14.37 ***
Dispersion	Standard deviation (months)	*LE* < *FE*	3.83	3.71	No	0.13
	Range (months)	*LE* < *FE*	14.57	16.64	Yes	2.07 *
	IQR (months)	*LE* < *FE*	4.07	6.21	Yes	2.14 ***
Skewness		*LE* > *FE*	0.599	0.401	Yes	0.198
Kurtosis		*LE* > *FE*	0.460	0.456	Yes	0.004

Note: [1] Single-tailed paired *t*-tests: * probably significant ($p = 0.05$), ** significant ($p = 0.01$), *** highly significant ($p = 0.001$). IQR = interquartile range.

A fast epidemic wave will also display low dispersion in time to district infection, with most districts infected within a short time of one another; a slow wave will display reverse characteristics. Here the evidence is less clear, with two of the three measures of dispersion calculated from the frequency distribution of number of infected districts against time (the non-parametric measures of range and inter-quartile range, *IQR*) showing statistically significant faster leading edges. The third measure, the standard deviation, shows little difference, possibly reflecting the influence of a few extreme observations.

A fast epidemic wave will have a positively skewed frequency distribution of infected districts because the majority of cases will occur in the early phases of an epidemic. In Table 10.6, both leading and following edges show positive values for the Pearson measure of skewness, b_1, but the differences between $b_1(LE)$ and $b_1(FE)$ are in the expected direction. Finally, a fast epidemic wave will have a high concentration (peaking) of infected districts around the mean, and vice versa for a slow-moving wave. The standard measure of peaking (Pearson kurtosis, b_2) shows that leading edges have, as expected, higher values than the following edges, but the differences are small and not statistically significant.

We conclude that, overall, the various measures of epidemic velocity suggest that the Icelandic waves we have studied have relatively faster leading edges and relatively slower following edges.

EPIDEMIOLOGICAL SIGNIFICANCE OF SWASH–BACKWASH STAGES

Identification of the swash and backwash stages for the 14 waves yields some interesting results, which are summarized in Figure 10.16. The duration of the stages averages around eight months for swash and 11 months for

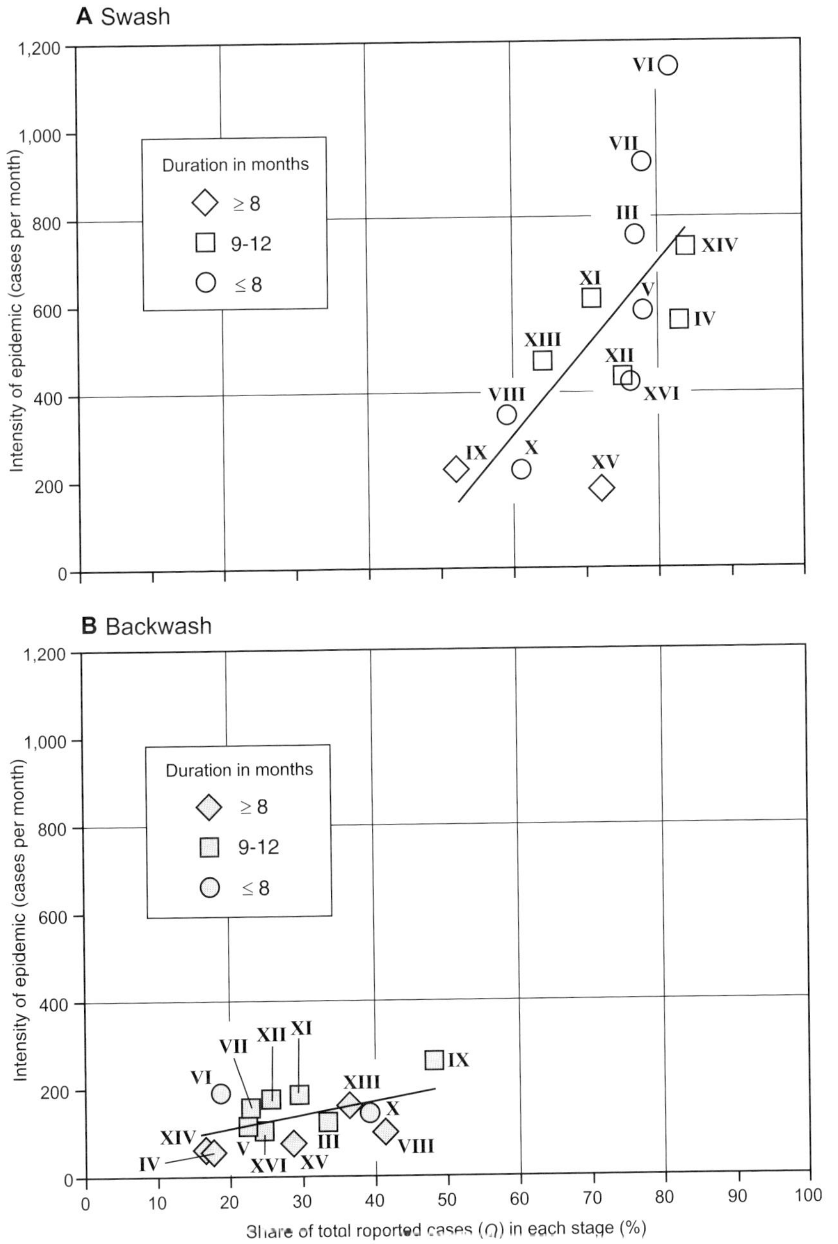

Fig. 10.16. Epidemiological implications of swash and backwash stages in the 14 Icelandic measles Waves III–XVI

The intensity of the epidemic (vertical axis) is plotted against the proportion of total cases recorded in each stage (horizontal axis). (A) Swash stage. (B) Backwash stage. Linear regression lines for each of the two clusters are shown.

Source: Cliff and Haggett (2006, fig. 11, p. 246).

backwash. Despite its shorter length, the share of reported cases is much greater in the swash period, averaging 72 per cent, with the balance of 28 per cent in the longer backwash stage. The intensity of cases is much greater in the swash period with 550 cases per month, four times greater than in the backwash stage (140 per month).

For the 14 Icelandic waves, the average value for R_{0A} was found to be 1.28. Values for individual waves ranged from 1.88 (Wave XIV) to 0.89 (Wave IX). For twelve of the waves, $R_{0A} \geq 1$. The two unexpected results were produced by Waves IX and XII, which were unusual in being negatively skewed, with a slow spatial build-up of infected districts.

10.5 Emergence Detection

Do the results we have presented for influenza and measles in Sections 10.3 and 10.4 imply that the swash–backwash model has a potential use as part of a disease early-warning system? As recent WHO reports have stressed, among the critical needs of any epidemic forecasting system are the ability (i) to predict an epidemic's likely spatial spread at some point relatively early in its unfolding history and (ii) to estimate the probable final size. Two simple examples of the possibilities and pitfalls are given in this section, using French influenza to illustrate capability (i) and Icelandic measles capability (ii).

10.5.1 French Influenza

The following experiment was devised using the French influenza data analysed in Section 10.3.1:

(i) In month 2 (August) of a given influenza season, the swash model parameters, R_{0A}, V_{LE}, and V_{FE}, defined in Appendix 10.1, equations 10.A2 and 10.A7, were calculated and plotted.

(ii) In each successive month through to the end of the influenza season, the data set was updated as new data arrived. The model parameters were recalculated and plotted.

(iii) The experiment was applied to the following groups of influenza seasons, each centred around a pandemic year(s): (*a*) 1887–92; (*b*) 1896–1902; (*c*) 1914–20; (*d*) 1955–9; (*e*) 1966–72.

By way of illustration, Figure 10.17 plots the results for R_{0A} when the approach was tested for the group (*c*) seasons, centred on the 1918 pandemic. This pandemic spread over three influenza seasons (Wave I in the spring of 1918 in the 1917–18 season, Wave II in the autumn of 1918 in the 1918–19

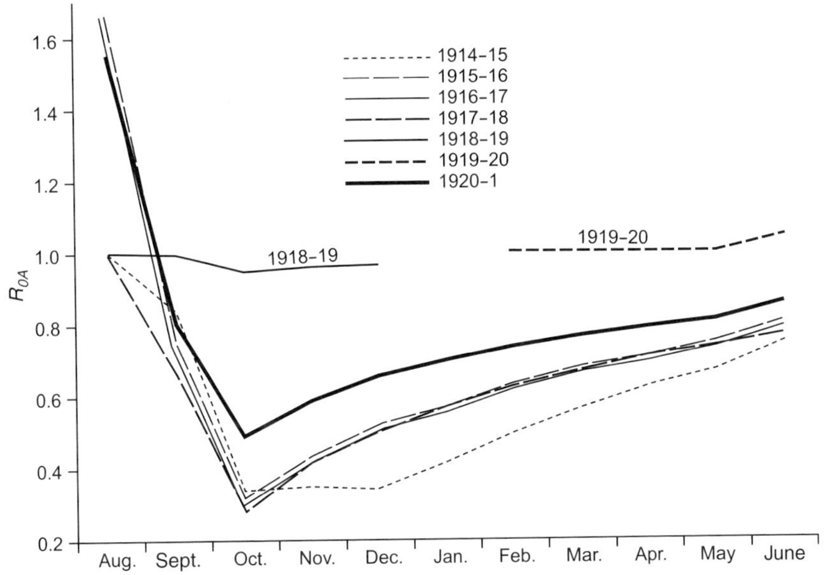

Fig. 10.17. Real-time detection of the 1918–1920 influenza pandemic in France Time series plot of the values of the spatial basic reproductive ratio, R_{0A}, for the swash–backwash model applied to continually updated influenza mortality reports in France for the 1914–20 influenza seasons.

season, and Wave III in the spring of 1919, affecting both the 1918–19 and 1919–20 seasons). The plots for R_{0A} show that, for the main part of the pandemic (Waves II and III), R_{0A} ran at a consistently higher level from September than in immediately preceding and succeeding seasons. From the viewpoint of online monitoring, public health officers would have had early warning from the beginning of the 1918–19 season that the impending influenza experience was likely to be unlike anything they had encountered in the war years.

Figure 10.18 summarizes the results of the experiment for all the pandemic seasonal groups, (*a*)–(*e*). Each chart plots the median values of the model parameters obtained in each seasonal group for (i) the virus shift season(s) and (ii) the non-shift seasons.

From October in the influenza seasons studied, this diagram shows that the spatial basic reproductive ratio, R_{0A}, was consistently greater in virus shift seasons than in other seasons. For the leading edge parameter, V_{LE}, velocity of spread was also greater in shift seasons than in other seasons except for 1889. For the following edge parameter, V_{FE}, no consistent picture emerges from Figure 10.18.

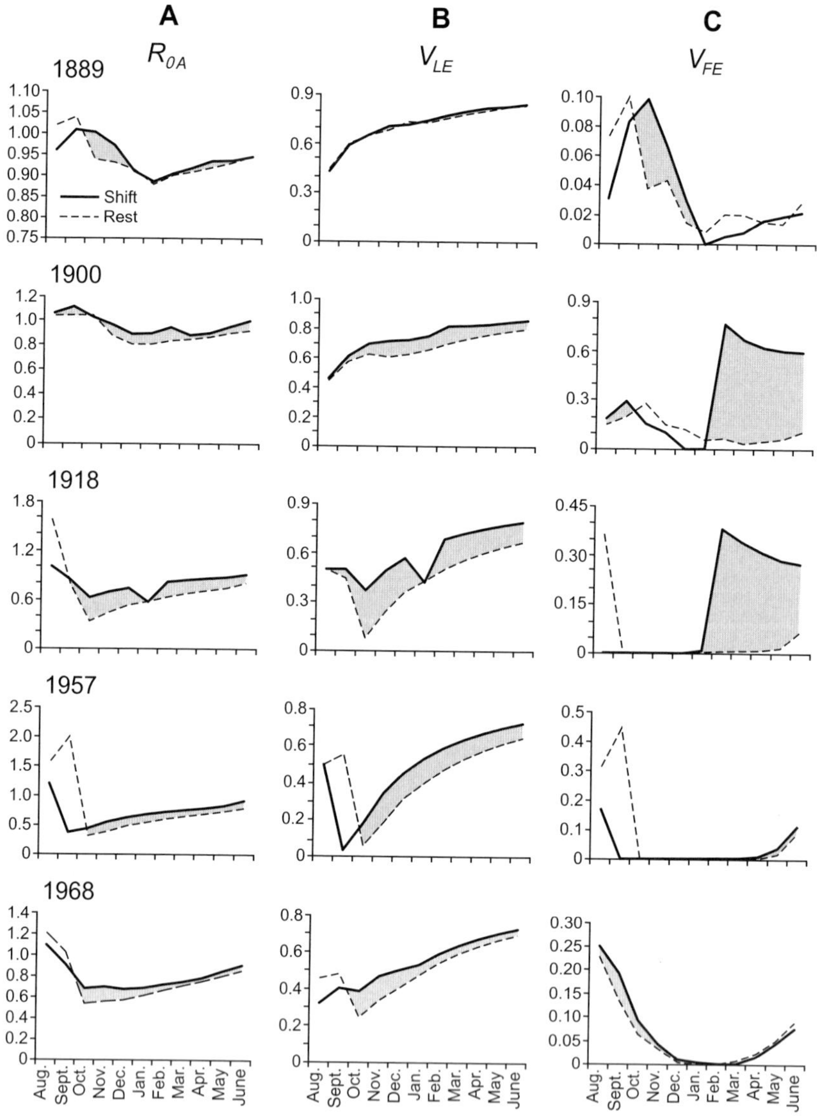

Fig. 10.18. Real-time detection of influenza pandemics in France, 1887–1999
Median values of (A) the spatial basic reproductive ratio, R_{0A}, (B) the leading edge parameter, V_{LE}, and (C) the following edge parameter, V_{FE}, for the swash–backwash model applied to continually updated influenza mortality reports in France for the following groups of influenza seasons: (*a*) 1887–92; (*b*) 1896–1902; (*c*) 1914–20; (*d*) 1955–9; (*e*) 1966–72. In each group, influenza seasons were classified as *shift* if they were affected by a new strain of influenza virus and *rest* otherwise. Months in which the parameter values for shift seasons exceeded those for rest are shaded.

DISCUSSION

When a new strain of human influenza A appears, the population will have at best limited natural resistance, resulting in a much larger stock of susceptibles for infection than normal. Under these circumstances, pandemic influenza may occur, with the new strain running rapidly through the population. *Ceteris paribus*, characteristic features of virus shift seasons are likely to be (i) high levels of morbidity and mortality compared with 'normal' influenza seasons, manifested in larger values of R_{0A}, and (ii) rapid geographical spread (large values for V_{LE}). The expected behaviour of the following edge parameter, V_{FE} is not clear. In shift seasons, long spatial occupancy would lead to a low value for V_{FE}, whereas rapid passage through and clearing of an area, which is feasible with a new virus strain, would yield a small value for V_{FE}. Indeed, the ambiguous behaviour of V_{FE} is confirmed by a correlation of 0.07 between R_{0A} and V_{FE} for the French data.

The results presented in this subsection broadly match expectation. Figure 10.19 shows that, in shift years, epidemics occurred earlier in the season and that they were, for the 1918, 1957, and 1968 shifts, more sharply peaked than in adjacent seasons. Figure 10.6A displays a long-term decline in the reproductive ratio for influenza which was linked to declining velocity of spread (the correlation coefficient between R_{0A} and V_{LE} is 0.77). The localized peaks in R_{0A} and in epidemic velocity set against the century-long falling trend all occurred in virus shift seasons and their immediate aftermath.

10.5.2 Icelandic Measles

In Figure 10.20 we have plotted the cumulative number of cases reported (vertical axis, on a logarithmic scale) for the 14 measles waves against the first 10 months of the epidemic outbreak (horizontal axis). The average trend is shown by the solid line, with the shaded area indicating the zone within which two-thirds of all waves occurred; the individual points mark the upper and lower extremes. The diagram shows that, on average, one half of all cases will have been recorded within the first six months of the measles epidemic and that this will rapidly rise to three-quarters within the next three months. Most infective activity falls in the swash stage of a wave, with many fewer cases in the long tail of the backwash stage. Against this positive indicator of eventual wave size, we have to stress that—probably unsurprisingly—relatively few reliable guides are given to the size of the approaching storm in the first three months of the epidemic.

10.6 Surveillance Systems

Integral to any real-time disease detection system is the capability to collect data which will enable public health assessments to be made. In this section,

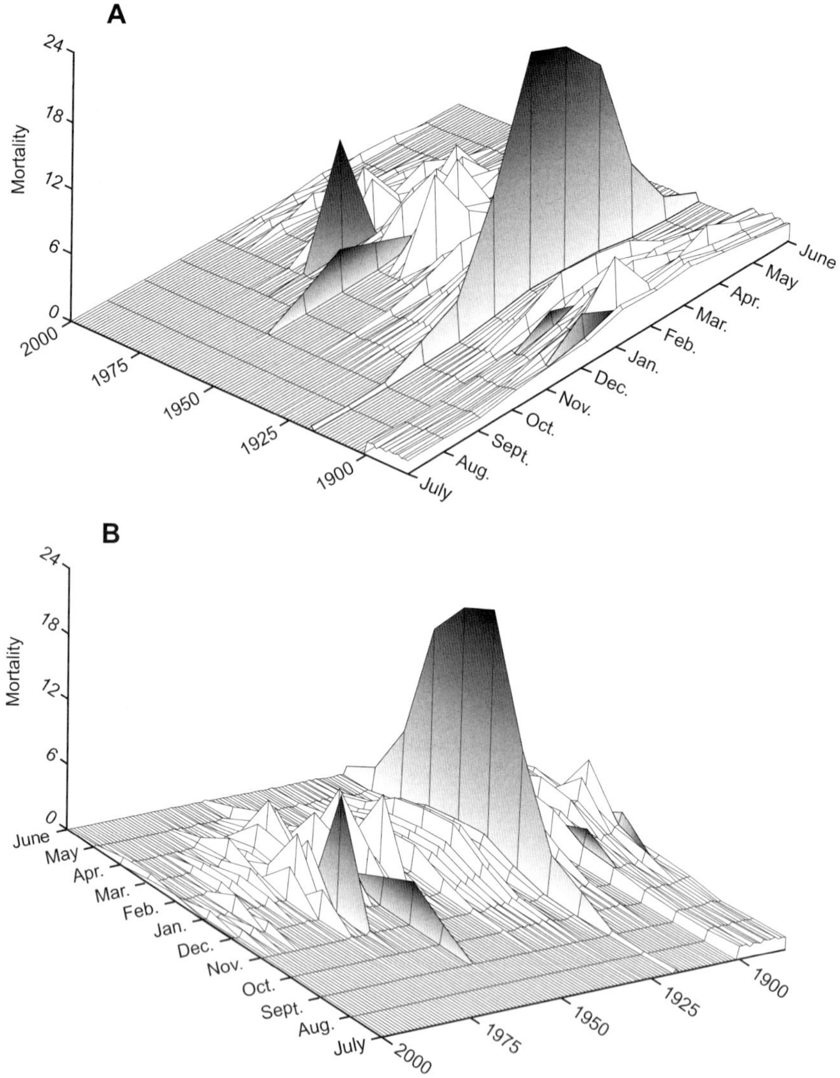

Fig. 10.19. Block diagram of influenza seasons in France, 1887–1999
The recorded monthly mortality from influenza in France is plotted by season. Viral shift years have been highlighted. Outbreaks in shift years generally start earlier and commonly had larger mortality than non-shift seasons. The block has been drawn from two different viewpoints to highlight these features.

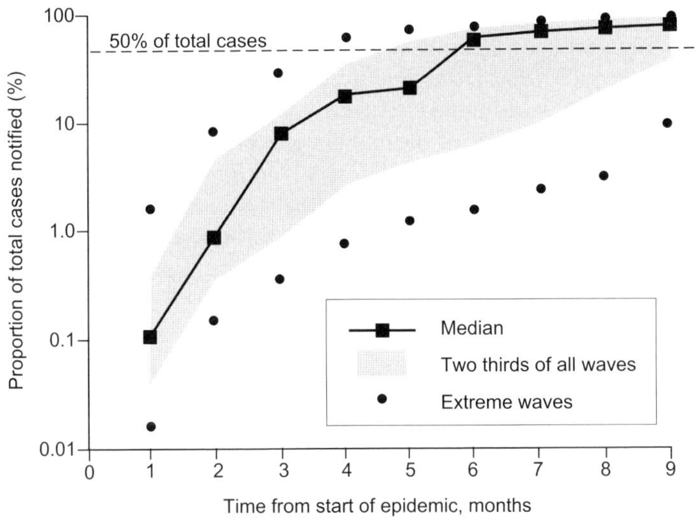

Fig. 10.20. Icelandic measles: cumulative distribution of reported cases plotted against time in months for the 14 Icelandic measles waves
The vertical axis is logarithmic with total epidemic size = 100. The median line shows that half of all measles cases were reported by the sixth month of an outbreak.

we look at surveillance systems as developed in the context of public health surveillance in the United States.

10.6.1 Public Health Surveillance in the United States

Public health surveillance is the ongoing, systematic collection, analysis, and interpretation of health data essential to both (i) the planning, implementation, and evaluation of public health practice and (ii) disease prevention and control (Brookmeyer and Stroup 2003). Public health surveillance data systems should have the capacity to collect and analyse data (Sonesson and Bock 2003), disseminate data to public health programmes (Langmuir 1963; McNabb *et al.* 2002), and regularly evaluate the effectiveness of the use of the disseminated data (Regidor *et al.* 2007; Miller, Roche, *et al.* 2004). More broadly, public health information systems may include data collected for other purposes but essential to public health and often used for surveillance, but perhaps lacking critical elements of surveillance systems (Choi *et al.* 2002). For example, vital statistics data are critical to surveillance (particularly for chronic conditions) but do not focus on specific outcomes, are collected for other purposes (for example, legal burial or cremation), and may not be timely (Stroup, Brookmeyer, *et al.* 2003).

Public health surveillance in the US was founded on the principles developed by Langmuir for infectious diseases (Langmuir 1963). National surveillance at the Centers for Disease Control and Prevention (CDC) relies on collaboration with various levels of government and other organizations. For example, surveillance of notifiable conditions involves reporting by physicians and laboratories, as well as local, county, and state health departments. There was limited expansion of the principles of infectious disease surveillance in the 1970s to other public health disciplines, most notably abortion and congenital malformations (Edmonds *et al.* 1981). In the 1980s and 1990s the CDC mission expanded into the broader areas of public health, and surveillance practice expanded into chronic disease (Thacker, Stroup, Rothenberg, *et al.* 1995), behavioural risk factors (Marks *et al.* 1985), unintentional injury (Graitcer 1988), violence (Ikeda *et al.* 1998), occupational (Baker *et al.* 1988) and environmental health (Thacker, Stroup, *et al.* 1996). Equally importantly, surveillance practice was approached as a science, and evaluation methods (Centers for Disease Control 1988) and analytic methods (Stroup and Thacker 1993) were enhanced. The introduction of the microcomputer and the Internet in the 1990s led to rapid electronic data collection and dissemination; the emergence of informatics as a science led to systems integration and to more strategic and effective surveillance practice. In the new century, the goal is situational awareness, knowing just what is needed to make the best decision. Innovations such as web-based query systems and distributed, grid computing in an open source environment have the potential to put principles of public health surveillance into a conceptual framework far beyond the tools used by Langmuir.

10.6.2 National Systems and Strategies

In many countries, notifiable disease surveillance systems have historically relied on reporting by physicians and laboratories (Krause *et al.* 2005). In the United States, notifiable disease reporting is mandated by state and local regulations (Roush *et al.* 1999) but is enhanced by national leadership in the development of case definitions (Centers for Disease Control and Prevention 1997*c*). Recent efforts to integrate data on reportable diseases, content of case definitions, and tables of coded observations have increased the sensitivity, timeliness, and quality of the data (Doyle *et al.* 2005).

In most countries, surveillance now encompasses non-infectious conditions, the recording of vital events, and the registration of health outcomes such as birth defects and cancer (McNabb *et al.* 2002). Indeed, the most helpful information for planning primary prevention programmes for non-communicable diseases and predicting future burden is currently the population distribution of major common (and, for the most part, modifiable) risk factors (Mokdad *et al.* 2004). Since 1994, the Behavioral Risk Factor

Surveillance System (BRFSS) (http://www.cdc.gov/brfss) has expanded to survey now approximately 200,000 adults in all US states and territories, and many counties and large metropolitan areas (Centers for Disease Control and Prevention 2003*c*). These data have been used to assess the epidemic of obesity (Wang and Beydoun 2007) and health problems among older adults (Brown, Balluz, *et al.* 2004) or among racial or ethnic groups (Gary *et al.* 2003). In addition, international consultation has resulted in modifications of the BRFSS in China, Australia, Canada, Russia, Brazil, Argentina, and Jordan (Holtzman 2003). Other chronic conditions are assessed through registries which assess risk factors useful for prevention (Truelson *et al.* 2001).

10.6.3 Real-Time Early Warning Systems

EXISTING APPROACHES

Recognized gaps in disease surveillance capacity, highlighted by emerging infections, antimicrobial resistance, bioterrorist threats, and pandemic influenza preparedness, have driven the development of efficient, real-time identification of diseases and early-warning systems (Mandl *et al.* 2003; Baxter *et al.* 2000). These systems use real-time electronic surveillance of non-specific disease indicators to provide early warnings of large intentional or natural outbreaks (Mostashari and Hartman 2003). Such systems take two basic approaches: facilitating clinicians' active reporting of cases of disease of interest, or using existing information captured in medical care delivery of administration of medical care benefits. For example, automated information about diagnoses assigned by clinicians during ambulatory care visits allows daily assessment of episodes of illness for which no aetiological agent may be identified (syndromic surveillance) (Lazarus *et al.* 2001; Centers for Disease Control and Prevention 2005*d*). The detection of an increased frequency of such events can trigger further analysis to reveal patterns that warrant ongoing investigation by public health officials (Najmi and Magruder 2005; Jackson *et al.* 2007; Wieland *et al.* 2007). Syndromic surveillance has proved to be especially useful in emergency situations (Fraser 2007).

The utility of these early-warning systems is dependent on three essential elements: data standards, a communications infrastructure, and policy-level agreements on data access, sharing, validity, and reduction of burden on data providers. Data standards require that users and providers agree on common definitions of data elements and terms, common classification systems, compatible telecommunication protocols, and other technical specifications that allow different systems to be compared, linked, and otherwise integrated (Humphreys 2007). In the development of electronic health records, attention to core functions of public health (assessment, policy development, and assurance) is critical (Broome, Horton, *et al.* 2003; Broome and Loonsk 2003). For example, to support public health's work on socio-behavioural factors for prevention, electronic health data standards models need to incorporate environmental, psychosocial, and other non-medical data elements (Kukafka *et al.* 2007).

Public health data are created in numerous locations. Therefore, an information network infrastructure is essential if the public health surveillance system is to be integrated (Parry *et al.* 2007). An integrated surveillance and information system requires major cultural change, financial investment, and logistical planning, balancing competition in the medical marketplace with fiscal pressures affecting providers and health systems (Shortliffe and Sondik 2006), as well as the constraints of many international settings (Morse 2007).

An integrated public health surveillance system is the result of agreements that exist between those who provide data and those who use the information. That agreement depends upon certain ethical assurances. Surveillance poses risks to privacy as governments collect sensitive health information from patients, travellers, and other vulnerable groups. The United States and the European Union both have data protection statutes, but both exclude surveillance activities from these regulations (Gostin 2007*a*). As a result, we see strategies that can result in important benefits to communities but produce fear and distrust in those same communities. For example, in response to the growing burden of diabetes in New York City, the Health Department implemented mandatory reporting of data for a registry of glycosolated haemoglobin test results containing names of patients and their physicians (Steinbrook 2006). The criticism surrounding this initiative springs from the claim that surveillance for diabetes, a chronic disease primarily affecting individuals without spillover to others, represents unjustified paternalism of government, overriding a social imperative (Gostin 2007*b*). Policies and legislation to prevent wrongful disclosures would address such controversy (Gostin *et al.* 2001).

Public health officials must evaluate the usefulness of the surveillance systems to make rational decisions about allocating limited resources (Centers for Disease Control and Prevention 2001*c*). Evaluation activities include a description of the preventability and public health importance of the event under surveillance, case definitions, and the specific components of data collection, analysis, and dissemination. Subsequently, an evaluation of a surveillance system should include assessment of system attributes: simplicity, flexibility (for example, can it adapt to changing disease characteristics and population structure?), and acceptability to both data collectors and users; see Romaguera *et al.* (2000). Evaluations internationally have shown areas where the system has met objectives and identified aspects for improvement (Miller, Roche, *et al.* 2004). Progress in syndromic surveillance has illustrated new methods for evaluation of quantitative attributes (Mostashari and Hartman 2003; Burr *et al.* 2006; Jackson *et al.* 2007).

An example of an effective laboratory-based surveillance system in the United States is PulseNet USA (Section 5.2.3). Since 1996, it has been instrumental in the detection, investigation, and control of numerous outbreaks caused by Shiga toxin-producing *Escherichia coli*, *Salmonella*, *Listeria monocytogenes*, *Shigella*, and *Campylobacter*. The network uses pulse-field gel electrophoresis (PFGE) for molecular subtyping of agents involved in foodborne outbreaks (Jones, Scallon, *et al.* 2007). For example, in 2006 a multistate outbreak of *E. coli* O157:H7 (one of 3,520 unique *E. coli* O157: H7 strains reported using PulseNet) was, for the first time, linked to consumption of fresh spinach (Table 5.5) (Centers for Disease Control and Prevention 2006*a*). Molecular subtyping of *L. monocytogenes* isolates reported through PulseNet assisted the investigation of outbreaks of listeriosis in ready-to-eat meat and unpasteurized cheese. Data from this system informed a national *Listeria* Action Plan to help guide control efforts by industry, regulators, and public health officials (Centers for Disease Control and Prevention 2003*e*).

SEVERE ACUTE RESPIRATORY SYNDROME (SARS)

Between late 2002 and mid-2003, a total of 8,098 probable SARS cases were reported to the World Health Organization (WHO) from 29 countries (Section 6.4.1). In the United States, only eight cases had laboratory evidence of infection with SARS-CoV. The key to controlling a SARS outbreak is prompt detection of cases and their contacts, followed by rapid implementation of control measures. Two features of SARS-CoV disease pose challenges for surveillance. First, the early signs and symptoms are not specific enough to distinguish SARS disease reliably from other common respiratory illnesses. Second, laboratory diagnostic tests are not adequately sensitive early in the course of illness. Therefore, there is risk of exposure to another case of SARS disease or to a setting where SARS transmission is occurring.

During the 2003 epidemic, CDC and the Council of State and Territorial Epidemiologists (CSTE) developed and modified surveillance criteria (Centers for Disease Control and Prevention 2003*d*). Data from SARS surveillance have been used in statistical models to evaluate the effectiveness of early intervention activities (Cauchemez *et al.* 2006).

10.7 Conclusion

In this chapter, we have reviewed spatial approaches in the SIR tradition to modelling the spread of infectious diseases in human populations. A robust swash–backwash model which focuses upon estimating the rate of spatial propagation of epidemic waves has been developed. The model has been applied to (i) influenza data for France, Iceland, and Cirencester and (ii) measles data for Iceland to evaluate the model at different spatial scales and in varied geographical settings. It has been shown that the model can readily separate pandemic years of influenza from 'normal' influenza seasons, as well as highlight the distinctive spread characteristics of large rather than small measles epidemics.

The swash model was then tested with influenza data for France and measles data for Iceland in a manner which simulated real-time surveillance. For influenza, it was shown that the model did give early warning of approaching pandemics. The Icelandic results for measles were consistent with this; major measles epidemics were distinguished from normal measles epidemics by their greater concentration of cases and infected districts in the swash stage of the epidemic curve. While the utility of the swash–backwash model in the context of real-time surveillance systems of the sort discussed in Section 10.6 requires further testing, if the early promise is confirmed in future studies, the question of epidemic control based upon early warning will naturally arise. It is to this topic that we turn in the next and final chapter of this book.

Appendix 10.1: Swash–Backwash Model Equations

Let the first month of an influenza season (July, say) be coded as $t = 1$. The subsequent months of the season are then coded serially as $t = 2, t = 3, \ldots, t = T$, where T is the number of monthly periods from the beginning to the end of the season (i.e. $T = 12$ in our yearly cycle). We call the month in which an influenza case is first recorded in a given geographical unit the leading edge (*LE*) of the outbreak in that unit, and the last month of record the following edge (*FE*). As described in Cliff and Haggett (2006), standard statistical analysis of the distribution of the two edges enables us to define a time-weighted arithmetic mean, $\bar{t}_{LE}$ and $\bar{t}_{FE}$ for each edge. For the leading edge, the equation is

$$\bar{t}_{LE} = \frac{1}{N}\sum_{t=1}^{T} t n_t \qquad (10.\text{A}1)$$

where N is the total number of units in the area under consideration (the 96 *départements* of France in the 1990s, for example), n_t is the number of units whose leading edge occurred in month t, and $N = \sum n_t$. The time-weighted mean is a useful measure of the velocity of the wave in terms of average time to unit infection. A similar equation can be written for *FE*, and higher-order moments can also be specified. To allow comparison between diseases with different wave characteristics, we convert these time-weighted means to a velocity ratio, V, $(0 \leq V \leq 1)$,

$$V_{LE} = 1 - \frac{\bar{t}_{LE}}{D} \qquad (10.\text{A}2)$$

where D is the duration of the wave. A similar equation can be written for V_{FE}.

The conventional *basic reproduction number* (or *rate* or *ratio*), R_0, is defined as the ratio between an infection rate (β) and a recovery rate (μ):

$$R_0 = \frac{\beta}{\mu}. \tag{10.A3}$$

In the spatial domain, A, the spatial reproduction number, R_{0A}, is the average number of secondary infected geographical units produced from one infected unit in a virgin area. In a given study area, the integral S_A (the proportion of the study area at risk of infection) is given by:

$$S_A = \frac{(\bar{t}_{LE} - 1)}{T}, \tag{10.A4}$$

while the proportion of the area which is infected (the infected area integral) is

$$I_A = \frac{\bar{t}_{FE}}{T} - S_A. \tag{10.A5}$$

The recovered area integral, R_A, is

$$R_A = 1 - (S_A + I_A). \tag{10.A6}$$

All three integrals are dimensionless numbers with values in the range [0, 1]. S_A parallels the reciprocal of β in that a small value indicates a very rapid spread while the integral R parallels the reciprocal of μ in that a small value indicates very rapid recovery. Since both are inversely related to their power, we suggest that their complement might be substituted in estimating a spatial version of R_0, namely,

$$R_{0A} = \frac{1 - S_A}{1 - R_A}. \tag{10.A7}$$

Such a spatial basic reproduction number would measure the propensity of an infected geographical unit to spawn other infected units in later time periods. In effect it provides an indicator of the tendency of an infected unit to produce secondaries. Values of R_{0A} calibrate the velocity of such spread (the larger the value, the greater the rate of spread).

It is important not to over-stretch the analogy between R_0 and R_{0A}. R_0 is defined for the hypothetical situation when a new case is introduced into a *wholly susceptible population*. While R_{0A} is defined for a virgin region, it is calculated using spatial data for the entire span of the outbreak. As a result, it is contaminated with data from the later phases of the outbreak when many spatial sub-areas are no longer virgin. This may account for the frequent small calculated values. Normal R_0 is useful because it distinguishes between situations where an epidemic can take off ($R_0 > 1$) and those where it cannot ($R_0 < 1$), and this is arguably the most important attribute of R_0 as a summary parameter in epidemiology. R_0's spatial cousin, R_{0A}, does not share this property—for example in Tables 10.2, 10.3, and 10.5 there are analyses of real epidemics that had sustained spread from one district to another in which $R_{0A} < 1$. But it does allow large numbers of spatial settings to be examined and the relative velocity at different stages of outbreaks to be assessed and compared. Finally, it should be noted that the parameters R_{0A}, LE, and FE are correlated, but each gives slightly different insights into the progress of an outbreak through a geographical area.

Appendix 10.2: French Monthly Influenza Time Series

This appendix summarizes how the monthly geographically disaggregated influenza time series for France, 1887–1999, were generated from data sources (1)–(4) described in Section 10.3.1.

1. 1887–1900

From data source (1), a temporally consistent set of 51 towns with populations in excess of 30,000 (mapped in Figure 10.4) was identified. For each of these towns, a monthly time series of influenza deaths was estimated as follows.

NOTATION

p_{iT} = the population of town i in year T;
P_T = the population of France in year T;
a_{it} = the monthly number of pneumonia and bronchopneumonia deaths *reported* in sources (1) and (2) for town i in month t;
$\hat{g}_{it}$ = the number of influenza deaths *estimated* for town i in month t;
G_t = the number of deaths from influenza *reported* for France in source (1) in month t.

Step 1. Estimate pro rata the monthly number of influenza deaths, $\hat{G}'_t$, attributable to the 51 towns as $\hat{G}'_t = G_t \times (\sum_{i=1}^{51} p_{iT}/P_T)$ to allow for the fact that the 51 towns represent only a proportion of the total population of France.
Step 2. Estimate g_{it}, the reported number of influenza deaths in town i during month t, as $\hat{g}_{it} = \hat{G}'_{it} \times (a_{it}/\sum_{i=1}^{51} a_{it})$. This distributes the influenza deaths attributed to the 51 towns in month t by the proportion of the pneumonia and bronchopneumonia deaths occurring in the 51 towns in month t which were *reported* from town i.

This approach assumes that the monthly distribution of pneumonia cases in a given town can be used to approximate the (unknown) monthly distribution of influenza cases. The resulting matrix is T (= 168) months × n (= 51) towns.

2. 1901–1905

For the 51 towns used to generate matrix (1), a T (= 60) months × n (= 51) towns matrix of reported influenza mortality was abstracted directly from source (2).

3. 1906–1968

Monthly influenza mortality counts for each *département* were formed by distributing the annual total for each *département* recorded in source (3) through the year according to the proportion of the year's total of cases recorded for France in month j. Between 1906 and 1942, when only annual influenza mortality data are available for France, the average monthly proportion of the year's total recorded for France, 1943–99, was used instead.

4. 1969–1999

Source (4) was used directly, generating a T (= 372) months × n (= 96) *départements* matrix of reported influenza mortality.

11

Controlling Re-emerging and Newly Emerging Diseases

11.1 Introduction

As earlier chapters in this book have shown, cyclically re-emerging old plagues and newly emerging scourges are, because of their multifactorial ecology, likely to be the enduring experience of the human race. And so, in this concluding chapter, we look at some of the broad ideas which lie behind disease control and which might be used to mitigate the impact of new or re-emerging infections. Linked to surveillance systems, *quarantine* and *vaccination* are currently the front-line approaches, and we discuss these in Sections 11.2 and 11.3. The chapter is concluded in Section 11.4 with an assessment of the twenty-first-century context within which containment of newly emerging and re-emerging diseases is likely to occur.

It is helpful to consider control strategies for communicable diseases by setting them within a modelling framework. A basic susceptible–infective–removed (SIR) epidemic model was described in Section 10.2.1. As shown in Figure 11.1, protection against the spread of infection can be undertaken at two points. The first method, (i), is to interrupt the mixing of infectives and susceptibles with protective spatial barriers. This may take the form of isolating an individual or a community, or of restricting the geographical movements of infected individuals by quarantine; another approach is by locating populations in supposedly safe areas. The historical use of quarantine in protecting communities against the plague and other diseases is considered in Section 11.2. For animal populations, there exists a third possibility: the creation of a disease-free buffer zone by the wholesale evacuation of areas or by the destruction of those infected.

The second method, (ii), is to short-circuit the route from susceptibles to removed by the establishment of immunity through some variant of immunization. Vaccination as a control strategy is discussed in Section 11.3.

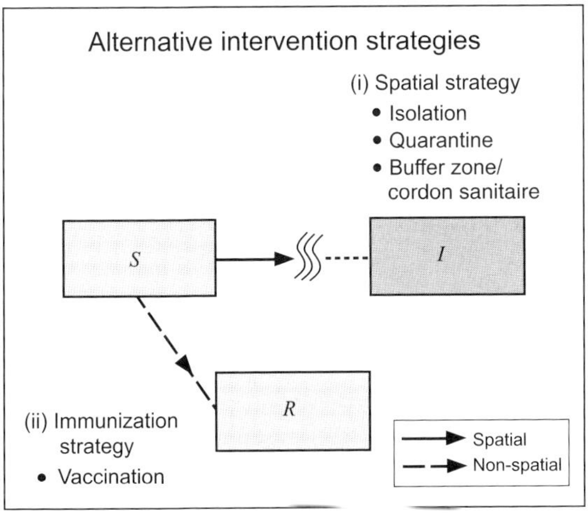

Fig. 11.1. Interrupting chains of infection
Alternative intervention strategies based on (i) *spatial strategy*, blocking links by isolation and quarantine between susceptibles and infectives, and (ii) *non-spatial vaccination strategy*, opening of new direct pathways from susceptible to recovered status through immunization. This outflanks the infectives (I) box.
Source: Cliff, Haggett, and Smallman-Raynor (1993, fig. 16.1, p. 414).

11.2 Spatial Barriers: Quarantine Strategies

Potential control strategies are illustrated schematically in Figure 11.2. In the two maps, infected areas have been shaded, while disease-free areas have been left blank. In Figure 11.2A, the disease-free areas need to be protected by isolation. Such *defensive isolation* entails the building of a spatial barrier (a quarantine ring, or cordon sanitaire) around the diseased area, the aim being to prevent infectious cases in the diseased area from gaining access to susceptibles in the disease-free area outside the ring. As an example, we describe in Section 11.2.1 the extraordinary lengths to which the Italian republics and principalities went over five centuries to try to protect themselves from the

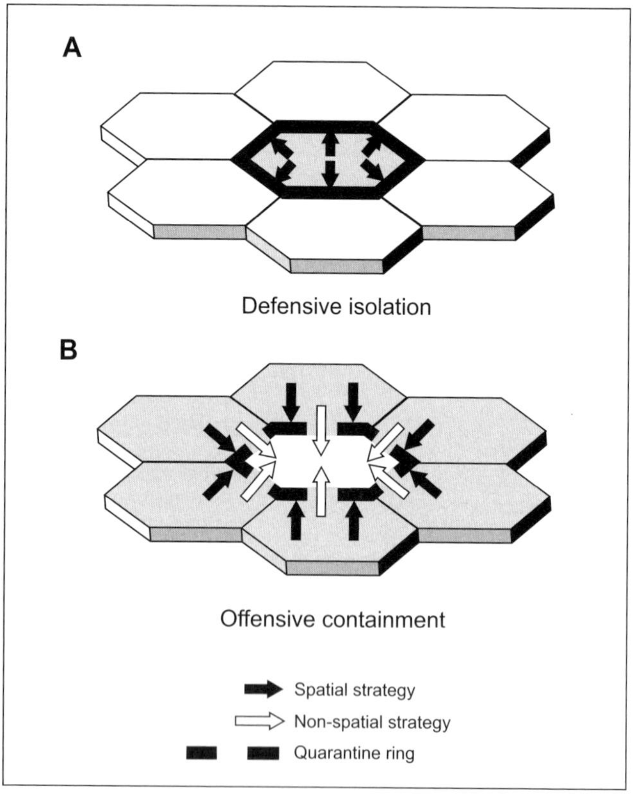

Fig. 11.2. Spatial control strategies
Schematic diagram of two spatial control strategies to prevent epidemic spread. (A) Defensive isolation. (B) Offensive containment. Infected areas are shaded; disease-free areas are left blank. Geographical areas are shown arbitrarily as hexagons. Non-spatial strategies are defined in Fig. 11.1.
Source: Cliff, Haggett, and Smallman-Raynor (1993, fig. 16.9, p. 423).

plague. As we shall see, their attempts had only limited success and are frequently impractical today except in particular circumstances; in general, twenty-first century-transport systems pose severe problems to the use of spatial isolation (see Chapter 6). An example of these difficulties, based upon attempts to control a 1994 plague outbreak in India, is described in Section 11.2.4.

An alternative approach to defensive isolation (Figure 11.2B) is *offensive containment*. This is the reverse of defensive isolation in that the spread of a disease from an infected region into a disease-free area is again halted by a quarantine ring around the perimeter of the disease-free area; the disease is then progressively eliminated from the infected region by a combination of (today) vaccination and (mainly historically) removal of infection by isolation in the case of human diseases. Offensive containment was also deployed in some Italian states alongside defensive isolation to control the plague. For disease in farm livestock, offensive containment usually involves removal by slaughter. During 2007, parts of England were affected by outbreaks of highly pathogenic avian influenza type H5N1 among turkeys in January, by foot and mouth disease among cattle in August, and by bluetongue among sheep from September. The nature of these outbreaks and their control by offensive containment is discussed in Section 11.2.4.

We now consider in more detail the articulation of these strategies.

11.2.1 Defensive Isolation: Italy and the Plague

CONTEXT

After the great pandemic of the Black Death which affected Europe for some seven years from 1346, plague became endemic in Europe (see Section 2.3.2). Italy was entrained in 1347–8, with outbreaks continuing there for the next four and a half centuries (Figures 11.3 and 11.4). The courses of the major epidemics are described in Scott and Duncan (2001: 303–18). The repeated outbreaks deeply affected culture, society, and economy at all levels. But, despite the threat posed by plague visitations, local patriotism was too strong to permit the growth of a national unity during the plague centuries. Instead three main groupings of states emerged (Scott and Duncan 2001: 303): (i) the city states of the north (particularly Venice, Milan, Genoa, and Florence), wealthy and jealous of each other; (ii) the Papal States; and (iii) in the south two very different and poor regions, the kingdoms of Naples and Sicily (eventually the kingdom of the Two Sicilies; see Figure 11.5).

It was the northern group of states which led the fight against the disease, gradually evolving a system of public health which, by the middle of the seventeenth century, had reached a high degree of sophistication. The northern Italian focus of this evolution was driven by the position of Italy at the interface of Europe and Asia, its location on arms of the Silk Road, and the

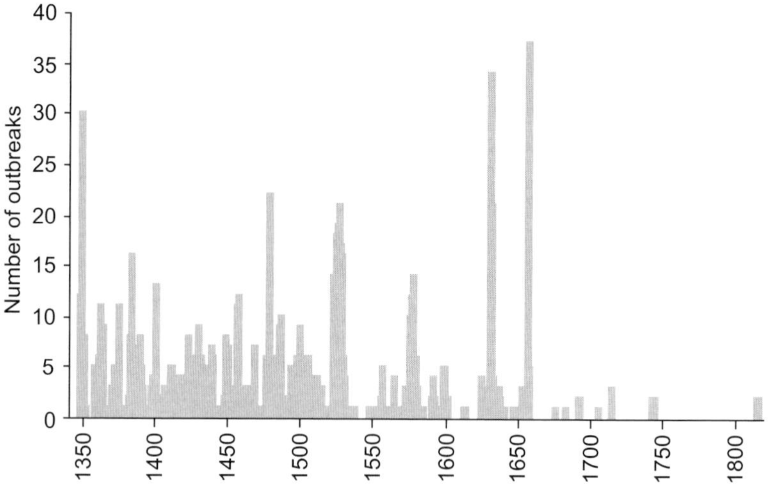

Fig. 11.3. Plague outbreaks in Italy, 1347–1816
Annual time series of number of localities reporting plague. The generalized epidemics of 1348, 1383, 1457, 1478, 1522–8, 1577, 1630, and 1656 stand out from the annual background of 4–5 outbreaks which occurred in one place or another throughout the period.

Source: Biraben (1975–6, annexes III and IV, pp. 363–74, 394–400).

dependence of the great republics like Venice and Genoa upon trade with Asia for their prosperity, factors which combined to ensure that importation of the plague, especially by ships returning from the Levant, was an ever-present threat. Similar developments to those in northern Italy took place north of the Alps but remained at a much more primitive level—as they did in Italy south of the dukedom of Tuscany (Cipolla 1981: 4–5).

As described in Kiple (1993: 198), the first rudimentary steps to curb the annual visitations were taken in 1377 when Venice attempted to place a moratorium on travel and trade upon its tiny Dalmatian colony of Ragusa (now Dubrovnik) to contain a plague outbreak. The system which evolved from this root over the next two centuries was based upon special magistracies, which, while they combined legislative, judicial, and executive powers in all matters pertaining to the public health, had as their prime focus prevention of the plague. By the middle of the sixteenth century, all major cities of northern Italy had permanent magistracies, reinforced in times of emergency by health boards set up in minor towns and rural areas. All boards were subordinate to and directly answerable to the central health magistracies of their respective capital cities (Cipolla 1981: 4). The magistracies stressed prevention rather than cure, and out of their organizational genius came the ideas of quarantine that have persisted to the present day. The Italian system had two main elements:

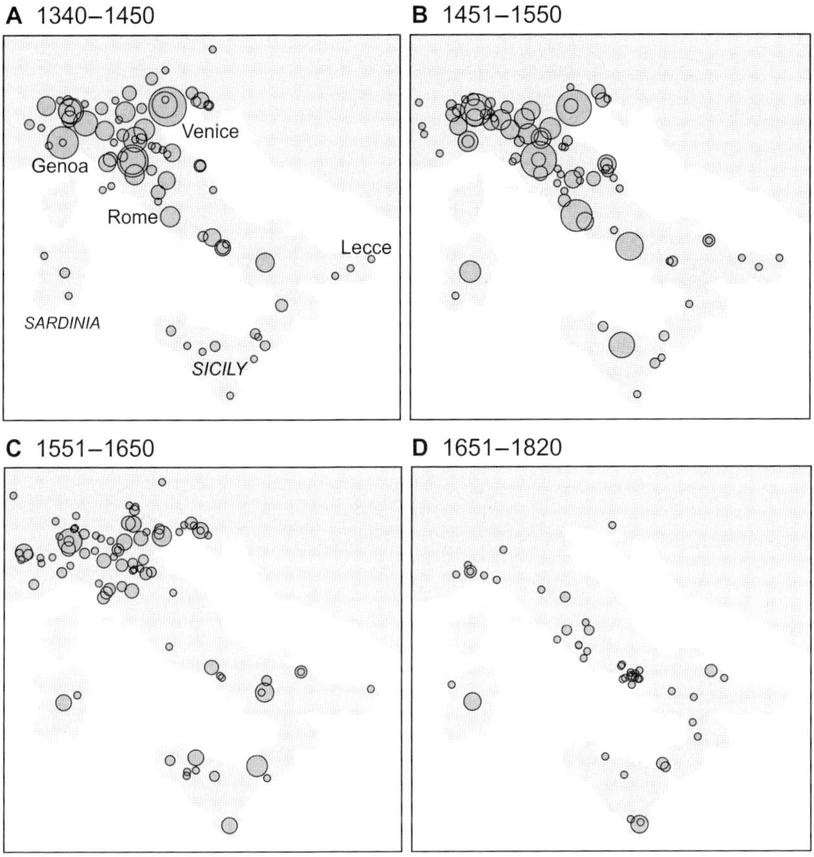

Fig. 11.4. Geographical distribution of number of recorded plague outbreaks in Italy, 1340–1820
(A) 1340–1450. (B) 1451–1550. (C) 1551–1650. (D) 1651–1820. Outbreaks declined in number and became more widely dispersed spatially over the period.
Source: Biraben (1975–6, annexe IV, pp. 394–400).

(1) Communication. The northern Italian cities kept each other informed of the believed state of health of other locations in the region. In the course of the sixteenth and seventeenth centuries the health magistracies of the capital cities of the republics and principalities of northern Italy had established the eminently civilized custom of regularly informing each other of all news they gathered on health conditions prevailing in various parts of Italy, the rest of Europe, North Africa, and the Middle East. Florence 'corresponded' regularly with Genoa, Venice, Verona, Milan, Mantua, Parma, Modena, Ferrara, Bologna, Ancona, and Lucca. The frequency of the correspondence

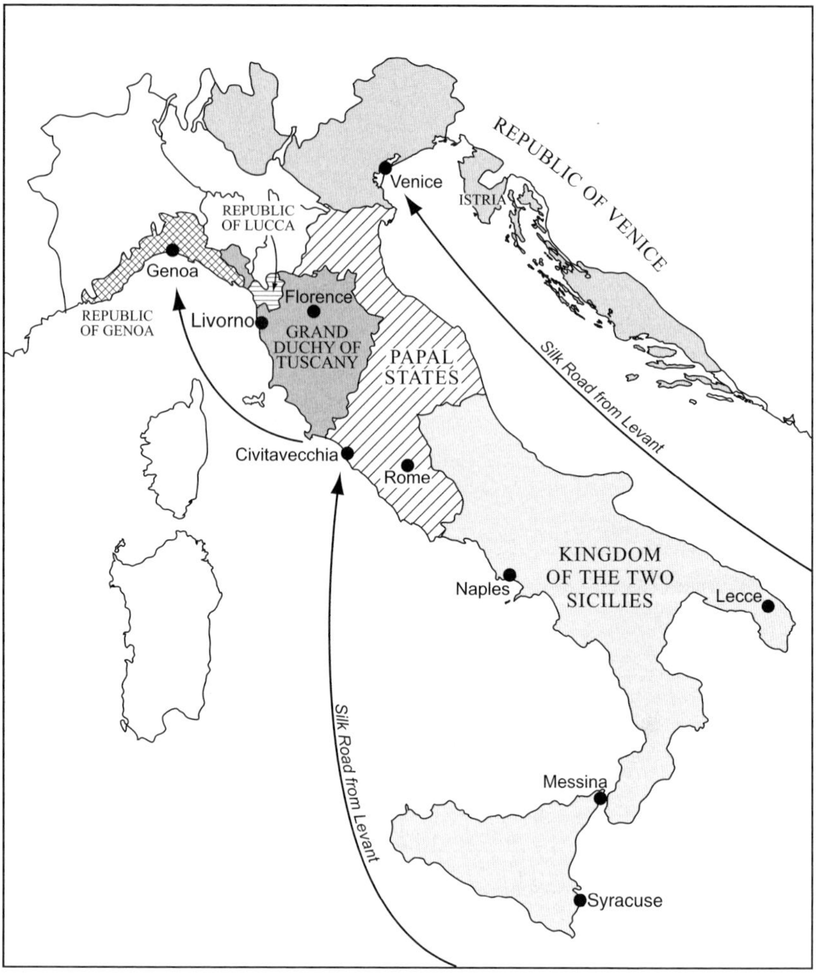

Fig. 11.5. Political divisions of Italy towards the end of the eighteenth century The Silk Road at the interface with the Mediterranean is marked.

with each of these places ranged from one letter every two weeks in periods of calm to several letters a week in times of emergency (Cipolla 1981: 21).

Spies and later official observers were also present in the major cities, who reported back to their employers on the state of health in the various republics and principalities. But it was the great plague epidemic of 1652 which ultimately led to agreed, coordinated and enforced action among the north Italian states in a Capitolazione (Convention) between Florence, Genoa, and the Holy See. The Convention bound the three powers to common practices and health measures in the principal ports of Genoa, Livorno, and Civitavecchia (see Figure 11.5). Each state agreed to allow

A

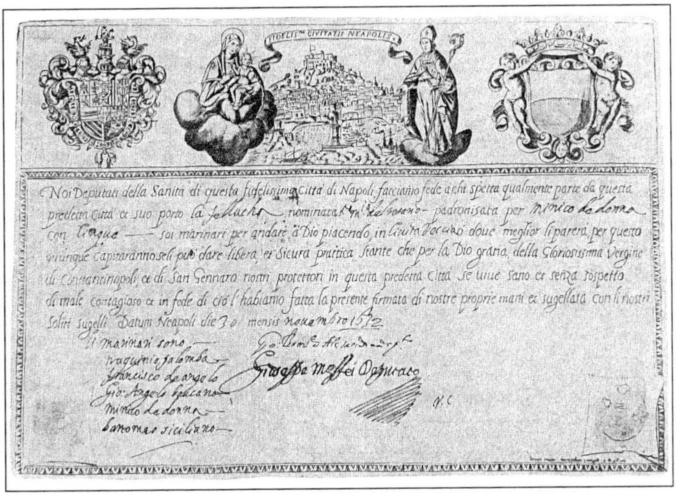

Noi Deputati della Sanità di questa fidelissima Città di Napoli facciamo fede à chi spetta qualmente parte da questa predetta Città et suo porto la felucha nominata S.ta M.a del Rosario padronisata per Minico da donna con Cinque soi marinari per andare à Dio piacendo in Civita Vecchia doue meglior li parerà, per questo ovunque capitaranno seli può dare libera, et sicura prattica stante che per la Dio gratia, della Gloriosissima Vergine di Constantinopoli, et di San Gennaro nostri protettori in questa predetta Città se viue sano et senza sospetto di male contagioso et in fede di ciò l'habiamo fatta la presente firmata di nostre proprie mani et sugellata con li nostri soliti sugelli. Datum Neapoli die 30 mensis novembro 1632

Li marinari sono
Inaquinio palomba
Francisco de angelo
Gio: Angelo bucano
Minico da donna
Santomas siciliano

Giuseppe Maffei Deputato

B

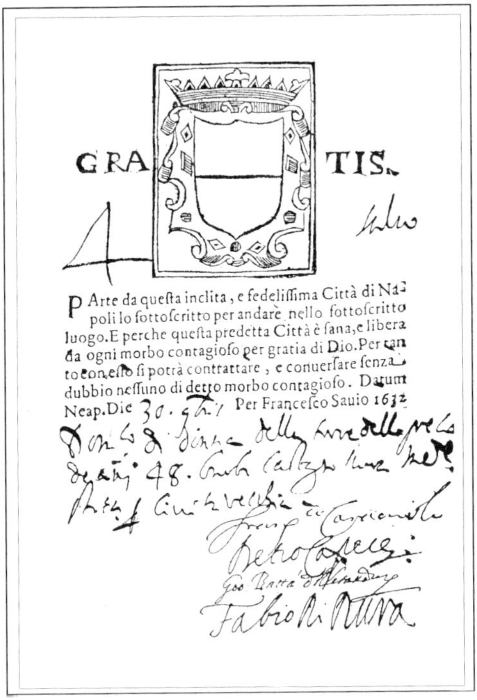

GRA TIS.

PArte da queſta inclita, e fedeliſſima Città di Napoli lo ſottoſcritto per andare nello ſottoſcritto luogo. E perche queſta predetta Città è ſana, e libera da ogni morbo contagioſo per gratia di Dio. Per tanto con eſſo ſi potrà contrattare, e conuerſare ſenza dubbio neſſuno di detto morbo contagioſo. Datum Neap. Die 30. 9bri Per Franceſco Sauio 1632

Fabio Ri[illegible]

Pl. 11.1. Certificates issued by the City of Naples in 1632

(A) This document, which measures 35 × 25 cm, is embossed with coats of arms and a panorama of Naples. It was issued to the captain of the *felucca* (a type of boat) named *Santa Maria del Rosario*, which was sailing from Naples to Civitavecchia, the port of Rome, with five sailors on board, whose names are listed at the end of the certificate. It declares Naples to be free of all infectious disease, and asks for unrestricted and secure *pratique* (*prattica*: a licence to deal with a port after quarantine or on producing a clean bill of health).

the other two to station one representative of their respective health boards in the main harbour—a forerunner of 'international controls and the voluntary relinquishment of discretionary powers by fully sovereign states in the matter of public health' (Cipolla 1981: 34). The *concerto* between Tuscany and Genoa came rapidly to pass, but attempts to bring in the state groupings (ii) and (iii) above (the Holy See and Naples) proved meagre. Even the *concerto* between Tuscany and Genoa collapsed a few years later, but it was a remarkable early attempt at international health collaboration not repeated for 200 years until the international control of the great nineteenth-century cholera pandemics became paramount.

(2) Defensive isolation. When contagious disease was uncovered anywhere by a particular magistracy, a proclamation of *ban* (when the presence of communicable disease was positively ascertained) or *suspension* (precaution because there was legitimate suspicion of disease) was issued. Bans were long-term, suspensions short-term. Bans and suspensions were used to denote the interruption of regular trade and communication. With banishment and suspension, no person, boat, merchandise, or letter could enter the state issuing the order except at a few well-specified ports or places of entrance where quarantine stations were set up. At the stations, incoming people, boats, and merchandise were subject to quarantine and disinfection even if they carried health certificates issued at the point of departure (Plate 11.1). The authorities also reserved the right to refuse access to anything or anybody from banished areas—even, if necessary, to the quarantine stations. People attempting to violate the ban or enter the territory of the banishing state were executed (Plate 11.2).

The ideas of banning and isolation were grounded in the prevailing beliefs as to how plague spread. The basic idea was that it originated with venomous

---

(B) This certificate, measuring 16 × 12 cm and embossed with the arms of the city of Naples, was given in plague periods to each traveller from the port of Naples at embarkation. It declares the city to be healthy and free of all morbid contagions. It also declares that it is safe to trade and negotiate with the bearer without fear of infection. The almost illegible handwriting gives the date (30 June or July), the name and a description of the bearer, his destination, as well as the signatures of the four representatives of the city authorities. The anonymous source author (p. 32) interprets the script as Giovanni Angelo Baucano, of the Greek Tower ('de la Torre dello Greco' barely recognizable at the end of line 1), aged 48 ('de anni 48', line 2), with a dark chestnut moustache ('castagno', middle of line 2) and a mole on the upper left cheek, travelling to Civitavecchia (line 3). The signatories are: Francesco Caracciolo, Delio Capece, Giov. Battista d'Alessandro, and Fabio di Ruvo. Such certificates were issued to try to guarantee free passage and continuance of travel in the face of bans and suspensions.

Source: Ministero dell'Interno, Direzione Generale della Sanità Pubblica, Napoli (1910, pls II and III following p. 32).

A

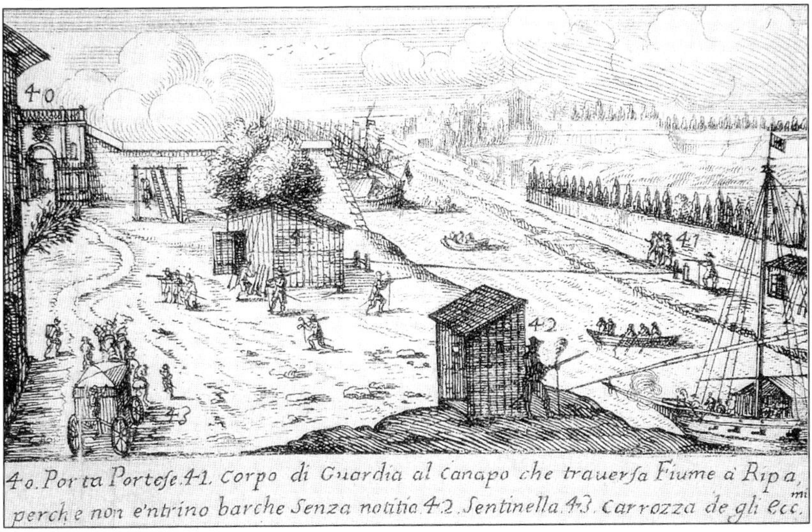

B

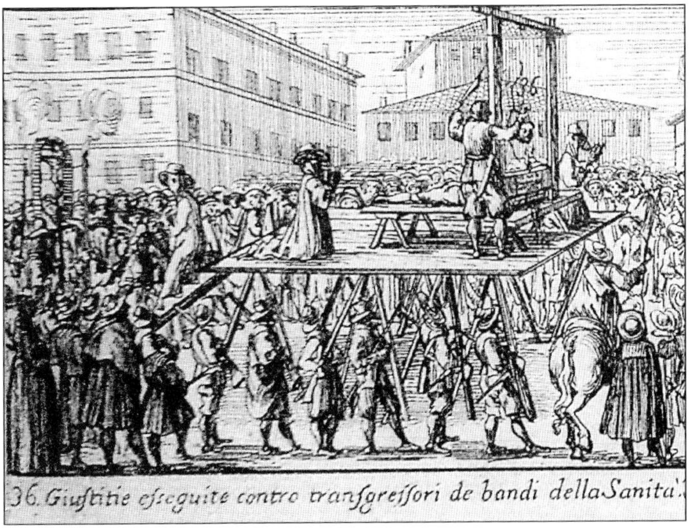

Pl. 11.2. The plague in Rome, 1656

Extracts from G. G. de Rossi's 1657 three-part etching of episodes of the 1656 outbreak of the plague in Rome. (A) Guarded river crossing point (41) to ensure boats did not land illegally with a sentry (42) at his post. (B) (36) Execution of persons who broke the quarantine rules.

Source: World Health Organization Library, Geneva.

atoms which infected the air and made it 'miasmic'. Besides being poisonous, the atoms were held to be sticky and would adhere to the surfaces of inanimate objects, animals, and people from which they would penetrate the body and cause death. A consequence of this belief system was that it was held that the only way to avoid the spreading of disease was 'to prevent all intercourse with people, animals, and objects coming from areas afflicted by the plague' (Cipolla 1981: 8).

Because doctors thought that human intercourse was primarily responsible for the propagation of plague (and indirectly it was, because it encouraged the dispersion of infected rat-fleas), when an epidemic occurred, most trade and communication was forbidden. And, when an epidemic gave signs of subsiding, it was customary for health authorities to decree a 'general quarantine' which meant as many people as possible were locked into their homes for a period of 40 days to reduce to a minimum all human intercourse (cf. Section 11.2.3 later).

To enforce bans and suspension, the republics and principalities established along the Mediterranean and Adriatic coasts, as well as along land borders with other countries, a complex network of forts, towers, and observation posts, organized by the military (coastal guards), to prevent both the landing of boats other than at authorized quarantine stations, and overland travel and intercourse. In terms of the model described earlier in Section 11.2, a ring quarantine system was established to maintain defensive isolation. Such was the importance of the system that maps were produced to show the location and manning of the sanitary observation and guard posts which comprised the rings. Some of these little-known maps, along with the associated records of manning and the day books of travellers through the posts, have survived in a number of Italian state archives; and it is to their analysis that we now turn. We consider first the general picture which emerges before examining in turn maps and prints for (i) two of the northern states (the republics of Venice and Genoa), (ii) the Papal States, and finally (iii) the Two Sicilies.

ITALY

Figure 11.6 shows the geographical distribution of maps traced which plot the guard/observation posts comprising the defensive cordon sanitaire. The strings of posts are denoted by the solid lines. The identity numbers correspond with the numbered list of sources given in Appendix 11.1.

The lines of posts ran round the entire sea coast of Italy, as well as down the Dalmatian coast. As we shall see from the examples which follow, the defensive system consisted of two elements: (i) in both the Adriatic and the Mediterranean, armed sailing boats (*feluccas*, *trabaccoli*, *baragozzi*) to stop illegal landings; and (ii) coastal observation towers and sentry boxes manned by armed infantry who stopped and recorded people and merchandise passing

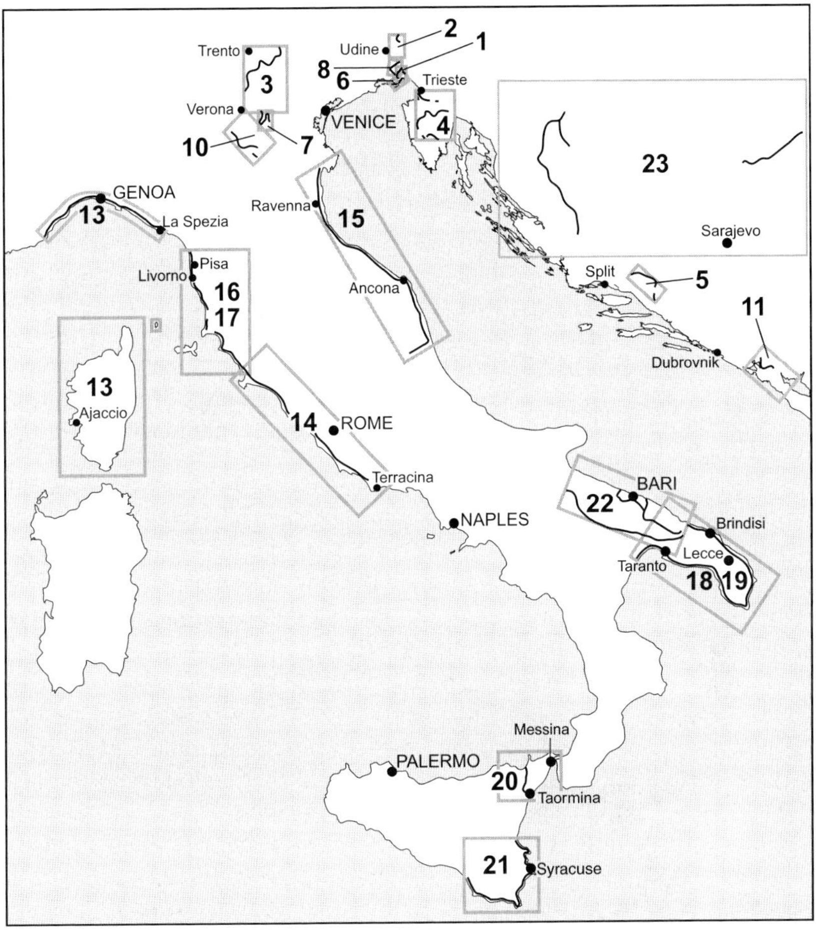

Fig. 11.6. Defensive containment and the plague in Italy in the eighteenth century Geographical locations of maps showing observation posts which comprised the defensive isolation ring maintained around Italy against the plague. Map extents are shown by boxes, and strings of posts by heavy lines. The identity numbers correspond with the sources listed in App. 11.1.

through the post. In addition, so-called 'flying corps' of cavalry were deployed in some locations in the rear of the observation posts. The role of the flying corps was to act as a rapid response force, mopping up sources of infection which penetrated the outer rings of boats and observation posts. The flying corps represent the offensive containment element of Figure 11.2B. Finally, within the overall ring, individual defensive quarantine rings were constructed

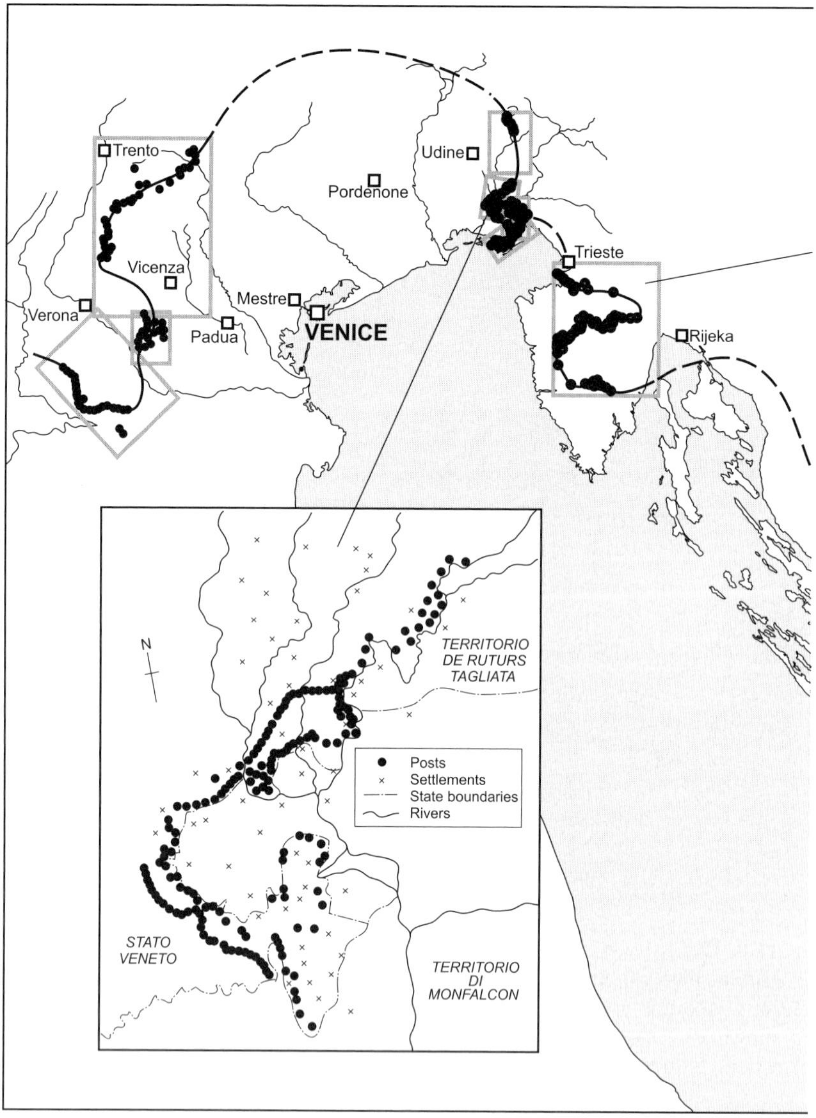

Fig. 11.7. Ring quarantine systems. I: Eighteenth-century Venice
This map shows the general shape of the ring of sanitary guard posts around the Venetian empire in thc 18th century, reconstructed from surviving maps (grey shaded boxes) in the Venice State Archives. Guard posts are plotted as solid black circles. Between surviving maps, the hypothesized general shape of the ring is sketched as a pecked line. The inset maps show two of the maps at a larger scale.

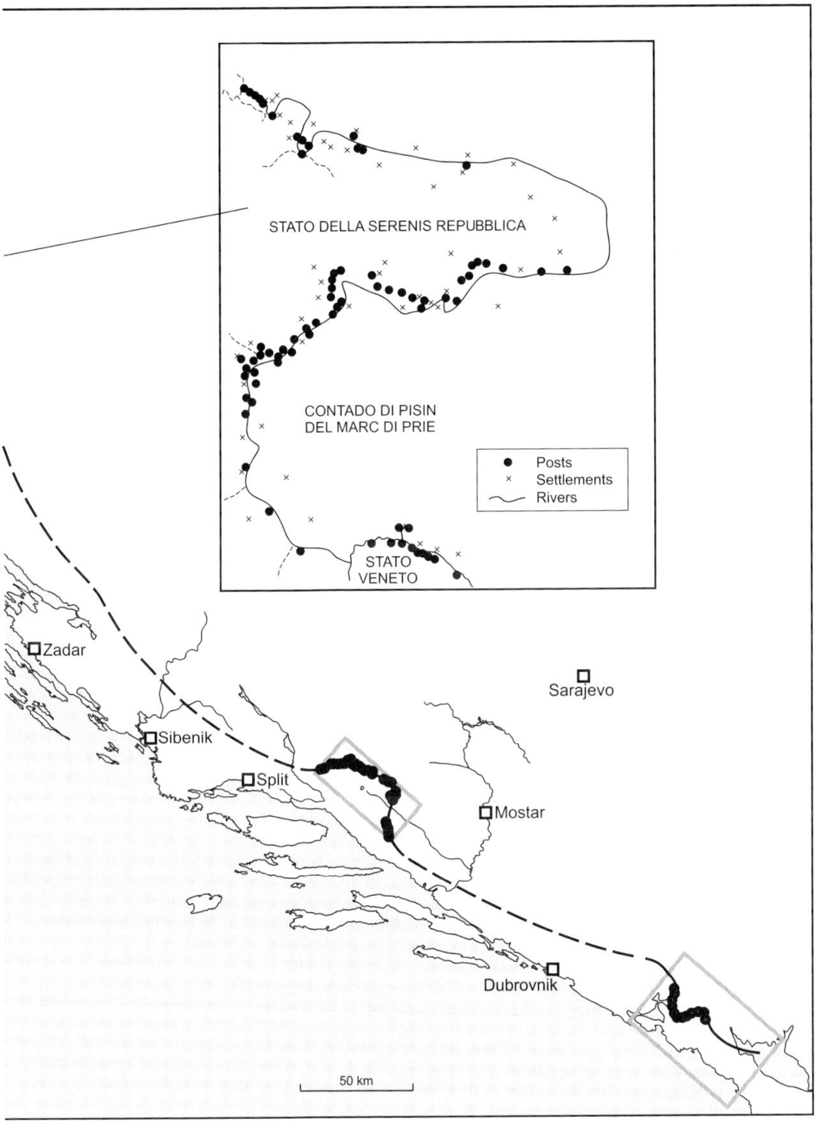
STATO DELLA SERENIS REPUBBLICA
CONTADO DI PISIN
DEL MARC DI PRIE
STATO
VENETO
Posts
Settlements
Rivers
Zadar
Sarajevo
Sibenik
Split
Mostar
Dubrovnik
50 km

from time to time along land borders and around individual towns as necessary to respond to local disease threats.

The observation posts were constructed within sighting distance of each other; communication between posts was primarily by semaphore (daylight) and beacon (night) signals. The reporting system was hierarchical: *local observation posts ⇒ district central command post ⇒ regional reporting centre*. Some of the maps give an indication of the manning—around 2–5 soldiers per observation post, with periodic forts of around 30–50 men. Observation posts not only recorded the traffic passing, but also tried to prevent illegal passage so that ships, goods, and travellers were routed into fixed quarantine stations.

THE NORTHERN STATES

Venice

Because of its maritime supremacy and trading connections, the Venetian republic was visited by plague at regular intervals over nearly five centuries. Accordingly, the republic established an extensive ring of sanitary guard posts around its borders from an early date. The locations of those known to have existed in the eighteenth century are plotted in Figure 11.7. As the figure shows, the guard posts swept in a large arc around the perimeter of the republic.

Plate 11.3 illustrates an extract from one of the surviving maps around Monfalcone. The individual guard posts appear as tents (see added enlarged inset in the bottom left corner), while the 76 posts (*cas*[*s*]*elli*) are named in the lower right entablature. Plate 11.4 illustrates the frontier ring erected along the borders of the territory of Friuli in 1713 at times of epidemics. This print shows the guard posts for the infantry (*appostamenti di infanteria*—see enlarged inset), as well as men in arms (element (i) in the defensive ring of Figure 11.2A) and supporting cavalry (the flying corps for the offensive containment of Figure 11.2B).

The guard posts were designed primarily to prevent the arrival of plague overland. The Ottoman dominions were regarded as the main threat. On arrival, persons and goods suspected of carrying disease were confined in one of the city's two *lazarettos* for a statutory quarantine period of 40 days.

Trying to prevent plague from arriving by sea was especially complex and is described in a mid-eighteenth-century booklet by Venice's Magistrato della sanità (1752).

> Experience has shewn, that in the *Ottoman* Dominions, the Plague is never utterly extinct: Hence it is an immutable Law with the Magistrate of the Office of Health, to consider the whole Extent of the *Ottoman* Dominions and every State dependent on it, as always to be suspected to be in an infected Condition, to such a Degree, as not to receive, in any Part of the Dominions of the Republick [Venice], either confining to or commercing with them, any Persons, Merchandizes, Animals, or any other Thing coming from thence, without the necessary Inspection of the Office of Health, and the previous purifications. (p. 4)

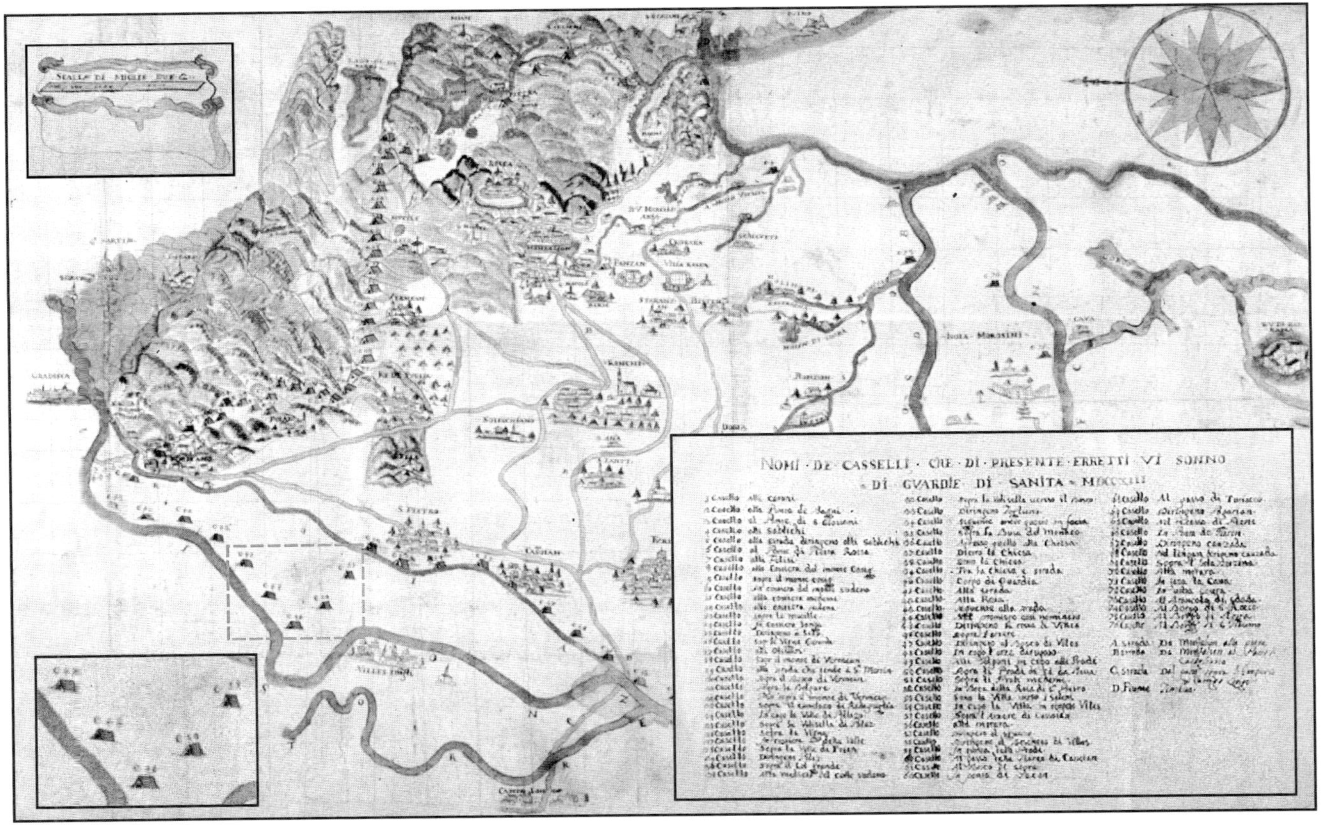

Pl. 11.3. Map of the territory of Monfalcone between the lake of Pietra Rossa and the river Isonzo, showing the towns, posts, and sanitary guard huts at the border with the Granducale (Tuscany)

Source: App. 11.1 (3).

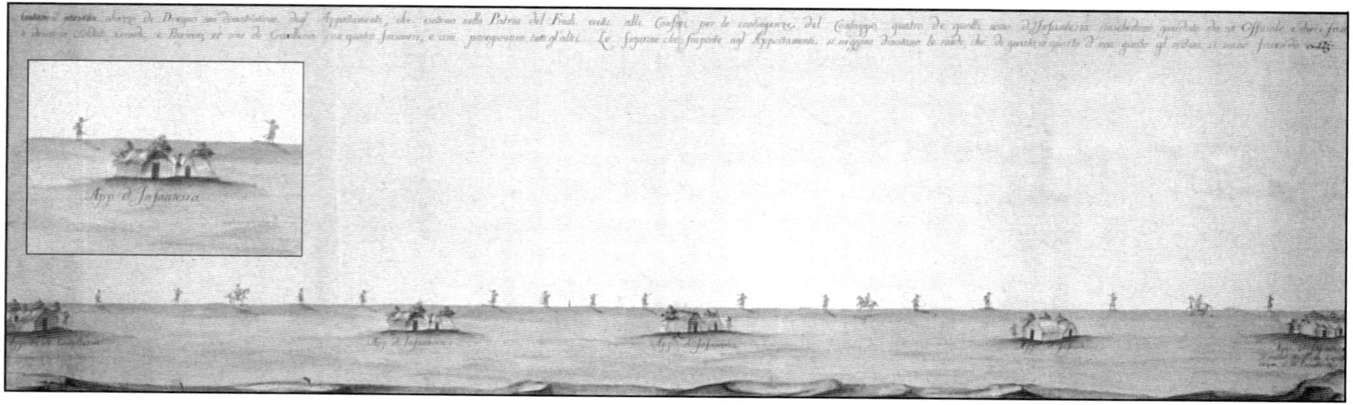

Pl. 11.4. Aquatint drawing of the infantry and cavalry posts erected along the borders of the territory of Friuli in times of epidemics The inset shows one of the infantry posts at a larger scale

Source: App. 11.1 (9).

Although the Ottoman dominions were perceived as the prime risk, the same procedures were followed for 'every Vessel, coming from any Part of the World, that is either infected, or suspected to be so' (p. 4). Vessels were normally expected to stop at Istria (located on Figure 11.5) to take on board a pilot, or were towed up to Venice. Spies were maintained on the high tower of San Marco to watch for approaching vessels. The Magistrate sent one of his 60 guardians to meet the ship, which was moored in distant canals up to 25 km from the city according to the level of perceived risk. Ships were guarded throughout the quarantine period. They were unloaded of goods and passengers and both were dispatched to one of the city's two *lazarettos*. Generally, unless they were afflicted with full-blown plague, new arrivals were confined in the Nuovo Lazaretto (New Lazaretto). The unfortunate creatures suffering from full plague either on arrival or during quarantine were dispatched to Lazaretto Vecchio (the Old Lazaretto); see Plate 11.5 for locations and descriptions. Only when the ship had been fully unloaded did the statutory 40-day quarantine period begin.

The Old and New Lazarettos were isolation hospitals on islands. The Old was 525 feet by 425 feet, the New 560 feet by 460 feet. Each was capable of holding 6,730 bales of merchandise. The Old could properly house about 300 passengers, the New 200. The *lazarettos* were not only externally isolated but constructed to provide internal isolation of goods and passengers to the individual level. Conditions were frequently appalling. It was not uncommon for people to die at the rate of 500 per day in Lazaretto Vecchio during plague outbreaks in the sixteenth century, while Lazaretto Nuovo was recorded as holding 8,000 inmates on one occasion, far beyond the capacities of either *lazaretto* to do anything worthwhile.

The captain of the vessel was taken ashore by a guarded way to a point of examination. The examination turned upon whence the vessel had come, duration of the journey, places visited and their health, visits ashore, contact with other vessels at sea, the health of the ship's crew and passengers, and the nature of the cargo. Account had to be rendered of any crew or passengers who had died on board or who had left the ship en route 'and particularly the Condition of that Person who is wanting' (p. 8). If the examining officer was satisfied 'if the Vessel really came from a place that is free, it [the vessel] is declared free; if from a suspected one [place], the ship was placed in quarantine'.

The principles of quarantine for goods were frequent handling, airing, and smoke fumigation with aromatic herbs. Cloth and untreated animal hides were regarded as especially risky. Although the procedure varied in detail by product, bales were generally opened, aired, rummaged, and cleaned up to twice a day, and moved from one location to another once a week. For people, social interaction was prevented, and each individual had his/her own cell, garden plot, and cooking facilities. Individuals who died in quarantine were checked for plague marks before being buried in lime in holes at least 12 feet deep. In the event that any disease broke out during a quarantine period,

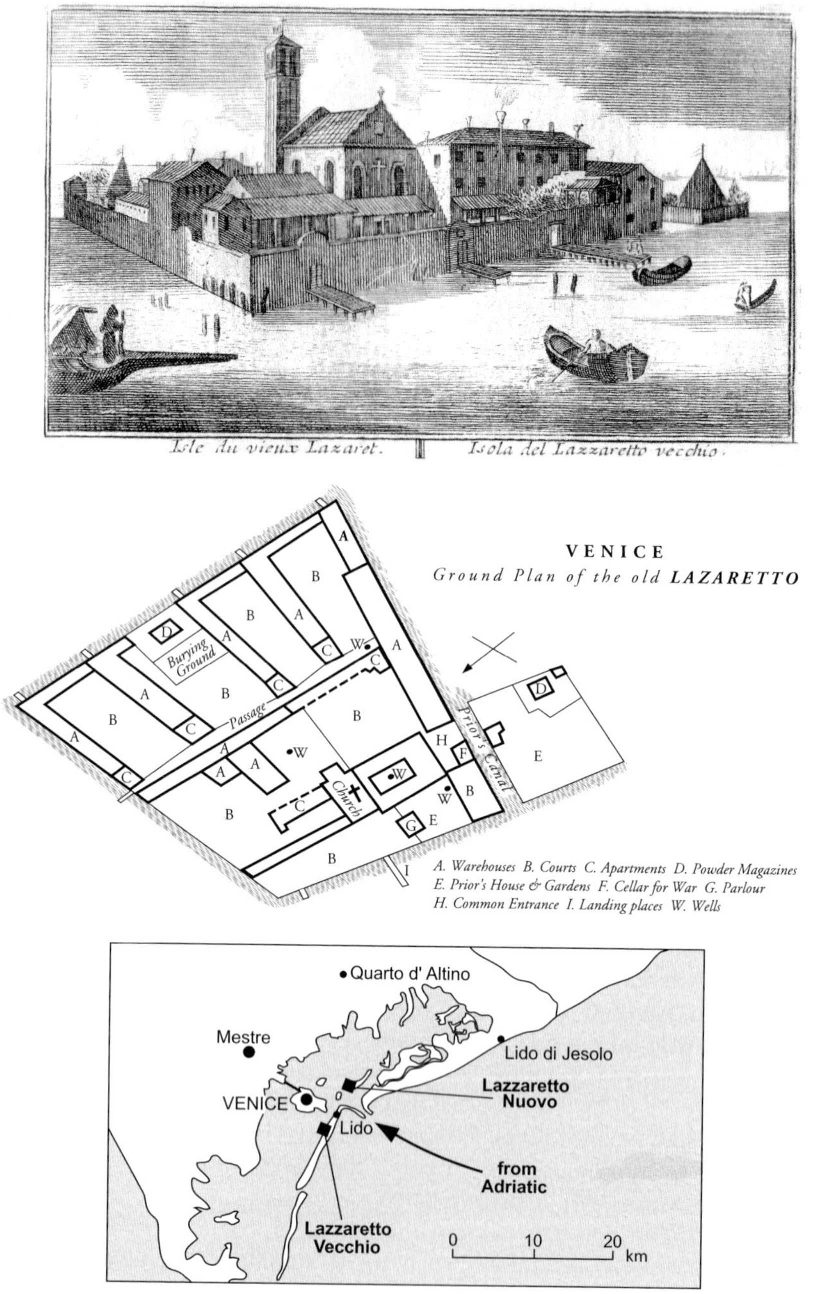

Pl. 11.5. *Lazarettos* of Venice

Location map of the Old (Lazzaretto Vecchio) and New (Lazzaretto Nuovo) Lazarettos of Venice. The engravings show the ground-floor plan of Lazzaretto Vecchio and a prospect of the *lazaretto* from the north-west corner. (The ground-floor plan has been distorted to conform with the prospect.) Lazzaretto Vecchio was established the process was repeated so that second and third quarantines were not unheard of for individual ships.

The Venetian example is important for illustrating certain repeating features of quarantine systems down the ages, namely: isolation of suspected goods/animals and travellers from the populus for a period long enough to reduce the risk of transmission of infection to the public at large; the idea of a ring system of health check posts around an area; isolation hospitals in which suspected individuals and chattels were housed until cleared; and identification of parts of the world where infection was likely to be found.

Genoa

The defensive quarantine ring, as well as the location of other infrastructure used to protect the public health of the republic of Genoa, was mapped in a remarkable atlas by Matteo Vinzoni in 1758 (Appendix 11.1 (13)). In the first half of the eighteenth century, Liguria was divided into 36 health districts, each overseen by a Commissioner for Health. Using one plate per district, Vinzoni charted the locations of the hospitals, *lazarettos*, and sanitary (health) observation posts serving each district. The manning information recorded by Vinzoni varied by health district and is of three types: (i) the complement by day and night at each of the guard posts; (ii) post complement plus information on the military support in the district; (iii) simple lists of the post names. From these data, Figure 11.8 maps the manning complement of each district using proportional circles, as well as the number of sanitary officers. In addition, the locations of the individual posts are marked as solid black dots.

Archival documents indicate how the system operated. Regular armed soldiers were assigned to the posts, supported by men from the local area on a rotation basis. Some posts were manned day and night while others were manned only at night. As Figure 11.8 indicates, nocturnal manning was more

---

in 1423 about 2 km from Venice on a small island then known as Santa Maria di Nazareth, close to modern Lido. It is generally regarded as the world's first fully functioning quarantine station. Lazzaretto Nuovo was established in 1468 on the island then known as Vigna Murada, separated by a navigable channel from the southern tip of the island of Sant' Erasmo, about 3 km from Venice. It occupied a strategic location at the entrance to the Venetian lagoon from the Adriatic and, when visited by John Howard in 1786, was used primarily to quarantine Turks, soldiers, and crews of plague-infected ships (Howard 1791: 11). By decree, ships, passengers, and goods were isolated for a limited period to allow for the manifestation of any disease and to dissipate imported infection. Originally the period was 30 days, *trentina*, but this was later extended to 40 days, *quarantina*. The choice of this period is said to be based on the period that Christ and Moses spent in isolation in the desert. The Venetian system became the model for other European countries and the basis for widespread quarantine control for several centuries.

Source: Ground-floor plan of Lazzaretto Vecchio from Howard (1791, pl. 12); prospect is a mid-18th-century copper engraving by the Venetian artist Giuseppe Filosi.

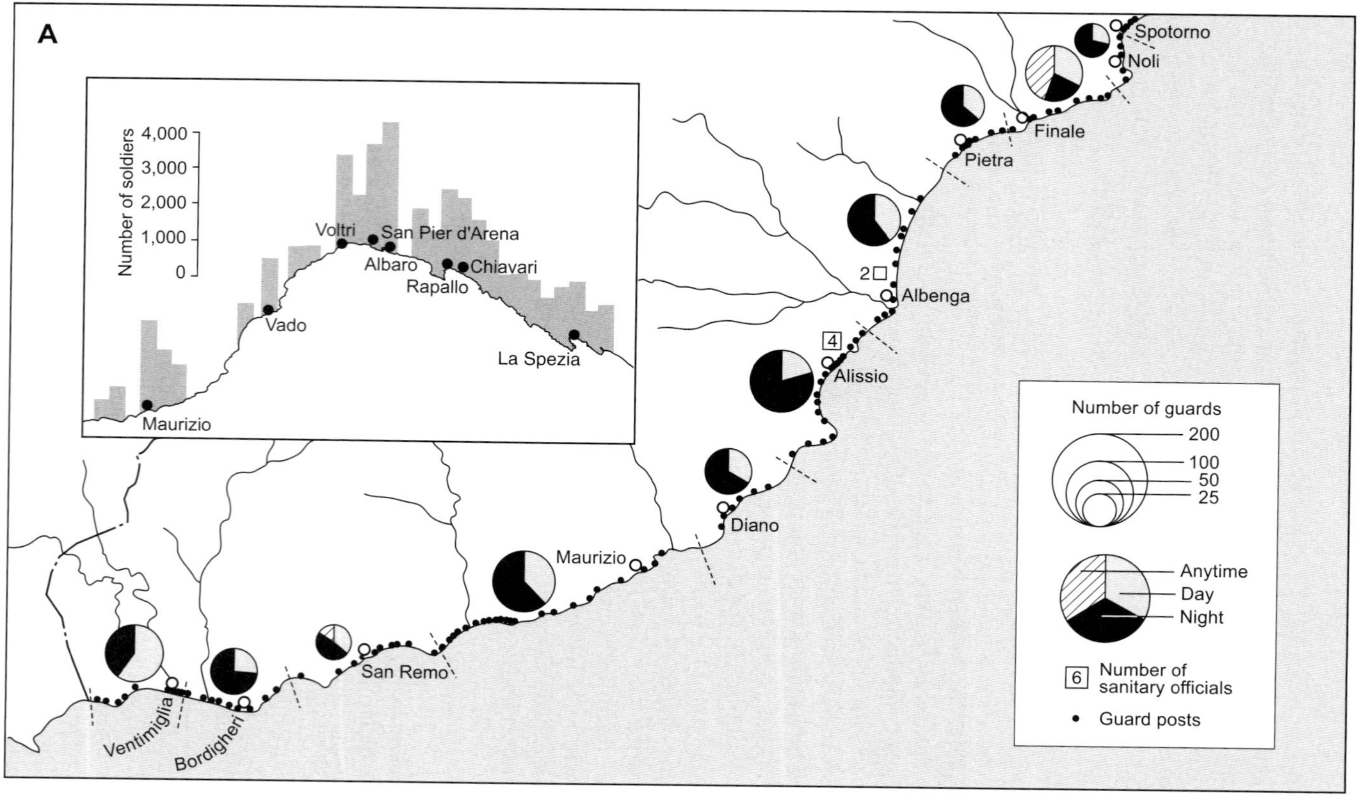

Fig. 11.8. Ring quarantine in Liguria

Compiled from information in Matteo Vinzoni's 1758 atlas of the public health of the republic of Genoa, the map plots the locations of the sanitary guard posts which comprised Liguria's defensive quarantine ring against disease. Posts are classified as sentry boxes, observation towers, and forts, while proportional circles show the manning complement by day and night.

Source: App. 11.1 (13).

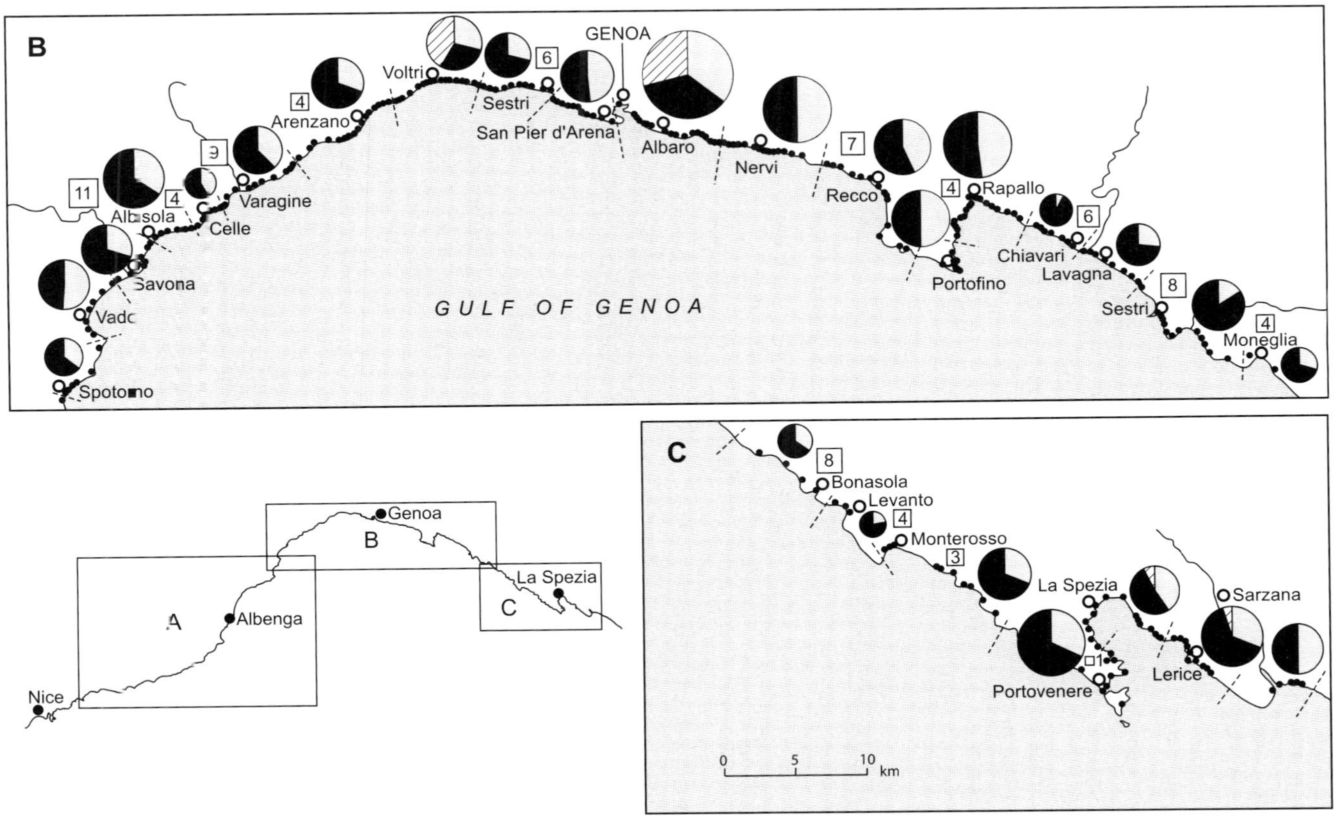

Fig. 11.8. (Continued)

intensive because inter-post communication and observation was restricted by darkness. Logs were kept at each post of the visitors passing through the post.

Plate 11.6 illustrates the map for the health district of San Pier d'Arena, which comprised the subdistricts of Cornigliano and Sampierdarena (*sic*). The plate shows that 10 smaller observation posts (*guardia*) were supported by a castle (*castello*) (site 9). Some of the accompanying text details the night patrols. The two for San Pier have been added to Plate 11.6. The guard posts of the two subdistricts were visited by three patrols nightly. Each patrol consisted of two men from the castle who had been collected by a patrol leader from each subdistrict. The first patrol ran between 01.00 and 05.00 hours, the second between 05.00 and 09.00 hours, and the third from 09.00 and 13.00 hours. At the conclusion of each patrol, the guard was returned to the castle by the patrol leader. This intensity was judged sufficient for the number of visitors to San Pier (90 per day).[1]

THE HOLY SEE (PAPAL STATES)

The geographical extent of the Papal States is illustrated in Figure 11.5. Two maps exist showing the defensive cordon sanitaire for the Papal States, one for the Mediterranean coast, and one for the Adriatic coast including the land border with the kingdom of Naples. We discuss each in turn.

Mediterranean Coast

This map plots and tabulates the military, sanitary, and customs posts along the 226 km Mediterranean coast of the Papal States from the border with the Grand Duchy of Tuscany to Graticciare on the border with the kingdom of Naples. The tabulation of the health observation posts which comprised the cordon is illustrated in Plate 11.7. Operationally, the coast was divided into four divisions, Civitavecchia (12 observation posts), Fiumicino (5 posts), Porto d'Anzio (7 posts), and Terracina (10 posts), at average spacing of 6.6 km. The table in Plate 11.7 is strongly geographical. The column

[1] 'Le distanze delle Ville, e luoghi da questi Posti di San Pier d'Arena, e Cornigliano sono notati in fine della presente diserizione. Tutti li detti Posti, e guardie avanzate, tanto di San Pier d'Arena, quanto di Cornigliano vengono visitati di notte da tre Ronde di due Uomini per ciascheduna, l'una sucessi-vaménte all' altra, cio e quei di San Pier d'Arena dalle tre Ronde loro destinate, e quei di Cornigliano da alter tre a cio destinate. Le dette Ronde tanto di San Pier d'Arena, che di Cornigliano anno obligo di girare di prima, cio e da un ora sino alle cinque, la seconda dalle cinque sino alle novo, la terza dalle nove sino alle tredici. Le dette Ronde sono composte, cio e quelle di San Pier d'Arena d'un Uomo di San Pier d'Arena, che all 'ora destinatale si fa dare una guardia dal Posto del Castello, e con essa di compagnia fa sua visita rimandando la guardia al suo Posto terminata la Visita, e cose succedendo altro per la seconDa, ed altro per la terza, pigliando anch' essi una guardia al detto Posto. Quelle di Cornigliano d'un Uomo di Cornigliano, che all 'ora destinatale piglia una guardia al posto di mezzo di Cornigliano, e fa il suo giro, rimanendo la guardia al suo Posto terminato detto giro, il simile il Visitator di seconda, e quello di terza, pigliando anch' essi a suo tempo una guardia al detto Posto. Li Visitatori di San Pier d'Arena sono in n° di 90, e a' tre per note supliscono per giorni n° 30, e cosi anno di respiro un mese a' ricomin ciare il loro giro' (App. 11.1 (13), p. 12).

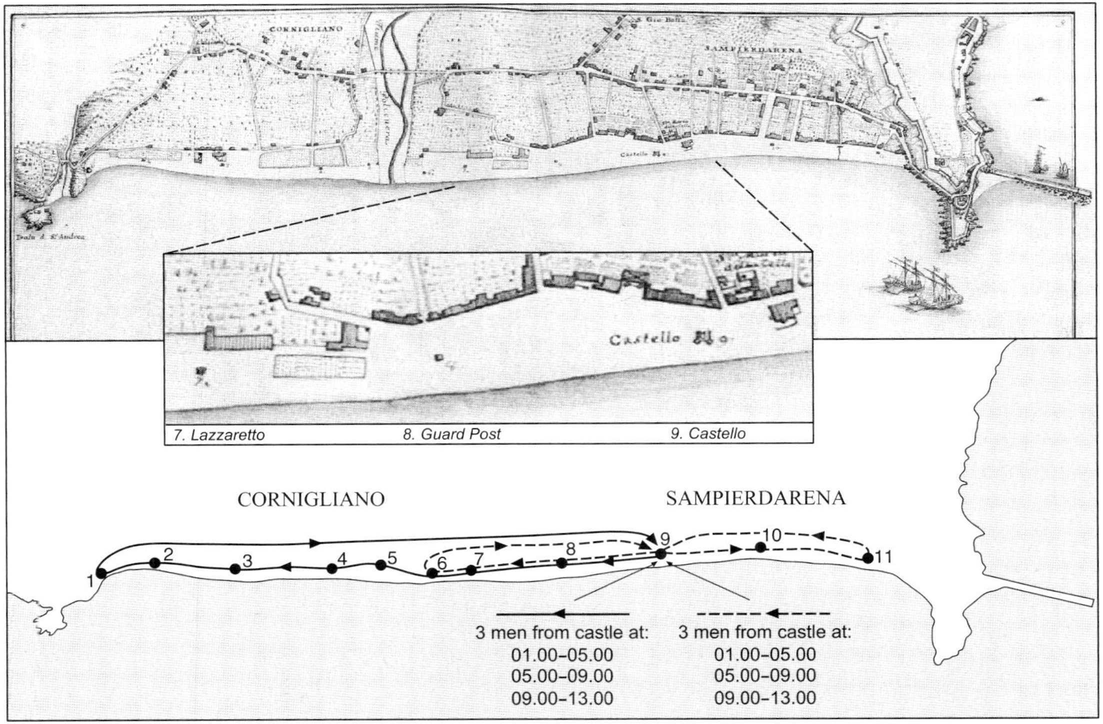

Pl. 11.6. Sanitary guard posts of Genoa

Extract from the map of the health district of San Pier d'Arena from Vinzoni's sanitary atlas of Genoa (1758) showing the guard posts (*guardia*) along the coast, along with the routes followed by the night patrols (added). The enlargement shows that Vinzoni numbered the posts serially on his maps, and this was linked to an account of the manning and nature of each guard post in his Atlas. See text for examples.

Source: App. 11.1 (13: 8–9).

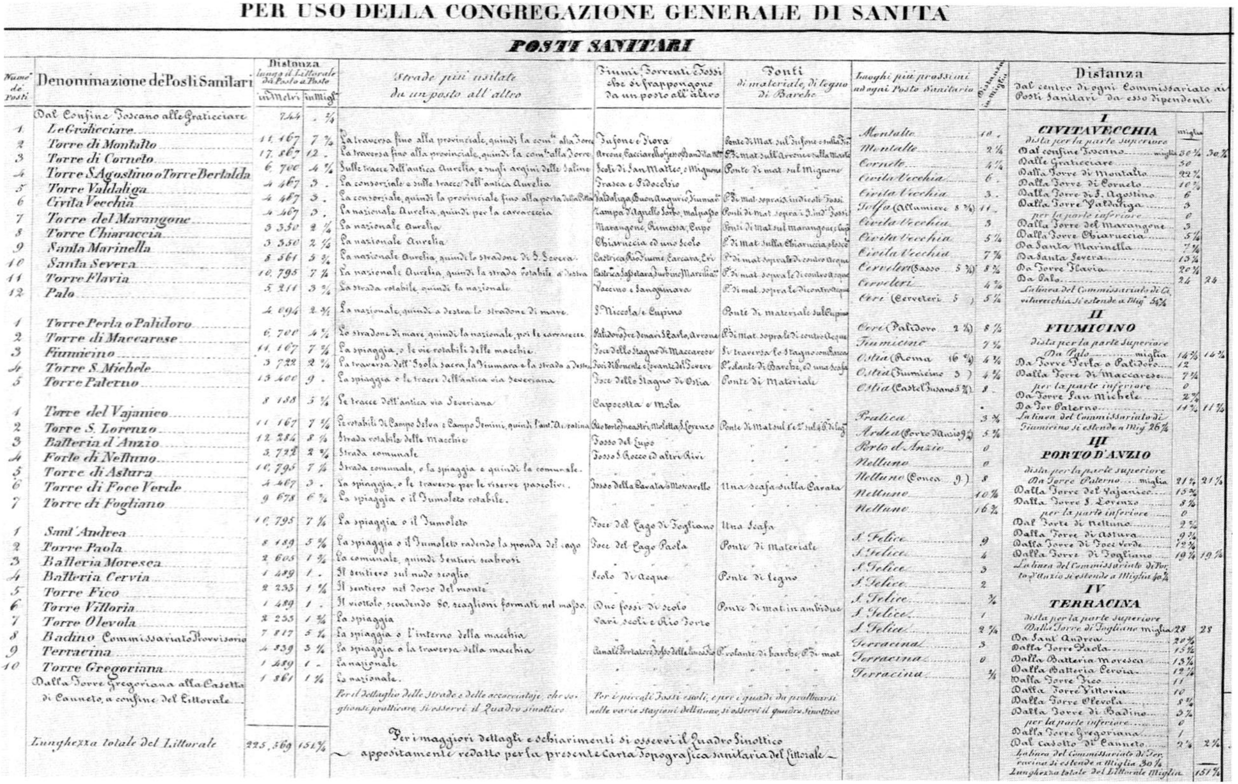

PER USO DELLA CONGREGAZIONE GENERALE DI SANITÀ

POSTI SANITARI

Num.ro de' Posti	Denominazione de' Posti Sanitari	Distanza lungo il Littorale da Posto a Posto in Metri	in Miglia	Strade più usitate da un posto all'altro	Fiumi, Torrenti, Fossi che si frappongono da un posto all'altro	Ponti di materiale, di legno di Barche	Luoghi più prossimi ad ogni Posto Sanitario	Distanza in miglia
	Dal Confine Toscano alle Graticciare	744	. ¾					
1	Le Graticciare						Montalto	10 .
2	Torre di Montalto	11.167	7 ½	La traversa fino alla provinciale, quindi la com.le alla Torre	Tufone e Fiora	Ponte di Mat. sul Tufone e sulla Fiora	Montalto	2 ¼
3	Torre di Corneto	17.867	12 .	La traversa fino alla provinciale, quindi la com.le alla Torre	Arrone, Cacciarello, e Banditaccia	P. di mat. sull'Arrone e sulla Marta	Corneto	4 ¼
4	Torre S. Agostino o Torre Bertalda	6.700	4 ½	Sulle tracce dell'antica Aurelia, e sugli argini delle Saline	Scoli di San Matteo, e Mignone	Ponte di mat. sul Mignone	Civita Vecchia	6 .
5	Torre Valdaliga	4.467	3 .	La consorziale e sulle tracce dell'antica Aurelia	Frasca e Pidocchio		Civita Vecchia	3 .
6	Civita Vecchia	4.467	3 .	La consorziale, quindi la provinciale fino alla porta della Città	Valdaliga, Buon Augurio, Fiumaretta	P. di mat. sopra gl'indicati Fossi	Tolfa (Allumiere 8 ¾)	11 .
7	Torre del Marangone	4.467	3 .	La nazionale Aurelia, quindi per la carrareccia	Zampa d'Agnello, Sorbo, malpasso	Ponti di mat. sopra i 3 ind.i Fossi	Civita Vecchia	3
8	Torre Chiaruccia	3.350	2 ¼	La nazionale Aurelia	Marangone, Rimessa, Cupo	Ponti di mat. sul Marangone e Cupo	Civita Vecchia	5 ¼
9	Santa Marinella	3.350	2 ½	La nazionale Aurelia	Chiaruccia ed uno scolo	P. di mat. sulla Chiaruccia e scolo	Civita Vecchia	7 ¾
10	Santa Severa	8.561	5 ¾	La nazionale Aurelia, quindi lo stradone di S. Severa	Castrica, Rio Fiume, Carcara, Eri	P. di mat. sopra le di contro Acque	Cerveteri (Sasso 5 ¾)	8 ¾
11	Torre Flavia	10.795	7 ¼	La nazionale Aurelia, quindi la strada rotabile a destra	Castrica, Sasso, Sanguinara	P. di mat. sopra le di contro Acque	Cerveteri	4 ¾
12	Palo	5.211	3 ¾	La strada rotabile, quindi la nazionale	Vaccino e Sanguinara	P. di mat. sopra le di contro Acque	Ceri (Cerveteri 5)	5 ¼
		4.094	2 ¾	La nazionale, quindi a destra lo stradone di mare.	S. Niccola e Cupino	Ponte di materiale sul Cupino		
1	Torre Perla o Palidoro						Ceri (Palidoro 2 ¼)	8 ½
2	Torre di Maccarese	6.700	4 ½	Lo stradone di mare, quindi la nazionale, poi le carrarecce.	Palidoro, tre denari, S. Carlo, Arrone	P. di mat. sopra le di contro Acque	Fiumicino	7 ¾
3	Fiumicino	11.167	7 ½	La spiaggia, o le vie rotabili delle macchie.	Foce dello Stagno di Maccarese	Si traversa lo Stagno con Barca	Ostia (Roma 16 ¼)	4 ¾
4	Torre S. Michele	3.722	2 ½	La traversa dell'Isola sacra, la Fiumara e la strada a destra	Foci di Ponente e Levante del Tevere	P. volante di Barche, ed una Scafa	Ostia (Fiumicino 3)	4 ¾
5	Torre Paterno	13.400	9 .	La spiaggia e le tracce dell'antica via Severiana	Foce dello Stagno di Ostia	Ponte di Materiale	Ostia (Castel Fusano 5 ¾)	8 .
		8.138	5 ½	Le tracce dell'antica via Severiana	Capocotta e Mola			.
1	Torre del Vajanico						Pratica	3 ¾
2	Torre S. Lorenzo	11.167	7 ½	Le rotabili di Campo Selva e Campo Jemini, quindi l'ant. di rotina	Rio torto, Incastri, Moletta, S. Lorenzo	Ponte di Mat. sul 1.e 2.e sul 4.e di leg.	Ardea (Porto d'Anzio 9 ½)	5 ¾
3	Batteria d'Anzio	12.284	8 ½	Strada rotabile delle Macchie	Fosso del Lupo	. .	Porto d'Anzio	0
4	Forte di Nettuno	3.722	2 ½	Strada comunale	Fosso S. Rocco ed altri Rivi	. .	Nettuno	0
5	Torre di Astura	10.795	7 ¼	Strada comunale, o la spiaggia e quindi la comunale.	.	. .	Nettuno (Conca 9)	8
6	Torre di Foce Verde	4.467	3 .	La spiaggia, o le traverse per le riserve pascolive.	Fosso della Carata o Moscarello	Una scafa sulla Carata	Nettuno	10 ¾
7	Torre di Fogliano	9.678	6 ½	La spiaggia e il Tumoleto rotabile.	.	. .	Nettuno	16 ¾
		10.795	7 ¼	La spiaggia o il Tumoleto	Foce del Lago di Fogliano	Una Scafa		
1	Sant'Andrea						S. Felice	9
2	Torre Paola	8.189	5 ½	La spiaggia o il Tumoleto radendo la sponda del Lago	Foce del Lago Paola	Ponte di Materiale	S. Felice	4
3	Batteria Moresca	2.605	1 ¾	La comunale, quindi Sentieri scabrosi	.	. .	S. Felice	3
4	Batteria Cervia	1.489	1 .	Il sentiero sul nudo scoglio	Scolo di Acque	Ponte di legno	S. Felice	2
5	Torre Fico	2.233	1 ½	Il sentiero nel dorso del monte	.	. .	S. Felice	¾
6	Torre Vittoria	1.489	1 .	Il viottolo, scendendo 80. scaglioni formati nel masso.	Due fossi di scolo	Ponte di mat. in ambidue	S. Felice	1
7	Torre Olevola	2.233	1 ½	La spiaggia	Vari scoli e Rio Torto	. .	S. Felice	2 ¾
8	Badino Commissariato Provvisorio	7.817	5 ¼	La spiaggia o l'interno della macchia	.	. .	Terracina	3
9	Terracina	4.839	3 ¼	La spiaggia o la traversa della macchia	Canale Portatore, Fosso della Linea, Pio	P. volante di barche, P. di mat.	Terracina	0
10	Torre Gregoriana	1.489	1 .	La nazionale	.	. .	Terracina	¾
	Dalla Torre Gregoriana alla Casetta di Canneto, a confine del Littorale	1.861	1 ¼	La nazionale.	.	. .		
				Per il dettaglio delle Strade e delle accorciatoje, che soglionsi praticare, si osservi il Quadro sinottico	Per i piccoli Fossi e scoli, e per i guadi da praticarsi nelle varie stagioni dell'anno, si osservi il Quadro sinottico			
	Lunghezza totale del Littorale	225.369	151 ¾	Per i maggiori dettagli e schiarimenti si osservi il Quadro Sinottico appositamente redatto per la presente Carta Topografica sanitaria del Littorale				

Distanza dal centro di ogni Commissariato ai Posti Sanitari da esso dipendenti	miglia	
I CIVITAVECCHIA		
dista per la parte superiore		
Dal confine Toscano ... miglia	30 ¾	30 ¾
Dalle Graticciare	30	
Dalla Torre di Montalto	22 ¾	
Dalla Torre di Corneto	10 ¾	
Dalla Torre di S. Agostino	6	
Dalla Torre Valdaliga	3	
per la parte inferiore	0	
Dalla Torre del Marangone	3	
Dalla Torre Chiaruccia	5 ¼	
Da Santa Marinella	7 ¾	
Da Santa Severa	13 ½	
Da Torre Flavia	20 ¾	
Da Palo	24	24
La linea del Commissariato di Civitavecchia si estende a Mig.a 54 ¾		
II FIUMICINO		
dista per la parte superiore		
Da Palo ... miglia	14 ¾	14 ¾
Da Torre Perla o Palidoro	12	
Dalla Torre di Maccarese	7 ¼	
per la parte inferiore	0	
Da Torre San Michele	2 ¾	
Da Tor Paterno	11 ½	11 ½
La linea del Commissariato di Fiumicino si estende a Mig.a 26 ¼		
III PORTO D'ANZIO		
dista per la parte superiore		
Da Torre Paterno ... miglia	21 ½	21 ½
Dalla Torre del Vajanico	15 ¾	
Dalla Torre S. Lorenzo	8 ½	
per la parte inferiore	0	
Dal Forte di Nettuno	2 ½	
Dalla Torre di Astura	9 ¾	
Dalla Torre di Foce Verde	12 ¾	
Dalla Torre di Fogliano	19 ¼	19 ¼
La linea del Commissariato di Porto d'Anzio si estende a Miglia 40 ¾		
IV TERRACINA		
dista per la parte superiore		
Dalla Torre di Fogliano miglia	28	28
Da Sant'Andrea	20 ¾	
Dalla Torre Paola	15 ½	
Dalla Batteria Moresca	13 ¾	
Dalla Batteria Cervia	12 ¾	
Dalla Torre Fico	11	
Dalla Torre Vittoria	10	
Dalla Torre Olevola	8 ½	
Dalla Torre di Badino	3 ½	
per la parte inferiore	0	
Dalla Torre Gregoriana	1	
Dal casotto di Canneto	2 ¼	2 ¼
La linea del Commissariato di Terracina si estende a Miglia 30 ¼		
Lunghezza totale del Littorale Miglia		151 ¾

Pl. 11.7. Mediterranean coast of the Papal States, 1843: tabulation of the sanitary observation posts giving distances between neighbouring posts, adjacent towns, and obstacles on the route between posts

Source: App. 11.1 (14).

headings give (from left to right): the superintending district within which the observation post lay; post number; post name; distance from post to post along the coast in metres and miles; rivers, streams, and ditches (gullies) between one post and the next; bridges (masonry, wood, boat); name of nearest town and distance in miles to each sanitary post; and the distance from the centre of each district to the sanitary posts within it.

The table emphasizes the geographical proximity of each sanitary observation post to its neighbours and the nearest town, and the water obstacles on the route between posts. It is about accessibility and communication to preserve the integrity of the cordon. The associated text with the map details the quality of the road and the terrain between observation posts.

Adriatic Coast, Ravenna to Ascoli

The map of this 80 km section of coast was divided into four geographical divisions, each under the command of an army captain and his adjutant. The extract in Plate 11.8 shows the First Division from Ancona to Ascoli, and the Fourth Division (the land border with the kingdom of Naples). Figure 11.9 identifies the key elements on the whole map. The divisions were divided into sections (for example, 10 in the case of the First Division). Within each section, observation or lookout posts were established at regular intervals, approximately 0.33 km apart. Nearly all sections had their own sanitary officer (marked with an asterisk). There was a reporting hierarchy; section lookout posts reported to a central lookout post occupied by the commander of the section and the sanitary superintendent. In their turn, the central lookout posts returned their data to divisional reporting lookout posts (hexagons in Figure 11.9) which were responsible for transmitting the information to the commander-in-chief of the cordon sanitaire (Captain Giuseppe Vaselli), whose seal appears in the lower right corner of Plate 11.8.

As Plate 11.8 shows, the map plots the location of each lookout post; these are serially numbered 1, 2, . . . , *n* within each division. Also given is the military complement of each post (italic script on the seaward side of each bar). In addition to the infantry, flying corps (cavalry; cf. Plate 11.4 for Venice) were based in Ascoli to support the lookout posts in maintaining the cordon along the land border with the kingdom of Naples. In terms of Figure 11.2B, the flying corps operated an offensive containment policy. The map includes a summary table of the manning of the cordon—for the four divisions, nearly 1,900 men; see Table 11.1. Armed sailing boats (*trabaccoli*) cruised the Adriatic and completed the protection ring (one appears in Plate 11.8). The area around Ravenna (Section 5 of the Third Division) must have been especially vulnerable, adjacent as it was to the great trading city of Venice, and with many inland rivers. Here the quarantine defences were reinforced by squadrons of 4–6 small sailing boats (*baragozzi*). Plate 11.9 is a detail from the map showing squadrons 1–3, each of which comprised six *baragozzi*.

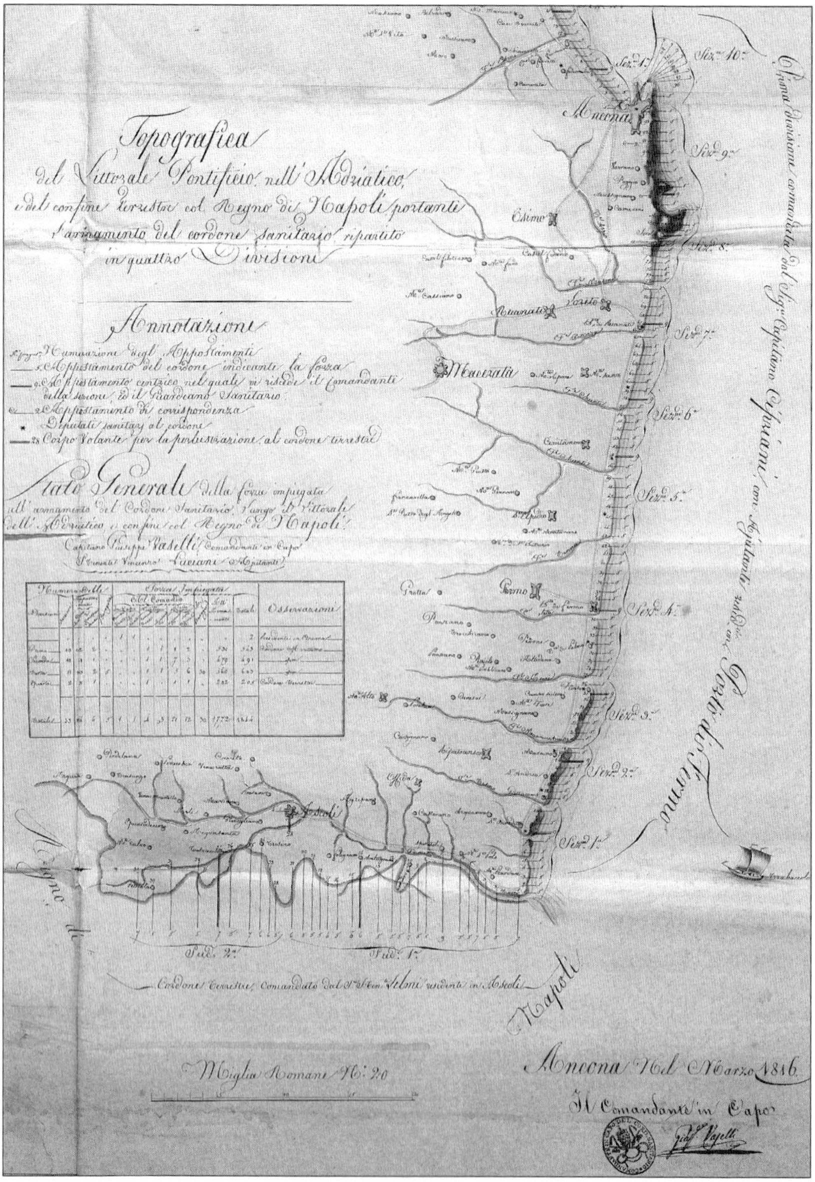

Pl. 11.8. Divisions 1 and 4 of the cordon sanitaire of the Adriatic coast of the Papal States, 1816
See text for a description of the map elements.
Source: App. 11.1 (15).

Table 11.1. Cordon sanitaire for the Adriatic coast of the Papal States, 1816: troop deployments and organization

					Forces being used									
					At the command post									
		Observation posts			Headquarters		In the divisions		In the sections					
Number of Division	Sections	In cordon	Reporting	*Baragozzi*	Commander	Adjutant	Commander	Adjutant	Officers	NCOs	*Baragozzi*	Men in arms	Total	Observations
					1	1							2	Resident in Ancona
First	10	112	2				1	1	8	2		531	543	Marine cordon
Second	10	18	1				1	1	7	3		479	491	Marine cordon
Third	11	103	2	5			1	1	5	6	30	560	603	Marine cordon
Fourth	2	31	1				1		1	1		202	205	Land cordon
TOTAL	33	264	6	5	1	1	4	3	21	12	30	1,772	1,844	

Source: App. 11.1 (15).

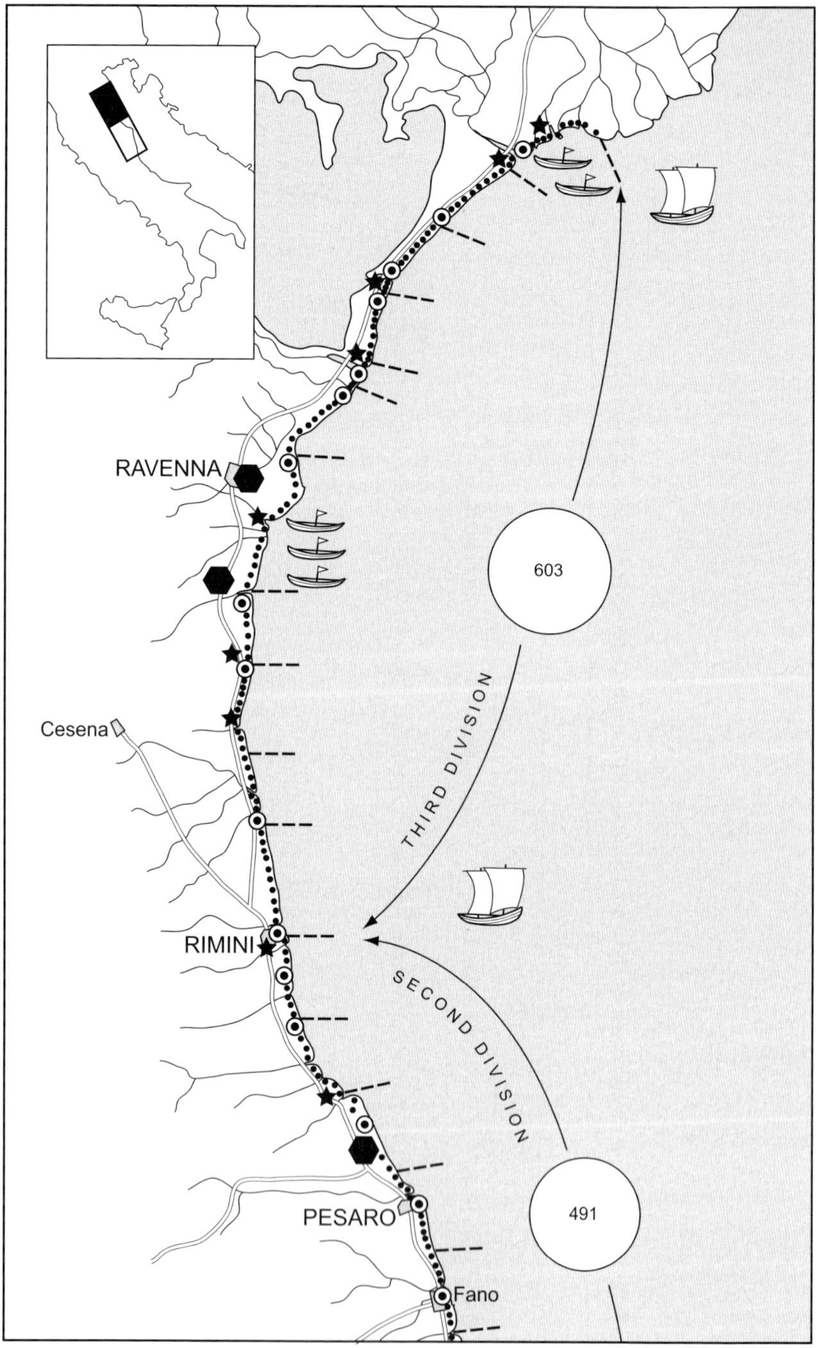

Fig. 11.9. Defensive isolation for the Adriatic coast of the Papal States, 1816
Compiled from Vaselli's map, the diagrams show the organization of the quarantine ring along this section of coast into four divisions with an upwards observation and reporting structure. The observation posts were supported on the seawards side by patrolling armed boats (*trabaccoli* and *baragozzi*), and on the landwards side by a rapid-response force of cavalry based in Ascoli.

Source: App. 11.1 (15).

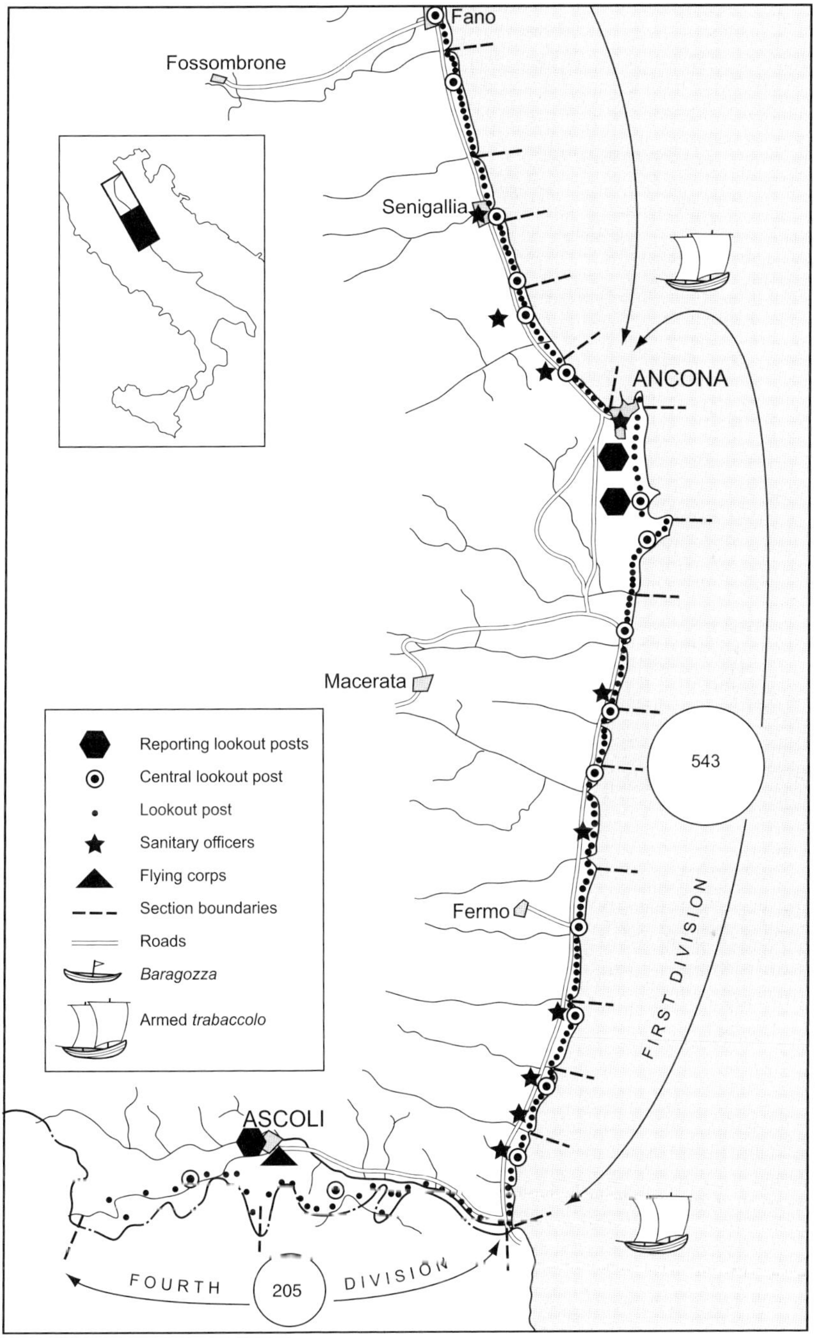

Fig. 11.9. (Continued)

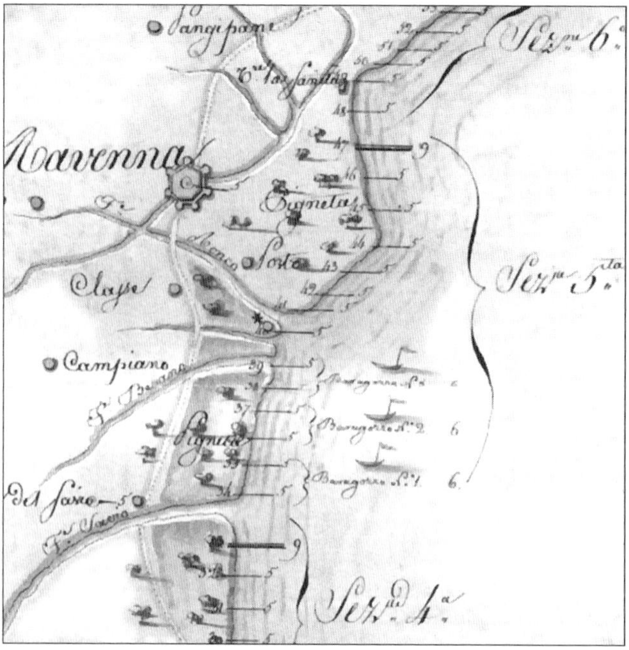

Pl. 11.9. Section 5 of Division 3 of the cordon sanitaire of the Adriatic coast of the Papal States, 1816
Detail showing three squadrons of armed *baragozzi* (small sailing boats) which patrolled the area.
Source: App. 11.1 (15).

Thus, consistent with the system around Venice, the quarantine ring was three layers deep; an outer ring of armed boats in the Adriatic, a middle ring of coastal observation posts manned by infantry, and an inner ring of what in modern terms would be called a rapid response force of cavalry providing additional offensive cover—here at the land frontier with the kingdom of Naples.

KINGDOM OF THE TWO SICILIES (NAPLES)

The regular attacks by Turks and Barbary Coast and Corsican pirates from the Middle Ages onwards upon the coastline of the provinces which ultimately comprised the kingdom of the Two Sicilies meant that the kingdom had an extensive system of coastal defensive towers which could be used and extended to provide a maritime cordon sanitaire in time of plague. The defensive system reached its final specification in the *Regolamento generale di servizio sanitario marittimo, sanzionato da S.M. il 1 gennajo 1820, in esecuzione dell'articolo 20 legge de' 20 ottobre 1819* (Petitti 1852). *Inter alia*, paragraphs 219–35 of the general service regulations specify the geographical structure of the cordon, its manning, operation, and reporting system. Table 11.2 lists the critical elements, while Figure 11.10 converts these into a schematic diagram; A shows the implied arrangement of guard posts along the coast and B illustrates the hierarchical reporting system. Many of the features of A and B—for example, the siting of posts within viewing distance of each other, the complement of three soldiers per post, and the reporting structure—have been noted earlier as the practice for the coastlines of the republic of Genoa and the Papal States.

A handful of maps of parts of the cordon sanitaire for the kingdom have survived in the State Archives of Naples and Palermo which show the realization of the 1819–20 legislation on the ground at the time of the Plague of Messina, 1743, and it is to these that we now turn.

Sicily, 1743: The Plague of Messina (North-East Sicily)

The Plague of Messina was the last major outbreak of plague in Europe. Messina had been free from plague since 1624, and the Sicilians prided themselves on the rigour of their quarantine laws, which they thought had preserved them. In May 1743 a Genoese vessel arrived in Messina from Morea (near Patras in the Little Dardanelles), on board which had occurred some suspicious deaths (plague was present in the Levant at this time). The ship and cargo were burnt, but, soon after, cases of a suspicious form of disease were observed in the hospital and in the poorest parts of the town. The Supremo Magistrato di Commercio preferred commercial expediency to rigorous enforcement of the sanitary laws and a major epidemic of plague developed, which killed an estimated 40,000–50,000 persons. It was this plague which led to the establishment of the island-wide permanent sanitary magistracy with jurisdiction over the pre-existing local health deputations which had existed for decades to control the importation of infectious diseases.

Once the epidemic began to rage in Messina, the sanitary magistrates of the republics and provinces across Italy activated their maritime cordons sanitaires and imposed suspensions upon contact with Messina. Plates 11.10A and B show the cordon sanitaire for the province of Lecce on the heel of Italy (see Figure 11.5 for location map) and adjacent to Messina. Consistent with the legislative framework summarized in Tables 11.2 and Figure 11.10, the plates show the division of the coastline into sections (pecked lines), with the regular and dense network of masonry towers (*torre*, housing the local sanitary official and section commander; large grey circles on Plate 11.10B) and guard huts (*barracca*, each housing three guards, or *uomini di guardia*; black lozenges on Plate 11.10B). An armed patrol boat (*felucca*) appears at D in the enlargement (Plate 11.10B and Article 235 in Table 11.2). The entablature gives the manning details for this cordon; 494 guard huts, 79 towers, 2,319 *uomini*, and 160 *cavallari* (horsemen) along

Table 11.2. Kingdom of the Two Sicilies: geographical structure of the cordon sanitaire specified in the general service regulations of 1820

Paragraph	Regulation	Cordon structure
Geographical features		
221	La distanza tra un posto e l'altro dev' esser tale, che l'uno sia sempre a vista dell' altro	Each guard post to be within sight of its neighbours
222	Quando in una provincia o valle vi sieno delle coste inaccessibili, per le quali vi ha bisogno di poca o niua custodia, l'Intendente deve impiegare questo risparmio di forze de cordone per assicurare le spiagge aperte, ed i siti più esposti a degli sbarchi furtive	Any economies in manpower from not having to patrol inaccessible coastal sections to be used to guard open beaches and places most available for clandestine landings
Integrity of the cordon		
229	Gli obblighi di tutti gl'individui destinati a formare il cordone, si riducono generalmente ad impedir nelle spiagge l'approdo di qualsivoglia legno, qualunque ne sia la provegnenza, obbligandolo a dirigersi ne'punti più vicini, ove risiede una deputazione de salute	All individuals in the cordon must act to prevent, through a general reduction of manpower, unauthorized beach landings by boat by funnelling those concerned towards the nearest points manned by sanitary officers
230	Ne' casi di burrasca, i legni amici o nemici possono, quando il naufragio è quasi sicuro, farsi approdare nelle spiagge, impiegando all' uopo tutte le cautele di custodia, ed un rigoroso cordone *parziale*, sino a che non accorrano i deputati di salute corrispondenti per applicarvi l'analogo trattamento sanitaria	Shipwrecks to be quarantined by a local cordon sanitaire until sanitary officers can attend
231	Se qualche posto fosse minacciato da gente, che volesse sbarcare a viva forza, ed alla quale non potesse resistere, il capo posto deve innalzare un bandiera di convenzione, ed a questo segnale deve accorrere subito la forza de' posti limitrofi. Avvenendo questo caso in tempo di notte, il segnale per aver soccorso sarà di due fuochi consecutive	Post heads must signal for support from neighbouring posts if a forced landing is threatened. Two consecutive fire signals used at night
232	In ogni posto devono farsi, durante la notte, de'fuochi convenuti di corrispondenza, a fin di assicurarsi della vigilanza de'posti limitrofi.	Fire signals to be agreed between adjacent posts for night communication
233	Nei tempi di cordone l'esercizio della pesca non è più libero. Le barche pescarecce possono uscire dal levare al tra montar del sole; ed in questo periodo è anche proibito loro di allontanarsi dal lido oltre le quattro miglia. I padroni di queste barche devono essere allora muniti di una *bolletta*, che i deputati di salute corrispondenti devono loro vistare giorno per giorno	A charge is made for fishing during times of cordon, collected daily by the sanitary inspectors from the boat captain. Fishing is permitted only during daylight hours and not more than 4 miles from the beach
235	I cordone sanitari marittimi possono anche stabilirsi per mezzo di altrettante crociere di barche armate, applicandosi a queste, sotto certe tali necessarie modificazioni, le norme di sopra indicate per la distribuzione, il servigio e la dipendenza de' posti situati a terra su i littorali	Armed boats (*felucca*) patrol the coastline

Manning		
223	In ogni posto devono montar di guardia tre individui ed un basse uffiziale, che farà le funzioni di capo posto. Quando le spiagge sieno aperte ed esposte in modo che non bastion a custodirle in quattro individui destinati per ciascun posto, può allora aumentarsene il numero a seconda del bisogno e delle circostanze	Normally three guards per post with a low-level official as head of post; four on open beaches difficult to guard, augmented if necessary to suit the conditions
224	La guardia dee recarsi al suo posto la mattina, ed esserne rilevata il domane alla stess'ora, durante il qual tempo è vietato agl'individui che la compongono, il potersi appatare dal posto sotto qualunque pretesto. Il capo-posto dee rimaner fisso per un'inera settimana, ad oggetto di conoscer bene le consegne e trasmetterle, e di conoscere i segnali e le pratische da osservarsi. Egli ha l'obbligo particolare d'invigilar sulla condotta de'suoi subaltern	Guards must be on station from daylight and relieved the following morning. The head guard has a one-week tour of duty; he has recording, reporting, and supervisory duties
225	Per ogni sei posti vi sarà un'Uffizial comandante, che dee rimaner distaccato per l'intera settimana, e tener presso di se una o più persone a cavallo per la sollecita diramazione degli ordini. La posizione da assegnarsi al suddetto Comandante sarà, per quanto è possible, la centrale. Egli avrà specialmente l'incarico d'invigilare all'adempimento dgli oblighi ingiunti a(i)l capi-posti	A sanitary official every six posts, centrally located, on a weekly tour of duty. The official is responsible for distributing orders rapidly using horsemen
226	Per ogni tre distaccamenti di sei posti l'uno, vi sarà un sottoispettore, che anche deve avere una situazione centrale. Il suo incarico è quello d'invigilare alla regolarità del servisio de'tre distaccameni che compongono la sua sotto-ispezione	Three detachments per six posts under the supervision of an under-inspector in a central position
Reporting system		
228	Tra tutt' i capi del cordone vi deve essere una corrispondenza giornaliera ed esatta, onde si rilevi il modo con cui si attende al servizio, e le novità che possono avervi luogo. Affinchè la corrispondenza suddetta proceda colla massima regolarità, e nel modo più celere, i capi-posti devono corrispondere coi rispettivi Comandanti di distaccamento, questi col sotto-ispettore, il sotto-ispettore col' Ispettore, l'Ispettore contemporaneamente coll' Intendente, e col Comandante militare della provincia o valle. Da siffatta regola sono eccettuati i casi di seria considerazione ne' quali, oltre del rapporto regolare da passarsi col cennato metodo, i Comandanti di distaccamento sono autorizzati di far rapporto straordinario, e spedirlo con espresso all' Intendente ed al Comandante della provincia o valle	Cordon commanding officers must communicate daily with each other. The normal upwards reporting system is from local guard post heads via intermediate officers to the provincial military commander and the sanitary superintendent (Figure 11.10B); the intermediate officers can be bypassed in an emergency

Source: Based on Petitti (1852: 318–55).

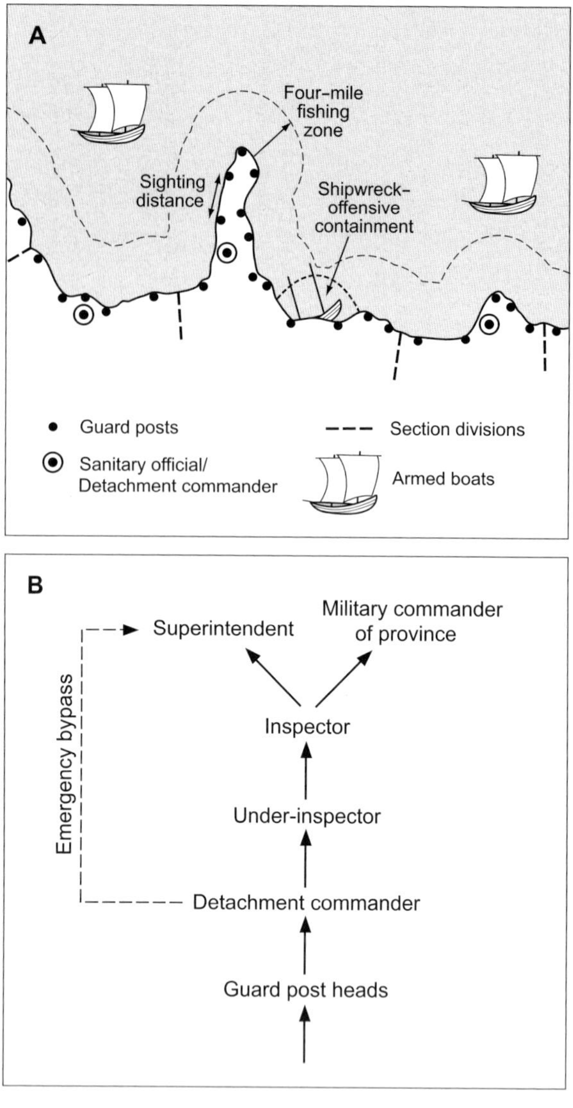

Fig. 11.10. Kingdom of the Two Sicilies: maritime cordon sanitaire
(A) Arrangement of guard posts along the coastline recommended in the general service regulations of 1819–20 (Table 11.2). (B) Reporting system for the cordon.

c.400 km of coast. During the epidemic, a Turkish ship was unfortunate enough to be shipwrecked off the port of Lecce. Following Article 230 of the General Regulations in Table 11.2, a local cordon was established around the wreck, and this is illustrated in Plate 11.11.

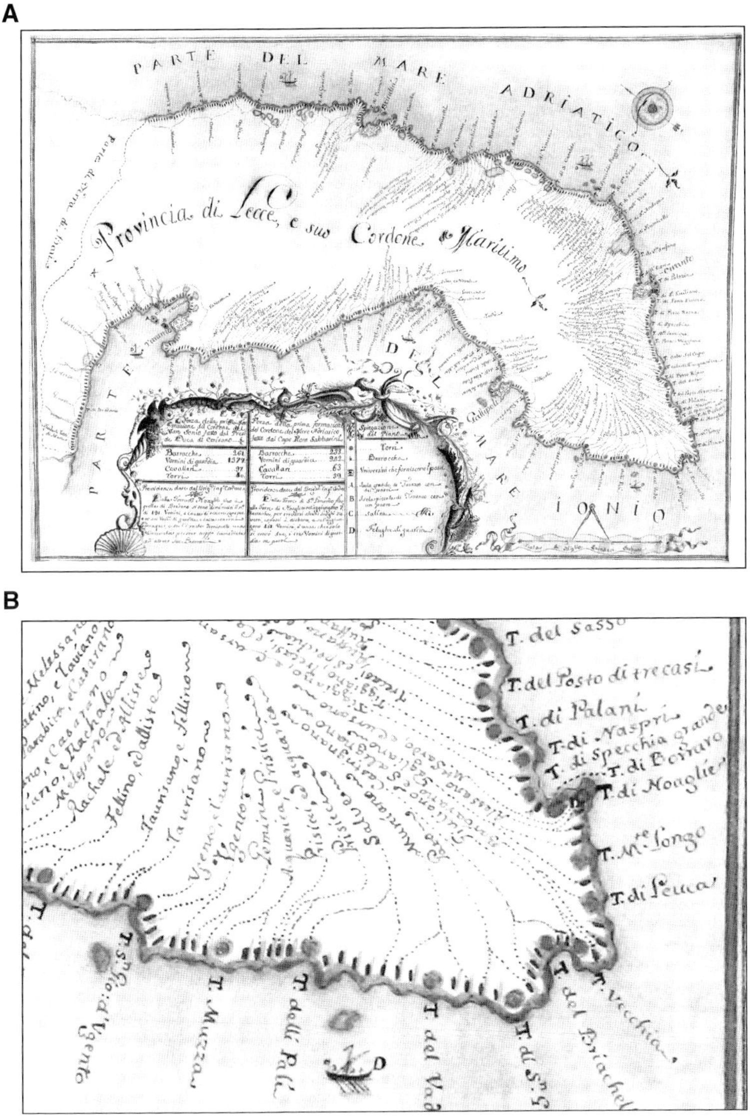

Pl. 11.10. Province of Lecce, 1743, cordon sanitaire
(A) Distribution of towers and guard huts comprising the cordon sanitaire. The entablature gives manning details. (B) Enlargement of the south-east tip showing the geographical congruence of the cordon with the legislative framework summarized in Table 11.2.
Source: App. 11.1 (18).

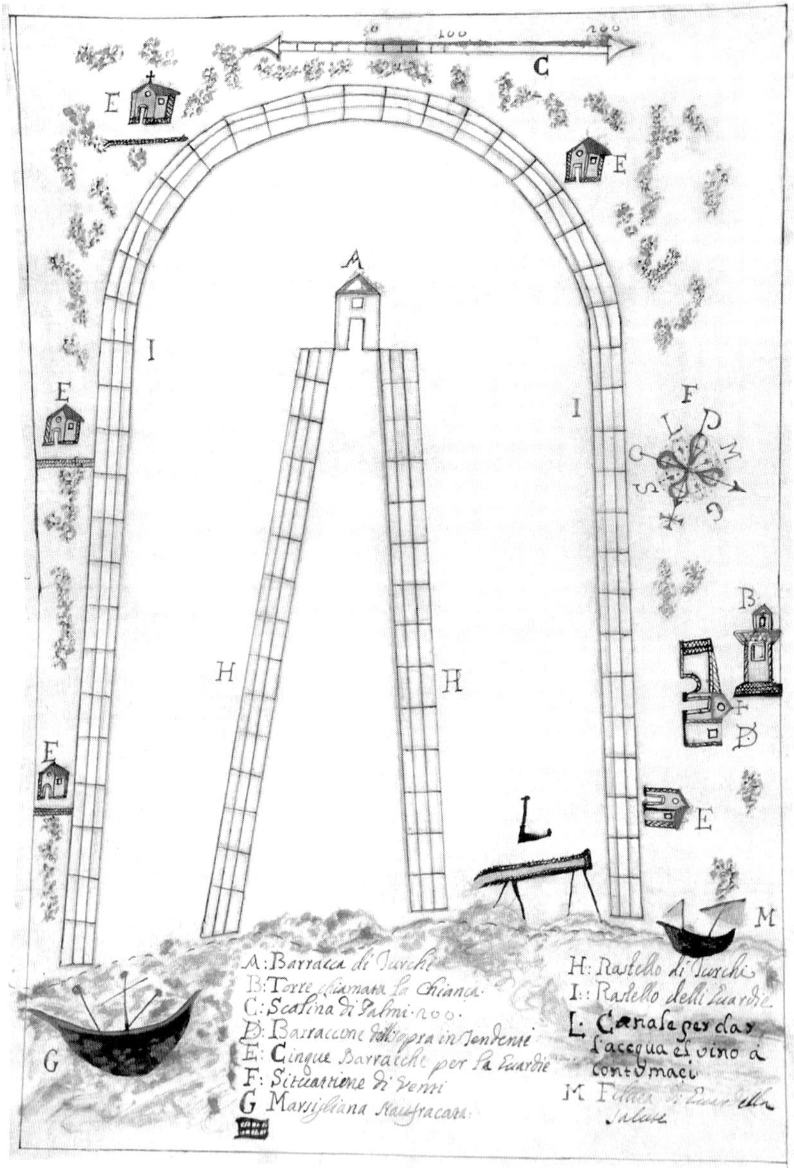

Pl. 11.11. Lecce, tower of Chianca, 1743: local cordon sanitaire
At the time of the Plague of Messina, a Turkish boat was unfortunate enough to be shipwrecked near the Tower of Chianca, Lecce harbour. The plate illustrates the local offensive containment cordon sanitaire erected around the wreck to prevent any risk of plague from being carried by the sailors into Lecce. It shows the hut for the Turks (A), Chianca tower (B), the five sanitary guard huts (E), the stockades used to separate the Turkish compound from the guards (H, I), an armed patrol boat (*felucca*, G), and the *felucca* with the public health officers on board (M).

Source: App. 11.1 (19).

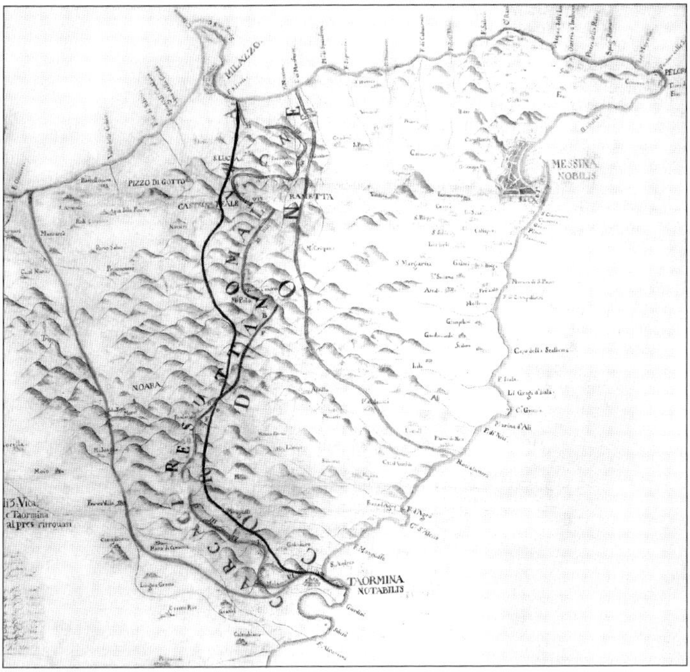

Pl. 11.12. Plague of Messina, 1743: offensive containment
Location of three internal cordon sanitaire lines running north–south used to isolate Messina from the rest of Sicily.
Source: App. 11.1 (20).

To prevent spread within Sicily, three internal cordon lines were established in August 1743 by the health officials in Palermo, stretching across the neck of land from Milazzo on the north coast to Taormina on the south (Plate 11.12). From east to west, the cordon lines were: (east) 26 miles (42 km) long, number of posts and men unrecorded; 23 miles (37 km), 152 posts, 700 men; 21 miles (34 km), 130 posts, 633 men (west). This offensive containment appears to have worked, for there is no surviving evidence that plague spread to other parts of the island. An external cordon was also maintained around Sicily during the epidemic, and this may account in part for the lack of spread beyond Messina.

Bari

Although we have focused upon the Plague of Messina in describing the cordon arrangements for the kingdom of the Two Sicilies, the system was in operation in earlier centuries. For example, the offensive containment of Bari is depicted cartographically in a monograph published at Naples in 1694 by Filippo de Arrieta, a professional administrator who served as Royal

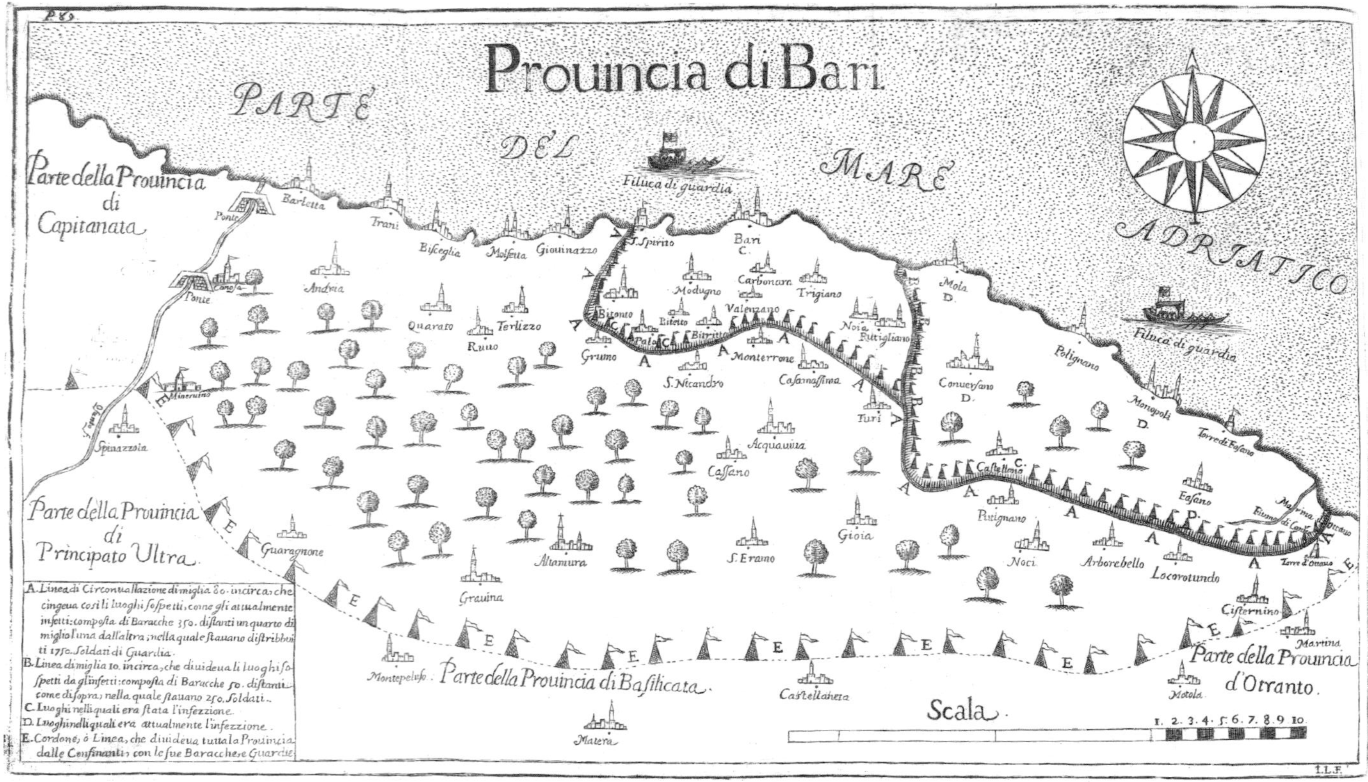

Pl. 11.13. Offensive containment for Bari, 1690–1692
See text for map description.

Auditor of the province of Bari in the domain of the kingdom of Naples. The English title is *Historical Report on the Contagion that Occurred in the Province of Bari in the Years 1690, 1691 and 1692*. As described in Jarcho (1981), de Arrieta's engraved map (Plate 11.13) shows about 170 km of the Adriatic coastline, almost from Manfredonia to Brindisi, and the terrain extending inward for a maximum of 50 km. Bari is shown as having been isolated from its neighbours by a cordon, depicted as a dashed line, along which are shown tents, each surmounted by a triangular pennant (cf. Plate 11.3 for Venice). Of the segregated terrain a small part along the Adriatic is marked off by a smaller and thicker border, which describes a circumvallation 125 km long. The thicker line was composed of 350 huts joined by a wall of living rock 4 to 5 palms high. The huts were an eighth of a league apart. Within the district cordoned off by heavy palisaded circumvallation are places marked by the letter D to indicate existing infection and places marked with a C to designate former infection. The segregation was completed on the Adriatic side by a row of guard boats, two of which are shown. Each has a cabin at its stern and a crew of seven or eight men.

11.2.2 Island Quarantine

We saw in Section 11.2.1 how Venice used island isolation for quarantine as one feature of its defensive disease protection policy. Initially it was the natural isolation of islands that was exploited to afford protection. By the late nineteenth century, the use of natural and man-made islands for quarantine had become widespread, particularly as filter points to prevent disease importation into (relatively) disease-free areas. Examples include the islands used by Fiji as an entry point for immigrant labour at the cusp of the twentieth century,[2] and the 'Marseilles Sieve' utilized in World War I as a gathering zone for troops on their way to the Western Front (Cliff, Haggett, and Smallman-Raynor 1993: 139, 148). But the greatest of all was Ellis Island, first employed by the US Marine Hospital Service in 1892 as part of an early-warning system against disease importation into the United States.

Ellis Island, located off New York City (Plate 11.14), operated for 62 years from 1892 to 1954. Over this period, more than 12 million immigrants—as many as 5,000 a day, with a record of nearly 13,000—underwent immigration processing at Ellis Island (Figure 11.11). This total represents more than 66 per cent of immigrants who came to America, and it is estimated that today

[2] During the period of indentured labour in the Fiji sugar cane plantations following the disastrous measles epidemic of 1875, quarantining of Indian passengers on immigrant boats became routine and persisted until the end of the period of indentured labour in 1916 (Section 6.3.1). The first quarantine station was established on Yamuca Levu island between Ovalau and Moturiki islands and was used by the first immigrants from the *Leonidas*. With the shift of the Fijian capital to Suva, the quarantine station was moved to the island of Nukulau on the reef about 10 km east of Suva harbour. Immigrants were usually detained for a 14-day period before being delivered to the plantation areas.

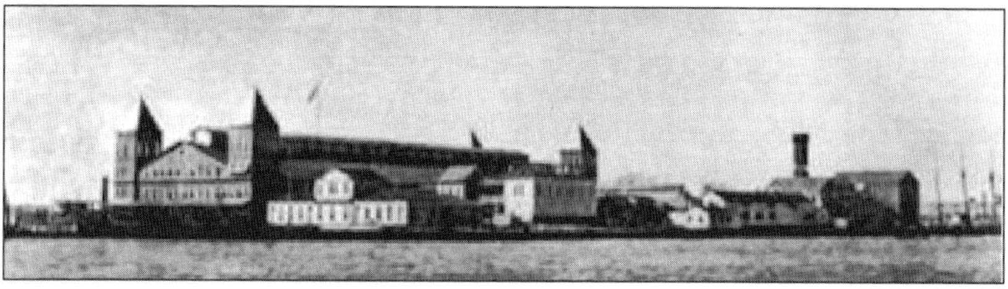

Pl. 11.14. Ellis Island Quarantine Station, New York City
The original Georgia-pine main building at Ellis Island, opened 1 Jan. 1892, destroyed by fire in 1897, and then rebuilt.
Sources: US National Park Service, Statue of Liberty National Monument web site, repr. in Cliff, Haggett, and Smallman-Raynor (2000, pl. 5.6, p. 200).

more than 100 million Americans can trace their roots to an ancestor who came through Ellis Island. As described in Coan (1997, p. xiii), the Federal Immigration and Naturalization Service (INS), which operated the station, enforced a number of Acts to exclude mentally disabled persons, paupers, and those who might become public charges. The INS also excluded those suffering from 'a loathsome or contagious disease', or convicted of various crimes. Over the life of the station, 82,199 potential immigrants were rejected as mental or physical defectives. Screening for disease was carried out by Ellis Island doctors in a set of 15 medical buildings (Plate 11.15) until 1932, when this task was transferred to American consulates in originating countries. Thereafter, the role of Ellis Island declined until final closure in 1954.

11.2.3 Estimating the Impact of Quarantine

Quarantine of the sort practised in Italy was a blunt instrument in that it attempted to limit the travel of people between communities (and often of goods as well) irrespective of their disease status. For humans, most quarantine efforts until the early years of the twentieth century focused upon controlling infection arising from maritime trade; Kilwein (1995*a*,*b*), Mafart and Perret (1998), Sattenspiel and Herring (2003), and Gensini *et al.* (2004) provide reviews of the literature. The general experience with quarantine and defensive isolation over this period was that it was more successful in reducing impact than in keeping areas disease-free—as in Italy with plague. But how successful was quarantine as an approach in the twentieth century as transport technology changed and the international flux of people multiplied exponentially year on year? And what are its prospects for the future? See, for example, Barbera *et al.* (2001). We consider these questions in this and the next subsection.

Quarantine can be enacted at two main spatial scales: (i) inter-community, to reduce interactions between communities, and (ii) within community, to inhibit mixing of disease carriers and susceptibles. We examine each in turn,

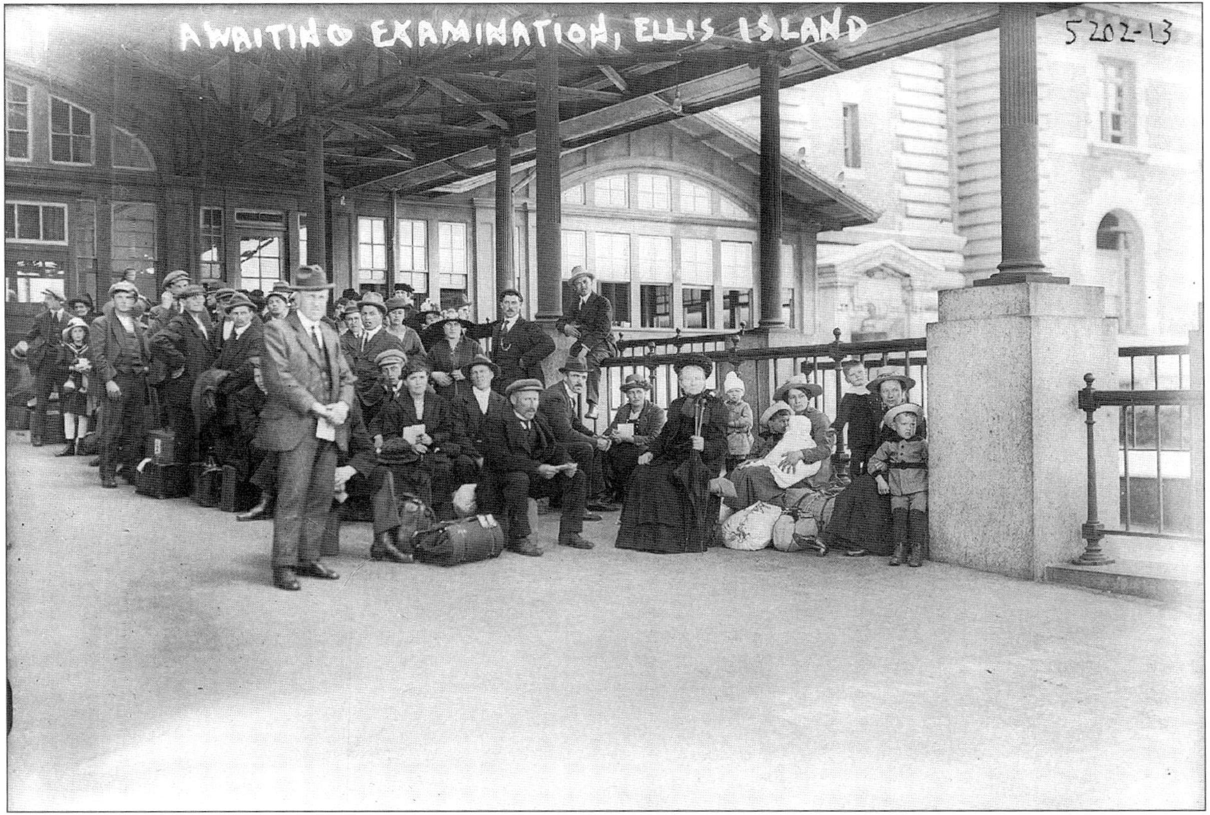

Pl. 11.15. Ellis Island—'Awaiting examination'

Source: US National Park Service, Statue of Liberty National Monument web site.

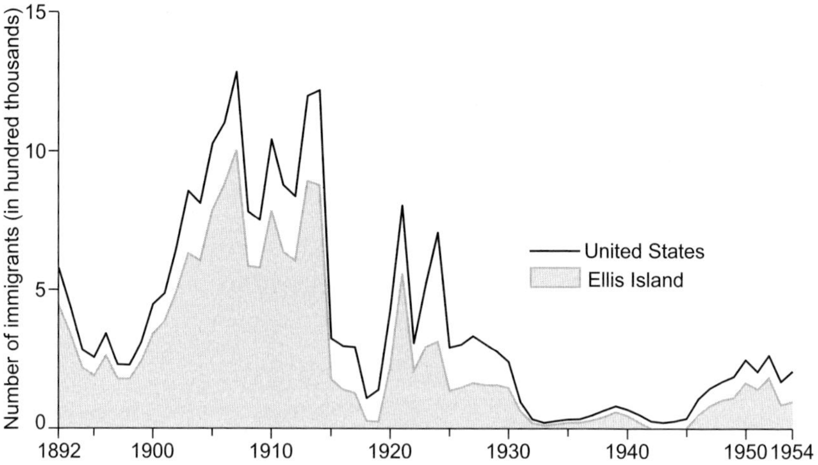

Fig. 11.11. Ellis Island immigration, 1892–1954
Number of immigrants passing through the Ellis Island station annually and the total number of arrivals in the US.
Source: Cliff, Haggett, and Smallman-Raynor (2000, fig. 5.10, p. 199).

using human influenza to give unity to the discussion. Australia and Canada are used to illustrate (i), and a small urban community in the United States to address (ii).

Australia, 1918–1919

The medical officer who successfully led the Australian fight against the 1918–19 influenza pandemic was J. H. L. Cumpston, Australia's first Commonwealth Director-General of Health. Australia's involvement in World War I was on a massive scale in relation to its small size. From a population of some 5 million, over 300,000 troops served in Europe, and the problems of bringing the survivors home in the midst of the pandemic after November 1918 was on a similar massive scale.

Records have survived for 228 vessels arriving in Australia between October 1918 and April 1919 (Cliff, Haggett, and Smallman-Raynor 2000: 192–7). Of these, 79 document cases of influenza, mostly on the larger and heavily crowded troopships coming from Europe via Suez or the Cape. The long journey from Europe gave Cumpston time to organize a quarantine system. Boats reporting influenza were isolated in harbour, and troops were not allowed ashore until they were free of the disease. Once soldiers were landed and returned to their homes, they found that interstate travel was also restricted to inhibit transmission—by armed guards in the case of the land border between Queensland and New South Wales. The effect of these

Table 11.3. Spanish influenza, 1918–1919: international maximum weekly death rates: the Australian experience compared with other countries

Location	Rate
US	
Philadelphia	261
San Francisco	135
South Africa[1]	>103[2]
New Zealand	>65[2]
Australia	
New South Wales	34
Victoria	19
Rest	<20[2]

Notes: [1] Europeans only. [2] Averaged from monthly values.

measures is seen in Table 11.3. Peak death rates in Australia were about an eighth of those in the US, and a quarter of those in South Africa and New Zealand.

Canada, 1918–1919

Sattenspiel and Herring (2003) used data from the Hudson's Bay Company records on the 1918–19 influenza pandemic among aboriginal fur trappers in three northern communities (Norway House, Oxford House, and God's Lake) in the Keewatin district of central Manitoba (Figure 11.12) to examine two topical questions relating to quarantine:

(i) What is the impact of varying the time during an epidemic at which intercommunity quarantine is implemented?
(ii) What is the effect of varying the duration of quarantine?

An SIR compartment model[3] was used with a 30-day quarantine period which was applied only at Norway House.

Figure 11.13A shows the impact upon case levels at Oxford House of varying the time on the epidemic curve at which quarantine measures were introduced at Norway House (question (i) above), with epidemic starts at Norway House and God's Lake. Caseload at the epidemic peak was minimized when quarantine was introduced well before the epidemic peaked, but

[3] See Section 10.2.1 for the specification of an SIR model. The compartment model allows the mixing parameter, β, to vary spatially, thus allowing inhomogeneous mixing of susceptibles and infectives. In their version of the model, Sattenspiel and Herring (2003) replaced β with two parameters: σ, the rate of travel out of communities, and ρ, the rate of return into communities. For a theoretical discussion of quarantine in infectious disease models, see Hethcote *et al.* (2002).

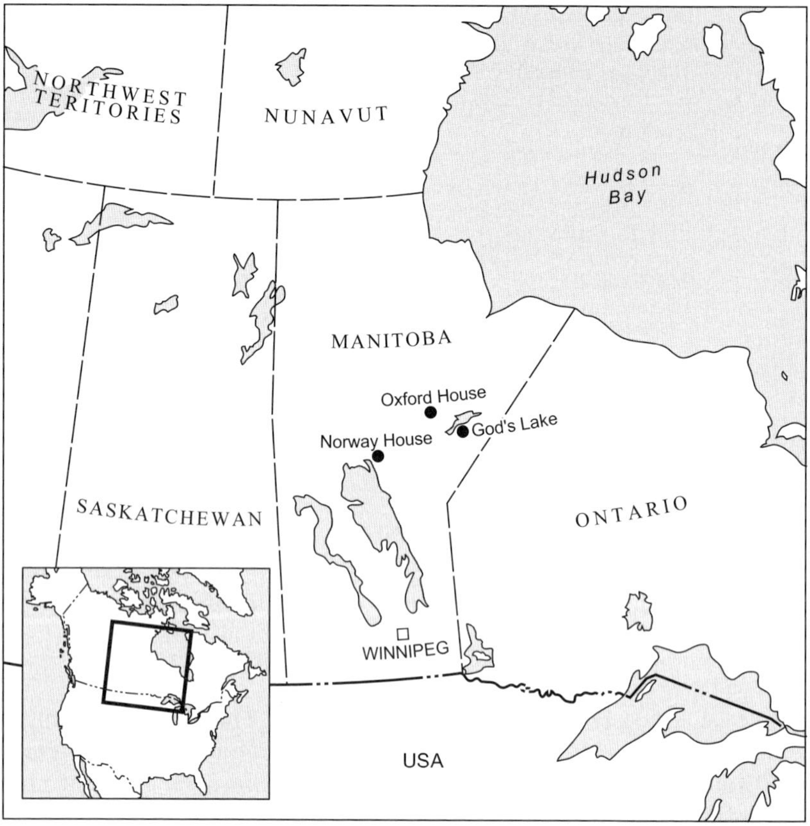

Fig. 11.12. Keewatin district of central Manitoba, Canada
Location map showing positions of the trading communities of Norway House, Oxford House, and God's Lake.

not right at the beginning of an epidemic. The maximum effect was felt when quarantine was started about halfway to the peak. Introduction of quarantine at this point on the epidemic curve also had the maximum delaying effect upon the epidemic peak. This is shown for God's Lake in Figure 11.13B. Such delay can buy public health authorities time to devise other control strategies.

Figure 11.13C shows the impact of quarantine periods of different lengths at Norway House upon the total number of cases estimated to occur at God's Lake. For quarantines of up to 30 days, the case total dropped sharply. There is no further benefit gained by quarantines of greater duration—although this will, of course, be affected by the serial interval of the disease (about 4–8 days for influenza), so that we might expected the optimal quarantine duration to be positively correlated with the serial interval of the disease.

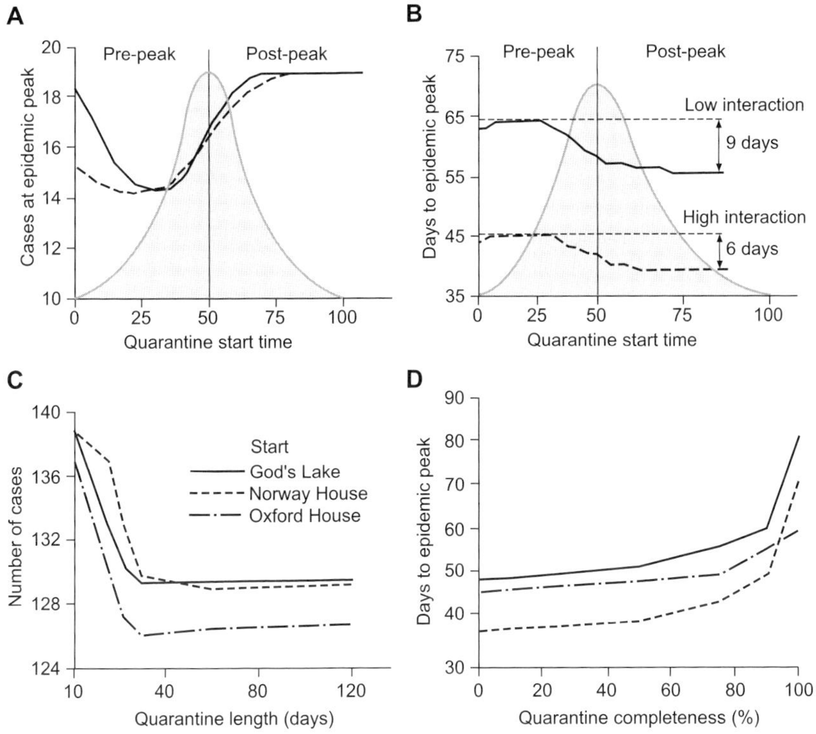

Fig. 11.13. Quarantine in Canada, 1918–1919

Estimated impact of inter-community quarantine upon the Spanish influenza pandemic in the Keewatin district of central Manitoba, Canada. (A) Oxford House (OH): estimated cases at epidemic peak as a function of the time on the epidemic curve at which quarantine was started at Norway House (NH). Maximum case reduction occurred for quarantine start times about a quarter of the way through the epidemic. There was no effect after the epidemic peak. Curves for epidemics starting in NH and God's Lake (GL) are shown. The hypothesized epidemic curve is shaded. (B) God's Lake: estimated delay in timing of the epidemic peak (in days) for different quarantine start times at NH and epidemics starting at NH and GL. Consistent with A, maximum delay is delivered by starting quarantine about a quarter way through the epidemic. Curves are shown for high and low rates of inter-community travel. (C) God's Lake: estimated size of epidemic (in cases) as a function of the quarantine period at NH and epidemic starts at NH, OH, and GL. No appreciable effect is felt with quarantines >30 days. (D) Oxford House: days to epidemic peak as function of quarantine completeness at NH on a scale from 0–100 per cent (no–complete quarantine), and epidemic starts at NH, OH, and GL.

Source: Based upon graphs in Sattenspiel and Herring (2003, figs 4–7, pp. 18–20).

The duration of quarantine will also be affected by its effectiveness. Figure 11.13D explores this for Oxford House. The curves show the time in days to the epidemic peak at Oxford House (vertical axis), against quarantine completeness at Norway House on the horizontal axis. The traces show that, once mobility goes above about 10 per cent (i.e. the quarantine is less than 90 per cent effective), quarantine did not delay the onset of the epidemic peak at Oxford House. Up to this threshold, the epidemic peak was delayed by several days. Sattenspiel and Herring also found a similar 10 per cent threshold for the ultimate size of the epidemic.

United States, 1918–1919 and 1957

Two studies, by Markel *et al.* (2007) and by Haber *et al.* (2007), have investigated the impact of various non-prophylactic techniques such as school closures as an approach to epidemic mitigation. Markel *et al.* used data from 43 cities in the continental United States for the 24-week period from 8 September 1918 to 22 February 1919, to determine whether city-to-city variations in mortality were associated with the timing, duration, and combination of various non-pharmaceutical interventions (school closures, cancellation of public gatherings, and isolation and quarantine); allowance was made for confounding variables like city size and population density. In a similar vein, but using simulation to evaluate different scenarios, Haber *et al.* (2007) estimated the impact upon the ultimate size of an influenza epidemic of reducing contact rates among specified classes of citizens in a hypothetical small urban community in the United States. The community was assumed to have a distribution of sizes of household ages and members following the 2000 US Census. The interventions they investigated were school closures, confinement of ill persons and their household contacts to their homes, and reduction in contact rates among residents of long-term care facilities. Interventions were implemented at the start of the outbreak. Data from the 1957–8 Asian influenza pandemic were used to test the model. A mixing matrix was devised with the following age categories and mixing groups: $<$1–4, 5–18, 19–64, $\geq$65 at home, $\geq$65 in long-term care; households, day-care centres, schools, workplaces, long-term care facilities, and the community.

Markel *et al.* took weekly excess death rate per 100,000 population (EDR) as a measure of the success of different interventions. Over the 24-week study period, there were 115,340 excess pneumonia and influenza deaths (EDR = 500) in the 43 cities analysed. Every city adopted at least one of the three non-pharmaceutical interventions: school closure, cancellation of public gatherings, and isolation/quarantine. School closure and public gathering bans was the most common intervention combination, implemented in 34 cities (79 per cent), with a median duration of 4 weeks (range, 1–10 weeks). The longer the period of non-pharmaceutical intervention, the lower was the EDR. This is illustrated in Figure 11.14A by comparing St Louis (143 days of non-pharmaceutical intervention) and New York City (73 days). The cities which implemented non-pharmaceutical interventions earlier also had greater delays in reaching peak mortality (Spearman $r = -0.74$, $p < 0.001$) and lower peak mortality rates (Spearman $r = 0.31$, $p = 0.02$); see Figure 11.14B. There was a statistically significant inverse correlation between duration of non-pharmaceutical interventions and total mortality (Spearman $r = -0.39$, $p = 0.005$) and, as noted, cities experienced lower total mortality when intervention started early (Spearman $r = 0.37$, $p = 0.008$); see Figure 11.14C.

Haber *et al.* used a different measure of the success of non-prophylactic interventions in their study, namely *effectiveness*, defined as:

$$\text{effectiveness} = (\text{baseline influenza rate} - \text{rate with intervention})/\text{baseline rate}.$$

Figure 11.14D and E show the estimated impact upon outbreak size of (D) school closures and (E) confinement of sick people to home. For schools, closure at around 10 per cent sick and for 14 days is the most effective compromise in the trade-off between reducing infection and increasing societal disruption. Striking early takes children incubating the disease out of circulation, while 14-day closure exceeds the serial interval of influenza. As graph D shows, delay (as measured by percentage illness required to trigger closure) allows incubators and infectives to produce secondary downstream cases, thus greatly reducing effectiveness. Within the family, chart E shows that the same principles apply. Confining sick individuals and their contacts to home with high isolation compliance greatly reduces the chances of community-wide contacts between infectives and susceptibles; it is a highly effective intervention. Haber *et al.* also found that, for long-term care facilities, reducing contacts of the healthy residents with sick co-residents has a significant impact upon illness levels. This is an important finding since residents of long-term care facilities respond poorly to vaccination and often escape vaccination entirely in the US.

The findings of the Markel and Haber studies are consistent with that of Sattenspiel: the application of non-pharmaceutical interventions which reduce mixing between infectives and susceptibles early in an epidemic has the capability of both reducing the ultimate size of an epidemic and delaying the peak of infection. It suggests, as do the recent studies by Davey and Glass (2008) and Meltzer (2008), that in planning for future severe influenza pandemics, non-pharmaceutical interventions should be considered for inclusion as companion measures to developing effective vaccines and medications for prophylaxis and treatment. Haber *et al.* estimate that, by combining these interventions, rates of illness and death in a community might be reduced by as much as 50 per cent. Such non prophylactic interventions are included in the current US Department of Health and Human Services Influenza Pandemic Plan (United States Department of Health and Human Services 2005, 2007). Similar findings have also been found for international travel. For example, Epstein *et al.* (2007) used a stochastic epidemic model to study

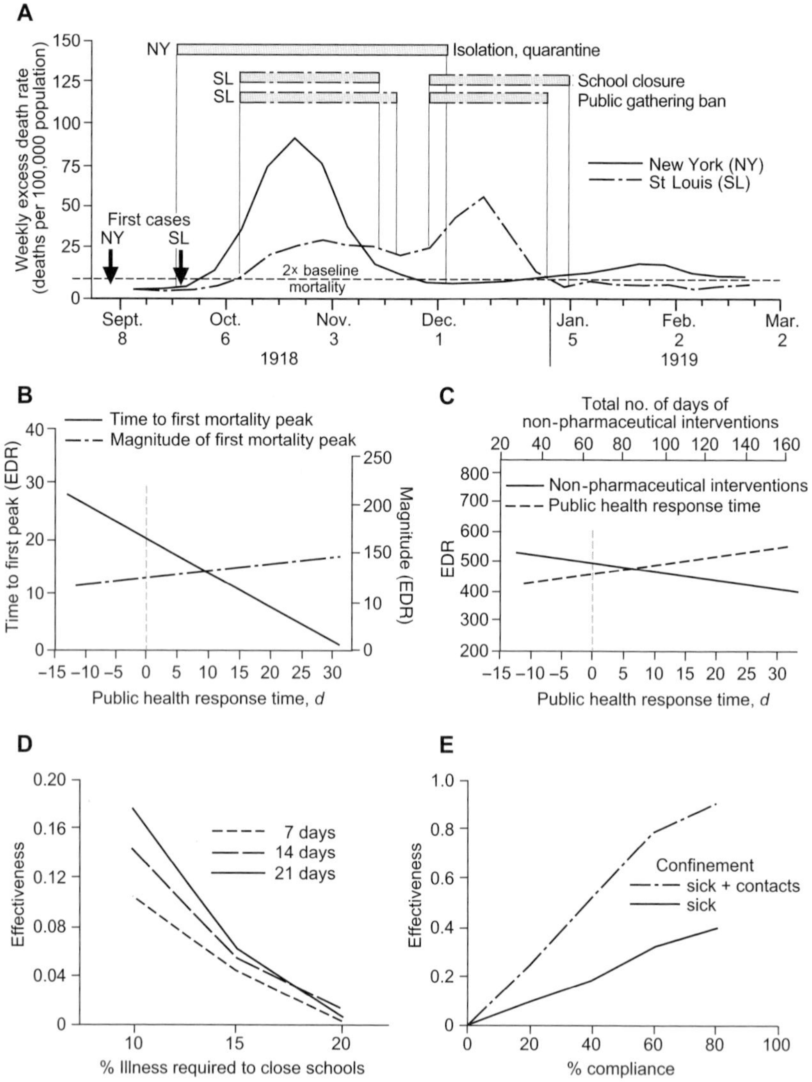

Fig. 11.14. United States: estimated impact of non-prophylactic interventions upon rates of illness and mortality in pandemic influenza in 1918 (A, B, and C) and 1957 (D and E) (A) Weekly excess death rate (EDR) in New York City and St Louis, Sept. 1918–Feb. 1919 in relation to the duration of non-pharmaceutical interventions. The lower excess mortality in St Louis may be attributed to the longer duration of intervention. (B) and (C), regression lines showing (B) the relationship between public health response time (PHRT) and the timing and magnitude of the first influenza peak in 43 cities and (C) weekly EDR in relation to timing and duration of non-prophylactic interventions. Vertical line indicates the day on which the pandemic accelerated in each city. An intervention introduced on this day was given a PHRT of zero; interventions introduced on days before acceleration have negative PHRTs and, on days after, positive PHRTs. (D) Impact of school closures for varying levels of sickness and closure periods. (E) Impact of home confinement of sick individuals and their contacts for varying levels of quarantine compliance. In D and E, *effectiveness* is defined as: *effectiveness* = (baseline rate − rate with intervention)/baseline rate, where the baseline rate is that for illness during the 1957–8 pandemic in the US.

Sources: A–C constructed from scattergraphs given in Markel *et al.* (2007, figs 1, 3, pp. 650, 652). D and E drawn from graphs and data in Haber *et al.* (2007, figs 1, 2, pp. 584–5).

global transmission of pandemic influenza, including the effects of travel restrictions and vaccination. They found that the distribution of first passage times to the United States and the numbers of infected persons in metropolitan areas worldwide could be slightly delayed by international air travel restrictions alone. When other local containment measures were applied at the source of infection, in conjunction with travel restrictions, delays could be much longer and caseload reduced (cf. Section 6.4.2).

11.2.4 Offensive Containment

We saw in Section 11.2.1 how Italian states like Venice and the Papal States used cavalry for the offensive containment of human diseases. In this subsection, a recent example in the airline era is outlined: a plague outbreak in India in 1994. This shows that, just as with plague in earlier centuries, offensive containment for infections in human populations only has limited success with modern transport. In contrast, in animal populations, offensive containment can be more efficacious because it is normally accompanied by mass slaughter of infected livestock. We illustrate containment with slaughter in this section, taking the 2007 outbreaks of avian influenza and foot-and-mouth and bluetongue diseases in the United Kingdom as examples.

OFFENSIVE CONTAINMENT FOR HUMAN DISEASES

Plague in India, August–October 1994

Beginning on 26 August 1994, outbreaks of bubonic and pneumonic plague began to be reported in south-central, south-western, and northern India. However, owing to the unconfirmed nature of many of the reports at the time, the actual extent of the outbreaks—and, indeed, if the disease really was plague at all—remained unclear at first. However, all doubt was finally removed by DNA analysis in 2000 (Dutt *et al.* 2006). The outbreak probably resulted in some 5,150 pneumonic or bubonic plague cases and 53 deaths in eight Indian states, with the majority from south-central and south-western regions. Of the 5,150 cases, the majority (2,793) were reported from Maharashtra state (including Bombay), with much of the balance from Gujarat state (1,391 cases) and Delhi (749 cases); the remaining 169 cases were from Andhra Pradesh, Haryana, Madhya Pradesh, Rajasthan, Uttar Pradesh, and West Bengal (Centers for Disease Control and Prevention 1994*a*,*c*). By 19 October, the outbreak was under control.

The space–time sequence of events was mapped by Dutt *et al.* in 2006; see Figure 11.15. These authors divided the spread into four phases: (i) Phase I, localized spread around the initial centre of Surat; (ii) Phase II, spread from Surat to the Delhi region; (iii) Phase III, spread from Surat to Calcutta and surrounding areas; (iv) Phase IV, spread from Surat to the vicinity of

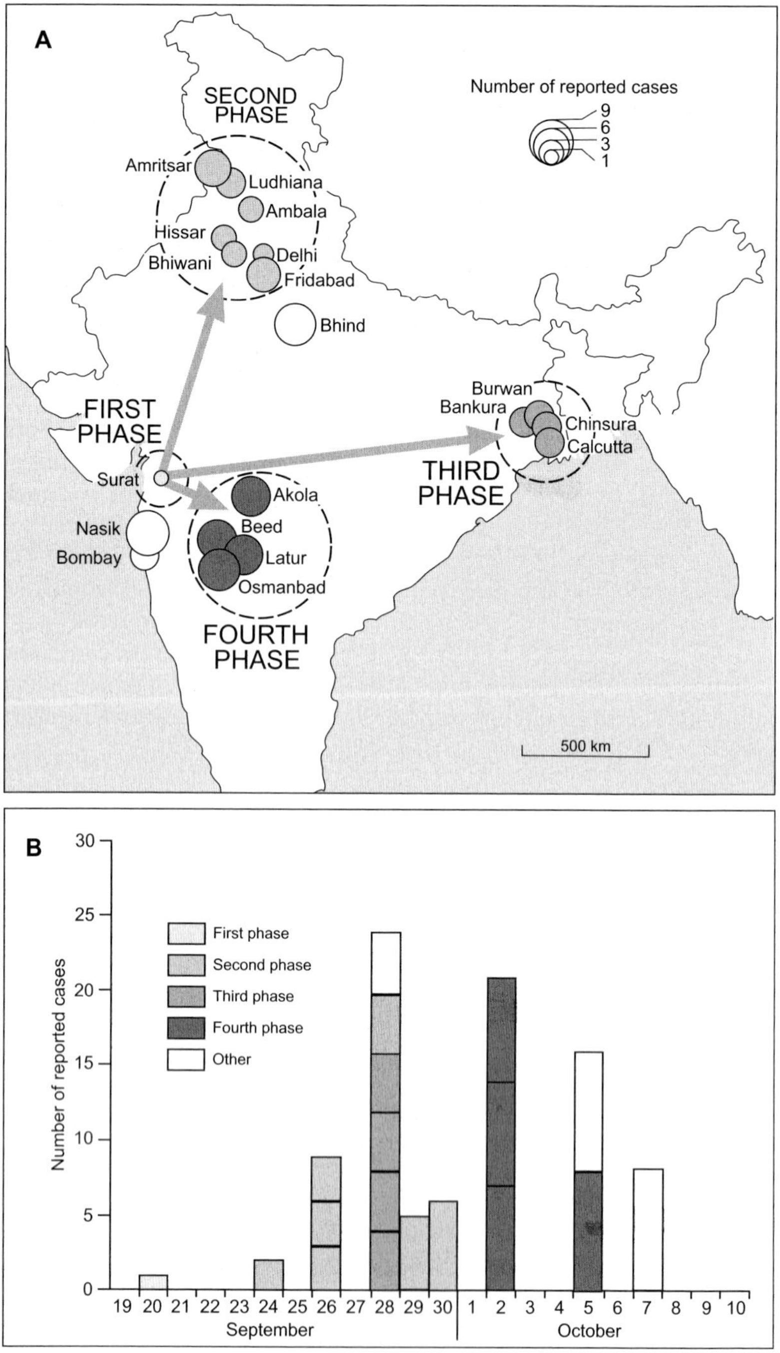

Fig. 11.15. Plague in India, 1994

Phases in the spread of the Surat plague outbreak to other Indian states. (A) Circle sizes are proportional to the number of reported cases and are shaded by phase. (B) Time series of reported cases, coded by outbreak phase. Phases are geographically rather than temporally distinct, especially in the second and third phases.

Source: Based on Dutt *et al.* (2006, fig. 2, p. 759).

Beed. In Phases II–IV, localized spread around the new main centres proceeded through the system of adjacent cities. In all instances, spread to new centres appears to have been caused by infected people travelling home by train.

As Madan (1995) and Fritz *et al.* (1996) observe, the initial reports of the 1994 outbreak caused considerable international concern, especially among countries which were uncertain of the effectiveness of their own public healthcare systems, over the possible importation of pneumonic plague from India by air travel. Official responses ranged from increased surveillance at airports to the embargo of flights to and from India—*offensive containment* in terms of Figure 11.2. For example, Indians travelling to the US from plague-affected areas had to fill out special forms upon arrival. Many countries, particularly in Asia, banned flights to and from India. For example, Saudi Arabian authorities refused a scheduled Air India flight from Bombay permission to land in Jeddah (Madan 1995). Air India aircraft were fumigated on arrival at airports in Rome and Milan and passengers were subjected to special health checks. In Moscow, authorities ordered six-day quarantines for passengers from India and banned travel to India. The response reflected recognition of the risk of transmission in the modern global community.

OFFENSIVE CONTAINMENT FOR EPIZOOTICS

During 2007, three epizootics occurred in livestock populations in England for which offensive containment was used to control spread.

Avian Influenza among Turkeys, Holton, Suffolk

The year began with an outbreak of highly pathogenic avian influenza (HPAI), strain H5N1, on a turkey finishing site at Holton in Suffolk, England (Figure 11.16A). The disease was suspected on 1 February 2007, culling of all birds (*c*.160,000) was completed on 2 February, and the strain of HPAI was confirmed as H5N1 on 3 February (DEFRA 2007*a*). The outbreak was confined to a single farm adjacent to a turkey factory which comprised a slaughterhouse and two processing plants. By the end of February, the event was over and normal operations resumed.

Investigation suggested infection was introduced into the turkey finishing site between 5 December 2006 and 25 January 2007. The virus was sequenced and shown to be almost 100 per cent homologous to that recovered from Hungarian outbreaks in geese in January 2007 and very similar (95 per cent homologous) to certain wild-bird isolates in Hungary and Scotland in 2006. Concurrent with the Holton outbreak, a similar outbreak occurred in Hungary at a turkey processing plant with which the Holton factory had links. DEFRA (2007*a*: 4) concluded that infection was probably introduced to the turkey factory via the importation of turkey meat from a subclinically infected turkey flock in Hungary which had been infected from a common

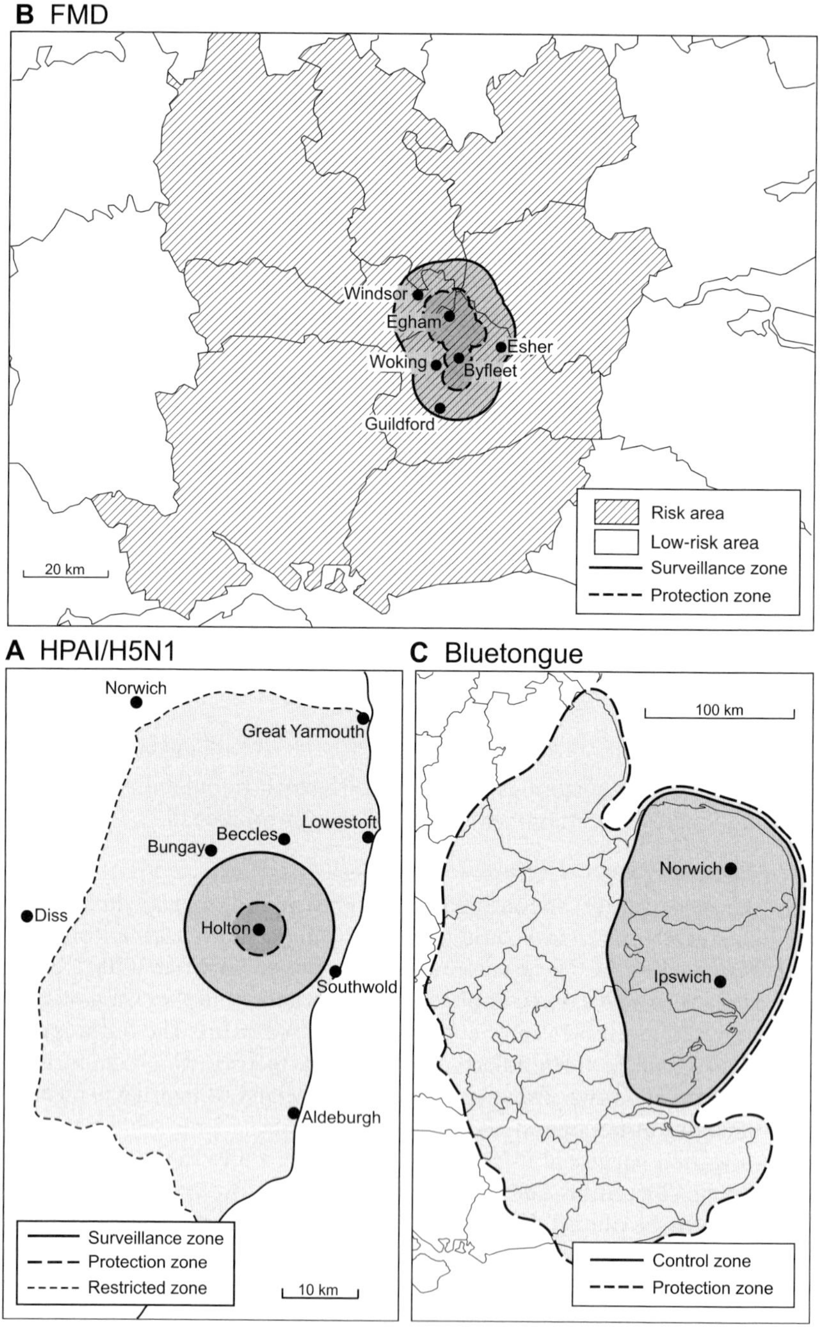

Fig. 11.16. Offensive containment and defensive isolation for epizootics
(A) Highly pathogenic avian influenza, Suffolk, 2007. Protected, surveillance and restricted zones around outbreak epicentre, Holton, Jan. 2007. (B) Foot and mouth disease (FMD), Surrey, July–Oct. 2007. Spatial configuration of the protected, surveillance, and risk zones in Sept. around the Pirbright locus. (C) Bluetongue disease, eastern England, 2007. Spatial configuration of the control and protection zones in Sept.
Sources: Maps based upon various maps on DEFRA web site (http://www.defra.gov.uk).

source, possibly wild birds, which may also have infected two goose farms in Hungary. How spread occurred from the factory to the adjacent farm at Holton remains uncertain but was probably via rats, mice, or gulls visiting bins containing waste material from processing of the Hungarian consignment at the factory.

Subsequent spread of the disease from Holton did not occur because offensive containment was rapidly implemented. As shown in Figure 11.16A, this consisted of a 3 km protection zone around the site, surrounded by a 10 km surveillance zone, which was itself enclosed in a *c*.2,000 km^2 restricted zone. Working from the restricted zone in towards the epicentre, each of these zones had increasingly severe restrictions upon bird flock movements. In general, movements could be inwards towards the epicentre but not outwards. The offensive containment was reinforced by culling of around 160,000 birds at the Holton site itself. Paralleling the movement restrictions, surveillance also increased inwards from the restricted zone towards the epicentre. For example, within the surveillance zone, all 70 commercial bird flocks were visited and swabbed at 23 sites carrying geese and ducks. Within the protection zone, repeated surveillance and swabbing of all 78 commercial bird flocks was undertaken until the end of February.

Foot and Mouth Disease, Pirbright, Surrey

The containment principles used at Holton were re-employed between August and November to contain an outbreak of foot and mouth disease (a virus disease of cloven-footed animals caused by the foot and mouth virus, FMDV) which occurred on two farms near Pirbright, Surrey, at the beginning of August. The farms were adjacent to a government facility at Pirbright. This site hosts the Institute for Animal Health (IAH) laboratories, which conduct research into animal diseases and potential vaccines including FMDV, and the Merial Animal Health vaccine production facility, which produces vaccines to assist in the control of FMD and bluetongue, a midge-borne virus disease of sheep (see below). These are the only two facilities in the United Kingdom authorized to work with live FMDV.

It was rapidly established that the initial outbreak was caused by FMDV of a strain not known to be circulating in nature (O_1 BFS 1860) but which was in use at IAH and Merial (Spratt 2007). The most likely source of the release of FMDV into the environment was an old, poorly maintained liquid effluent system shared by the two facilities and in an area of the Pirbright site liable to flooding, associated with heavy rains on 20 July 2007. This probably led to release of infectious virus from one or both of the facilities into or onto the surrounding soil. There was recent contractor activity at IAH, including around the area above the defective effluent pipes, so that mechanical spread by virus-contaminated contractors' vehicles to the first outbreak farm is considered the most likely cause.

To contain the outbreak, an extensive risk area was established across southern England (Figure 11.16B), containing nested surveillance and protection zones, with, as at Holton, restrictions on animal movements becoming more severe towards the epicentre (offensive containment). Slaughter of infected and suspected animals was used as part of the offensive policy. The outbreak finally expired having reached eight farms in the general area (Surrey, Windsor, and Maidenhead).

Bluetongue Disease in East Anglia

Bluetongue is a disease of animals affecting all ruminants. Although sheep are the most severely affected, cattle are the main mammalian reservoir. The causative agent is a virus (bluetongue virus, BTV) spread by certain biting midges of the genus *Culicoides*. In Europe since 1999, there have been widespread outbreaks in Greece, Italy, Corsica, and the Balearic Islands. Cases have also occurred in Bulgaria, Croatia, Macedonia, Kosovo, and Yugoslavia. The virus appears to have spread from both Turkey and North Africa (DEFRA 2007*b*,*c*).

In 2007, a new serotype, 8, appeared and spread rapidly in Germany, Belgium, France, Luxembourg, the Netherlands, and Denmark. All cases are within existing livestock movement restriction zones, implying that BTV has survived in the zones over winter; peak populations of the vector midges occur in late summer and autumn.

The vector midge can travel up to 1.5–2 km per day in a local area. However, if caught in suitable meteorological conditions, midges can be carried up to 200 km over water masses. Such conditions prevailed in September 2007, when winds blew infected midges from continental Europe into East Anglia, where the first case of bluetongue was confirmed on 22 September. The disease has subsequently spread across large parts of east and south-east England and is ongoing. When disease is confirmed, a 20 km control zone (offensive containment) and a wider 100–50 km protection zone (100 km protection + optional additional 50 km surveillance) is established around the infected premises. Figure 11.16C shows these zones in England in September 2007; further westerly extension of the protection zone has already occurred. Within the control zone, control is mainly effected by restrictions on animal movements, housing animals indoors, and vaccination (where vaccine effective against the serotype is available). In the protection zone, surveillance and communication are the main weapons for containment.

11.3 Aspatial Barriers: Vaccination Strategies

In Section 10.2.1, we showed how natural breaks in chains of infection for a specific disease can occur depending upon the sizes of the communities in which the disease agent is circulating. This gave rise to the notion of critical

Table 11.4. Critical community size and disease properties: Icelandic evidence, 1888–1988

Disease	Transmission	Immunity	Critical community size (thousands): Quoted[1]	Critical community size (thousands): Estimated *CCS*: Iceland	Normal infectious period in days (rank, 1 = shortest)
Scarlet fever	Intimate contact	Some repeat cases		48	15 (3)
Diphtheria	Normal contact	Usually lasting		67	21 (5)
Whooping cough	Airborne droplet	Lasting		106	18 (4)
Rubella	Airborne droplet	Lasting	132	151	7 (2=)
Measles	Airborne droplet	Lasting	250–500	259	7 (2=)
Influenza	Airborne droplet	None	1,000,000	102	5 (1)

Note: [1] Ramsay and Emond (1978); Yorke *et al.* (1979); Cliff, Haggett, and Ord (1986); and Cliff and Haggett (1990).

community size (CCS)—the population size of a community above which a sufficiently large stock of susceptibles will exist to enable the disease to be endemic, and below which the stock of susceptibles will not be large enough to maintain continuous chains of infection. In studies of the CCS, total population of a community is generally used as a convenient correlate of the difficult-to-estimate true susceptible population. Many studies have attempted to estimate the CCS for a range of common infectious diseases, and the results of these are summarized in Table 11.4, while Cliff, Haggett, and Smallman-Raynor (2000: 85–117) have shown how the CCS is affected by factors such as geographical isolation and population density.

The basic notion of a threshold population below which an infectious disease becomes naturally self-extinguishing is paramount in articulating aspatial control strategies (Figure 11.2B). It implies that vaccination may be employed to reduce the susceptible population below some critical mass so that the chains of infection are broken. Once the susceptible population size of an area falls below the threshold, then, when the disease concerned is eventually eliminated, it can only recur by reintroduction from other reservoir areas. In the remainder of this section, we review the theoretical work on vaccination and its impact upon CCS.

11.3.1 Vaccination Impact on Epidemic Cycles

In theory, provided an appropriate vaccine is available, control of a new or re-emerging disease should be straightforward for sicknesses caused by stable disease agents. Here we show that this is far from the case using the two childhood diseases of measles and poliomyelitis as examples.

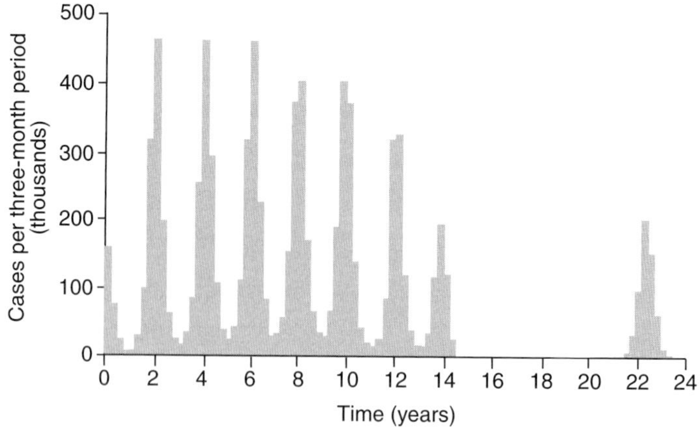

Fig. 11.17. Predicted effect of widespread immunization
Predicted effects of widespread measles immunization. Application of the SIR model with the level of immunization held constant for 15 years at 80 per cent of 1- to 2-year-olds.
Source: Adapted from Cutts (1990, fig. 10, p. 23).

As shown in Table 11.4, the CCS for measles in an unvaccinated population is generally estimated to be around 250,000, above which the continuous epidemic chains displayed by community A in Figure 10.2 occur. In 1973, Griffiths showed that, if x denotes the proportion of children not immunized by vaccination, the CCS required to sustain endemic measles is multiplied by $1/x^2$. Thus, 50 per cent immunization increases the critical community size from 250,000 to 1 million, while 90 per cent immunization increases the threshold to 25 million. So, for all practical purposes, when the percentage of the population vaccinated reaches the mid-1990s, *herd immunity* is established and major epidemics will not occur; 100 per cent vaccination is impossible to achieve because there always exist subgroups in a population who are inaccessible for any number of reasons (for example, objection to vaccination on religious grounds and inaccurate demographic recording).

But levels of vaccination well below herd immunity will also severely disrupt chains of infection. Figure 11.17 shows the predicted effect of partial immunization, sustained over 15 years, at 80 per cent of the 1–2-year-olds in a theoretical population. The slow damping of epidemic amplitude is evident as the cumulative impact of vaccination is felt. Eventually the endemic cycle is broken and whole epidemics are missed. Thus, natural fade-out becomes very widespread, enhancing the possibility of local elimination and long-run global eradication of a disease.

The use of vaccination to establish a containing 'quarantine ring' around outbreaks has been considered by a number of workers. See, for example, Cliff and Haggett (1989) for a review and Greenhalgh (1986). The main focus of this work has been to use simulation models to establish the optimal width

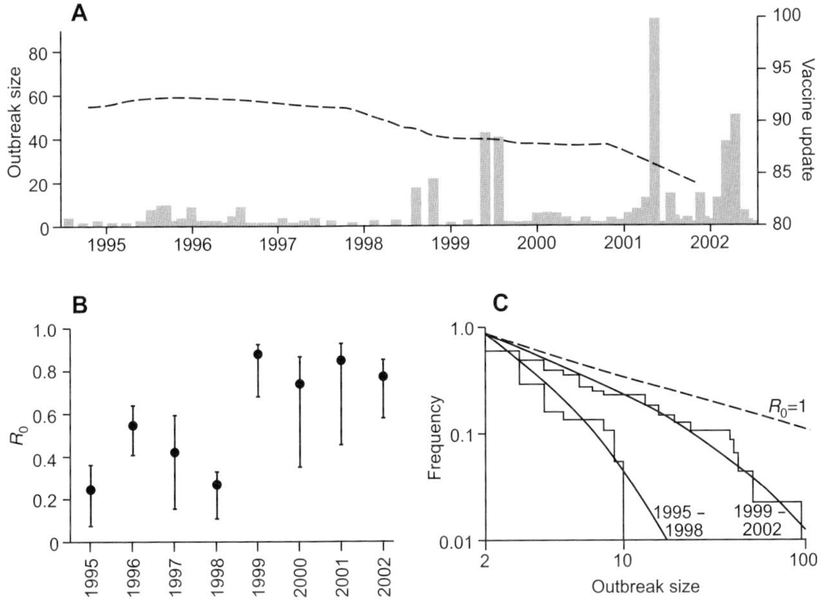

Fig. 11.18. England and Wales measles outbreaks, 1995–2002
(A) Monthly time series of outbreaks (bar chart) and per cent vaccine coverage (pecked line). (B) Estimated reproductive ratio, R_0, given by equation 10.A3 in App. 10.1 shown as solid circles with 90 per cent confidence intervals as bars. (C) Frequency distributions of outbreaks of a certain size and larger (stepped lines), 1995–8 and 1999–2002 with fitted trend lines. Distribution for $R_0 = 1$ is shown as a pecked line. Note from A and B how estimates of R_0 increased as vaccination coverage fell.
Source: Redrawn from Jansen *et al.* (2003, fig. 1, p. 804).

of any vaccine-induced quarantine ring and the distance at which it should be placed from the epicentre of the outbreak for maximum containment. Maintenance in the population of high levels of vaccination against a particular agent is essential when vaccination is used as a control strategy until the disease is eradicated (see, for example, the studies by Cullen and Walker (1996) of measles outbreaks in New Zealand, 1949–91, and by MacIntyre *et al.* (2002) on the Australian Measles Control Campaign).

Figure 11.18 shows what can happen when vaccination levels fall away. In the United Kingdom, protection levels against measles achieved by administration of the triple MMR (measles, mumps, and rubella) vaccine had reached 91 per cent by 1998 (Jansen *et al.* 2003). However, the unfounded controversy which surrounded the safety of the vaccine led to a fall in vaccination uptake, with herd immunity falling as low as 60 per cent in some geographical localities in England. As Figure 11.18A shows, the predictable increase in measles outbreaks occurred from 2000, leading to the possibility, if current vaccination levels cannot be improved, that endemic measles will become re-established in the UK. Indeed, in June 2008, the UK Department of Health declared provisionally that this had occurred.

The facility with which a disease can re-establish itself when vaccination levels fall carries important implications for the control of new and re-emerging diseases by vaccination (see, for example, Wallinga *et al.* 2005). It implies that disease surveillance systems (Section 10.6) should ideally incorporate components which can accurately estimate the fraction of susceptible individuals over time—by demographic assessment of birth, death, and migration patterns among communities, and by serosurveys to estimate changes in immunity. Only by including these items will appropriate assessments of the health risks posed by a new or re-emerging disease be possible.

11.3.2 Vaccine Failure

A problematic, but fortunately rare, feature of vaccination as a control strategy is the risk of vaccine failure. We illustrate what may happen using the well-known Cutter incident, which occurred in the early history of the US poliomyelitis vaccination campaigns which were based upon Salk's inactivated poliovirus vaccine.

SALK'S INACTIVATED POLIOVIRUS VACCINE

As described in Smallman-Raynor, Cliff, Trevelyan, *et al.* (2006: 437–41), an inactivated poliovirus vaccine had been undergoing clinical trials in the United States during 1954. The trial revealed the vaccine to be 60–70 per cent effective against type 1 poliovirus and 90 per cent effective against type 2 and 3 polioviruses. While batches of the vaccine were found to vary in quality, with some being wholly impotent, there was no suggestion of any danger associated with the vaccine.

The official response to the announcement of the trial results in April 1955 was immediate. Within two hours, the US Public Health Service had issued a licence for the production and application of Salk's vaccine, while the National Foundation for Infantile Paralysis—having already underwritten the production costs of the requisite vaccine—mobilized plans for a national immunization programme. As a result, between 12 April and 7 May 1955, approximately 4 million doses of vaccine, manufactured by five different pharmaceutical companies, were administered to first- and second-grade children across the Union (Paul 1971; Blume and Geesink 2000).

THE CUTTER INCIDENT

The nascent vaccination programme was called to a sudden halt in early May 1955. Between 18 and 27 April, some 400,000 inoculations with batches of vaccine manufactured by Cutter Laboratories of Berkeley, California, had been administered to the general public, of which an estimated 120,000 were drawn from production pools that contained residual live poliovirus. When cases of poliomyelitis began to appear among recipients of the defective vaccine, Leonard A. Scheele, Surgeon General, requested the manufacturer to recall all outstanding lots of vaccine on Wednesday 27 April. Ten days later, on Saturday 7 May, Scheele recommended a complete suspension of the vaccination programme pending a full assessment of the safety of the vaccines (Langmuir *et al.* 1956; Nathanson and Langmuir 1963*a*,*b*).

Temporal Course

According to Langmuir *et al.* (1956), the Cutter incident was associated with 158 notified cases of paralytic poliomyelitis and 46 cases of non-paralytic poliomyelitis in three exposure categories: (i) recently vaccinated children; (ii) family contacts of recently vaccinated children; and (iii) community contacts of (i) and (ii). To illustrate the temporal course of the outbreak, the histograms in Figure 11.19 are drawn from evidence relating to the 158 paralytic cases and plot the daily incidence of paralysis in each of the three exposure categories. Inspection of the histograms reveals a time-ordered sequence to the population-based progression of the Cutter outbreak, with the first appearance of paralysis among vaccine recipients on 23 April (graph 11.19A), family contacts on 30 April (11.19B), and community contacts on 12 May (11.19C). As the histograms show, the majority of cases of paralysis occurred within a month of the recall of defective vaccine (27 April), but the long tail of the outbreak extended to late June (Langmuir *et al.* 1956).

Spatial Dimension

Figure 11.20 plots, as proportional circles, the state-wise distribution of cases of paralytic and non-paralytic poliomyelitis associated with the defective Cutter vaccine. The Pacific and Mountain states of California (57 paralytic cases) and Idaho (49 paralytic cases) dominate the distribution; with the exception of Nevada (7 paralytic cases) and Washington (6 paralytic cases), all other states recorded ≤5 paralytic cases. The focus on California and Idaho reflected the unwitting distribution of defective vaccine by the National Foundation for Infantile Paralysis to school clinics in these states. Defective lots of Cutter vaccine were also used in school clinics in Nevada, Arizona, New Mexico, and Hawaii, while the remaining scattered cases were associated with vaccine that had been distributed through commercial channels (Langmuir *et al.* 1956).

Poliomyelitis Associated with Other Vaccine Manufacturers

Cutter Laboratories was not the only manufacturer to experience difficulties in the production of Salk vaccine. Coincidental with the Cutter outbreak, a small number of poliomyelitis cases were reported among Pennsylvanian children in receipt of vaccine manufactured by Wyeth Inc. of Philadelphia;

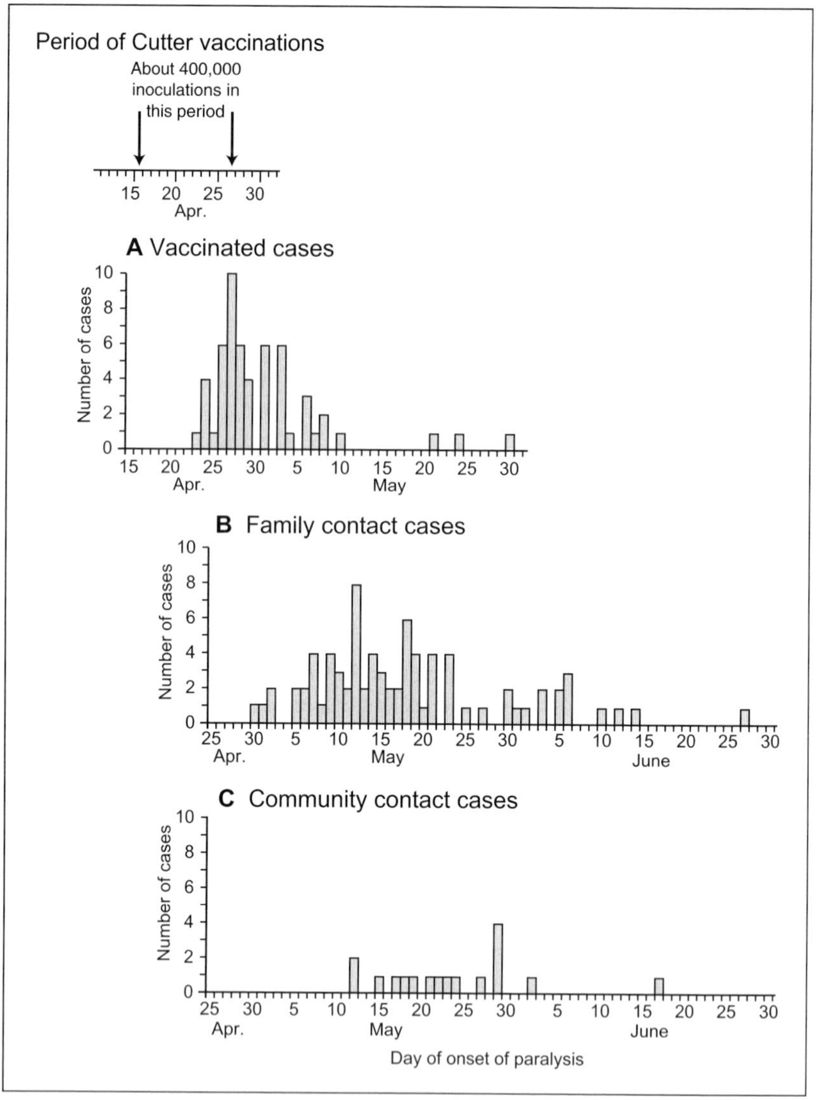

Fig. 11.19. Time series of paralytic poliomyelitis associated with the Cutter incident, April–June 1955

Histograms plot, by day of onset of paralysis, the number of recorded cases of poliomyelitis associated with the administration of vaccine manufactured by Cutter Laboratories, California. (A) Cases among vaccine recipients. (B) Cases among family contacts of vaccine recipients. (C) Cases among community contacts of vaccine recipients and their family contacts.

Sources: Smallman-Raynor, Cliff, Trevelyan, *et al.* (2006, fig. 10.2, p. 439), originally redrawn from Langmuir *et al.* (1956, fig. 1, p. 80).

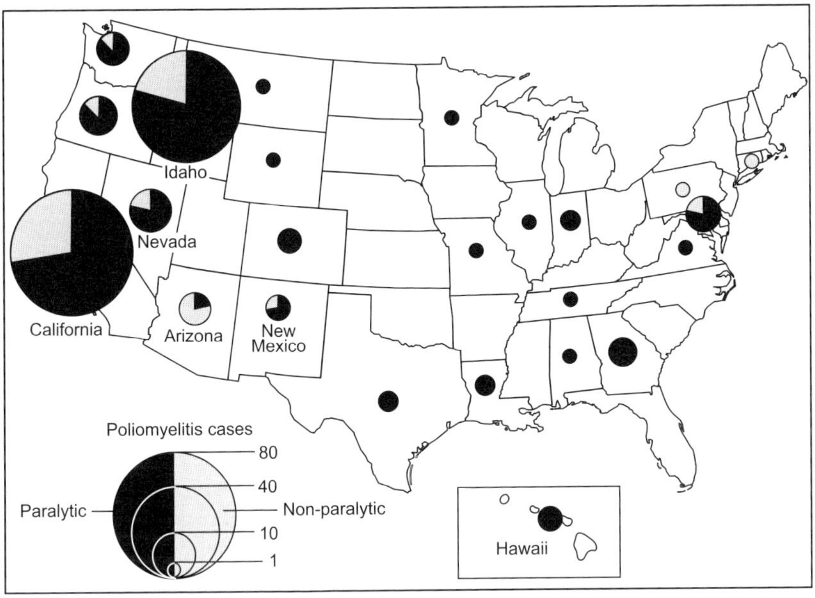

Fig. 11.20. The geographical distribution of cases of poliomyelitis associated with the Cutter incident, April–June 1955
Circle areas are drawn proportional to the total number of cases of poliomyelitis recorded in a given state. The proportion of cases in which paralysis was observed is indicated by the shaded sectors.
Sources: Smallman-Raynor, Cliff, Trevelyan, *et al.* (2006, fig. 10.3, p. 440), drawn from Langmuir *et al.* (1956, table 1, p. 77).

subsequent studies revealed additional cases of the disease in family and community contacts of the vaccine recipients. At about the same time, an outbreak of poliomyelitis among schoolchildren and others in Maryland was also traced to the administration of defective Wyeth vaccine. Vaccine produced by other manufacturers, by contrast, appeared to present no significant hazard to the general public (Langmuir *et al.* 1956).

11.4 Epilogue

The final chapter of this book has touched upon some of the approaches used historically to control resurging or 'new' diseases when they emerged in different places and times—a mixture of quarantine and isolation (Section 11.2), immunization (Section 11.3), and, in the case of epizootics, slaughter (Section 11.2.4). The ways in which these approaches will have to be integrated and deployed to contain future disease patterns as the twenty-first century unrolls will change, but it is certain that continued vigilance and application of early-warning systems (Section 10.6) will be at the leading edge of global preparedness. We therefore conclude by identifying six trends which will affect this surveillance process.

1. EPIDEMIC DISEASE CONTROL WILL NEED CONTINUOUS ADJUSTMENT

One of the world's greatest bacteriologists, Louis Pasteur, was asked in his later years whether he was optimistic or pessimistic about disease control. He replied that he expected microbes to prove formidable, resilient, and persistent enemies. The ability of microbiological entities to change (Chapter 4) is one of their greatest weapons. We have noted the effects of recurring shifts in the influenza A virus and the challenges they pose for anticipating pandemic influenza (Section 10.3). Equally, tuberculosis (Section 4.3.2) is an example where apparent early successes in treatment and control have proved short-lived. Today tuberculosis annually continues to kill about 4 million people worldwide. With tuberculosis, resistance to single drugs (e.g. isoniazid, rifampin) has, since the late 1980s, been further complicated by resistance to multidrug treatments. Despite extensive publicity about the renewed danger of multidrug-resistant tuberculosis (MDR-TB) and WHO's major DOTS (directly observed treatment short course) campaign, a disease which was once considered to be in retreat has shown a major resurgence.

Tuberculosis is not alone in resurging. As we have seen in Section 4.3.1, resistance due to the use and misuse of antibiotics is reported for a wide range of bacterial diseases, with methicillin-resistant *Staphylococcus aureus* (MRSA) as an outstanding example of a nosocomial disease of growing importance. Malaria, a disease against which DDT control of breeding grounds for malarious mosquitoes was so successful, is again a significant global hazard. Resistance of *falciparum* to chloroquine (the old drug of choice) occurs in many areas of the world and is having to be replaced by more costly drug-combination therapies with repeated courses of treatment. Although the geographical area affected by malaria has shrunk dramatically over the last 60 years, the gains produced by chloroquine are now being eroded with increasing evidence of drug resistance. Figure 11.21 illustrates this for Ethiopia, 1996–8, by mapping, for 18 towns, against a backcloth of the population density in persons per km^2, the failure rates for chloroquine among patients. Circles have been drawn proportional to the number of patients sampled, while the divisions show the share of this total whose treatment with chloroquine failed in different ways. Early treatment failure approached 50 per cent of patients across the country; once the failure rate reaches 25 per cent, the drug should be replaced.

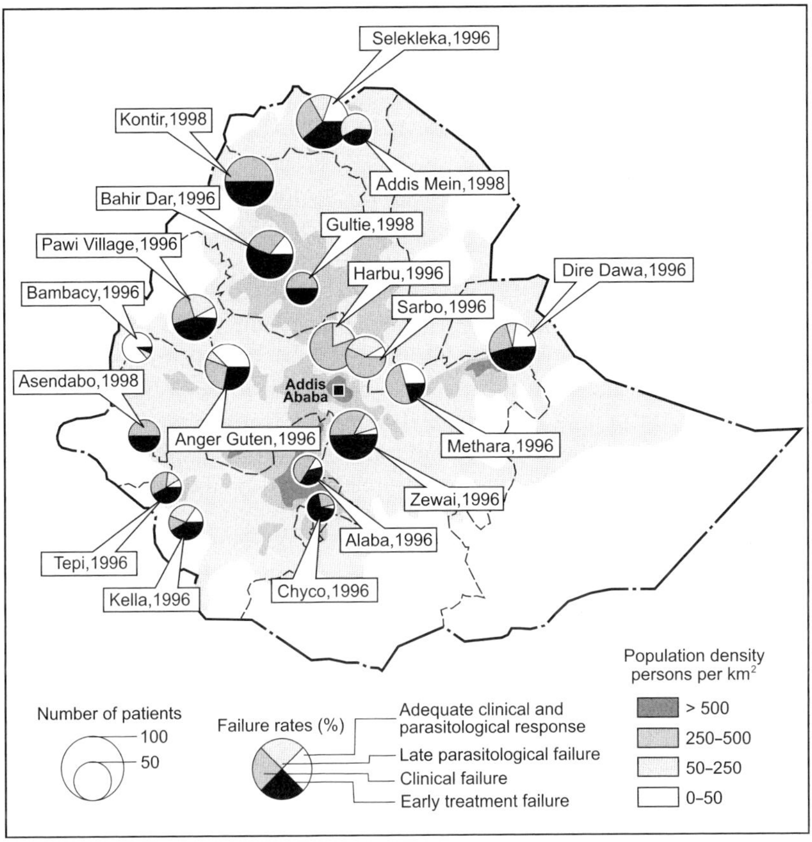

Fig. 11.21. Monitoring malaria drug resistance
Chloroquine failure rates in Ethiopia, 1996–8. Circles give proportion of failures at different treatment stages.
Source: World Health Organization (2007*g*: 37).

2. SPATIAL BARRIERS TO INFECTION ARE INCREASINGLY INEFFECTIVE

We noted in Section 6.4 that the speed of modern air transport was changing the spatial relations of infectious diseases. Most of the world's great cities are now within 36 hours' travel of each other. The complexity of air connections (there are now over 4,000 airports in the world with regular scheduled services) makes the traditional 'drawbridge' or quarantine strategy increasingly difficult to apply. The quarantine barriers first used as a defence against the plague and enshrined in the International Sanitary Regulations in the nineteenth century were modelled to fit a slower mode of travel (ships and railroads) and far fewer connection points. While the incubation times of disease agents remain constant, the movements of infectives become ever faster. Such rapid movements intensify the practical and legal problems associated with vaccination, identification, and constraints on freedom of movement.

3. RAPID REPORTING AND CONSTANT SURVEILLANCE REMAIN CRITICAL TO CONTROL

Although individual cities and countries gradually introduced the systematic recording of disease data from the middle of the nineteenth century, it was the widespread occurrence of diseases like typhus among the legions of displaced persons after World War I which provoked the systematic international surveillance of disease with control in mind (see Section 3.2.1). Today, the use of electronic publication allows disease outbreaks to be reported through the Internet. Because disease is no respecter of national boundaries, maintaining international reporting through the WHO and its agencies is essential. Electronic communication and the ready availability of findings and advice from both international and national centres (such as the Centers for Disease Control and Prevention in Atlanta) has tilted the balance back towards disease detection and defence since 1990. Central elements in the disease reporting network are, at the local spatial scale, the doctors who treat patients. The records produced by individual doctors make their way up through a hierarchy of reporting, to finish eventually in the global network of specialist centres to which infected material and DNA samples can be sent. In the developing world, the WHO devotes substantial resources to the assessment of healthcare coverage through Service Availability Mapping (SAM). Figure 11.22 has been generated by SAM and illustrates the uneven coverage of doctors per 100,000 people, and of antiretroviral therapy and TB diagnosis sites in Zambia. Such unevenness impacts upon both data recording and treatment. At national and international scales, Figure 11.23 illustrates a global laboratory network of the type used by the WHO as its first line of defence in the early detection of disease outbreaks.

4. WIDENING RANGES OF COMMUNICABLE DISEASES AND HIGH SURVEILLANCE COSTS MAKE SAMPLING ESSENTIAL

We noted in Section 1.2.1 and 1.5.3 that the number of identified infectious diseases multiplied hugely as the twentieth century progressed. Wilson's *World Guide to Infections* (1991) covers 230 different diseases. But, if one includes the hundreds of arboviruses and the many sub-varieties of standard diseases, that number soars above 1,000. Until recently, the number of diseases for which case reporting was universally required by the International Health Regulations 1992 was just three (cholera, plague, yellow fever), although, as noted in Benenson (1995, p. xxiv), another five were under surveillance by the WHO (louse-borne typhus fever, relapsing fever, paralytic poliomyelitis, malaria, and influenza). The most recent (2005)

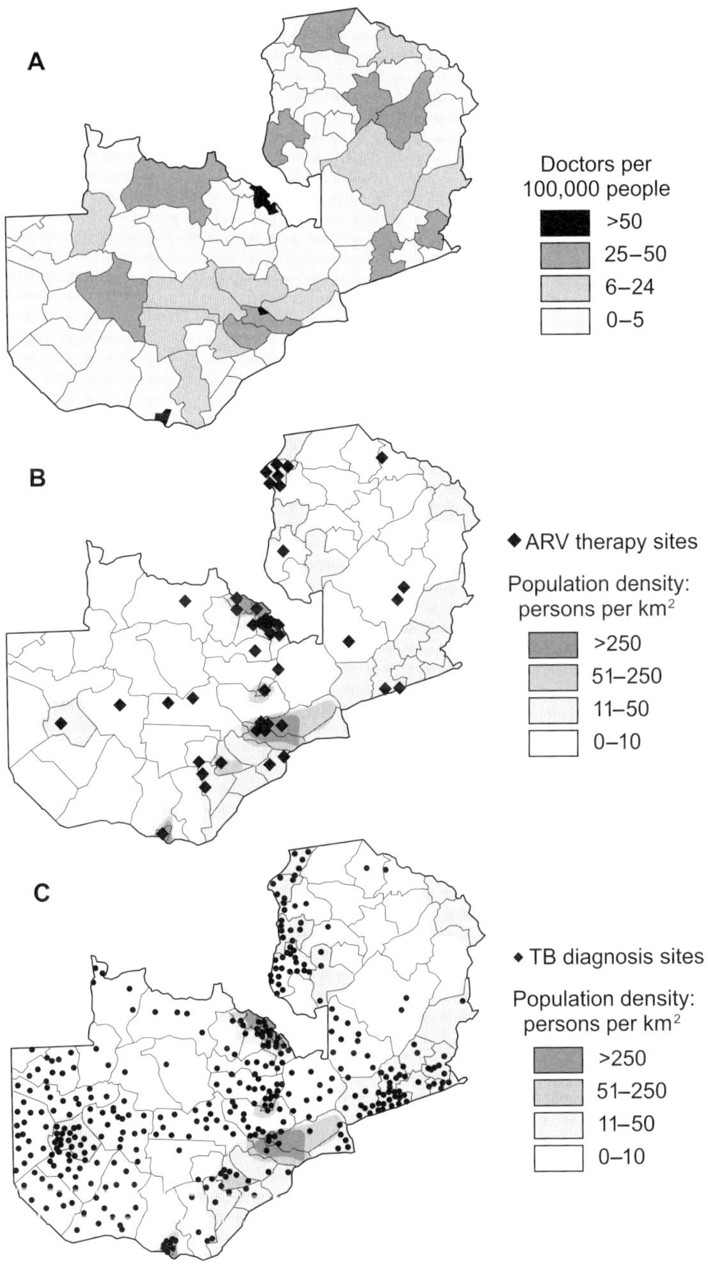

Fig. 11.22. Service availability mapping (SAM) in Zambia, 2004
(A) Number of doctors per 100,000 people. (B) Location of antiretroviral (ARV) therapy sites. (C) Location of sites providing tuberculosis diagnosis.
Source: World Health Organization (2007*g*: 16–17).

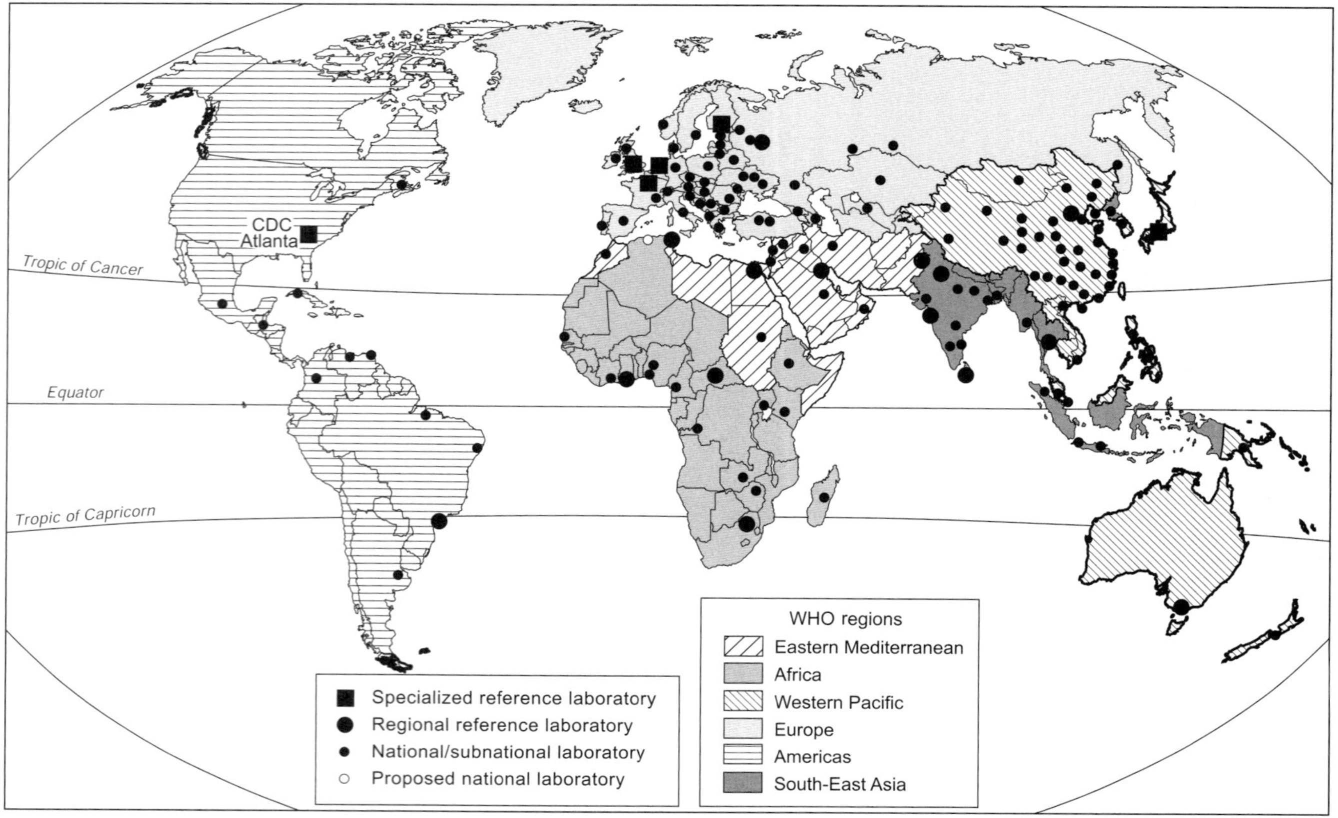

Fig. 11.23. An example of a global laboratory network used by WHO Location of laboratories, 2000, by laboratory type and WHO region.
Source: World Health Organization (2000*a*, map 1, p. 71).

revision of the International Health Regulations has ushered in a new global public health surveillance regime which, as noted in Section 8.5, requires member states to notify the WHO of all events which may constitute a public health emergency of international concern. The reporting requirement covers communicable and non-communicable disease events of natural or intentional origin (Baker and Fidler 2006).

The legal requirements to notify critical infectious diseases are tending to be left behind by the reality of disease proliferation. As a result, regular reporting is increasingly replaced by sampling systems in which sentinel practices are used to pick up trends in disease prevalence (Section 10.6). Some cities have pioneered local monitoring; the Seattle Virus Watch Program is an outstanding example. In the developing world, sentinel surveillance is the only cost-effective way of monitoring population health. As an example, Figure 11.24 maps the HIV sentinel surveillance rates for pregnant women in Botswana, 2002–5.

5. AUTOMATIC MONITORING OF EPIDEMIOLOGICAL RECORDS TO PROVIDE EARLY WARNINGS OF EPIDEMICS

Improvements in computer software now allow continuous scanning of epidemiological reports. There is a need regularly to scan the torrent of international and local data for 'aberrant' behaviour. Historical records provide an insight into 'normal' behaviour and can be modelled mathematically to estimate a benchmark against which newly received data can be checked. Such models are used regularly in the developed nations for influenza monitoring so that early warning of epidemic behaviour can be provided (Choi and Thacker 1981*a*,*b*; Stroup, Wharton, *et al.* 1993). In the less developed world, other diseases are similarly assessed. Figure 11.25 illustrates a West African example. Geographical information systems are employed to define alert and epidemic thresholds for meningitis and to identify districts which, under enhanced surveillance, cross these thresholds—here, during the 2006 meningitis season.

Automatic monitoring of epidemic data allows other anomalous events to be highlighted for the epidemiologist to consider. Figure 11.26 shows a world map of selected subnational disease outbreaks in 2005–6 which were in some sense unexpected; many of these diseases have been discussed earlier in this book. In each case epidemiologists and public health officials are alerted to potential threats.

6. REAL-TIME MAPPING OF DISEASE CAN NOW BE ACHIEVED RAPIDLY USING GIS METHODS

Epidemiological data can now be stored in computer memories together with relevant demographic or environmental information. A Geographical

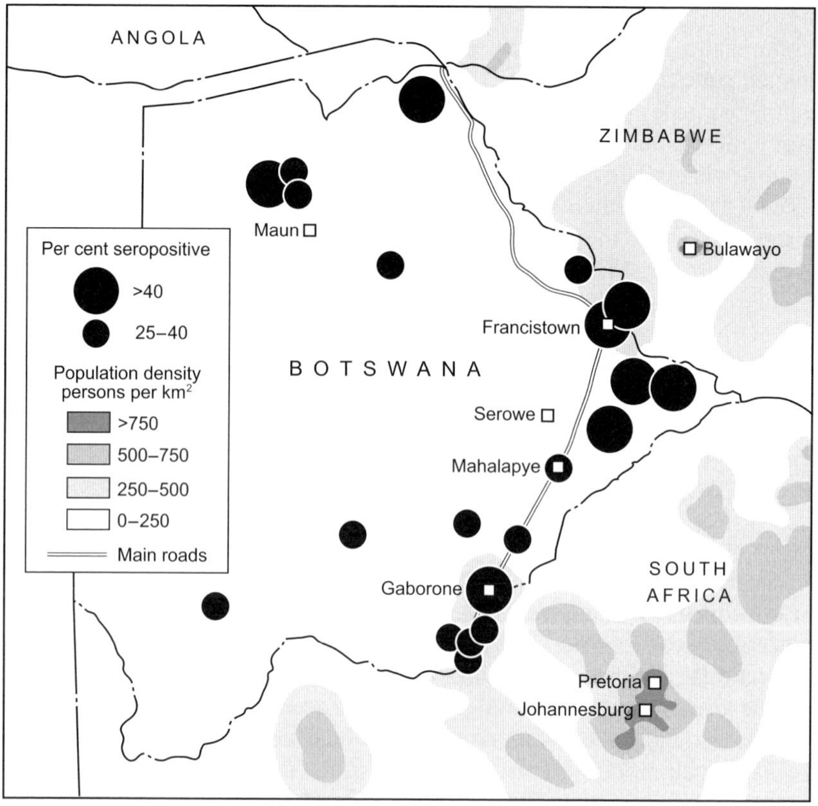

Fig. 11.24. Botswana: HIV sentinel surveillance rates among pregnant women, 2002–2005

Source: World Health Organization (2007*g*: 12).

Information System, or GIS, provides a framework for the display, manipulation, and analysis of such data if the positions of the data points in time and space are known. When applied to disease data, GIS enables the data to be displayed at different spatial scales, often against backcloth maps of associated demographic and environmental variables. Such displays may throw up unrecognized disease clusters or suggest underlying processes for the epidemiologist to investigate. Associations between diseases and their environmental matrix can be rapidly scanned and mapped. Figure 11.27 illustrates this integrated view of disease, environment, and society for the Mexican state of Querétaro. Here, the Pan American Health Organization (PAHO) has used its own GIS-based public health mapping tool, SIGEpi, to identify the populations at highest risk of environmental disasters (earthquakes, floods, land subsidence in relation to oil and gas pipelines). The risk assessment helped to identify poor marginalized populations in 242 settlements in

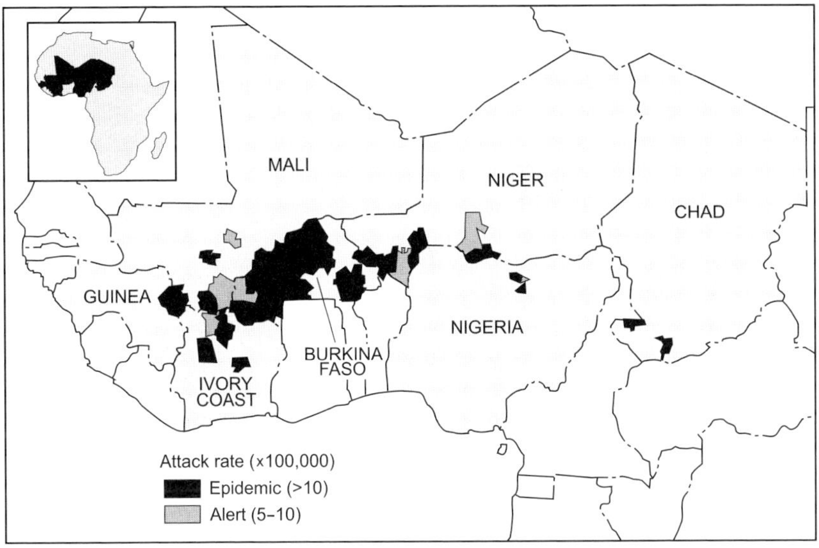

Fig. 11.25. Meningitis in West Africa
Districts identified under enhanced surveillance during the 2006 meningitis epidemic season as crossing the alert (5–10 cases per 100,000 population) and epidemic (≥10 cases per 100,000 population) thresholds defined from historic data.
Source: World Health Organization (2007*g*: 7).

the north-east of the state with low levels of health coverage and the highest exposure to health hazards.

The above six are some of the more important contexts of change against which spatial control of newly emerging and re-emerging diseases is likely to be set. Each century, public health has had to fight disease with the tools available and the constraints imposed at the time. The twenty-first century will be no exception as it prepares to fight both old diseases causing old problems, old diseases causing new problems (for example, drug resistance), as well as wholly new diseases.

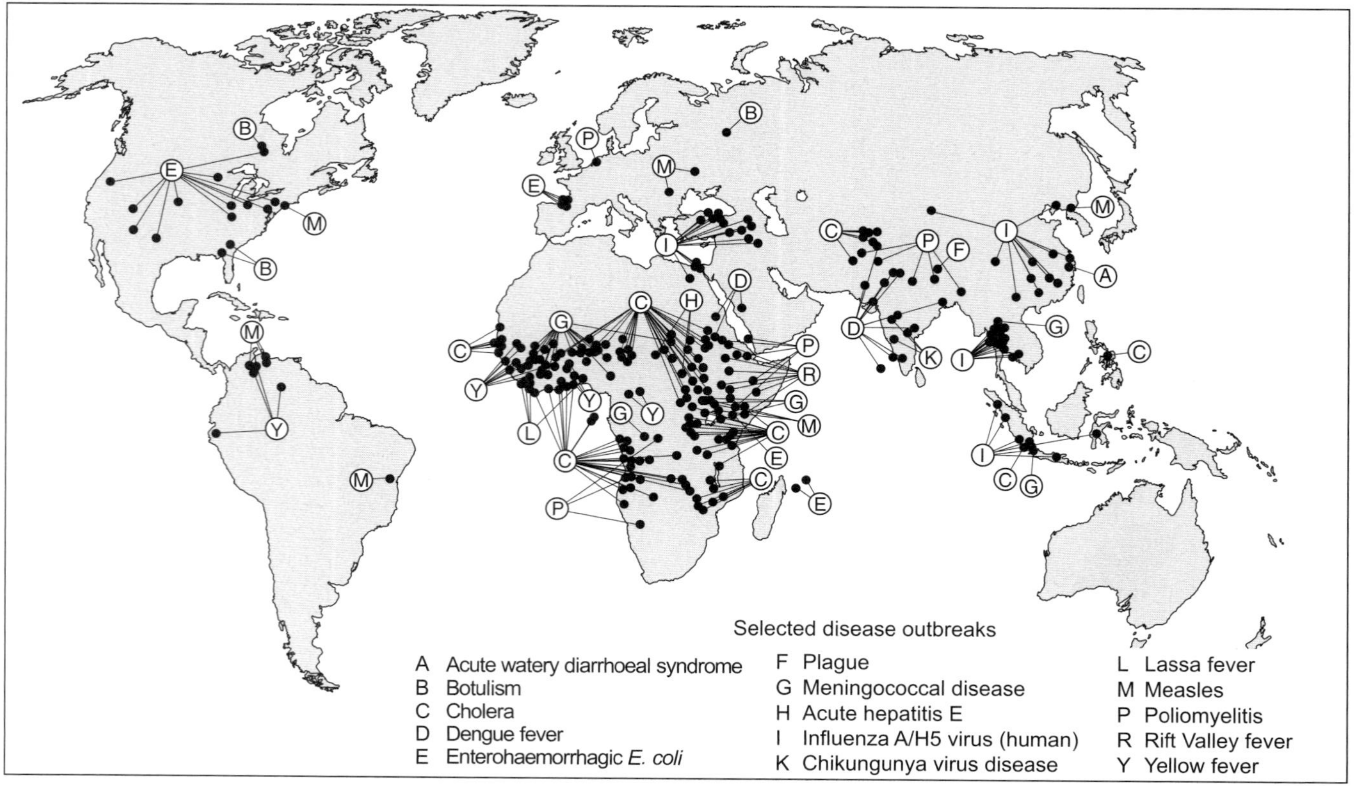

Fig. 11.26. Unexpected disease outbreaks, 2005–2006

Selected disease outbreaks at the subnational level reported to the WHO, June 2005–Dec. 2006. Human cases of highly pathogenic influenza A/H5 are but the latest in a line of unexpected epidemic events.

Source: World Health Organization (2007*g*: 52–3).

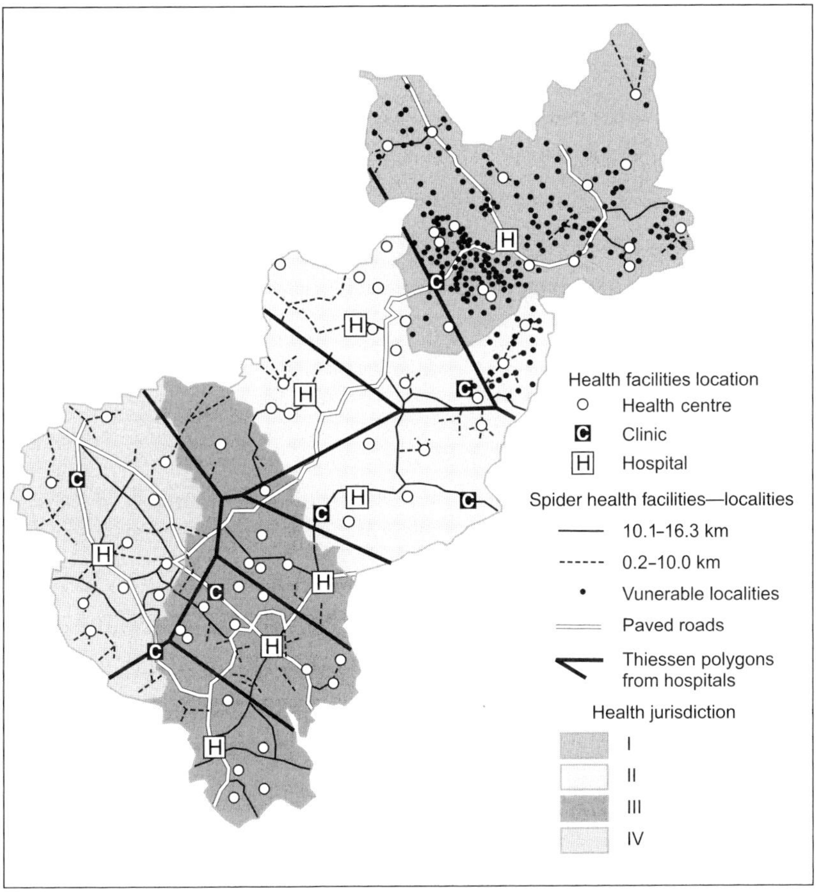

Fig. 11.27. Mapping health risks in Querétaro, Mexico
The Geographical Information System (GIS) maps disease incidence against a backcloth, shown here, in which Thiessen polygons identify the nearest hospital for each community, the location of health centres and clinics, spider facilities (outreach extents from health centres), paved roads, and vulnerable localities.
Source: World Health Organization (2007*g*: 10).

Appendix 11.1: Map Sources

This appendix gives the sources of the maps used in Section 11.2.1. The item numbers correspond with the key map shown in Figure 11.6. All plates with sources cross-referenced to this appendix have been reproduced by kind permission of the directors of the state archives and libraries cited.

Venice

Archivio di Stato di Venezia (ASV)

1. Giacomo Binard

Mappa del territorio del basso Friuli compreso tra Palma la linea formata dal- l'Iudri, il Torre e l'Isonzo e Cervignano, con l'indicazione delle postazioni sanitarie. 4 marzo in Udine; scala di miglia 3 = mm 30; dim mm 940 × 650. Disegno a mano, su carta, con colorazioni ad acquarello. ASV. Provveditori alla Sanità, Disegni, B2N8.

2. Iacopo Spinelli

Mappa con parte del corso del fiume Natisone e tracciate le postazioni di guardia al confine tra il Friuli e la Schiavonia veneta in caso di epidemie. 1714; scala di miglia = mm 90; dim mm 1,025 × 720. Disegno a mano, su carta, con colorazioni ad acquarello. ASV. Provveditori alla Sanità, Disegni, B3N12.

3. Tommaso Pedrinelli

Mappa comprendente parte del territorio Vicentino dei Settecommni e Bassanese al cinfine con il Trentino e con l'indicazione dei posti e guardie sanitarie. 28 febbraio 1739, Bassano; scala di miglia italiane 5 = mm 155; dim mm 1,140 × 975. Disegno a mano, su carta, con colorazioni ad acquarello. ASV. Provveditori alla Sanità, Disegni, B3N16.

4. P. Giuseppe di San Francesco

Mappa con la linea di confine tra l'Istria veneta ed il territorio austriaco e gli appostamenti sanitari posti da Zaule, territorio di Muia e Fiauona, territorio d'Albona. 1712; scala di miglia italiane 5 = mm 162; dim mm 1,230 × 1,305. Disegno a mano, su carta, con colorazioni ad acquarello. ASV. Provveditori alla Sanità, Disegni, B1N16.

5. Pietro Soranzo

Mappa del territorio di Imoschi (Dalmazia veneta) confine con l'Impero Ottomano, con il territorio Sign, di Duare e di Vergoraz ed i caselli ed appostamenti sanitari. 18 novembre 1783; scala passi veneti 2400 = mm 130; dim mm 1,570 × 765. Disegno a mano, su carta, con colorazioni ad acquarello. ASV. Provveditori alla Sanità, Disegni, B4N21.

6. Giacomo Pellegrini

Mappa con il litorale di Monfalcone da Porto Anfora al castello di Duino e con l'indicazioni dei posti di guardia sanitari al confine con gli arciducali. 13 novembre 1713, Monfalcone; scala miglia Quattro = mm 140; dim mm 1,430 × 675. Disegno a mano, su carta di più pezzi uniti insieme e riforzati con tela, con colorazioni ad acquerello. ASV. Provveditori alla Sanità, Disegni, B1N3.

7. Unknown
Colognese (territorio)
Mappa del territorio colognese, al confine con le province di Padova e Vicenza, con i castelli e le separazioni stabilite dal Provv. Gen. in T.F. in occasione di una epidemia bovina. 10 guigno 1747; dim mm 420 × 340. Disegno a mano, su carta, con colorazioni ad acquarello. ASV. Provveditori alla Sanità, Disegni, B4N19.

8. Gio. Giacomo pellegrini
Monfalcone (territorio)
Mappa del territorio di Monfalcone compreso tra il lago di Pietra Rossa e il corso del fiume Isonzo con l'indicazione delle ville, posti e caselli di guardia sanitari al confine con il granducale. 1713; di miglia due = mm 123; dim mm 1,400 × 700. Disegno a mano, su carta, di due pezzi uniti insieme rinforzati con tela, con colorazioni ad acquarello. ASV. Provveditori alla Sanità, Disegni, B5N26.

9. Bartolo Riviera
Friuli
Disegni con raffigurati gli appostamenti di cavalleria e di fanteria creati ai confini del Friuli in occasione di epidemie. (Att. Linea di confine per contaggio dei Bovini fatta nel Friuli—87). Sec. 18; dim mm 1,040 × 395. Disegno a mano, su carta di due pezzi uniti insieme, con colorazioni ad acquarello. ASV. Provveditori alla Sanità, Disegni, B5N27.

10. Gio Batta Cavalcaselle
Veronese (territorio)
Mappa con parte del territorio veronese al confine con il mantovano e il ferrarese e con la descrizione di vari caselli sanitari. Sec 18; scala di miglia di circa = mm 125; mm 958 × 730. Disegno a mano, su carta rinforzata su tela con colorazioni ad acquarello. ASV. Provveditori alla Sanità, Disegni, B5N29.

11. Unknown
Budua (territorio di)
Mappa comprendente un tratto di mare tra Porto Rose e Castel di Lastva ed i territori di Cattaro Zupa, Budua, Maini e Pastroviech con l'indicazione dei posti di confine. Sec 18; dim mm 785 × 580. Disegno a mano, su carta di due pezzi uniti insieme e rinforzata con tela, con colorazioni ad acquarello. ASV. Provveditori alla Sanità, Disegni, B6N34.

12. Vicenzo Bernardi
Adige (fiume)
Parte del corso del fiume Adige all'altezza di Ossevigo in territorio veronese, con l'indicazione degli appostamenti al confine, lungo la strada postale. Sec 18; scala pertiche veronesi 100 = mm 180; dim mm 1,260 × 720. Disegno a mano, su carta di più pezzi uniti insieme, con colorazioni ad acquarello. ASV. Provveditori alla Sanità, Disegni, B7N43.

Genoa
Biblioteca Civica Berio
13. Matteo Vinzoni
Piante delle due Riviere della Serenissima Repubblica di Genova. Divise Ne. Commissariati di Sanita. Cavate Dal M. Col. Ing. Matteo Vinzoni. Per Ordine Dell' Ill Mag. di

Sanita. 1758; mm 528 × 355; cc. 119 complessive, num nel sec XVIII per pagg 230 (escluso il foglio di guardia ant. e il front.). Mostra di manoscritti e libri rari della Biblioteca Civica Berio, Genova.

Holy See
Archivio di Stato di Roma (ASR)
14. Gaspare Grassellini
Carta topografica sanitaria del littorale del Mediterraneo nello Stato Pontificio dal confine del Gran Ducato di Toscana quello del Regno di Napoli nel rapporto di 1 a 1000000. Compilata nel Dicastero Generale del Censo essendo Pro Presidente sua eccnza RMA Monsignor Gaspare Grassellini per uso della Congregazione Generale di Sanità. 9 decembre 1843. Scala 1:100,000; dim mm 2,790 × 415; disegno a penna su carta, colorato. ASR. Disegni, Coll I cart 106f, 215.

15. Giuseppe Vaselli
Topografica del Littorale Pontificio, nell' Adriatico, e del confine terrestre col Regno di Napoli portante l'armamento del cordone sanitario, ripartito in quattro Divisioni (Stato generale della forza impiegata dell' Adriatico, e confine col Regno di Napoli). Ancona, marzo 1816. dim mm 550 × 1,580; disegno a penna su carta, colorato. ASR. Disegni, Coll I cart 106f, 218.

Tuscany
Archivio di Stato di Firenze (ASF)
16. Unknown
Livorno (torri costiere)
Piano specificazione e stato delle Torri e Posti che sono situati sul Lido del Mare da Livorno fino a Torre Nuova, aumentati in occasione della contumacia della Città di Messina dell'anno MDCC XLIII (1743). 1743. Scala di miglia italiane 10 = mm 215; dim mm 435 × 1,385; disegno a penna su carta, colorato. ASF. Miscellanea di piante 5/20, 38.

17. P. Giovanni Fabbroni
Toscana (torri costiere)
Pianta della costa del Mare Toscano guarnita con tutte le sue Torri e Casotti fatta in occasione della Peste di Messina l'anno MDCCXXXXIII principiando dalla Torre del Cinquale fino alla Torre di Cala del Forno che confina con lo Stato di Orbetello. 1754. Scala di miglia 6 = mm 76; dim mm 770 × 2,110; disegno à penna su carta telata, colorato. ASF. Disegni, Miscellanea di piante 5/20, 258.

Naples
Archivio di Stato di Napoli (ASN)
18. Augustin de Bargas Machuco
Lecce
Piano dimostrativo della marina di Lecce e del suo cordone marittimo. 1743. Scala di miglia quindici italiane pari a mm 95; dim mm 355 × 485 (350 × 480); disegno a inchiostro acquerellato. Segreteria di Stato d'Azienda, fs. 253, fascic. 20.

19. Soprintendenza Generale della Salute
Lecce, Chianca di
Pianta delle baracche e rastelli fatti costruire per la custodia dei Turchi naufragati nella marina della torre della Chianca di Lecce. 1743. Scala di palmi 200 pari a mm 110; dim

mm 415 × 285 (385 × 265); disegno a inchiostro acquerellato. Segreteria di Stato d'Azienda, fs. 252, fascic. 38.

20. Vicari Generali (Vicars General)
Messina, 1743
Relazione topografica dell' intèro cordone, commandato dalli 3: Vica[j] Gener[i] il quale hà li suoi termini nelli due mari di Milazzo, e Taormina che per linea retta saria miglia so mà per tortuosa come al pres ritrouasi si estende a miglia. Dim mm 910 × 920; disegno a inchiostro acquerellato. Piante e disegni, busta XXXIII, 8.

Palermo
Archivio di Stato di Palermo (ASP)
21. Alì Innocenzo: Ministero e Real Segreteria di Stato Presso il Luotenente Generale in Sicilia, Ripartiment Lavori Pubblica
Pianta topografica del littorale della valle di Siracusa distinto nei littorali rispettivi di ogni comune e con l'indicazione dei posti di cordone sanitario terrestre. Siracusa 30 April 1837. Miglia siciliani; dim mm 920 × 1,310; disegno a penna su carta, colorato.

Bari
Wellcome Trust Medical Photographic Library, London
22. F. de Arrieta
Raguaglio historico del contaggio occorso nella provincial di Bari negli anni 1690, 1691, *e* 1692. (Naples, Parrino, and Mucii, 1694). 324 × 180 mm. Scale ≈1:500,000. The map is on p. 183.

University of Bologna
Library of the University of Bologna
23. L. F. Marsili
Mappa geographica, qua praecautio contra pestem post factam locorum, juxta pacis instrumentum, evacuationem ac demolitonem in confinibusistis Cis Danubialibus instituenda ostenditur. See L. Frati (1928). *Catalogo dei Manoscritti di Luigi Ferdinando Marsili Conservati nella Biblioteca Universitaria di Bologna*, p. 213, entry 25 (Firenze: Olschki). A manuscript map prepared by or for Marsili and dated April, 1700. Dimensions: mm 224 × 130, Scale ≈1:500,000.

Appendix 11.2: Vaccination and Critical Community Size

The minimum population size of a community required to sustain an infectious disease endemically is called the *critical community size*. For measles, this is conventionally taken as *c*.250,000 in an unvaccinated population; see Bartlett (1957, 1960*b*), Black (1966), and Schenzle and Dietz (1987). Griffiths (1973) has studied the impact of vaccination upon the critical community size. To follow his arguments, we define the following terms:

S = the number of individuals susceptible to the measles virus;

I = the number of individuals actively infective with measles;

ν = the birth rate;

λ = the infection rate;

μ = the recovery rate.

In the absence of vaccination, equilibrium is achieved when $S = \mu/\lambda = n$, and $I = \nu/\mu = m$, and the expected time, T, to the fade-out of infection, with $n \gg m$, is given by

$$T(m,n) \sim \frac{(2\pi n)^{1/2}}{\mu m} \exp\left\{ \frac{\left(m + \frac{n}{m}\right)^2}{2n} \right\}. \tag{11.A1}$$

Now suppose that a proportion $(1-x)$ of people is vaccinated each quarter. Then $m' = xm$ is the number of people infective post-vaccination and $n' = n$ is the number of people susceptible post-vaccination. This causes a change in the fade-out time, T, such that

$$T(m,n) \rightarrow T(m',n') = T(xm,n) \sim T\left(m, n/x^2\right). \tag{11.A2}$$

Thus, the effect on the critical community size is to multiply it by a factor of $1/x^2$.

References

Numbers in square brackets after references indicate the sections in the text where the item is cited.

A

Abramson, G., Kenkre, V. M., Yates, T. L., and Parmenter, R. R. (2003). 'Travelling waves of infections in the Hantavirus epidemics'. *Bulletin of Mathematical Biology*, 65: 519–34. [10.2.1]

Acuna-Soto, R., Romero, L. C., and Maguire, J. H. (2000). 'Large epidemics of hemorrhagic fevers in Mexico 1545–1815'. *American Journal of Tropical Medicine and Hygiene*, 62: 733–9. [2.3.5]

—— Stahle, D. W., Cleaveland, M. K., and Therrell, M. D. (2002). 'Megadrought and megadeath in 16th century Mexico'. *Emerging Infectious Diseases*, 8: 360–2. [2.3.5]

—— —— —— Griffin, R. D., and Cleaveland, M. K. (2004). 'When half the population died: The epidemic of hemorrhagic fevers of 1576 in Mexico'. *FEMS Microbiology Letters*, 240: 1–5. [2.3.5]

—— —— Therrell, M. D., Chavez, S. G., and Cleaveland, M. K. (2005). 'Drought, epidemic disease, and the fall of classic period cultures in Mesoamerica (AD 750–950). Hemorrhagic fevers as a cause of massive population loss'. *Medical Hypotheses*, 65: 405–9. [2.3.5]

Adams, M. S., Croft, A. M., Winfield, D. A., and Richards, R. (1997). 'An outbreak of rubella in British troops in Bosnia'. *Epidemiology and Infection*, 118: 253–7. [8.4.3]

Adamson, B. (1980). 'Death from disease in Ancient Mesopotamia'. In B. Alster (ed.), *Death in Mesopotamia: Papers Read at the XXVIe Rencontre Assyriologique Internationale*. Copenhagen: Akademisk Forlag, 187. [2.2]

Agri-Food and Veterinary Authority (2008). *'Poultry is safe for consumption' Poster for Supermarkets and Hawkers*. Singapore: AVA. http://www.ava.gov.sg, accessed 21 July 2008. [4.2.4]

Aguilera, J.-F., Perrocheau, A., Meffre, C., Hahné, S., and the W135 Working Group (2002). 'Outbreak of serogroup W135 meningococcal disease after the Hajj pilgrimage, Europe, 2000'. *Emerging Infectious Diseases*, 8: 761–7. [6.5.2]

Ahern, M., Kovats, R. S., Wilkinson, P., Few, R., and Matthies, F. (2005). 'Global health impacts of floods: Epidemiologic evidence'. *Epidemiologic Reviews*, 27: 36–46. [7.6.3]

Ahmad, K. (2002). 'Norwalk like virus attacks troops in Afghanistan'. *Lancet Infectious Diseases*, 2: 391. [8.4.2]

Alderson, M. (1981). *International Mortality Statistics*. London: Macmillian. [9.3, 9.3.1]

Alexander, D. (1997). 'The study of natural disasters, 1977–1997: Some reflections on a changing field of knowledge'. *Disasters*, 21: 284–304. [7.6]

Allison, M. J. (1993). 'Leishmaniasis'. In K. F. Kiple (ed.), *The Cambridge World History of Human Disease*. Cambridge: Cambridge University Press, 832–4. [8.4.1]

Allukian, M. and Atwood, L. (1997). 'Public health and the Vietnam War'. In B. S. Levy and V. W. Sidel (eds), *War and Public Health*. Oxford: Oxford University Press, 215–37. [8.2.2]

Alvarado de la Barrera, C. and Reyes-Terán, G. (2005). 'Influenza: Forecast for a pandemic'. *Archives of Medical Research*, 36: 628–36. [4.2.4]

Amábile-Cuevas, C. F. (ed.) (2007). *Antimicrobial Resistance in Bacteria*. Wymondham: Horizon Bioscience. [4.3.1]

Ambrosio, A. M., Saavedra, M. del C., Riera, L. M., and Fassio, R. M. (2006). 'La producción nacional de vacuna a virus Junín vivo atenuado (Candid #1) anti-fiebre hemorrágica Argentina'. ['The national production of a live attenuated Junín virus vaccine (Candid #1) anti-Argentine haemorrhagic fever']. *Acta Bioquímica Clínica Latinoamericana*, 40: 5–17. [7.2.1]

Anderson, A. D., Garrett, V. D., Sobel, J., Monroe, S. S., Fankhauser, R. L., Schwab, K. J., Bresee, J. S., Mead, P. S., Higgins, C., Campana, J., Glass, R. I., and the Outbreak Investigation Team (2001). 'Multistate outbreak of Norwalk-like virus gastroenteritis associated with a common caterer'. *American Journal of Epidemiology*, 154: 1013–19. [5.2.3]

Anderson, R. M. and May, R. (1991). *Infectious Diseases of Humans: Dynamics and Control*. Oxford: Oxford University Press. [4.4.1, 10.2]

—— Donnelly, C. A., Ferguson, N. M., Woolhouse, M. E. J., Watt, C. J., Udy, H. J., MaWhinney, S., Dunstan, S. P., Southwood, T. R. E., Wilesmith, J. W., Ryan, J. B. M., Hoinville, L. J., Hillerton, J. E., Austin, A. R., and Wells, G. A. H. (1996). 'Transmission dynamics and epidemiology of BSE in British cattle'. *Nature*, 382: 779–88. [5.2.5]

Anonymous (1894). '*A History of Epidemics in Britain*. By Charles Creighton, M.A., M.D., *Vol. II. From the Extinction of the Plague to the Present Time*'. *Lancet*, 2: 1541–3. [2.4.1]

Anonymous (1953). 'Government services'. *Journal of the American Medical Association*, 152: 1448–50. [8.2.1]

Anyamba, A., Chretien, J.-P., Small, J., Tucker, C. J., and Linthicum, K. J. (2006). 'Developing global climate anomalies suggest potential disease risks for 2006–2007'. *International Journal of Health Geographics*, 5/60. doi:10.1186/1476-072X-5-60. [7.5.2]

Appleby, A. B. (1980). 'The disappearance of plague: A continuing puzzle'. *Economic History Review*, 33: 161–73. [2.3.2]

Aronson, N. E., Sanders, J. W., and Moran, K. A. (2006). 'In harm's way: Infections in deployed American military forces'. *Clinical Infectious Diseases*, 43: 1045–51. [8.4.2]

Arribalzaga, R. A. (1955). 'Una nueva enfermedad a gérman desconocido: Hipertermia nefrotóxica, leucopénica y enantemántica'. ['New epidemic disease due to unidentified germ: Nephrotoxic, leukopenic and enanthematous hyperthermia']. *El Día Médico*, 27: 1204–10. [7.2.1]

Arthur, R. R., El-Sharkawy, M. S., Cope, S. E., Botros, B. A., Oun, S., Mourill, J. C., Shope, R. E., Hibbs, R. G., Darwish, M. A., and Imam, I. Z. E. (1993). 'Recurrence of Rift Valley fever in Egypt'. *Lancet*, 342: 1149–50. [7.3.1]

ASNIS, D. S., CONETTA, R., TEIXEIRA, A. A., WALDMAN, G., and SAMPSON, B. A. (2000). 'The West Nile virus outbreak of 1999 in New York: The Flushing Hospital experience'. *Clinical Infectious Diseases*, 30: 413–18. [6.5.3]

AUFDERHEIDE, A. C., SALO, W., MADDEN, M., STEITZ, J., BUIKSTRA, J., GUHL, F., ARRIAZA, B., RENIER, C., WITTMERS, L. E., FORNACIARI, G., and ALLISON, M. (2004). 'A 9,000-year record of Chagas' disease'. *Proceedings of the National Academy of Sciences USA*, 101: 2034–9. [1.3.3]

B

BAILEY, M. S., BOOS, C. J., VAUTIER, G., GREEN, A. D., APPLETON, H., GALLIMORE, C. I., GRAY, J. J., and BEECHING, N. J. (2005). 'Gastroenteritis outbreak in British troops, Iraq'. *Emerging Infectious Diseases*, 11: 1625–8. [8.4.2]

BAILEY, N. T. J. (1975). *The Mathematical Theory of Infectious Diseases*. London: Griffin. [10.2]

BAKER, E. L., MELIUS, J. M., and MILLAR, J. D. (1988) 'Surveillance of occupational illness and injury in the United States'. *Journal of Public Health Policy*, 9: 198–221. [10.6.1]

BAKER, M. G. and FIDLER, D. P. (2006). 'Global public health surveillance under new International Health Regulations'. *Emerging Infectious Diseases*, 12: 1058–65. [11.4]

BALMER, B. (2002). 'Biological warfare: The threat in historical perspective'. *Medicine, Conflict and Survival*, 18: 120–37. [8.5.2]

BANGS, M. and SUBIANTO, D. B. (1999). 'El Niño and associated outbreaks of severe malaria in highland populations in Irian Jaya, Indonesia: A review and epidemiological perspective'. *Southeast Asian Journal of Tropical Medicine and Public Health*, 30: 608–19. [7.5.2]

BANNISTER, B. A. (ed.) (1991). *Report of a Think Tank on the Potential Effects of Global Warming and Population Increase on the Epidemiology of Infectious Diseases*. Colindale: Public Health Laboratory Service. [7.5.1]

BARBERA, J., MACINTYRE, A., GOSTIN, L., INGLESBY, T., O'TOOLE, T., DEATLEY, C., TONAT, K., and LAYTON, M. (2001). 'Large scale quarantine following biological terrorism in the United States'. *Journal of the American Medical Association*, 286, 2711–17. [11.2.3]

BARBOUR, A. G. and FISH, D. (1993). 'The biological and social phenomenon of Lyme disease'. *Science*, 260: 1610–16. [7.4.2]

BARRAT, A., BARTHÉLEMY, M., and VESPIGNANI, A. (2004). 'Modeling the evolution of weighted networks'. *Physical Review*, E70. doi:10.1103/PhysRevE.70.066149. [6.4.2]

BARRETT, O., SKRZYPEK, G., DATEL, D., and GOLDSTEIN, J. D. (1969). 'Malaria imported to the United States from Vietnam: Chemoprophylaxis evaluated in returning soldiers'. *American Journal of Tropical Medicine and Hygiene*, 18: 495–9. [8.2.2]

BARTLETT, M. S. (1957). 'Measles periodicity and community size'. *Journal of the Royal Statistical Society A*, 120: 48–70. [6.2.1, 10.2.1, App. 11.2]

—— (1960*a*). 'The critical community size of measles in the United States'. *Journal of the Royal Statistical Society A*, 123: 37–44. [6.2.1]

Bartlett, M. S. (1960*b*). *Stochastic Population Models.* Andover: Methuen. [App. 11.2]

Barua, D. (1992). 'History of cholera'. In D. Barua and W. B. Greenough (eds), *Cholera.* New York: Plenum, 1–36. [2.3.4, 9.2, 9.2.1, 9.2.2, 9.3.2]

—— and Greenough, W. B. (1992). *Cholera.* New York: Plenum. [2.3.4, 9.2.2]

Baxter, R., Rubin, R., Steinberg, C., Carroll, C., Shapiro, J., and Yang, A. (2000). *Assessing Core Capacity for Infectious Disease Surveillance.* Final Report. Prepared for the Office of the Assistant Secretary for Planning and Evaluation, US Department of Health and Human Services. Falls Church, Va.: Lewin Group [10.6.3]

Beadle, C. and Hoffman, S. L. (1993). 'History of malaria in the United States naval forces at war: World War I through the Vietnam conflict'. *Clinical Infectious Diseases*, 16: 320–9. [8.2.2]

Beaman, M. H. (1997). 'Emerging infections in Australia'. *Annals of the Academy of Medicine, Singapore*, 26: 609–15. [9.4.2]

Benach, J. L., Bosler, E. M., Hanrahan, J. P., Coleman, J. L., Habicht, G. S., Bast, T. F., Cameron, D. J., Ziegler, J. L., Barbour, A. G., Burgdorfer, W., Edelman, R., and Kaslow, R. A. (1983). 'Spirochetes isolated from the blood of two patients with Lyme disease'. *New England Journal of Medicine*, 308: 740–2. [7.4.2]

Benenson, A. S. (ed.) (1995). *Control of Communicable Diseases in Man.* Washington, DC: American Public Health Association. [11.4]

Benin, A. L., Benson, R. F., and Besser, R. E. (2002). 'Trends in Legionnaires' disease, 1980–1998: Declining mortality and new patterns of diagnosis'. *Clinical Infectious Diseases*, 35: 1039–46. [5.3.3]

Beović, B. (2006). 'The issue of antimicrobial resistance in human medicine'. *International Journal of Food Microbiology*, 112: 280–7. [4.3.1]

Berrang Ford, L. B. (2007). 'Civil conflict and sleeping sickness in Africa in general and Uganda in particular'. *Conflict and Health*, 1/6. doi:10.1186/1752–1505–1–6, accessed 5 Feb. 2008. [8.1, 8.4]

Beuchat, L. R. and Ryu, J.-H. (1997). 'Produce handling and processing practices'. *Emerging Infectious Diseases*, 3: 459–65. [5.2.1]

Bhattacharya, S., Sharma, C., Dhiman, R. C., and Mitra, A. P. (2006). 'Climate change and malaria in India'. *Current Science*, 90: 369–75. [7.5.1]

Binson, G. (1936). *État sanitaire des grandes lignes aériennes mondiales et convention sanitation international pour la navigation aérienne.* Lyon: Berthod. [6.5.3]

Biraben, J. N. (1975–6). *Les Hommes et la peste en France et dans les pays européens et Méditerranéens.* Paris: Mouton. [11.2.1]

Bise, G. and Coninx, R. (1997). 'Epidemic typhus in a prison in Burundi'. *Transactions of the Royal Society of Tropical Medicine and Hygiene*, 91: 133–4. [8.3.1]

Black, F. L. (1966). 'Measles endemicity in insular populations: Critical community size and its evolutionary implication'. *Journal of Theoretical Biology*, 11: 207–11. [10.2.1, App. 11.2]

Black, J. (2000). *War: Past, Present and Future.* Stroud: Sutton. [8.4]

Blume, S. and Geesink, I. (2000). 'A brief history of polio vaccines'. *Science*, 288: 1593–4. [11.3.1]

Boccia, D., Guthmann, J.-P., Klovstad, H., Hamid, N., Tatay, M., Ciglenecki, I., Nizou, J.-Y., Nicand, E., and Guerin, P. J. (2006). 'High mortality associated with an outbreak of hepatitis E among displaced persons in Darfur, Sudan'. *Clinical Infectious Diseases*, 42: 1679–84. [8.4.1]

BOUMA, M. J. and DYE, C. (1997). 'Cycles of malaria associated with El Niño in Venezuela'. *Journal of the American Medical Association*, 278: 1772–4. [7.5.2]

—— —— and VAN DER KAAY, H. J. (1996). 'Falciparum malaria and climate change in the Northwest Frontier Province of Pakistan'. *American Journal of Tropical Medicine and Hygiene*, 55: 131–7. [7.5.2]

BOX, G. E. P., JENKINS, G. M., and REINSEL, G. C. (1994). *Time Series Analysis: Forecasting and Control*, 3rd edn. Upper Saddle River, NJ: Prentice-Hall International. [2.4.2, 7.5.3]

BRADEN, C. R. and TAUXE, R. V. (2006). 'Surveillance for emerging pathogens in the United States'. In Y. Motarjemi and M. Adams (eds) (2006). *Emerging Foodborne Pathogens*. Cambridge: Woodhead, 23–49. [5.2.3]

BRADLEY, D. J. (1989). 'The scope of travel medicine'. In R. Steffen (ed.), *Travel Medicine: Proceedings of the First Conference on International Travel Medicine*. Berlin: Springer Verlag, 1–9. [6.4.1, 6.5.1]

BREED, A., FIELD, H., and PLOWRIGHT, R. (2005). 'Volant viruses: A concern to bats, humans and other animals'. *Microbiology Australia*, 26: 59–62. [9.4.2]

BREIMAN, R. F. (1996). 'Impact of technology on the emergence of infectious diseases'. *Epidemiologic Reviews*, 18: 4–9. [5.1, 5.3.2]

BREUER, T., BENKEL, D. H., SHAPIRO, R. L., HALL, W. N., WINNETT, M. M., LINN, M. J., NEIMANN, J., BARRETT, T. J., DIETRICH, S., DOWNES, F. P., TONEY, D. M., PEARSON, J. L., ROLKA, H., SLUTSKER, L., GRIFFIN, P. M., and the Investigation Team (2001). 'A multistate outbreak of *Escherichia coli* O157:H7 infections linked to alfalfa sprouts grown from contaminated seeds'. *Emerging Infectious Diseases*, 7: 977–82. [5.2.3]

BRIDGES, J. R. (1973). 'A study of malaria rates in the Que Son Mountains of Vietnam'. *Military Medicine*, 138: 413–17. [8.2.2]

BRITISH BROADCASTING CORPORATION (2002). 'Food safety given thumbs up'. London: BBC. http://news.bbc.co.uk/1/hi/scotland/2561269.stm, accessed 21 July 2008. [5.2.4]

BROCK, T. D. (ed.) (1990). *Microorganisms: From smallpox to Lyme disease*. New York: Freeman. [2.3.2, 5.3.3]

BROGDON, W. G. and MCALLISTER, J. C. (1998). 'Insecticide resistance and vector control'. *Emerging Infectious Diseases*, 4: 605–13. [4.4.1, 4.5]

BROOKMEYER, R. and STROUP, D. F. (eds) (2003). *Monitoring the Health of Populations: Statistical Principles and Methods of Public Health Surveillance*. New York: Oxford University Press. [10.6.1]

BROOME, C. V. and LOONSK, J. W. (2003). 'A standards-based approach to integrated information systems for bioterrorism preparedness and response'. US Department of Health and Human Services Data Council Meeting, February 13, 2003. Atlanta, Georgia: CDC. [10.6.3]

—— GOINGS, S. A. J., THACKER, S. B., VOGT, R. L., BEATTY, H. N., FRASER, D. W., and the Field Investigation Team (1979). 'The Vermont epidemic of Legionnaires' disease'. *Annals of Internal Medicine*, 90: 573–7. [5.3.3]

—— HORTON, H. H., TRESS, D., LUCIDO, S. J., and KOO, D. (2003). 'Statutory basis for public health reporting beyond specific diseases'. *Journal of Urban Health*, 80, suppl. 1, 14–22. [10.6.3]

BROWN, D., BALLUZ, L., GILES, W., BECKLES, G., MORIARTY, D., FORD, E., and MOKDAD, A. (2004). 'Diabetes mellitus and health-related quality of life among older adults'. *Diabetes Research and Clinical Practice*, 65: 105–15. [10.6.2]

BROWN, P., WILL, R. G., BRADLEY, R., ASHER, D. M., and DETWILER, L. (2001). 'Bovine spongiform encephalopathy and variant Creutzfeldt–Jakob disease: Background, evolution and current concerns'. *Emerging Infectious Diseases*, 7: 6–16. [5.2.5]

BROWN, V., REILLEY, B., FERRIR, M.-C., GABALDON, J., and MANONCOURT, S. (1997). 'Cholera outbreak during massive influx of Rwandan returnees in November, 1996'. *Lancet*, 349: 212. [8.3.2]

BROWNSTEIN, J. S., WOLFE, C. J., and MANDL, K. D. (2006). 'Empirical evidence for the effect of airline travel on inter-regional influenza spread in the United States'. *PLoS Medicine*, 3/10: e401. doi:10.1371/journal.pmed.0030401. [6.4.3]

BRUCE-CHWATT, L. J. (1987). 'Malaria and its control: Present situation and future prospects'. *Annual Review of Public Health*, 8: 75–110. [4.4.3]

BRYANT, G. and MONK, P. (2001). *Summary of the Final Report of the Investigation into the North Leicestershire Cluster of Variant Creutzfeldt–Jakob Disease*. Leicester: Leicestershire NHS Health Authority. [5.2.5]

BURGDORFER, W., BARBOUR, A. G., HAYES, S. F., BENACH, J. L., GRUNWALDT, E., and DAVIS, J. P. (1982). 'Lyme disease—A tickborne spirochetosis?' *Science*, 216: 1319–20. [7.4.2]

BURNET, F. M. (1945). *Virus as Organism: Evolutionary and Ecological Aspects of Some Human Virus Diseases*. Cambridge, Mass.: Harvard University Press. [1.3]

—— (1979). 'Portraits of viruses: Influenza virus A'. *Intervirology*, 11: 201–14. [4.2.2]

—— and WHITE, D. O. (1972). *Natural History of Infectious Disease*, 4th edn. Cambridge: Cambridge University Press. [1.3]

BURNHAM, G., LAFTA, R., DOOCY, S., and ROBERTS, L. (2006). 'Mortality after the 2003 invasion of Iraq: A cross-sectional cluster sample survey'. *Lancet*, 368: 1421–8. [8.4.2]

BURR, T., GRAVES, T., KLAMANN, R., MICHALAK, S., PICARD, R., and HENGARTNER, N. (2006). 'Accounting for seasonal patterns in syndromic surveillance data for outbreak detection'. *BMC Medical Informatics and Decision Making*, 6/40. doi:10.1186/1472–6947–6–40. [10.6.3]

BUSH, L. M., ABRAMS, B. H., BEALL, A., and JOHNSON, C. C. (2001). 'Index case of fatal inhalational anthrax due to bioterrorism in the United States'. *New England Journal of Medicine*, 345: 1607–10. [8.5.3]

BUTLER, D. (2006*a*). 'Family tragedy spotlights flu mutations'. *Nature*, 442: 114–15. [4.2.4]

—— (2006*b*). 'Thai dogs carry bird-flu virus, but will they spread it?' *Nature*, 439: 773. [4.2.3]

BUTLER, J. C. and BREIMAN, R. F. (1998). 'Legionellosis'. In A. S. Evans and P. S. Brachman (eds), *Bacterial Infections of Humans: Epidemiology and Control*, 3rd edn. New York: Plenum Medical Book Company, 355–75. [5.3.1, 5.3.3]

C

CAIRNS, J. (1975). *Cancer, Science and Society*. San Francisco: W. H. Freeman. [1.4.2]

CALDWELL, J. C. (1982). *Theory of Fertility Decline*. London: Academic Press. [1.4.1]

CAMPANELLA, N. (1999). 'Infectious diseases and natural disasters: The effects of Hurricane Mitch over Villanueva municipal area, Nicaragua'. *Public Health Reviews*, 27: 311–19. [7.6.1]

Campbell-Lendrum, D. H., Corvalán, C. F., and Prüss-Ustün, A. (2003). 'How much disease could climate change cause?' In A. J. McMichael, D. H. Campbell-Lendrum, C. F. Corvalán, K. L. Ebi, A. Githeko, J. D. Scheraga, and A. Woodward (eds), *Climate Change and Human Health: Risks and Responses*. Geneva: WHO, 133–58. [7.5.1]

Capua, I. and Alexander, D. J. (2004). 'Avian influenza: Recent developments'. *Avian Pathology*, 33: 393–404. [4.2.2, 4.2.3]

Carballal, G., Videla, C. M., and Merani, M. S. (1988). 'Epidemiology of Argentine hemorrhagic fever'. *European Journal of Epidemiology*, 4: 259–74. [7.2.1]

Carlson, J. R. and Hammond, W. (1999). 'The English sweating sickness (1485–*c*.1551): A new perspective on disease etiology'. *Journal of the History of Medicine and Allied Sciences*, 54: 23–54. [2.3.5]

Carmichael, A. G. (1993*a*). 'Bubonic plague'. In K. F. Kiple (ed.), *Cambridge World History of Human Disease*. Cambridge: Cambridge University Press, 628–31. [2.3.1]

—— (1993*b*). 'Diphtheria'. In K. F. Kiple (ed.), *Cambridge World History of Human Disease*. Cambridge: Cambridge University Press, 680–3. [2.3.1]

—— (1993*c*). 'Plague of Athens'. In K. F. Kiple (ed.), *Cambridge World History of Human Disease*. Cambridge: Cambridge University Press, 934–7. [2.2.2]

Carter, R. and Mendis, K. N. (2002). 'Evolutionary and historical aspects of the burden of malaria'. *Clinical Microbiology Reviews*, 15: 564–94. [2.1]

Castiglioni, A. (1947). *A History of Medicine*, 2nd edn. London: Routledge & Kegan Paul. [2.2.2]

Cauchemez, S., Boëlle, P.-Y., Donnelly, C. A., Ferguson, N. M., Thomas, G., Leung, G. M., Hedley, A. J., Anderson, R. M., and Valleron, A. J. (2006). 'Real-time estimates in early detection of SARS'. *Emerging Infectious Diseases*, 12: 110–13. [10.6.3]

Cavanaugh, D. C., Dangerfield, H. G., Hunter, D. H., Joy, R. J. T., Marshall, J. D., Quy, D. V., Vivona, F., and Winter, E. (1968). 'Some observations on the current plague outbreak in the Republic of Vietnam'. *American Journal of Public Health*, 58: 742–52. [8.2.2]

Cello, J., Paul, A. V., and Wimmer, E. (2002). 'Chemical synthesis of poliovirus cdna: Generation of infectious virus in the absence of natural template'. *Science*, 297: 1016–18. [8.5.4]

Centers for Disease Control (1988). 'Guidelines for evaluating surveillance systems'. *Morbidity and Mortality Weekly Report*, 37/S-5: 1–18. [10.6]

—— (1990*a*). 'Epidemic meningococcal disease—Kenya and Tanzania: Recommendations for travelers, 1990'. *Morbidity and Mortality Weekly Report*, 39: 13–14. [9.3.2]

—— (1990*b*). 'Update: Filovirus infections among persons with occupational exposure to nonhuman primates'. *Morbidity and Mortality Weekly Report*, 39: 266–7, 273. [9.3.2]

Centers for Disease Control and Prevention (1992). 'Surveillance in evacuation camps after the eruption of Mt. Pinatubo, Philippines'. *Morbidity and Mortality Weekly Report Surveillance Summaries*, 41: 9–12. [7.6.1]

—— (1993*a*). 'Update: Multistate outbreak of *Escherichia coli* O157:H7 infections from hamburgers—western United States, 1992–1993'. *Morbidity and Mortality Weekly Report*, 42: 258–63. [5.2.3, 5.2.4]

Centers for Disease Control and Prevention (1993*b*). 'Update: Hantavirus pulmonary syndrome—United States, 1993'. *Morbidity and Mortality Weekly Report*, 42: 816–20. [7.5.3]

—— (1994*a*). 'Human plague—India, 1994'. *Morbidity and Mortality Weekly Report*, 43: 689–91. [11.2.4]

—— (1994*b*). 'Health status of displaced persons following civil war—Burundi, December 1993–January 1994'. *Morbidity and Mortality Weekly Report*, 43: 701–3. [8.3.1]

—— (1994*c*). 'Update: Human plague—India, 1994'. *Morbidity and Mortality Weekly Report*, 43: 722–3. [11.2.4]

—— (1994*d*). 'Dengue fever among US military personnel—Haiti, September–November, 1994'. *Morbidity and Mortality Weekly Report*, 43: 845–8. [8.4.3]

—— (1994*e*). *Addressing Emerging Infectious Disease Threats: A Prevention Strategy for the United States*. Atlanta: CDC. [1.5.2]

—— (1996*a*). 'History of CDC'. *Morbidity and Mortality Weekly Report*, 45: 526–30. [3.3.2]

—— (1996*b*). 'Surveillance for foodborne-disease outbreaks—United States, 1988–1992'. *MMWR Surveillance Summary*, 45/SS-5. [5.2.1, 5.2.3, 5.2.4]

—— (1997*a*). 'Outbreaks of *Escherichia coli* O157:H7 infection associated with eating alfalfa sprouts—Michigan and Virginia, June–July 1997'. *Morbidity and Mortality Weekly Report*, 46: 741–4. [5.2.4]

—— (1997*b*). 'Isolation of avian influenza A (H5N1) viruses from humans—Hong Kong, May–December 1997'. *Morbidity and Mortality Weekly Report*, 46: 1204–7. [4.2.3]

—— (1997*c*). 'Case definitions for infectious conditions under public health surveillance'. *Morbidity and Mortality Weekly Report*, 46/RR-10: 1–55. [10.6.2]

—— (1998*a*). 'Cholera outbreak among Rwandan refugees—Democratic Republic of Congo, April 1997'. *Morbidity and Mortality Weekly Report*, 47: 389–91. [8.3.2]

—— (1998*b*). 'Multistate outbreak of *Salmonella* serotype Agona infections linked to toasted oats cereal—United States, April–May, 1998'. *Morbidity and Mortality Weekly Report*, 47: 462–4. [5.2.3]

—— (1998*c*). 'Update: Isolation of avian influenza A (H5N1) viruses from humans—Hong Kong, 1997–1998'. *Morbidity and Mortality Weekly Report*, 45: 1245–7. [4.2.3]

—— (1998*d*). 'Preventing emerging infectious diseases: A strategy for the 21st century. Overview of the updated CDC plan'. *Morbidity and Mortality Weekly Report*, 47/RR-15: 1–14. [1.5.2]

—— (1999). 'Update: Outbreak of Nipah virus—Malaysia and Singapore, 1999'. *Morbidity and Mortality Weekly Report*, 48: 335–7. [7.4.1]

—— (2000*a*). 'Outbreak of *Escherichia coli* O157:H7 infection associated with eating fresh cheese curds—Wisconsin, June 1998'. *Morbidity and Mortality Weekly Report*, 49: 911–13. [5.2.4]

—— (2000*b*). 'Surveillance for foodborne-disease outbreaks—United States, 1993–1997'. *MMWR Surveillance Summary*, 49/SS-1. [5.2.3, 5.2.4]

—— (2001*a*). 'Update: Investigation of bioterrorism-related anthrax and interim guidelines for clinical evaluation of persons with possible anthrax'. *Morbidity and Mortality Weekly Report*, 50: 941–8. [8.5.3]

—— (2001*b*). 'Update: Investigation of bioterrorism-related anthrax and adverse events from antimicrobial prophylaxis'. *Morbidity and Mortality Weekly Report*, 50: 973–6. [8.5.3]

—— (2001*c*). 'Updated guidelines for evaluating public health surveillance systems'. *Morbidity and Mortality Weekly Report*, 50/RR-13: 1–35. [10.6.3]

—— (2002). 'Outbreak of acute gastroenteritis associated with Norwalk-like viruses among British military personnel—Afghanistan, May 2002'. *Morbidity and Mortality Weekly Report*, 51: 477–9. [8.4.2]

—— (2003*a*). 'Multistate outbreak of *Salmonella* serotype Typhimurium infections associated with drinking unpasteurized milk—Illinois, Indiana, Ohio, and Tennessee, 2002–2003'. *Morbidity and Mortality Weekly Report*, 52: 613–15. [5.2.3]

—— (2003*b*). 'Cutaneous leishmaniasis in US military personnel—Southwest/Central Asia, 2002–2003'. *Morbidity and Mortality Weekly Report*, 52: 1009–12. [8.4.2]

—— (2003*c*). 'Notice to readers: SMART BRFSS provides data comparisons by metropolitan and micropolitan statistical area (MMSA)'. *Morbidity and Mortality Weekly Report*, 52: 1106. [10.6.2]

—— (2003*d*). 'Revised US surveillance case definition for severe acute respiratory syndrome (SARS) and update on SARS cases—United States and worldwide, December 2003'. *Morbidity and Mortality Weekly Report*, 52: 1202–6. [10.6.3]

—— (2003*e*). *Reducing the risk of Listeria monocytogenes: FDA/CDC 2003 update of the Listeria Action Plan*. Food and Drug Adminstration/Center for Food Safety and Applied Nutrition/Centers for Disease Control. [10.6.3]

—— (2004*a*). 'Update: Cutaneous leishmaniasis in US military personnel—Southwest/Central Asia, 2002–2004'. *Morbidity and Mortality Weekly Report*, 12: 264–5. [8.4.2]

—— (2004*b*). 'Two cases of visceral leishmaniasis in US military personnel—Afghanistan, 2002–2004'. *Morbidity and Mortality Weekly Report*, 12: 265–8. [8.4.2]

—— (2004*c*). '*Acinetobacter baumannii* infections among patients at military medical facilities treating injured US service members, 2002–2004'. *Morbidity and Mortality Weekly Report*, 53: 1063–6. [8.4.2]

—— (2005*a*). 'Outbreaks of *Salmonella* infections associated with eating Roma tomatoes—United States and Canada, 2004'. *Morbidity and Mortality Weekly Report*, 54: 325–8. [5.2.3]

—— (2005*b*). 'Infectious disease and dermatologic conditions in evacuees and rescue workers after Hurricane Katrina—multiple states, August–September, 2005'. *Morbidity and Mortality Weekly Report*, 54: 961–4. [7.6.3]

—— (2005*c*). 'Norovirus outbreak among evacuees from Hurricane Katrina—Houston, Texas, September 2005'. *Morbidity and Mortality Weekly Report*, 54: 1016–18. [7.6.3]

—— (2005*d*). 'Syndromic surveillance: Reports from a national conference, 2004. *Morbidity and Mortality Weekly Report*, 54, suppl. [10.6.3]

—— (2005*e*). *Epidemic Intelligence Service*. Atlanta, Ga.: CDC. http://www.cdc.gov/eis, accessed 21 July 2008. [3.4.1]

—— (2006*a*). 'Ongoing multistate outbreak of *Escherichia coli* serotype O157:H7 infections associated with consumption of fresh spinach—United States, September 2006'. *Morbidity and Mortality Weekly Report*, 55: 1–2, Dispatch. [5.2.3, 10.6.3]

—— (2006*b*). 'Public health response to Hurricanes Katrina and Rita—Louisiana, 2005'. *Morbidity and Mortality Weekly Report*, 55: 29–30. [7.6.3]

—— (2006*c*). 'Two cases of toxigenic *Vibrio cholerae* O1 infection after Hurricanes Katrina and Rita—Louisiana, October 2005'. *Morbidity and Mortality Weekly Report*, 55: 31–2. [7.6.3]

CENTERS FOR DISEASE CONTROL AND PREVENTION (2006*d*). 'Surveillance in hurricane evacuation centers—Louisiana, September–October 2005'. *Morbidity and Mortality Weekly Report*, 55: 32–5. [7.6.3]

—— (2006*e*). 'Emergence of *Mycobacterium tuberculosis* with extensive resistance to second-line drugs—worldwide, 2000–2004'. *Morbidity and Mortality Weekly Report*, 55: 301–5. [4.3.2]

—— (2006*f*). 'Morbidity surveillance after Hurricane Katrina—Arkansas, Louisiana, Mississippi, and Texas, September 2005'. *Morbidity and Mortality Weekly Report*, 55: 727–31. [7.6.3]

—— (2006*g*). 'Surveillance for foodborne-disease outbreaks—United States, 1998–2002'. *MMWR Surveillance Summary*, 55/SS-10. [5.2.3, 5.2.4]

—— (2007*a*). 'Summary of notifiable diseases—United States, 2005'. *Morbidity and Mortality Weekly Report*, 56: 1–92. [5.3.3, 7.4.2]

—— (2007*b*). 'Multistate outbreak of *Salmonella* serotype Tennessee infections associated with peanut butter—United States, 2006–2007'. *Morbidity and Mortality Weekly Report*, 56: 521–4. [5.2.3]

—— (2008*a*). *All About Hantaviruses*. Atlanta, Ga.: CDC. http://www.cdc.gov/ncidod/diseases/hanta/hps, accessed 21 July 2008. [7.5.3]

—— (2008*b*). *Bioterrorism Agents/Diseases*. Atlanta, Ga.: CDC. http://www.bt.cdc.gov, accessed 21 July 2008. [8.5.3]

—— (2008*c*). *Morbidity and Mortality Weekly Report*, 57: 681–6, Editorial Note. [9.2.3]

CHADHA, M. S., COMER, J. A., LOWE, L., ROTA, P. A., ROLLIN, P. E., BELLINI, W. J., KSIAZEK, T. G., and MISHRA, A. (2006). 'Nipah virus-associated encephalitis outbreak, Siliguri, India'. *Emerging Infectious Diseases*, 12: 235–40. [7.4.1]

CHANDLER, T. (1987). *Four Thousand Years of Urban Growth: An Historical Census*. LEWISTON, NY: St David's University Press. [6.2.1]

CHANTEAU, S., RATSIFASOAMANANA, L., RASOAMANANA, B., RAHALISON, L., RANDRIAMBELOSOA, J., ROUX, J., and RABESON, D. (1998). 'Plague, a reemerging disease in Madagascar'. *Emerging Infectious Diseases*, 4: 101–4. [1.5.2, 9.2.1]

CHAPIN, G. and WASSERSTROM, R. (1983). 'Pesticide use and malaria resurgence in Central America and India'. *Social Science and Medicine*, 17: 273–90. [4.4.3]

CHATFIELD, C. (2003). *The Analysis of Time Series: An Introduction*, 6th edn. Boca Raton, Fla.: Chapman and Hall. [2.4.2]

CHEN, H., LI, Y., LI, Z., SHI, J., SHINYA, K., DENG, G., QI, Q., TIAN, G., FAN, S., ZHAO, H., SUN, Y., and KAWAOKA, Y. (2006). 'Properties and dissemination of H5N1 viruses isolated during an influenza outbreak in migratory waterfowl in western China'. *Journal of Virology*, 80: 5976–83. [4.2.3]

—— SMITH, G. J. D., LI, K. S., WANG, J., FAN, X. H., RAYNER, J. M., VIJAYKRISHNA, D., ZHANG, J. X., ZHANG, L. J., GUO, C. T., CHEUNG, C. L., XU, K. M., DUAN, L., HUANG, K., QIN, K., LEUNG, Y. H. C., WU, W. L., LU, H. R., CHEN, Y., XIA, N. S., NAIPOSPOS, T. S. P., YUEN, K. Y., HASSAN, S. S., BAHRI, S., NGUYEN, T. D., WEBSTER, R. G., PEIRIS, J. S. M., and GUAN, Y. (2006). 'Establishment of multiple sublineages of H5N1 influenza virus in Asia: Implications for pandemic control'. *Proceedings of the National Academy of Sciences USA*, 103: 2845–50. [4.2.3]

CHOI, B. C. K., PAK, A. W. P., and OTTOSON, J. M. (2002). 'Understanding the basic concepts of public health surveillance'. *Journal of Epidemiology and Community Health*, 56: 402–11. [10.6.1]

Choi, K. and Thacker, S. B. (1981*a*). 'An evaluation of influenza mortality surveillance, 1962–1979: (I) Time series forecasts of expected pneumonia and influenza deaths'. *American Journal of Epidemiology*, 113: 215–26. [11.4]

—— —— (1981*b*). 'An evaluation of influenza mortality surveillance, 1962–1979: (II) Percentage of pneumonia and influenza deaths as an indicator of influenza activity'. *American Journal of Epidemiology*, 113: 227–35. [11.4]

Christopher, G. W., Cieslak, T. J., Pavlin, J. A., and Eitzen, E. M. (1997). 'Biological warfare: A historical perspective'. *Journal of the American Medical Association*, 278: 412–17. [8.5.2]

Chua, K. B. (2003). 'Nipah virus outbreak in Malaysia'. *Journal of Clinical Virology*, 26: 265–75. [7.4.1]

—— Bellini, W. J., Rota, P. A., Harcourt, B. H., Tamin, A., Lam, S. K., Ksiazek, T. G., Rollin, P. E., Zaki, S. R., Shieh, W. J., Goldsmith, C. S., Gubler, D. J., Roehrig, J. T., Eaton, B., Gould, A. R., Olson, J., Field, H., Daniels, P., Ling, A. E., Peters, C. J., Anderson, L. J., and Mahy, B. W. J. (2000). 'Nipah virus: A recently emergent deadly paramyxovirus'. *Science*, 288: 1432–5. [7.4.1]

Cipolla, C. M. (1981). *Fighting the Plague in Seventeeth-Century Italy*. Madison: University of Wisconsin Press. [11.2.1]

Claas, E. C., de Jong, J. C., van Beek, R., Rimmelzwaan, G. F., and Osterhaus, A. D. M. E. (1998). 'Human influenza virus A/Hong Kong/156/97 (H5N1) infection'. *Vaccine*, 16: 977–8. [4.2.3]

Clemow, F. G. (1889–90). 'Epidemic influenza'. *Public Health* (London), 2: 358–67. [2.3.1, 2.3.3]

—— (1903). *The Geography of Disease*. Cambridge: Cambridge University Press. [6.3.2]

Cliff, A. D. and Haggett, P. (1981). 'Methods for the measurement of epidemic velocity from time-series data'. *International Journal of Epidemiology*, 11: 82–9. [10.2.2]

—— —— (1985). *The Spread of Measles in Fiji and the Pacific: Spatial Components in the Transmission of Epidemic Waves through Island Communities*. Department of Human Geography publication no. HG/18. Canberra: Research School of Pacific Studies, Australian National University. [6.3.1]

—— —— (1988). *Atlas of Disease Distributions: Analytic Approaches to Epidemiological Data*. Oxford: Blackwell Reference. [2.3.4, 3.5, 9.2.2, 10.2.1]

—— —— (1989). 'Spatial aspects of epidemic control'. *Progress in Human Geography*, 13, 315–47. [11.3.1]

—— —— (1990). 'Epidemic control and critical community size: Spatial aspects of eliminating communicable diseases in human populations'. In R. W. Thomas (ed.), *Spatial Epidemiology*. London Papers in Regional Science, 21. London: Pion, 93–110. [11.3]

—— —— (2004). 'Time, travel and infection'. *British Medical Bulletin*, 69: 87–99. [6.3.1, 6.3.2, 6.4.3, 6.5.1]

—— —— (2006). 'A swash–backwash model of the single epidemic wave'. *Journal of Geographical Systems*, 8: 227–52. [10.2.2, 10.4, 10.4.1, App. 10.1]

—— —— and Ord, J. K. (1979). 'Graph theory and geography'. In R. J. Wilson and L. W. Beineke (eds), *Applications of Graph Theory*. New York: Academic Press, 293–326. [6.4.2]

CLIFF, A. D., HAGGETT, P., and ORD, J. K. (1986). *Spatial Aspects of Influenza Epidemics*. London: Pion. [4.2.2, 4.2.3, 4.2.4, 6.4.2, 10.3.2, 10.3.3, 11.3]

—— —— —— and VERSEY, G. R. (1981). *Spatial Diffusion: An Historical Geography of Epidemics in an Island Community*. Cambridge: Cambridge University Press. [3.3.5, 10.4.1]

—— —— and SMALLMAN-RAYNOR, M. R. (1993). *Measles: An Historical Geography of a Major Human Viral Disease from Global Expansion to Local Retreat, 1840–1990*. Oxford: Blackwell Reference. [2.3.1, 9.3.1, 10.2, 11.1, 11.2, 11.2.2]

—— —— —— (1998). *Deciphering Global Epidemics: Analytical Approaches to the Disease Records of World Cities, 1888–1912*. Cambridge: Cambridge University Press. [2.3.2, 3.2.1, 6.3.1]

—— —— —— (2000). *Island Epidemics*. Oxford: Oxford University Press. [2.3.1, 6.2.1, 6.2.3, 6.4.3, 11.2.2, 11.2.3, 11.3]

—— —— —— (2004). *World Atlas of Epidemic Diseases*. London: Arnold. [2.3.2, 4.3.2, 5.2.5, 5.3.3, 7.3.1, 7.4, 7.4.2, 7.5.1, 8.5.3, 9.2.2, 9.2.3, 9.3.2, 10.3.1]

—— —— —— (2008). 'An exploratory method for estimating the changing speed of epidemic waves from historical data'. *International Journal of Epidemiology*, 37: 106–12. [10.3.2]

CLIVER, D. O. (2002). 'Infrequent microbial infections'. In D. O. Cliver and H. P. Riemann (eds), *Foodborne Diseases*, 2nd edn. Amsterdam: Academic Press, 151–9. [5.2, 5.2.1]

COAN, P. M. (1997). *Ellis Island Interviews: In Their Own Words*. New York: Facts on File, Inc. [11.2.2]

COHEN, M. L. (1992). 'Epidemiology of drug resistance: Implications for a post-antimicrobial era'. *Science*, 257: 1050–5. [4.3.1]

—— (1998). 'Resurgent and emergent disease in a changing world'. *British Medical Bulletin*, 54: 523–32. [4.2.1]

COLCHESTER, A. C. F. and COLCHESTER, N. T. H. (2005). 'The origin of bovine spongiform encephalopathy: The human prion disease hypothesis'. *Lancet*, 366: 856–61. [5.2.5]

COLIZZA, V., BARRAT, A., BARTHÉLEMY, M., and VESPIGNANI, A. (2006*a*). 'The role of the airline transportation network in the prediction and predictability of global epidemics'. *Proceedings of the National Academy of Sciences USA*, 103: 2015–20. [6.4.2]

—— —— —— —— (2006*b*). 'The modeling of global epidemics: Stochastic dynamics and predictability'. *Bulletin of Mathematical Biology*, 68: 1893–1921. [6.4.2]

—— —— —— VALLERON, A. J., and VESPIGNANI, A. (2007). 'Modeling the worldwide spread of pandemic influenza: Baseline case and containment interventions'. *PLoS Medicine*, 4/1: e13. doi:10.1371/journal.pmed.0040013. [6.4.2]

COLLEE, J. G., BRADLEY, R., and LIBERSKI, P. P. (2006). 'Variant CJD (vCJD) and bovine spongiform encephalopathy (BSE): 10 and 20 years on: Part 2'. *Folia Neuropathologica*, 44: 102–10. [5.2.5]

COMMUNICABLE DISEASES WORKING GROUP ON EMERGENCIES (2006). *Communicable Diseases Following Natural Disasters: Risk Assessment and Priority Interventions*. Geneva: WHO (WHO/CDS/NTD/DCE/2006.4). [7.6.1]

CONWAY, D. J. and ROPER, C. (2000). 'Micro-evolution and the emergence of pathogens'. *International Journal for Parasitology*, 30: 1423–30. [1.3.3, 1.5.1]

Cooper, B. S., Pitman, R. J., Edmunds, W. J., and Gay, N. J. (2006). 'Delaying the international spread of pandemic influenza'. *PLoS Medicine*, 3/6: e212. doi:10.1371/journal.pmed.0030212. [6.4.2]

Cordes, L. G., Goldman, W. D., Marr, J. S., Friedman, S. M., Band, J. D., Rothschild, E. O., Kravitz, H., Feeley, J. C., Fraser, D. W., and the Field Investigation Team (1980). 'Legionnaires' disease in New York City, August–September 1978'. *Bulletin of the New York Academy of Medicine*, 56: 467–82. [5.3.3]

Corwin, E. H. L. (1949). *Ecology of Health*. New York: Commonwealth Fund. [1.3.1]

Cousens, S., Smith, P. G., Ward, H., Everington, D., Knight, R. S. G., Zeidler, M., Stewart, G., Smith-Bathgate, E. A. B., Macleod, M. A., MacKenzie, J., and Will, R. G. (2001). 'Geographical distribution of variant Creutzfeldt–Jakob disease in Great Britain, 1994–2000'. *Lancet*, 357: 1002–7. [5.2.5]

Cowley, R. G. (1970). 'Implications of the Vietnam War for tuberculosis in the United States'. *Archives of Environmental Health*, 21: 479–80. [8.2.2]

Cramer, E. H., Blanton, C. J., Blanton, L. H., Vaughan, G. H., Jr, Bopp, C. A., Forney, D. L., and the Vessel Sanitation Program Environmental Health Inspection Team (2006). 'Epidemiology of gastroenteritis on cruise ships, 2001–2004'. *American Journal of Preventive Medicine*, 30: 252–7. [6.3.1]

Crawfurd, R. (1914). *Plague and Pestilence in Literature and Art*. Oxford: Clarendon Press. [2.2.2]

Creighton, C. (1891–4). *A History of Epidemics in Britain*, i: *From A.D. 664 to the Great Plague*; ii: *From the Extinction of the Plague to the Present Time*. Cambridge: Cambridge University Press. [2.3.1, 2.3.5, 2.4.1, 2.4.2, 9.5.1]

Croft, A. M. J. and Creamer, I. S. (1997). 'Health data from Operation Resolute (Bosnia). Part 1: Primary care data'. *Journal of the Royal Army Medical Corps*, 143: 13–18. [8.4.3]

Crosby, A. W. (1993*a*). 'Influenza'. In K. F. Kiple (ed.), *The Cambridge World History of Human Disease*. Cambridge: Cambridge University Press, 807–11. [2.3.1, 2.3.3]

—— (1993*b*). 'Smallpox'. In K. F. Kiple (ed.), *The Cambridge World History of Human Disease*. Cambridge: Cambridge University Press, 1008–13. [2.3.1]

Cullen, R. M. and Walker, W. J. (1996). 'Measles epidemics 1949–91: The impact of mass immunization in New Zealand'. *New Zealand Medical Journal*, 109: 400–2. [11.3.1]

Cummings, K., Barrett, E., Mohle-Boetani, J. C., Brooks, J. T., Farrar, J., Hunt, T., Fiore, A., Komatsu, K., Werner, S. B., and Slutsker, L. (2001). 'A multistate outbreak of *Salmonella enterica* serotype Baildon associated with domestic raw tomatoes'. *Emerging Infectious Diseases*, 7: 1046–8. [5.2.3]

Cumpston, J. H. L. (1919). *Influenza and Maritime Quarantine in Australia*, Service Publication no. 18. Melbourne: Quarantine Service, Commonwealth of Australia. [6.3.1]

—— (1927). *The History of Diphtheria, Scarlet Fever, Measles and Whooping Cough in Australia*, Service Publication no. 37. Canberra: Department of Health, Commonwealth of Australia. [6.3.1]

—— and McCallum, F. (1927). *The History of the Intestinal Infections (and Typhus fever) in Australia, 1788–1923*, Service Publication no. 36. Melbourne: Department of Health, Commonwealth of Australia. [6.3.1]

Cutts, F. T. (1990). *Measles Control in the 1990s: Principles for the Next Decade*. Geneva: WHO Expanded Programme on Immunization. [11.3.1]

D

Dall'Asta, L., Barrat, A., Barthélemy, M., and Vespignani, A. (2006). 'Vulnerability of weighted networks'. *Journal of Statistical Mechanics: Theory and Experiment*. doi:10.1088/1742–5468/2006/04/Po4006. [6.4.2]

Dando, M. (1994). *Biological Warfare in the 21st Century: Biotechnology and the Proliferation of Biological Weapons*. London: Brassey's. [8.5, 8.5.1]

Davey, V. J. and Glass, R. I. (2008). 'Rescinding community mitigation strategies in an influenza pandemic'. *Emerging Infectious Diseases*, 14: 365–72. [11.2.3]

Davies, R. E. G. (1964). *A History of the World's Airlines*. London: Oxford University Press. [6.3.1, 6.3.2, 6.4, 6.4.1]

Davis, K. (1969). *World Urbanization, 1950–70*. Berkeley: Institute of International Studies, University of California. [6.2.2]

Dechet, A. M., Scallan, E., Gensheimer, K., Hoekstra, R., Gunderman-King, J., Lockett, J., Wrigley, D., Chege, W., Sobel, J., and the Multistate Working Group (2006). 'Outbreak of multidrug-resistant *Salmonella enterica* serotype Typhimurium Definitive Type 104 infection linked to commercial ground beef, northeastern United States, 2003–2004'. *Clinical Infectious Diseases*, 42: 747–52. [5.2.3]

DEFRA (Department for Environment, Food, and Rural Affairs) (2007*a*). *Outbreak of Highly Pathogenic H5N1 Avian Influenza in Suffolk in January 2007. A Report of the Epidemiological Findings by the National Emergency Epidemiology Group*. London: DEFRA. http://www.defra.gov.uk/animalh/diseases/notifiable/ai/pdf/epid_findings070405.pdf, accessed 26 Jan. 2009. [11.2.4]

—— (2007*b*). *Bluetongue Disease: Contingency Plans for Great Britain*. London: DEFRA. http://www.defra.gov.uk/animalh/diseases/pdf/bluetongue-contplan.pdf, accessed 21 July 2008. [11.2.4]

—— (2007*c*). *UK Bluetongue Control Strategy*. London: DEFRA. http://www.defra.gov.uk/animalh/diseases/notifiable/pdf/bluetongue-control-strategy0807.pdf, accessed 21 July 2008. [11.2.4]

de Jong, M. D. and Hien, T. T. (2006). 'Avian influenza A (H5N1)'. *Journal of Clinical Virology*, 35: 2–13. [4.2.2, 4.2.3]

—— Simmons, C. P., Thanh, T. T., Hien, V. M., Smith, G. J. D., Chau, T. N. B., Hoang, D. M., Chau, N. V. V., Khanh, T. H., Dong, V. C., Qui, P. T., Cam, B. V., Ha, D. Q., Guan, Y., Peiris, J. S. M., Chinh, N. T., Hien, T. T., and Farrar, J. (2006). 'Fatal outcome of human influenza A (H5N1) is associated with high viral load and hypercytokinemia'. *Nature Medicine*, 12: 1203–7. [4.2.4]

Dennis, D. T. (1998). 'Plague as an emerging disease'. In W. M. Scheld, W. A. Craig, and J. M. Hughes, *Emerging Infections 2*. Washington, DC: ASM Press, 169–83. [9.2.1]

Department of Commerce, Bureau of the Census (1952–2007). *Statistical Abstract of the United States*. Washington, DC: Government Printing Office. [3.4.3]

Department of Health and Health Protection Agency (2008). *Health Effects of Climate Change in the UK 2008: An Update of the Department of Health Report 2001/2002*. London: Department of Health and Health Protection Agency. [7.5.1]

Department of Livestock Development (2008). สรุป รายงาน ผลการดำเนินงาน ควบคุม โรคไข้หวัด นก [*Summary Report of Work Undertaken to Control Avian Influenza*]. Bangkok: Department of Livestock Development, Ministry of Agriculture and Cooperatives. http://www.dld.go.th/home, accessed 21 July 2008. [4.2.3]

Derraik, J. G. B. (2004). 'Exotic mosquitoes in New Zealand: A review of species intercepted, their pathways and ports of entry'. *Australian and New Zealand Journal of Public Health*, 28: 433–44. [6.5.3]

Desenclos, J. C., Klontz, K. C., Wilder, M. H., Nainan, O. V., Margolis, H. S., and Gunn, R. A. (1991). 'A multistate outbreak of hepatitis A caused by the consumption of raw oysters'. *American Journal of Public Health*, 81: 1268–72. [5.2.3]

Desselberger, U. (2000). 'Emerging and re-emerging infectious diseases'. *Journal of Infection*, 40: 3–15. [1.5.3]

Deuel, R. E., Bawell, M. B., Matsumoto, M., and Sabin, A. B. (1950). 'Status and significance of inapparent infection with virus of Japanese B encephalitis in Korea and Okinawa in 1946'. *American Journal of Hygiene*, 51: 13–20. [8.2.1]

de Ville de Goyet, C. (2000). 'Stop propagating disaster myths'. *Lancet*, 356: 762–4. [7.6.1]

de Wet, N., Ye, W., Hales, S., Warrick, R. A., Woodward, A., and Weinstein, P. (2001). 'Use of a computer model to identify potential hotspots for dengue fever in New Zealand'. *New Zealand Medical Journal*, 11: 420–2. [7.5.1]

Dewing, H. B. (1914). *Procopius: History of the Wars, Books I and II*. London: William Heinemann. [2.3.2]

Dietz, K. (1993). 'The estimation of the basic reproduction number for infectious diseases'. *Statistical Methods in Medical Research*, 2: 23–41. [10.2.2]

Doherr, M. G. (2007). 'Brief review on the epidemiology of transmissible spongiform encephalopathies (TSE)'. *Vaccine*, 25: 5619–24. [5.2.5]

Domingo, M., Ferrer, L., Pumarola, M., Marco, A., Plana, J., Kennedy, S., McAliskey, M., and Rima, B. K. (1990). 'Morbillivirus in dolphins'. *Nature*, 348: 21. [7.4.1]

Dowdle, W. R. (1999). 'Influenza A virus recycling revisited'. *Bulletin of the World Health Organization*, 77: 820–8. [4.2.2, 10.3.1]

Downs, W. G. (1993). 'Arenaviruses'. In K. F. Kiple (ed.), *The Cambridge World History of Human Disease*. Cambridge: Cambridge University Press, 595–9. [7.2.1]

Doyle, T. J., Ma, H., Groseclose, S. L., and Hopkins, R. S. (2005). 'PHSkb: A knowledgebase to support notifiable disease surveillance'. *BMC Medical Informatics and Decision Making*, 5/27. doi:10.1186/1472–6947–5–27. [10.6.2]

Drabick, J. J., Gambel, J. M., Gouvea, V. S., Caudill, J. D., Sun, W., Hoke, C. H., and Innis, B. L. (1997). 'A cluster of acute hepatitis E infection in United Nations Bangladeshi peacekeepers in Haiti'. *American Journal of Tropical Medicine and Hygiene*, 57: 449–54. [8.4.3]

Draief, M. (2006). 'Epidemic processes on complex networks: The effect of topology on the spread of epidemics'. *Physica A: Statistical Mechanics and its Applications*, 363: 120–31. [6.4.2]

Drancourt, M., Aboudharam, G., Signoli, M., Dutour, O., and Raoult, D. (1998). 'Detection of 400-year old *Yersinia pestis* DNA in human dental pulp. An approach to the diagnosis of ancient septicaemia'. *Proceedings of the National Academy of Sciences USA*, 95: 12637–40. [1.3.3]

Drudy, D., Harnedy, N., Fanning, S., Hannan, M., and Kyne, L. (2007). 'Emergence and control of fluoroquinolone-resistant, toxin A-negative, toxin B-positive *Clostridium difficile*'. *Infection Control and Hospital Epidemiology*, 28: 932–40. [4.3.1]

Duncan, C. J., Duncan, S. R., and Scott, S. (1996*a*). 'Oscillatory dynamics of smallpox and the impact of vaccination'. *Journal of Theoretical Biology*, 183: 447–54. [2.4.2]

—— —— —— (1996*b*). 'Whooping cough epidemics in London, 1701–1812: Infection dynamics, seasonal forcing and the effects of malnutrition'. *Proceedings of the Royal Society of London B*, 263: 445–50. [2.4.2]

—— —— —— (1997). 'The dynamics of measles epidemics'. *Theoretical Population Biology*, 52: 155–63. [2.4.2]

Dunn, F. L. (1993). 'Malaria'. In K. F. Kiple (ed.), *Cambridge World History of Human Disease*. Cambridge: Cambridge University Press, 855–62. [2.2.2, 2.3.1]

Dutt, A. K., Akhtar, R., and McVeigh, M. (2006). 'Surat plague of 1994 re-examined'. *Southeast Asian Journal of Tropical Medicine and Public Health*, 37: 755–8. [11.2.4]

E

Eckert, E. A. (2000). 'The retreat of plague from Central Europe, 1640–1720: A geomedical approach'. *Bulletin of the History of Medicine*, 74: 1–28. [2.3.2]

Edmonds, L. D., Layde, P. M., James, L. M., Flynt, J. W., Erickson, J. D., and Godfrey, P. O. (1981). 'Congenital malformations surveillance: Two American systems'. *International Journal of Epidemiology*, 10: 247–52. [10.6.1]

Eitrem, R., Vene, S., and Niklasson, B. (1990). 'Incidence of sand fly fever among Swedish United Nations soldiers in Cyprus during 1985'. *American Journal of Tropical Medicine and Hygiene*, 43: 207–11. [8.4.3]

El-Akkad, A. M. (1978). 'Rift Valley fever outbreak in Egypt, October–December 1977'. *Journal of the Egyptian Public Health Association*, 53: 123–8. [7.3.1]

Endy, T. P. and Nisalak, A. (2002). 'Japanese encephalitis virus: Ecology and epidemiology'. *Current Topics in Microbiology and Immunology*, 267: 11–48. [8.2.1]

Engelthaler, D. M., Mosley, D. G., Cheek, J. E., Levy, C. E., Komatsu, K. K., Ettestad, P., Davis, T., Tanda, D. T., Miller, L., Frampton, J. W., Porter, R., and Bryan, R. T. (1999). 'Climatic and environmental patterns associated with hantavirus pulmonary syndrome, Four Corners region, United States'. *Emerging Infectious Diseases*, 5: 87–94. [7.5.3]

Enria, D. A., Briggiler, A. M., and Sánchez, Z. (2008). 'Treatment of Argentine hemorrhagic fever'. *Antiviral Research*, 78: 132–9. [7.2.1]

Epstein, J. M., Goedecke, D. M., Yu, F., Morris, R. J., Wagener, D. K., and Bobashev, G. V. (2007). 'Controlling pandemic flu: The value of international air travel restrictions'. *PloS ONE*, 2/5: e401. doi:10.1371/journal.pone.0000401. [6.4.2, 11.2.3]

EPSTEIN, P. R. (1995). 'Emerging diseases and ecosystem instability: New threats to public health'. *American Journal of Public Health*, 85: 168–72. [7.5.3]

ESPINAL, M. A. (2003). 'The global situation of MDR-TB'. *Tuberculosis*, 83: 44–51. [4.3.2]

ETHERIDGE, E. W. (1992). *Sentinel for Health: A History of the Centers for Disease Control*. Berkeley: University of California Press. [3.3.2]

EUROPEAN AND ALLIED COUNTRIES COLLABORATIVE STUDY GROUP OF CJD (2008). *Variant Creutzfeldt–Jakob Disease: Current Data (February 2008)*. Edinburgh: EUROCJD. http://www.eurocjd.ed.ac.uk, accessed 21 July 2008. [5.2.5]

EVERITT, B. S., LANDAU, S., and LEESE, M. (2001). *Cluster Analysis*, 4th edn. London: Arnold. [9.3.1]

EWAN, C., BRYANT, E., and CALVERT, D. (1990). *Health Implications of Long Term Climate Change*. Canberra: National Health and Medical Research Council of Australia. [7.5.1]

F

FARR, W. (1861). 'Letter to the Registrar General on Causes of Death in England'. In *Twenty-Second Annual Report of the Registrar General of Births, Deaths, and Marriages in England 1859*. London: HMSO, 183–95. [1.1]

—— (1874). 'Letter to the Registrar General on Causes of Death in England'. In *Thirty-Fifth Annual Report of the Registrar General of Births, Deaths, and Marriages in England 1872*. London: HMSO, 219–29. [1.1]

FARRINGTON, C. P., KANAAN, M. N., and GAY, N. J. (2001). 'Estimation of the basic reproduction number for infectious diseases from age-stratified serological survey data'. *Journal of the Royal Statistical Society C*, 50: 251–92. [10.2.2]

FARUQUE, S. M., CHOWDHURY, N., KAMRUZZAMAN, M., AHMAD, Q. S., FARUQUE, A. S., SALAM, M. A., RAMAMURTHY, T., NAIR, G. B., WEINTRAUB, A., and SACK, D. A. (2003). 'Reemergence of epidemic *Vibrio cholerae* O139, Bangladesh'. *Emerging Infectious Diseases*, 9: 1116–22. [9.2.2]

FAUCI, A. S. (2006). 'Emerging and re-emerging infectious diseases: Influenza as a prototype of the host–pathogen balancing act'. *Cell*, 124: 665–70. [4.2.1, 4.5]

FEDSON, D. S. (2003) 'Pandemic influenza and global vaccine supply'. *Clinical Infectious Diseases*, 36: 1552–61. [10.2.1]

FERGUSON, N. M., CUMMINGS, D. A. T., FRASER, C., CAJKA, J. C., COOLEY, P. C., and BURKE, D. S. (2006). 'Strategies for mitigating an influenza pandemic'. *Nature*, 442: 448–52. [4.2.4]

FERSON, M. J. and RESSLER, K. A. (2005). 'Bound for Sydney town: Health surveillance on international cruise vessels visiting the Port of Sydney'. *Medical Journal of Australia*, 182: 391–4. [6.3.1]

FIELDS, B. S., BENSON, R. F., and BESSER, R. E. (2002). '*Legionella* and Legionnaires' disease: 25 years of investigation'. *Clinical Microbiology Reviews*, 15: 506–26. [5.3.3]

Flahault, A., Deguen, S., and Valleron, A. J. (1994). 'A mathematical model for the European spread of influenza'. *European Journal of Epidemiology*, 10: 471–4. [6.4.2]

—— Letrait, S., Blin, P., Hazout, S., Ménarés, J., and Valleron, A. J. (1988). 'Modelling the 1985 influenza epidemic in France'. *Statistics in Medicine*, 7: 1147–55. [6.3.2]

Fletcher, R. A. (1910). *Steamships: The Story of Their Development to the Present Day*. London: Sidgwick and Jackson. [6.3.1]

Floret, N., Viel, J.-F., Mauny, F., Hoen, B., and Piarroux, R. (2006). 'Negligible risk for epidemics after geophysical disasters'. *Emerging Infectious Diseases*, 12: 543–8. [7.6.1, 7.6.2, 7.6.3]

Food and Agriculture Organization (2004). 'Update on the avian influenza situation (as of 15/6/2004)'. *FAO AIDE News*, 16: 1–10. [4.2.3]

—— (2005). 'A review of highly pathogenic avian influenza in Asia and FAO's response to the disease'. *FAO AIDE News*, 29: 2–29. [4.2.3]

Fornaciari, G., Zavaglia, K., Giusti, L., Vultaggio, C., and Ciranni, R. (2003). 'Human papillomavirus in a 16th century mummy'. *Lancet*, 362: 1160. [1.3.3]

Fox, W., Ellard, G. A., and Mitchison, D. A. (1999). 'Studies on the treatment of tuberculosis undertaken by the British Medical Research Council Tuberculosis Units, 1946–1986, with relevant subsequent publications'. *International Journal of Tuberculosis and Lung Disease*, 3, suppl. 2, S231–79. [4.3.2]

Frampton, J. W., Lanser, S., and Nichols, C. R. (1995). 'Sin Nombre virus infection in 1959'. *Lancet*, 346: 781–2. [7.5.3]

Fraser, M. R. (2007). 'After 5 years of public health preparedness, are we ready yet?' *Journal of Public Health Management and Practice*, 13: 3–6. [10.6.3]

Fraser, W. D., Tsai, T. R., Orenstein, W., Parkin, W. E., Beecham, H. J., Sharrar, R. G., Harris, J., Mallison, G. F., Martin, S. M., McDade, J. E., Shepard, C. C., Brachman, P. S., and the Field Investigation Team (1977). 'Legionnaires' disease: Description of an epidemic of pneumonia'. *New England Journal of Medicine*, 297: 1189–97. [5.3.3]

Fratamico, P. M., Smith, J. L., and Buchanan, R. L. (2002). 'Infrequent microbial infections'. In D. O. Cliver and H. P. Riemann (eds), *Foodborne Diseases*, 2nd edn. Amsterdam: Academic Press, 79–101. [5.2.4]

Fryauff, D. J., Modi, G. B., Mansour, N. S., Kreutzer, R. D., Soliman, S., and Youssef, F. G. (1993). 'Epidemiology of cutaneous leishmaniasis at a focus monitored by the Multinational Force and Observers in the northeastern Sinai Desert of Egypt'. *American Journal of Tropical Medicine and Hygiene*, 49: 598–607. [8.4.3]

Frey, W. H. and Zimmer, Z. (2001). 'Defining the city'. In R. Paddison (ed.), *Handbook of Urban Studies*. London: Sage Publications, 14–35. [6.2.2]

Fricker, E. J., Spigelman, M., and Fricker, C. R. (1997). 'The detection of *Escherichia coli* DNA in the ancient remains of Lindow Man using polymerase chain reaction'. *Letters in Applied Microbiology*, 24: 351–4. [1.3.3]

Fritz, C. L., Dennis, D. T., Tipple, M. A., Campbell, G. L., McCance, C. R., and Gubler, D. J. (1996). 'Surveillance for pneumonic plague in the United States during an international emergency: A model for control of imported emerging diseases'. *Emerging Infectious Diseases*, 2: 30–6. [11.2.4]

G

GAD, A. M., FEINSOD, F. M., ALLAM, I. H., EISA, M., HASSAN, A. N., SOLIMAN, B. A., EL SAID, S., and SAAH, A. J. (1986). 'A possible route for the introduction of Rift Valley fever virus into Egypt during 1977'. *Journal of Tropical Medicine and Hygiene*, 89: 233–6. [7.2.1]

GAJDUSEK, D. C. (1956). 'Hemorrhagic fevers in Asia: A problem in medical ecology'. *Geographical Review*, 46: 20–42. [8.1, 8.1.1, 8.2.1]

GALIMAND, M., CARNIEL, E., and COURVALIN, P. (2006). 'Resistance of *Yersinia pestis* to antimicrobial agents'. *Antimicrobial Agents and Chemotherapy*, 50: 3233–6. [9.2.1]

GALLO, R. C. (1987). 'The AIDS virus'. *Scientific American*, 256: 39–48. [9.2.3]

GAO, F., BAILES, E., ROBERTSON, D. L., CHEN, Y., RODENBURG, C. M., MICHAEL, S. F., CUMMINS, L. B., ARTHUR, L. O., PEETERS, M., SHAW, G. M., SHARP, P. M., and HAHN, B. H. (1999). 'Origin of HIV-1 in the chimpanzee *Pan troglodytes troglodytes*'. *Nature*, 397: 436–41. [9.2.3]

—— YUE, L., ROBERTSON, D. L., HILL, S. C., HUI, H., BIGGAR, R. J., NEEQUAYE, A. E., WHELAN, T. M., HO, D. D., SHAW, G. M., SHARP, P. M., and HAHN, B. H. (1994). 'Genetic diversity of human immunodeficiency virus type 2: Evidence for distinct sequence subtypes with differences in virus biology'. *Journal of Virology*, 68: 7433–47. [9.2.3]

—— —— WHITE, A. T., PAPPAS, P. G., BARCHUE, J., HANSON, A. P., GREENE, B. M., SHARP, P. M., SHAW, G. M., and HAHN, B. H. (1992). 'Human infection by genetically diverse SIV_{SM}-related HIV-2 in West Africa'. *Nature*, 358: 495–9. [9.2.3]

GARCÍA, J. B., MORZUNOV, S. P., LEVIS, S., ROWE, J., Calderón, G., ENRÍA, D., SABATTINI, M., BUCHMEIER, M. J., BOWEN, M. D., and ST JEOR, S. C. (2000). 'Genetic diversity of the Junin virus in Argentina: Geographic and temporal patterns'. *Virology*, 272: 127–36. [7.2.1]

GARY, T. L., NARAYAN, K. M., GREGG, E. W., BECKELS, G. L., and SAADDINE, J. B. (2003). 'Racial/ethnic difference in the healthcare experience (coverage, utilization, and satisfaction) of US adults with diabetes'. *Ethnicity and Disease*, 13: 47–54. [10.6.2]

GEISBERT, T. W., and JAHRLING, P. B. (2004). 'Exotic emerging viral diseases: Progress and challenges'. *Nature Medicine*, 10, suppl., S110–S121. [7.2.1]

GENSINI, G. F., YACOUB, M. H., and CONTI, A. A. (2004). 'The concept of quarantine in history: From plague to SARS'. *Journal of Infection*, 49: 257–61. [11.2.3]

GERDES, G. H. (2004). 'Rift Valley fever'. *Revue Scientifique et Technique (International Office of Epizootics)*, 23: 613–23. [7.3.1]

GETIS, A. and ORD, J. K. (1992). 'The analysis of spatial association by use of distance statistics'. *Geographical Analysis*, 24: 189–206. [4.2.3]

GHANI, A. C., DONNELLY, C. A., FERGUSON, N. M., and ANDERSON, R. M. (2003). 'Updated projections of future vCJD deaths in the UK'. *BMC Infectious Diseases*, 3/4. doi:10.1186/1471–2334–3–4. [5.2.5]

GHONEIM, N. H. and WOODS, G. T. (1983). 'Rift Valley fever and its epidemiology in Egypt: A review'. *Journal of Medicine*, 15: 55–79. [7.3.1]

GIBBS, E. P. J. (2005). 'Emerging zoonotic epidemics in the interconnected global community'. *Veterinary Record*, 157: 674–9. [6.5, 6.5.3]

Gibson, C. (1998). *Population of the 100 Largest Cities and Other Urban Places in the United States: 1790–1990.* US Bureau of the Census, Working Paper, 27. [6.2.1]

Gibson, J. J., Brodsky, R. E., and Schultz, M. G. (1974). 'Changing patterns of malaria in the United States'. *Journal of Infectious Diseases*, 130: 553–5. [8.2.2]

Giladi, M., Metzkor-Cotter, E., Martin, D. A., Siegman-Igra, Y., Korczyn, A. D., Rosso, R., Berger, S. A., Campbell, G. L., and Lanciotti, R. S. (2001). 'West Nile encephalitis in Israel, 1999: The New York connection'. *Emerging Infectious Diseases*, 7: 659–61. [6.5.3]

Gilbert, D. N., Moore, W. L., Hedberg, C. L., and Sanford, J. (1968). 'Potential medical problems in personnel returning from Vietnam'. *Annals of Internal Medicine*, 68: 662–78. [8.2.2]

Gilbert, M., Chaitaweesub, P., Parakamawongsa, T., Premashthira, S., Tiensin, T., Kalpravidh, W., Wagner, H., and Slingenbergh, J. (2006). 'Free-grazing ducks and highly pathogenic avian influenza, Thailand'. *Emerging Infectious Diseases*, 12: 227–34. [4.2.3]

Gilbert, M. T., Rambaut, A., Wlasiuk, G., Spira, T. J., Pitchenik, A. E., and Worobey, M. (2007). 'The emergence of HIV/AIDS in the Americas and beyond'. *Proceedings of the National Academy of Sciences USA*, 104: 18566–70. [9.2.3]

Gilsdorf, A., Boxall, N., Gasimov, V., Agayev, I., Mammadzade, F., Ursu, P., Gasimov, E., Brown, C., Mardel, S., Jankovic, D., Pimentel, G., Amir Ayoub, I., Maher Labib Elassal, E., Salvi, C., Legros, D., Pessoa da Silva, C., Hay, A., Andraghetti, R., Rodier, G., and Ganter, B. (2006). 'Two clusters of human infection with influenza A/H5N1 virus in the Republic of Azerbaijan, February–March 2006'. *Eurosurveillance*, 11: 122–6. [4.2.4]

Githeko, A. K. and Woodward, A. (2003). 'International consensus on the science of climate and health: The IPCC Third Assessment Report'. In A. J. McMichael, D. H. Campbell-Lendrum, C. F. Corvalan, K. L. Ebi, A. Githeko, J. D. Scheraga, and A. Woodward (eds), *Climate Change and Human Health: Risks and Responses.* Geneva: WHO, 43–60. [7.5.1]

—— Lindsay, S. W., Confalonieri, U. E., and Patz, J. (2000). 'Climate change and vector-borne diseases: A regional analysis'. *Bulletin of the World Health Organization*, 78: 1136–47. [7.5.1]

Glass, G. E., Yates, T. L., Fine, J. B., Shields, T. M., Kendall, J. B., Hope, A. G., Parmenter, C. A., Peters, C. J., Ksiazek, T. G., Li, C.-S., Patz, J. A., and Mills, J. N. (2002). 'Satellite imagery characterizes local animal reservoir populations of Sin Nombre virus in the southwestern United States'. *Proceedings of the National Academy of Sciences USA*, 99: 16817–22. [7.5.3]

Glezen, W. P. and Couch, R. B. (1997). 'Influenza viruses'. In A. S. Evans and R. A. Kaslow (eds), *Viral Infections of Humans: Epidemiology and Control*, 4th edn. New York: Plenum Medical Book Company, 473–505. [2.3.3, 4.2.2, 4.2.4]

Glick, T. H., Gregg, M. B., Berman, B., Mallison, G., Rhodes, W. W., Jr, and Kassanoff, I. (1978). 'Pontiac fever: An epidemic of unknown etiology in a health department. I: Clinical and epidemiologic aspects'. *American Journal of Epidemiology*, 107: 149–60. [5.3.3]

Global Polio Eradication Initiative (2003). *Global Polio Eradication Initiative: Strategic Plan 2004–2008.* Geneva: WHO. [8.5.4]

Goh, K. J., Tan, C. T., Chew, N. K., Tan, P. S., Kamarulzaman, A., Sarji, S. A., Wong, K. T., Abdullah, B. J., Chua, K. B., and Lam, S. K. (2000). 'Clinical features of Nipah virus encephalitis among pig farmers in Malaysia'. *New England Journal of Medicine*, 342: 1229–35. [7.4.1]

Goma Epidemiology Group (1995). 'Public health impact of Rwandan refugee crisis: What happened in Goma, Zaire, in July, 1994?' *Lancet*, 345: 339–44. [8.1.2, 8.3.2]

González Ittig, R. E. and Gardenal, C. N. (2004). 'Recent range expansion and low levels of contemporary gene flow in *Calomys musculinus*: Its relationship with the emergence and spread of Argentine haemorrhagic fever'. *Heredity*, 93: 535–41. [7.2.1]

Goodman, R. A., Bauman, C. F., Gregg, M. B., Videtto, J. F., Stroup, D. F., and Chalmers, N. P. (1990). 'Epidemiologic field investigations by the Centers for Disease Control and Epidemic Intelligence Service, 1946–87'. *Public Health Reports*, 105: 604–10. [3.4.1, 3.4.2, 3.4.4]

Gostin, L. O. (2007*a*). 'Public health strategies for pandemic influenza'. *Journal of the American Medical Association*, 295: 1700–3. [10.6.3]

—— (2007*b*). 'Police Powers and Public Health Paternalism: HIV and Diabetes Surveillance'. *Hastings Center Report*, 37: 9–10. [10.6.3]

—— Hodge, J. G., and Valdiserri, R. O. (2001). 'Informational privacy and the public's health: The Model State Public Health Privacy Act'. *American Journal of Public Health*, 91: 1388–92. [10.6.3]

Gottlieb, S. (2003). 'US army investigates unrelated pneumonia cases in troops in Iraq'. *British Medical Journal*, 327: 358. [8.4.2]

—— Newbern, E. C., Griffin, P. M., Graves, L. M., Hoekstra, R. M., Baker, N. L., Hunter, S. B., Holt, K. G., Ramsey, F., Head, M., Levine, P., Johnson, G., Schoonmaker-Bopp, D., Reddy, V., Kornstein, L., Gerwel, M., Nsubuga, J., Edwards, L., Stonecipher, S., Hurd, S., Austin, D., Jefferson, M. A., Young, S. D., Hise, K., Chernak, E. D., Sobel, J., and the Listeriosis Outbreak Working Group (2006). 'Multistate outbreak of listeriosis linked to turkey deli meat and subsequent changes in US regulatory policy'. *Clinical Infectious Diseases*, 42: 29–36. [5.2.3]

Gould, P. (1993). *The Slow Plague: A Geography of the AIDS Pandemic*. Oxford: Blackwell. [6.3.2]

Gould, R. and Connell, N. D. (1997). 'The public health effects of biological weapons'. In B. S. Levy and V. W. Sidel (eds), *War and Public Health*. Oxford: Oxford University Press, 98–116. [8.5.2]

Grabenstein, J. D., Pittman, P. R., Greenwood, J. T., and Engler, R. J. M. (2006). 'Immunization to protect the US Armed Forces: Heritage, current practice, and prospects'. *Epidemiologic Reviews*, 28: 3–26. [8.4.2]

Grais, R. F., Ellis, J. H., and Glass, G. E. (2003). 'Assessing the impact of airline travel on the geographic spread of pandemic influenza'. *European Journal of Epidemiology*, 18: 1065–72. [6.4.2]

Graitcer, P. L. (1988). 'The development of state and local injury surveillance systems'. *Journal of Safety Research*, 13: 191–8. [10.6.1]

Grandesso, F., Sanderson, F., Kruijt, J., Koene, T., and Brown, V. (2005). 'Mortality and malnutrition among populations living in South Darfur, Sudan:

Results of 3 surveys, September 2004'. *Journal of the American Medical Association*, 293: 1490–4. [8.4.1]

Gratz, N. G., Steffen, R., and Cocksedge, W. (2000). 'Why aircraft disinsection?' *Bulletin of the World Health Organization*, 78: 995–1004. [6.5.3]

Graves, L. M., Hunter, S. B., Ong, A. R., Schoonmaker-Bopp, D., Hise, K., Kornstein, L., DeWitt, W. E., Hayes, P. S., Dunne, E., Mead, P., and Swaminathan, B. (2005). 'Microbiological aspects of the investigation that traced the 1998 outbreak of listeriosis in the United States to contaminated hot dogs and establishment of molecular subtyping-based surveillance for *Listeria monocytogenes* in the PulseNet network'. *Journal of Clinical Microbiology*, 43: 2350–5. [5.2.3]

Green, T., Talbot, M. D., and Morton, R. S. (2001). 'The control of syphilis, a contemporary problem: A historical perspective'. *Sexually Transmitted Infections*, 77: 214–17. [9.5.1]

Greenberg, J. H. (1969). 'Public health problems relating to the Vietnam returnee'. *Journal of the American Medical Association*, 207: 697–702. [8.2.2]

Greenhalgh, D. (1986). 'Optimal control of an epidemic by ring vaccination'. *Stochastic Models*, 2: 339–63. [11.3.1]

Greenwood, B. (2006). '100 years of epidemic meningitis in West Africa—has anything changed?' *Tropical Medicine and International Health*, 11: 773–80. [9.3.2]

Grenfell, B. T., Bjørnstad, O. N., and Kappy, J. (2001). 'Travelling waves and spatial hierarchies in measles epidemics'. *Nature*, 414: 716–23. [10.2.1]

Griffin, P. M. and Boyce, T. G. (1998). '*Escherichia coli* O157:H7'. In W. M. Scheld, D. Armstrong, and J. M. Hughes (eds), *Emerging Infections 1*. Washington, DC: ASM Press, 137–45. [5.2.4]

—— and Tauxe, R. V. (1991). 'The epidemiology of infections caused by *Escherichia coli* O157:H7, other enterohemorrhagic *E. coli*, and the associated hemolytic uremic syndrome'. *Epidemiologic Reviews*, 13: 60–98. [5.2.4]

Griffiths, D. A. (1973). 'The effect of measles vaccination on the incidence of measles in the community'. *Journal of the Royal Statistical Society A*, 136: 441–9. [11.3.1, App. 11.2]

Gubler, D. J. (1998). 'Resurgent vector-borne diseases as a global health problem'. *Emerging Infectious Diseases*, 4: 442–50. [4.4.1]

—— Reiter, P., Ebi, K. L., Yap, W., Nasci, R., and Patz, J. A. (2001). 'Climate variability and change in the United States: Potential impacts on vector- and rodent-borne diseases'. *Environmental Health Perspectives*, 109, suppl. 2, 223–33. [7.5.1]

Guhl, F., Jaramillo, C., Vallejo, G. A., Yockteng, R., Cardenas-Arroyo, F., Fornaciari, G., Arriaza, B., and Aufderheide, A. R. (1999). 'Isolation of *Trypanosoma cruzi* DNA in 4,000-year-old mummified human tissue from Northern Chile'. *American Journal of Physical Anthropology*, 108: 401–7. [1.3.3]

Guimera, R., Mossa, S., Turtschi, A., and Amaral, L. A. N. (2005). 'The worldwide air transportation network: Anomalous centrality, community structure, and cities' global roles'. *Proceedings of the National Academy of Sciences USA*, 102: 7794–9. [6.4.2]

Gurley, E. S., Montgomery, J. M., Hossain, M. J., Bell, M., Azad, A. K., Islam, M. R., Molla, M. A., Carroll, D. S., Ksiazek, T. G., Rota, P. A., Lowe, L., Comer, J. A., Rollin, P., Czub, M., Grolla, A., Feldmann, H., Luby, S. P., Woodward, J. L., and Breiman, R. F. (2007). 'Person-to-person transmission of

Nipah virus in a Bangladeshi community'. *Emerging Infectious Diseases*, 13: 1031–7. [7.4.1]

GUST, I. D., HAMPSON, A. W., and LAVANCHY, D. (2001). 'Planning for the next pandemic of influenza'. *Reviews in Medical Virology*, 11: 59–70. [4.2.2]

GUTHMANN, J.-P., KLOVSTAD, H., BOCCIA, D., HAMID, N., PINOGES, L., NIZOU, J.-Y., TATAY, M., DIAZ, F., MOREN, A., GRAIS, R. F., CIGLENECKI, I., NICAND, E., and GUERIN, P. J. (2006). 'A large outbreak of hepatitis E among a displaced population in Darfur, Sudan, 2004: The role of water treatment methods'. *Clinical Infectious Diseases*, 42: 1685–91. [8.4.1]

H

HAAS, C. J., ZINK, A., PÁLFI, G. Y., SZEIMIES, U., and NERLICH, A. G. (2000). 'Detection of leprosy in ancient human skeletal remains by molecular identification of *Mycobacterium leprae*'. *American Journal of Clinical Pathology*, 114: 428–36. [1.3.3]

HABER, M. J., SHAY, D. K., DAVIS, X. M., PATEL, R., JIN, X., WEINTRAUB, E., ORENSTEIN, E., and THOMPSON, W. W. (2007). 'Effectiveness of interventions to reduce contact rates during a simulated influenza pandemic'. *Emerging Infectious Diseases*, 13: 581–9. [11.2.3]

HAESER, H. (1882). *Lehrbuch der Geschichte der Medizin und der Epidemischen Krankheiten. III*, 3rd edn. Basel: Jena. [2.3.4]

HAGGETT, P. (2000). *The Geographical Structure of Epidemics*. Oxford: Clarendon Press. [6.2.1, 6.5.1]

—— (2001). *Geography: A Global Synthesis*. London: Pearson. [7.4.2]

—— and CHORLEY, R. J. (1969). *Network Analysis in Geography*. London: Arnold. [6.4.2]

—— CLIFF, A. D., and FREY, A. E. (1977). *Locational Analysis in Human Geography*, 2nd edn. London: Arnold. [6.2.1, 6.2.3]

HAHNÉ, S. J., GRAY, S. J., AGUILERA, J.-F., CROWCROFT, N. S., NICHOLS, T., KACMARSKI, E. B., and RAMSAY, M. E. (2002). 'W135 meningococcal disease in England and Wales associated with Hajj 2000 and 2001'. *Lancet*, 359: 582–3. [6.5.2]

HALES, S., DE WET, N., MAINDONALD, J., and WOODWARD, A. (2002). 'Potential effect of population and climate changes on global distribution of dengue fever: An empirical model'. *Lancet*, 360: 830–4. [7.5.1]

—— EDWARDS, S. J., and KOVATS, R. S. (2003). 'Impacts on health of climatic extremes'. In A. J. McMichael, D. H. Campbell-Lendrum, C. F. Corvalan, K. L. Ebi, A. Githeko, J. D. Scheraga, and A. Woodward (eds), *Climate Change and Human Health: Risks and Responses*. Geneva: WHO, 79–102. [7.5.2]

HALL, R. (1993). *Notifiable Disease Surveillance, 1917–1991*. Computer spreadsheet. Canberra: Department of Health, Housing, Local Government and Community Services. [9.1, 9.4.1]

HANNA, J. N., RITCHIE, S. A., RICHARDS, A. R., TAYLOR, C. T., PYKE, A. T., MONTGOMERY, B. L., PIISPANEN, J. P., MORGAN, A. K., and HUMPHREYS, J. L. (2006). 'Multiple outbreaks of dengue serotype 2 in north Queensland, 2003/04'. *Australian and New Zealand Journal of Public Health*, 30: 220–5. [9.4.2]

HARB, M., FARIS, R., GAD, A. M., HAFEZ, O. N., RAMZY, R., and BUCK, A. A. (1993). 'The resurgence of lymphatic filariasis in the Nile delta'. *Bulletin of the World Health Organization*, 71: 49–54. [7.2]

HARDEN, V. A. (1993). 'Typhus, epidemic'. In K. F. Kiple (ed.), *The Cambridge World History of Human Disease*. Cambridge: Cambridge University Press, 1080–6. [2.3.1]

HARDY, A. (1983). 'Smallpox in London: Factors in the decline of the disease in the nineteenth century'. *Medical History*, 27: 111–38. [2.4.2]

—— (1993*a*). 'Scarlet fever'. In K. F. Kiple (ed.), *The Cambridge World History of Human Disease*. Cambridge: Cambridge University Press, 990–2. [2.3.1]

—— (1993*b*). 'Whooping cough'. In K. F. Kiple (ed.), *The Cambridge World History of Human Disease*. Cambridge: Cambridge University Press, 1094–6. [2.3.1]

—— (1993*c*). *The Epidemic Streets: Infectious Disease and the Rise of Preventive Medicine, 1856–1900*. Oxford: Clarendon Press. [2.4.2]

—— (1994). '"Death is the cure of all diseases": Using the General Register Office cause of death statistics for 1837–1920'. *Social History of Medicine*, 7: 472–92. [2.4.2]

HARRUS, S. and BANETH, G. (2005). 'Drivers for the emergence and re-emergence of vector-borne protozoal and bacterial diseases'. *International Journal for Parasitology*, 35: 1309–18. [7.3]

HARTZELL, J. D., PENG, S. W., WOOD-MORRIS, R. N., SARMIENTO, D. M., COLLEN, J. F., ROBBEN, P. M., and MORAN, K. A. (2007). 'Atypical Q fever in US soldiers'. *Emerging Infectious Diseases*, 13: 1247–9. [8.4.2]

HAY, A. J., GREGORY, V., DOUGLAS, A. R., and LIN, Y. P. (2001). 'The evolution of human influenza viruses'. *Philosophical Transactions of the Royal Society of London, B Biological Sciences*, 356: 1861–70. [10.2.1]

HEALTH ORGANIZATION OF THE LEAGUE OF NATIONS (1931). *Health*. Geneva: Information Section, League of Nations. [3.2.1]

HEALTH SECTION OF THE LEAGUE OF NATIONS (1922). 'Introductory note'. *Epidemiological Intelligence: Eastern Europe in 1921*, E.I.1, 3. [3.2.1]

HECKER, J. F. C. (1859). *The Epidemics of the Middle Ages (Third Edition, Completed by the Author's Treatise on Child-Pilgrimages)*. Trans. B. G. Babington. London: Trübner. [2.3.5]

HEMINGWAY, J. and RANSON, H. (2000). 'Insecticide resistance in insect vectors of human disease'. *Annual Review of Entomology*, 45: 371–91. [4.4.1]

HENDERSON, D. A. (1999). 'The looming threat of bioterrorism'. *Science*, 283: 1279–82. [8.5.1, 8.5.2]

—— (2000). 'Weapons for the future'. *Lancet*, 354, suppl. IV, 64. [8.5, 8.5.2]

HENIPAVIRUS ECOLOGY COLLABORATIVE RESEARCH GROUP (2005). *Nipah Virus*. Queensland: Henipavirus Ecology Collaborative Research Group. http://www.henipavirus.org, accessed 21 July 2008. [7.4.1]

HENNESSY, T. W., HEDBERG, C. W., SLUTSKER, L., WHITE, K. E., BESSER-WIEK, J. M., MOEN, M. E., FELDMAN, J., COLEMAN, W. W., EDMONSON, L. M., MACDONALD, K. L., and OSTERHOLM, M. T. (1996). 'A national outbreak of *Salmonella enteritidis* infections from ice cream'. *New England Journal of Medicine*, 334: 1281–6. [5.2.3]

HERMANN, W. (1973). *Die El-Tor-Cholera-Pandemie 1961 bis 1968*. Leipzig: Johann Ambrosius Barth. [9.2.2]

Hesla, P. E. (1992). 'Hepatitis A in Norwegian troops'. *Vaccine*, 10, suppl. 1, S80–1. [8.4.3]

Hethcote, H., Zhien, M., and Shengbing, L. (2002). 'Effects of quarantine in six endemic models for infectious diseases'. *Mathematical Biosciences*, 180: 141–60. [11.2.3]

Heymann, D. L. (ed.) (2004). *Control of Communicable Diseases Manual*, 18th edn. Washington, DC: American Public Health Association. [2.3.2, 2.3.3, 2.3.4, 4.3.2, 5.2.4, 5.2.5, 5.3.1, 7.2.1, 7.3.1, 7.4.1, 7.4.2, 7.5.3, 8.2.1, 8.3.1, 8.4.1, 8.5, 8.5.3, 8.6, 9.2.2, 9.2.3, 9.3.2, 9.4.2]

Hilborn, E. D., Mermin, J. H., Mshar, P. A., Hadler, J. L., Voetsch, A., Wojtkunski, C., Swartz, M., Mshar, R., Lambert-Fair, M. A., Farrar, J. A., Glynn, M. K., and Slutsker, L. (1999). 'A multistate outbreak of *Escherichia coli* O157:H7 infections associated with consumption of mesclun lettuce'. *Archives of Internal Medicine*, 159: 1748–64. [5.2.3]

Hirsch, A. (1883–6). *Handbook of Geographical and Historical Pathology*, i: *Acute Infective Diseases*; ii: *Chronic Infective, Toxic, Parasitic, Septic and Constitutional Diseases*; iii: *Diseases of Organs and Parts*. Trans. from the second German edn by C. Creighton. London: The New Sydenham Society. [2.1, 2.3, 2.3.1, 2.3.2, 2.3.3, 2.3.4, 2.3.5, 4.2.2, 9.3.2]

Hirst, F. L. (1953). *The Conquest of Plague*. Oxford: Clarendon Press. [2.2.1]

Hjelle, B. and Glass, G. E. (2000). 'Outbreak of hantavirus infection in the Four Corners region of the United States in the wake of the 1997–1998 El Niño–Southern Oscillation'. *Journal of Infectious Diseases*, 181: 1569–73. [7.5.3]

Hoaglin, D. C., Mosteller, F., and Tukey, J. W. (eds) (1983). *Understanding Robust and Exploratory Data Analysis*. New York: Wiley. [10.2.1]

Holladay, A. J. (1986). 'The Thucydides syndrome: Another view'. *New England Journal of Medicine*, 315: 1170–3. [2.2.2]

Hollingsworth, T. D., Ferguson, N. M., and Anderson, R. M. (2006). 'Will travel restrictions control the international spread of pandemic influenza?' *Nature Medicine*, 12: 497–9. [6.4.2]

Holty, J.-E. C., Bravata, D. M., Liu, H., Olshen, R. A., McDonald, K. M., and Owens, D. K. (2006). 'Systematic review: A century of inhalational anthrax cases from 1900 to 2005'. *Annals of Internal Medicine*, 144: 271–80. [8.5.3]

Holtzman, D. (2003). 'Analysis and interpretation of data from the US Behavioral Risk Factor Surveillance System (BRFSS)'. In D. V. McQueen and P. Puska (eds), *Global Behavioral Risk Factor Surveillance*. New York: Kluwer Academic/Plenum Publishers. [10.6.2]

Hoogstraal, H. (1978). 'Rift Valley fever: An historical perspective'. *Journal of the Egyptian Public Health Association*, 53: 129–35. [7.3.1]

—— Meegan, J. M., Khalil, G. M., and Adham, F. K. (1979). 'The Rift Valley fever epizootic in Egypt 1977–78. 2. Ecological and entomological studies'. *Transactions of the Royal Society of Tropical Medicine and Hygiene*, 73: 624. [7.2.1]

Hooper, E. (1999). *The River: A Journey Back to the Source of HIV and AIDS*. Harmondsworth: Penguin. [9.2.3]

Horimoto, T. and Kawaoka, Y. (2001). 'Pandemic threat posed by avian influenza viruses'. *Clinical Microbiology Reviews*, 14: 129–49. [4.2.2, 4.2.3]

HOWARD, D., CORDELL, R., MCGOWAN, J. E., JR, PACKARD, R. M., SCOTT, R. D., II, and SOLOMON, S. L. (2001). 'Measuring the economic costs of antimicrobial resistance in hospital settings: Summary of the Centers for Disease Control and Prevention–Emory Workshop'. *Clinical Infectious Diseases*, 33: 1573–8. [4.3.1]

HOWARD, J. (1791). *An Account of the Principal Lazarettos in Europe; with Various Papers Relative to the Plague: Together with Further Observations on some Foreign Prisons and Hospitals; and Additional Remarks on the Present State of Those in Great Britain and Ireland*, 2nd edn. London: Johnson, Dilly and Cadell. [11.2.1]

HSU, V. P., HOSSAIN, M. J., PARASHAR, U. D., ALI, M. M., KSIAZEK, T. G., KUZMIN, I., NIEZGODA, M., RUPPRECHT, C., BRESEE, J., and BREIMAN, R. F. (2004). 'Nipah virus encephalitis reemergence, Bangladesh'. *Emerging Infectious Diseases*, 10: 2082–7. [7.4.1]

HUFNAGEL, L., BROCKMANN, D., and GEISEL, T. (2004). 'Forecast and control of epidemics in a globalized world'. *Proceedings of the National Academy of Sciences USA*, 101: 15124–9. [6.4.2]

HUGHES, J. M. (1999). 'The emerging threat of bioterrorism'. *Emerging Infectious Diseases*, 5: 494–5. [8.5.3]

—— PETERS, C. J., COHEN, M. L., and MAHY, B. W. (1993). 'Hantavirus pulmonary syndrome: An emerging infectious disease'. *Science*, 262: 850–1. [7.5.3]

HUI, E. K.-W. (2006). 'Reasons for the increase in emerging and re-emerging viral infectious diseases'. *Microbes and Infection*, 8: 905–16. [7.2.1]

HUKIC, M., KURT, A., TORSTENSSON, S., LUNDKVIST, Å., WIGER, D., and NIKLASSON, B. (1996). 'Haemorrhagic fever with renal syndrome in north-east Bosnia'. *Lancet*, 347: 56–7. [8.4]

HULSE, E. V. (1971). 'Joshua's curse and the abandonment of ancient Jericho: Schistosomiasis as a possible medical explanation'. *Medical History*, 15: 376–86. [2.2.1]

HUMPHREYS, B. L. (2007). 'Building better connections: The National Library of Medicine and public health'. *Journal of the Medical Library Association*, 95: 293–300. [10.6.3]

HUNTER, G. W. (1953). 'Local health hazards among US army troops returning from Korea'. *American Journal of Public Health and the Nation's Health*, 43: 1408–17. [8.2.1]

HUNTER, J. M. and YOUNG, J. C. (1971). 'Diffusion of influenza in England and Wales'. *Annals of the Association of American Geographers*, 61: 637–53. [4.2.3]

HUNTER, R. (1991). 'The English sweating sickness, with particular reference to the 1551 outbreak in Chester'. *Reviews of Infectious Diseases*, 13: 303–6. [2.3.5]

HYAMS, K. C., BOURGEOIS, A. L., MERRELL, B. R., ROZMAJZL, P., ESCAMILLA, J., THORNTON, S. A., WASSERMAN, G. M., BURKE, A., ECHEVERRIA, P., GREEN, K. Y., KAPIKIAN, A. Z., and WOODY, J. N. (1991). 'Diarrheal disease during Operation Desert Shield'. *New England Journal of Medicine*, 325: 1423–8. [8.4.2]

—— WIGNALL, F. S., and ROSWELL, R. (1996). 'War syndromes and their evaluation: From the US Civil War to the Persian Gulf War'. *Annals of Internal Medicine*, 125: 398–405. [8.4.3, 8.4.4]

I

IKEDA, R. M., MERCY, J. A., and TERET, S. P. (1998). 'Firearm-related injury surveillance'. *American Journal of Preventive Medicine*, 15, suppl., 6–16. [10.6.1]

INGHAM, F. J. (1953). 'Discussion on military medical problems in Korea: Army health problems'. *Proceedings of the Royal Society of Medicine, United Services Section*, 46: 1041–6. [8.2.1]

INTERGOVERNMENTAL PANEL ON CLIMATE CHANGE (2007*a*). *Climate Change 2007: Fourth Assessment Report. Working Group I Report, The Physical Science Basis*. Cambridge: Cambridge University Press. [7.5.1]

—— (2007*b*). *Climate Change 2007: Fourth Assessment Report. Working Group II Report, Impacts, Adaptation and Vulnerability*. Cambridge: Cambridge University Press. [7.5.1]

INTERNATIONAL COMMISSION (1978). 'Ebola haemorrhagic fever in Zaire, 1976'. *Bulletin of the World Health Organization*, 56: 271–93. [9.3.2]

INTERNATIONAL FEDERATION OF RED CROSS AND RED CRESCENT SOCIETIES (2007). *World Disaster Report 2007: Focus on Discrimination*. Geneva: International Federation of Red Cross and Red Crescent Societies. [7.6]

ISAKBAEVA, E. T., WIDDOWSON, M.-A., BEAR, R. S., BULENS, S. N., MULLINS, J., MONROE, S. S., BRESEE, J., SASSANO, P., CRAMER, E. H., and GLASS, R. I. (2005). 'Norovirus transmission on cruise ship'. *Emerging Infectious Diseases*, 11: 154–7. [6.3.1]

J

JACKSON, M. L., BAER, A., PAINTER, I., and DUCHIN, J. (2007). 'A simulation study comparing aberration detection algorithms for syndromic surveillance'. *BMC Medical Informatics and Decision Making*, 7/6. doi:10.1186/1472–6947–7–6. [10.6.3]

JAHRLING, P. B. (1997). 'Arenaviruses'. In A. S. Evans and R. A. Kaslow (eds), *Viral Infections of Humans: Epidemiology and Control*, 4th edn. London: Plenum Medical Book Company, 185–209. [7.2.1]

JANSEN, V. A. A., STOLLENWERK, N., JENSEN, H. J., RAMSAY, M. E., EDMUNDS, W. J., and RHODES, C. J. (2003). 'Measles outbreaks in a population with declining vaccine uptake'. *Science*, 301: 804. [11.3.1]

JARCHO, S. (1983). 'Some early Italian epidemiological maps'. *Imago Mundi*, 35: 9–19. [11.2.1]

JEZEK, Z., SZCZENIOWSKI, M. Y., MUYEMBE-TAMFUM, J. J., MCCORMICK, J. B., and HEYMANN, D. L. (1999). 'Ebola between outbreaks: Intensified Ebola haemorrhagic fever surveillance in the Democratic Republic of the Congo, 1981–1985'. *Journal of Infectious Diseases*, 179, suppl. 1, S60–4. [9.3.2]

JOHNSON, N. P. A. S. and MUELLER, J. (2002). 'Updating the accounts: Global mortality of the 1918–1920 "Spanish" influenza pandemic'. *Bulletin of the History of Medicine*, 76: 105–15. [4.2.2]

JOHNSON, R. T. (2003). 'Emerging viral infections of the nervous system'. *Journal of NeuroVirology*, 9: 140–7. [6.5.3]

JOHNSTON, W. D. (1993). 'Tuberculosis'. In K. F. Kiple (ed.), *The Cambridge World History of Human Disease*. Cambridge: Cambridge University Press, 1059–68. [2.3.1]

JONES, A., MORGAN, D., WALSH, A., TURTON, J., LIVERMORE, D., PITT, T., GREEN, A., GILL, M., and MORTIBOY, D. (2006). 'Importation of multidrug-resistant

Acinetobacter spp. infections with casualties from Iraq'. *Lancet Infectious Diseases*, 6: 317–18. [8.4.2]

JONES, E. and WESSELY, S. (1999). 'Case of chronic fatigue syndrome after Crimean War and Indian Mutiny'. *British Medical Journal*, 319: 1645–7. [8.4.4]

—— HODGINS-VERMAAS, R., MCCARTNEY, H., EVERITT, B., BEECH, C., POYNTER, D., PALMER, I., HYAMS, K., and WESSELY, S. (2002). 'Post-combat syndromes from the Boer War to the Gulf War: A cluster analysis of their nature and attribution'. *British Medical Journal*, 324: 321–4. [8.4.4]

JONES, T. F., SCALLON, E., and ANGULO, F. J. (2007). 'FoodNet: Overview of a decade of achievement'. *Foodborne Pathogenic Diseases*, 4: 60–6. [10.6.3]

JORDAN, E. O. (1927). *Epidemic Influenza: A Survey*. Chicago: American Medical Association. [4.2.2]

JOWETT, B. (1900). *Thucydides*, i: *Essay on Inscriptions and Books I–III*, 2nd edn, rev. Oxford: Clarendon Press. [2.2.2]

JUSATZ, H. J. (1954–61). 'Cerebrospinal meningitis, 1927–1958'. In E. Rodenwaldt and H. J. Jusatz (eds), *World-Atlas of Epidemic Diseases. Parts II and III*. Hamburg: Falk-Verlag, III/43–44b. [9.3.2]

K

KÄFERSTEIN, F. K., MOTARJEMI, Y., and BETTCHER, D. W. (1997). 'Foodborne disease control: A transnational challenge'. *Emerging Infectious Diseases*, 3: 503–10. [5.2.1]

KALIPENI, E. and OPPONG, J. (1998). 'The refugee crisis in Africa and implications for health and disease: A political ecology approach'. *Social Science and Medicine*, 46: 1637–53. [8.3]

KANESA-THASAN, N., IACONO-CONNORS, L., MAGILL, A., SMOAK, B., VAUGHN, D., DUBOIS, D., BURROUS, J., and HOKE, C. (1994). 'Dengue serotypes 2 and 3 in US forces in Somalia'. *Lancet*, 343: 678. [8.4.3]

KANSKY, K. J. (1963). *Structure of Transport Networks: Relationships between Network Geometry and Regional Characteristics*. University of Chicago, Department of Geography, Research Papers, 84. [6.4.2]

KAPER, J. B., MORRIS, J. G., JR, and LEVINE, M. M. (1995). 'Cholera'. *Clinical Microbiology Reviews*, 8: 48–86. [2.3.4, 9.2.2]

KASH, J. C., TUMPEY, T. M., PROLL, S. C., CARTER, V., PERWITASARI, O., THOMAS, M. J., BASLER, C. F., PALESE, P., TAUBENBERGER, J. K., GARCÍA-SASTRE, A., SWAYNE, D. E., and KATZE, M. G. (2006). 'Genomic analysis of increased host immune and cell death responses induced by the 1918 influenza virus'. *Nature*, 443: 578–81. [4.2.4]

KAZAKOVA, S. V., WARE, K., BAUGHMAN, B., BILUKHA, O., PARADIS, A., SEARS, S., THOMPSON, A., JENSEN, B., WIGGS, L., BESSETTE, J., MARTIN, J., CLUKEY, J., GENSHEIMER, K., KILLGORE, G., and MCDONALD, L. C. (2006). 'A hospital outbreak of diarrhea due to an emerging epidemic strain of *Clostridium difficile*'. *Archives of Internal Medicine*, 166: 2518–24. [4.3.1]

KEAWCHAROEN, J., ORAVEERAKUL, K., KUIKEN, T., FOUCHIER, R. A. M., AMONSIN, A., PAYUNGPORN, S., NOPPORNPANTH, S., WATTANODORN, S., THEAMBOON-

LERS, A., TANTILERTCHAROEN, R., PATTANARANGSAN, R., ARYA, N., RATANAKORN, P., OSTERHUAS, A. D. M. E., and POOVORAWAN, Y. (2004). 'Avian H5N1 in tigers and leopards'. *Emerging Infectious Diseases*, 10: 2189–91. [4.2.3]

KEELE, B. F., Van HEUVERSWYN, F., LI, Y., BAILES, E., TAKEHISA, J., SANTIAGO, M. L., BIBOLLET-RUCHE, F., CHEN, Y., WAIN, L. V., LIEGEOIS, F., LOUL, S., NGOLE, E. M., BIENVENUE, Y., DELAPORTE, E., BROOKFIELD, J. F., SHARP, P. M., SHAW, G. M., PEETERS, M., and HAHN, B. H. (2006). 'Chimpanzee reservoirs of pandemic and nonpandemic HIV-1'. *Science*, 313: 523–6. [9.2.3]

KEELING, M. J. and GRENFELL, B. T. (1997). 'Disease extinction and community size: Modeling the persistence of measles'. *Science*, 275: 65–7. [10.2.1]

KENNEDY, S., SMYTH, J. A., CUSH, P. F., MCCULLOUGH, S. J., ALLAN, G. M., and MCQUAID, S. (1988). 'Viral distemper now found in porpoises'. *Nature*, 336: 21. [7.4.1]

KESHAVJEE, S. and BECERRA, M. C. (2000). 'Disintegrating health services and resurgent tuberculosis in post-Soviet Tajikistan: An example of structural violence'. *Journal of the American Medical Association*, 283: 1201. [8.1]

KHAN, I. A. (2004). 'Plague: The dreadful visitation occupying the human mind for centuries'. *Transactions of the Royal Society of Tropical Medicine and Hygiene*, 98: 270–7. [9.2.1]

KHLAT, M. and KHOURY, M. (1991). 'Inbreeding and diseases: Demographic, genetic and inbreeding perspectives'. *Epidemiologic Reviews*, 13: 28–41. [6.5.1]

KILBOURNE, E. D. (1973). 'The molecular epidemiology of influenza'. *Journal of Infectious Diseases*, 127: 478–87. [4.2.2]

KILONZO, B. S., MAKUNDI, R. H., and MBISE, T. J. (1992). 'A decade of plague epidemiology and control in the western Usambara mountains, north-east Tanzania'. *Acta Tropica*, 50: 323–9. [9.2.1]

KILWEIN, J. H. (1995*a*). 'Some historical comments on quarantine: Part one'. *Journal of Clinical Pharmacy and Therapeutics*, 20: 185–7. [11.2.3]

—— (1995*b*). 'Some historical comments on quarantine: Part two'. *Journal of Clinical Pharmacy and Therapeutics*, 20: 249–52. [11.2.3]

KIM-FARLEY, R. J. (1993*a*). 'Measles'. In K. F. Kiple (ed.), *Cambridge World History of Human Disease*. Cambridge: Cambridge University Press, 871–5. [2.3.1]

—— (1993*b*). 'Mumps'. In K. F. Kiple (ed.), *Cambridge World History of Human Disease*. Cambridge: Cambridge University Press, 887–9. [2.2.2]

KIMURA, A. C., JOHNSON, K., PALUMBO, M. S., HOPKINS, J., BOASE, J. C., REPORTER, R., GOLDOFT, M., STEFONEK, K. R., FARRAR, J. A., VAN GILDER, T. J., and VUGIA, D. J. (2004). 'Multistate shigellosis outbreak and commercially prepared food, United States'. *Emerging Infectious Diseases*, 10: 1147–9. [5.2.3]

KIPLE, K. F. (ed.) (1993). *The Cambridge World History of Human Disease*. Cambridge: Cambridge University Press. [11.2.1]

KLEIN, E., SMITH, D. L., and LAXMINARAYAN, R. (2007). 'Hospitalizations and deaths caused by methicillin-resistant *Staphylococcus aureus*, United States, 1999–2005'. *Emerging Infectious Diseases*, 1840–6. [4.3.1]

KNABB, R. D., RHOME, J. R., and BROWN, D. P. (2006*a*). *Tropical Cyclone Report: Hurricane Katrina, 23–30 August 2005. Updated 10 August 2006 for Tropical Wave History, Storm Surge, Tornadoes, Surface Observations, Fatalities, and Damage Cost Estimates*. Miami: National Hurricane Center. http://www.nhc.noaa.gov/pdf/TCR-AL122005_Katrina.pdf, accessed 21 July 2008. [7.6.3]

KNABB, R. D., RHOME, J. R., and BROWN, D. P. (2006*b*). *Tropical Cyclone Report: Hurricane Rita, 18–26 September 2005. Updated 14 August 2006 for Updated Damage Cost Estimates and for a Few Storm Surge Observations*. Miami: National Hurricane Center. http://www.nhc.noaa.gov/pdf/TCR-AL182005_Rita.pdf, accessed 21 July 2008. [7.6.3]

KOHL, P. A., O'ROURKE, A. P., SCHMIDMAN, D. L., DOPKIN, W. A., and BIRNBAUM, M. L. (2005). 'The Sumatra–Andaman earthquake and tsunami of 2004: The hazards, events, and damage'. *Prehospital and Disaster Medicine*, 20: 355–63. [7.6.2]

KOHN, G. C. (1998). *Encyclopedia of Plague and Pestilence*. Ware: Wordsworth. [2.2, 2.2.2, 2.3.1, 2.3.2, 2.3.5, 8.2.2]

KOLLE, W. and PRIGGE, R. (1928). 'Cholera asiatica'. In W. Kolle, R. Kraus, and P. Uhlenhuth (eds) (1928–31), *Handbuch der Pathogenen Mikroorganismen*, 3rd edn, iv. Jena: Gustav Fischer. [2.3.4]

KOLMAN, C. J., CENTURION-LARA, A., LUKEHART, S. A., OWSLEY, D. W., and TUROSS, N. (1999). 'Identification of *Treponema pallidum* subspecies *pallidum* in a 200-year-old skeletal specimen'. *Journal of Infectious Diseases*, 180: 2060–3. [1.3.3]

KONDO, H., SEO, N., YASUDA, T., HASIZUME, M., KOIDO, Y., NINOMIYA, N., and YAMAMOTO, Y. (2002). 'Post-flood—infectious diseases in Mozambique'. *Prehospital Disaster Medicine*, 17: 126–33. [7.6.1]

KOPLAN, J. P. and THACKER, S. B. (2001). 'Fifty years of epidemiology at the Centers for Disease Control and Prevention: Significant and consequential'. *American Journal of Epidemiology*, 154: 982–4. [3.4.1]

KOTWAL, R. S., WENZEL, R. B., STERLING, R. A., PORTER, W. D., JORDAN, N. N., and PETRUCELLI, B. P. (2006). 'An outbreak of malaria in US Army Rangers returning from Afghanistan'. *Journal of the American Medical Association*, 293: 212–16. [8.4.2]

KOUMARÉ, B., OUEDRAOGO-TRAORÉ, R., SANOU, I., YADA, A. A., SOW, I., LUSAMBA, P.-S., TRAORÉ, E., DABAL, M., SANTAMARIA, M., HACEN, M.-M., KABORÉ, A. B., and CAUGANT, D. A. (2007). 'The first large epidemic of meningococcal disease caused by serogroup W135, Burkina Faso, 2002'. *Vaccine*, 25, suppl. 1, A37–41. [9.3.2]

KOVATS, R. S. (2000). 'El Niño and human health'. *Bulletin of the World Health Organization*, 78: 1127–35. [7.5.2]

—— BOUMA, M. J., HAJAT, S., WORRALL, E., and HAINES, A. (2003). 'El Niño and health'. *Lancet*, 362: 1481–9. [7.5.2]

—— CAMPBELL-LENDRUM, D. H., MCMICHAEL, A. J., WOODWARD, A., and COX, J. ST H. (2001). 'Early effects of climate change: Do they include changes in vector-borne disease?' *Philosophical Transactions of the Royal Society of London B*, 356: 1057–68. [7.5.1]

KRAUSE, G., ROPERS, G., and STARK, K. (2005). 'Notifiable disease surveillance and practicing physicians'. *Emerging Infectious Diseases*, 11: 442–5. [10.6.2]

KRAUSE, R. M. (ed.) (1998). *Emerging Infections*. San Diego: Academic Press. [1.5.2]

KRISHNAMOORTHY, K., JAMBULINGAM, P., NATARJAN, R., SHRIRAM, A. N., DAS, P. K., and SEHGAL, S. C. (2005). 'Altered environment and risk of malaria outbreak in South Andaman, Andaman & Nicobar Islands, India affected by tsunami disaster'. *Malaria Journal*, 4/32. doi:10.1186/1475–2875–4–32. [7.6.2]

KUHN, K., CAMPBELL-LENDRUM, D., and DAVIES, C. R. (2002). 'A continental risk map for malaria mosquito (Diptera: *Culicidae*) vectors in Europe'. *Journal of Medical Entomology*, 39: 621–30. [7.5.1]

KUKAFKA, R., ANCKER, J. S., CHAN, C., CHELICO, J., KHAN, S., MORTOTI, S., NATARJAN, K., PRESLEY, K., and STEPHENS, K. (2007). 'Redesigning electronic health record systems to support public health'. *Journal of Biomedical Informatics*, 40: 398–409. [10.6.3]

KUNZ, J. (1979). '*Index Medicus*: A century of medical citation'. *Journal of the American Medical Association*, 241: 387–90. [1.2.1]

L

LAM, S. K. and CHUA, K. B. (2002). 'Nipah virus encephalitis outbreak in Malaysia'. *Clinical Infectious Diseases*, 34, suppl. 2, S48–51. [7.4.1]

LANCASTER, H. O. (1967). 'The infections and population size of Australia'. *Bulletin of the International Statistical Institute*, 42: 459–71. [6.3.1]

—— (1990). *Expectations of Life: A Study in the Demography, Statistics, and History of World Mortality*. New York: Springer-Verlag. [6.3.1, 9.3.1]

LANCIOTTI, R. S., ROEHRIG, J. T., DEUBEL, V., SMITH, J., PARKER, M., STEELE, K., CRISE, B., VOLPE, K. E., CRABTREE, M. B., SCHERRET, J. H., HALL, R. A., MACKENZIE, J. S., CROPP, C. B., PANIGRAHY, B., OSTLUND, E., SCHMITT, B., MALKINSON, M., BANET, C., WEISSMAN, J., KOMAR, N., SAVAGE, H. M., STONE, W., MCNAMARA, T., and GUBLER, D. J. (1999). 'Origin of the West Nile virus responsible for an outbreak of encephalitis in the northeastern United States'. *Science*, 286: 2333–7. [6.5.3]

LANDERS, J. (1993). *Death and the Metropolis: Studies in the Demographic History of London 1670–1830*. Cambridge: Cambridge University Press. [2.4.2]

LANGMUIR, A. D. (1963). 'The surveillance of communicable diseases of national importance'. *New England Journal of Medicine*, 288: 182–92. [10.6.1]

—— (1980). 'The Epidemic Intelligence Service of the Centers for Disease Control'. *Public Health Reports*, 95: 470–7. [3.4.1]

—— NATHANSON, N., and HALL, W. J. (1956). 'Surveillance of poliomyelitis in the United States in 1955'. *American Journal of Public Health*, 46: 75–88. [11.3.1, 11.3.2]

LAPEYSSONNIE, L. (1963). 'La Méningite cérébro-spinale en Afrique'. *Bulletin of the World Health Organization*, 28, suppl., 3–114. [9.3.2]

LAWRENCE, J. (2005). 'Tsunami in South Asia and East Africa—infectious disease update'. *Eurosurveillance*, 10/4: pii=2630. http://www.eurosurveillance.org/ViewArticle.aspx?ArticleId=2630, accessed 21 July 2008. [7.6.2]

LAZARUS, R., KLEINMAN, K. P., DASHEVSKY, I., DEMARIA, A., and PLATT, R. (2001). 'Using automated medical records for rapid identification of illness syndromes (syndromic surveillance): The example of lower respiratory infection'. *BMC Public Health*, 1/9. doi:10.1186/1471–2458–1–9. [10.6.3]

LEARMONTH, A. (1988). *Disease Ecology: An Introduction*. Oxford: Blackwell. [4.4.3]

LECLERC, J. E., LI, B., PAYNE, W. L., and CEBULA, T. A. (1999). 'Promiscuous origin of a chimeric sequence in the *Escherichia coli* O157:H7 genome'. *Journal of Bacteriology*, 181: 7614–17. [5.2.4]

LEDERBERG, J. (1998). 'Emerging infections: An evolutionary perspective'. *Emerging Infectious Diseases*, 4: 366–71. [1.5.2]

—— SHOPE, R. E., and OAKS, S. C. (eds) (1992). *Emerging Infections: Microbial Threats to Health in the United States*. Washington, DC: National Academy Press. [1.2, 1.5.2, 8.1.1, 8.2.2]

LEE, H. W. (1989). 'Hemorrhagic fever with renal syndrome in Korea'. *Reviews of Infectious Diseases*, 11, suppl. 4, S864–76. [8.2.1]

—— (1994). *Hemorrhagic Fever with Renal Syndrome (Korean Hemorrhagic Fever, Epidemic Hemorrhagic Fever)*, i: *Letters and Annual Research Report, 1959–1993*. Institute of Viral Diseases, Korea University, Seoul: Ho Wang Lee. [8.2.1]

LEETE, R. (1985). 'Increased survival in East and South-East Asia: Towards new outer limits to life'. In *Proceedings, International Union for the Scientific Study of Population, International Population Conference, Florence*, 429–42. [1.4.1]

LEFF, R. D. (1993). 'Lyme borreliosis (Lyme disease)'. In K. F. Kiple (ed.), *Cambridge World History of Human Disease*. Cambridge: Cambridge University Press, 852–5. [7.4.2]

LEROY, E. M., ROUQUET, P., FORMENTY, P., SOUQUIÈRE, S., KILBOURNE, A., FROMENT, J.-M., BERMEJO, M., SMIT, S., KRESH, W., SWANEPOEL, R., ZAKI, S. R., and ROLLIN, P. E. (2004). 'Multiple Ebola transmission events and rapid decline of Central African wildlife'. *Science*, 303: 387–90. [9.3.2]

LEUNG-SHEA, C. and DANAHER, P. J. (2006). 'Q fever in members of the United States Armed Forces returning from Iraq'. *Clinical Infectious Diseases*, 43: e77–e82. [8.4.2]

LEVINE, M. M. (1991). 'South America: The return of cholera'. *Lancet*, 338: 45–6. [6.3.1]

LEVY, S. B. (1997). 'Antibiotic resistance: An ecological imbalance'. In D. J. Chadwick and J. Goode (eds), *Antibiotic Resistance: Origins, Evolution, Selection and Spread*. Chichester: John Wiley and Sons, 1–14. [4.3.1]

LI, H.-C., FUJIYOSHI, T., LOU, H., YASHIKI, S., SONODA, S., CARTIER, L., NUNEZ, I., MUNOZ, I., HORAI, S., and TAJIMA, K. (1999). 'The presence of ancient human T-cell lymphotropic virus type I provirus DNA in an Andean mummy'. *Nature Medicine*, 5: 1428–32. [1.3.3]

LI, K. S., GUAN, Y., WANG, J., SMITH, G. J. D., XU, K. M., DUAN, L., RAHARDJO, A. P., PUTHAVATHANA, P., BURANATHAI, C., NGUYEN, T. D., ESTOEPANGESTIE, A. T. S., CHAISINGH, A., AUEWARAKUL, P., LONG, H. T., HANH, N. T. H., WEBBY, R. J., POON, L. L. M., CHEN, H., SHORTRIDGE, K. F., YUEN, K. Y., WEBSTER, R. G., and PEIRIS, J. S. M. (2004). 'Genesis of a highly pathogenic and potentially pandemic H5N1 influenza virus in eastern Asia'. *Nature*, 430: 209–13. [4.2.4]

LI, W. H., TANIMURA, M., and SHARP, P. M. (1988). 'Rates and dates of divergence between AIDS virus nucleotide sequences'. *Molecular Biology and Evolution*, 5: 313–30. [9.2.3]

LI, Y. S., RASO, G., ZHAO, Z. Y., HE, Y. K., ELLIS, M. K., and MCMANUS, D. P. (2007). 'Large water management projects and schistosomiasis control, Dongting Lake Region, China'. *Emerging Infectious Diseases*, 13: 973–9. [7.3]

Lien-Teh, W. (1936). 'Historical aspects'. In W. Lien-Teh, J. W. H. Chun, R. Pollitzer, and C. Y. Wu (eds), *Plague: A Manual for Medical and Public Health Workers*. Shanghai: National Quarantine Service, 1–53. [2.3.2]

Ligon, B. L. (2006). 'Infectious diseases that pose specific challenges after natural disasters: A review'. *Seminars in Pediatric Infectious Diseases*, 17: 36–45. [7.6.1]

Lincoln, A. F. and Sivertson, S. E. (1952). 'Acute phase of Japanese B encephalitis: Two hundred and one cases in American soldiers, Korea, 1950'. *Journal of the American Medical Association*, 150: 268–73. [8.1.2, 8.2.1]

Lindblade, K. A., Walker, E. D., Onapa, A. W., Katungu, J., and Wilson, M. L. (1999). 'Highland malaria in Uganda: Prospective analysis of an epidemic associated with El Niño'. *Transactions of the Royal Society of Tropical Medicine and Hygiene*, 93: 480–7. [7.5.2]

Lindsay, M., Johansen, C., Broom, A. K., Smith, D. W., and MacKenzie, J. S. (1995). 'Emergence of Barmah Forest virus in Western Australia'. *Emerging Infectious Diseases*, 1: 22–6. [9.4.2]

Lindsay, S. W., Bodker, R., Malima, R., Msangeni, H. A., and Kisinza, W. (2000). 'The effect of the 1997–98 El Niño on highland malaria in Tanzania'. *Lancet*, 355: 989–90. [7.5.2]

Lingappa, J. R., Al-Rabeah, A. M., Hajjeh, R., Mustafa, T., Fatani, A., Al-Bassam, T., Badukhan, A., Turkistani, A., Makki, S., Al-Hamdan, N., Al-Jeffri, M., Al Mazrou, Y., Perkins, B. A., Popovic, T., Mayer, L. W., and Rosenstein, N. E. (2003). 'Serogroup W-135 meningococcal disease during the Hajj, 2000'. *Emerging Infectious Diseases*, 9: 665–71. [6.5.2, 9.3.2]

Liu, J., Xiao, H., Lei, F., Zhu, Q., Qin, K., Zhang, X.-w., Zhang, X.-l., Zhao, D., Wang, G., Feng, Y., Ma, J., Liu, W., Wang, J., and Gao, G. F. (2005). 'Highly pathogenic H5N1 influenza virus in migratory birds'. *Science*, 309: 1206. [4.2.3]

Locking, M., Allison, L., Rae, L., Pollock, K., and Hanson, M. (2006). 'VETC in Scotland 2004: Enhanced surveillance and reference laboratory data'. *HPS Weekly Report*, 39: 290–5. [5.2.4]

Loevinsohn, M. E. (1994). 'Climatic warming and increased malaria incidence in Rwanda'. *Lancet*, 343: 714–18. [7.5.2]

Louisiana Department of Health and Hospitals (2006). *Hurricane Katrina. Deceased Reports: Reports of Missing and Deceased Aug. 2, 2006*. Baton Rouge: Louisiana Department of Health and Hospitals. http://www.dhh.louisiana.gov, accessed 21 July 2008. [7.6.3]

Luby, J., Schultz, M. G., Nowosiwsky, T., and Kaiser, R. L. (1967). 'Introduced malaria at Fort Benning, Georgia, 1964–1965'. *American Journal of Tropical Medicine and Hygiene*, 16: 146–53. [8.2.2]

M

McArthur, N. (1967). *Island Populations of the Pacific*. Canberra: Australian National University. [6.3.1]

McDade, J. E., Brenner, D. J., and Bozeman, F. M. (1979). 'Legionnaires' disease bacterium isolated in 1947'. *Annals of Internal Medicine*, 90: 659–61. [5.3.3]

MacDonald, D. M., Fyfe, M., Paccagnella, A., Trinidad, A., Louie, K., and Patrick, D. (2004). '*Escherichia coli* O157:H7 outbreak linked to salami, British Columbia, Canada, 1999'. *Epidemiology and Infection*, 132: 283–9. [5.2.4]

McEvedy, C. (1988). 'The bubonic plague'. *Scientific American*, 254: 3–12. [2.3.2]

McGowan, J. E., Jr (2001). 'Economic impact of antimicrobial resistance'. *Emerging Infectious Diseases*, 7: 286–92. [4.3.1]

MacIntyre, C. R., Gay, N. J., Gidding, H. F., Hull, B. P., Gilbert, G. L., and MacIntyre, P. B. (2002). 'A mathematical model to measure the impact of the Measles Control Campaign on the potential for measles transmission in Australia'. *International Journal of Infectious Diseases*, 6: 277–82. [11.3.1]

McKarthy, S. A. and Khambaty, F. M. (1985). 'International dissemination of *Vibrio cholerae* by cargo ship ballast and other nonpotable waters'. *Applied Environmental Microbiology*, 121: 791–6. [6.3.1]

MacKenzie, J. S. (1999). 'Emerging virus diseases: An Australian perspective'. *Emerging Infectious Diseases*, 5: 1–8. [9.4.2]

—— Chua, K. B., Daniels, P. W., Eaton, B. T., Field, H. E., Hall, R. A., Halpin, K., Johanse, C. A., Kirkland, P. D., Lam, S. K., McMinn, P., Nisbet, D. J., Paru, R., Pyke, A. T., Ritchie, S. A., Siba, P., Smith, D. W., Smith, G. A., van den Hurk, A. F., Wang, L. F., and Williams, D. T. (2001). 'Emerging viral diseases of Southeast Asia and the Western Pacific'. *Emerging Infectious Diseases*, 7, suppl., 497–504. [9.4.2]

MacKenzie, J. S., Gubler, D. J., and Petersen, L. R. (2004). 'Emerging flaviviruses: The spread and resurgence of Japanese encephalitis, West Nile and dengue viruses'. *Nature Medicine*, 10, suppl., S98–S109. [8.2.1]

MacKenzie, W. R., Hoxie, N. J., Proctor, M. E., Gradus, M. S., Blair, K. A., Peterson, D. E., Kazmierczak, J. J., Addiss, D. G., Fox, K. R., Rose, J. B., and Davis, J. P. (1994). 'A massive outbreak in Milwaukee of cryptosporidium infection transmitted through the public water supply'. *New England Journal of Medicine*, 331: 161–7. [5.1]

McKeown, T. (1988). *The Origins of Human Disease*. Oxford: Blackwell. [1.3.2]

McMichael, A. J. (2001). 'Human culture, ecological change, and infectious disease: Are we experiencing history's fourth great transition?' *Ecosystem Health*, 7: 107–15. [7.2.1]

—— (2003). 'Global climate change and health: An old story writ large'. In A. J. McMichael, D. H. Campbell-Lendrum, C. F. Corvalan, K. L. Ebi, A. Githeko, J. D. Scheraga, and A. Woodward (eds), *Climate Change and Human Health: Risks and Responses*. Geneva: WHO, 1–17. [7.5.1]

—— (2004). 'Environmental and social influences on emerging infectious diseases: Past, present and future'. *Philosophical Transactions of the Royal Society B*, 359: 1049–58. [1.5.1, 1.5.2, 2.1, 2.3.3, 6.1, 7.1, 7.2]

—— Campbell-Lendrum, D. H., Corvalan, C. F., Ebi, K. L., Githeko, A., Scheraga, J. D., and Woodward, A. (eds) (2003). *Climate Change and Human Health: Risks and Responses*. Geneva: WHO. [7.5.1]

—— —— Kovats, S., Edwards, S., Wilkinson, P., Wilson, T., Nicholls, R., Hales, S., Tanser, F., Le Sueur, D., Schlesinger, M., and Andronova, N. (2004). 'Global climate change'. In M. Ezzati, A. D. Lopez, A. Rodgers, and C. J. L. Murray (eds), *Comparative Quantification of Health Risks: Global and*

Regional Burden of Disease Attributable to Selected Major Risk Factors, ii. Geneva: WHO, 1543–1651. [6.2.3]

McNabb, S. J. N., Chungong, S., Ryan, M., Wuhib, T., Nsubuga, P., Alemu, W., Carande-Kulis, V., and Rodier, G. (2002). 'Conceptual framework of public health surveillance and action and its application in health sector reform'. *BMC Public Health*, 2/2. doi:10.1186/1471–2458–2–2. [10.6.1, 10.6.2]

MacNamara, C. (1876). *A History of Asiatic Cholera*. London: Macmillan. [2.3.1, 2.3.4]

McNeill, W. H. (1976). *Plagues and Peoples*. Oxford: Blackwell. [2.2.2]

McNinch, J. H. (1953). 'Far East Command Conference on Epidemic Hemorrhagic Fever: Introduction'. *Annals of Internal Medicine*, 38: 53–60. [8.2.1]

Macpherson, J. (1884). *Annals of Cholera from the Earliest Periods to the Year 1817*. London: H. K. Lewis. [2.3.1, 2.3.4]

Macpherson, W. G., Herringham, W. P., Elliott, T. R., and Balfour, A. (eds) (1922–3). *History of the Great War Based on Official Documents: Medical Services, Diseases of the War*, 2 vols. London: HMSO. [8.1]

McSweegan, E. (2004). 'Anthrax and the etiology of the English sweating sickness'. *Medical Hypotheses*, 62: 155–7. [2.3.5]

Madan, T. N. (1995). 'The plague in India, 1994'. *Social Science and Medicine*, 40: 1167–8. [11.2.4]

Mafart, B. and Perret, J.-L. (1998). 'Histoire du concept de quarantaine'. *Médecine Tropicale*, 58: 14S–20S. [11.2.3]

Magistrato della sanità, Venice. (1752). *An Authentick Account of the Measures and Precautions used at Venice, by the Magistrate of the Office of Health, for the Preservation of the Publick Health*. London: Edward Owen, 32. [11.2.1]

Maguire, T. (1994). 'Do Ross River and dengue viruses pose a threat to New Zealand?' *New Zealand Medical Journal*, 107: 448–50. [6.5.3]

Mahar, D. J. (1989). *Government Policies and Deforestation in Brazil's Amazon Region*. Washington, DC: World Bank. [6.3.2, 7.4]

Maiztegui, J. (1975). 'Clinical and epidemiological patterns of Argentine haemorrhagic fever'. *Bulletin of the World Health Organization*, 52: 567–75. [7.2.1]

—— Feuillade, M., and Briggiler, A. (1986). 'Progressive extension of the endemic area and changing incidence of Argentine Hemorrhagic Fever'. *Medical Microbiology and Immunology*, 175: 149–52. [7.2.1]

Major, R. (1940). *War and Disease*. London: Hutchinson. [2.2.2]

Malek, E. A. (1975). 'Effect of the Aswan High Dam on prevalence of schistosomiasis in Egypt'. *Tropical and Geographical Medicine*, 27: 359–64. [7.2, 7.3]

Malloy, C. D. and Marr, J. S. (2001). 'Evolution of the *Control of Communicable Diseases Manual*: 1917 to 2000'. *Journal of Public Health Management and Practice*, 7: 97–104. [1.5.3]

Mamolen, M., Breiman, R. F., Barbaree, J. M., Gunn, R. A., Stone, K. M., Spika, J. S., Dennis, D. T., Mao, S. H., and Vogt, R. L. (1993). 'Use of multiple molecular subtyping techniques to investigate a Legionnaires' disease outbreak due to identical strains at two tourist lodges'. *Journal of Clinical Microbiology*, 31: 2584–8. [5.3.3]

Mandl, K. D., Overhage, J. M., Wagner, M. M., Lober, W. B., Mostashari, F., Pavlin, J. A., Treadwell, T., Koski, E., Buckeridge, D. L., Aller, R. D., and GRANNIS, S. (2003). 'Implementing syndromic surveillance: A practical guide informed by the early experience'. *Journal of the American Medical Informatics Association*, 11: 141–50. [10.6.3]

MANZIONE, N. DE, SALAS, R. A., PAREDES, H., GODOY, O., ROJAS, L., ARAOZ, F., FULHORST, C. F., KSIAZEK, T. G., MILLS, J. N., ELLIS, B. A., PETERS, C. J., and TESH, R. B. (1998). 'Venezuelan hemorrhagic fever: Clinical and epidemiological studies of 165 cases'. *Clinical Infectious Diseases*, 26: 308–13. [7.2.1]

MARKEL, H., LIPMAN, H. B., NAVARRO, J. A., SLOAD, A., MICHALSEN, J. R., and STERN, A. (2007). 'Nonpharmaceutical interventions implemented by US cities during the 1918–1919 influenza pandemic'. *Journal of the American Medical Association*, 298: 644–54. [11.2.3]

MARKS, J. S. HOGELIN, G. C., GENTRY, E. M., JONES, J. T., GAINES, K. L., FORMAN, M. R., and TROWBRIDGE, F. L. (1985). 'The behavioral risk factor surveys. I. State-specific prevalence estimates of behavioral risk factors'. *American Journal of Preventive Medicine*, 1: 1–8. [10.6.1]

MARR, J. S. and KIRACOFE, J. B. (2000). 'Was the *huey cocoliztli* a haemorrhagic fever?' *Medical History*, 44: 341–62. [2.3.5]

—— and MALLOY, C. D. (1996). 'An epidemiologic analysis of the Ten Plagues of Egypt'. *Caduceus*, 12: 7–24. [2.2, 2.2.1]

MARSHALL, I. H. (1954). 'Hemorrhagic fever. I. Epidemiology'. *American Journal of Tropical Medicine and Hygiene*, 3: 587–600. [8.2.1]

MARSHALL, J. D., JOY, R. J. T., AI, N. V., QUY, D. V., STOCKARD, J. L., and GIBSON, F. L. (1967). 'Plague in Vietnam 1965–66'. *American Journal of Epidemiology*, 86: 603–16. [8.1.2, 8.2.2]

MARTENS, P. and HUYNEN, M. (2003). 'A future without health? Health dimension in global scenario studies'. *Bulletin of the World Health Organization*, 81: 896–901. [1.4.2]

MASKEY, M., SHASTRI, J. S., SARASWATHI, K., SURPAM, R., and VAIDYA, N. (2006). 'Leptospirosis in Mumbai: Post-deluge outbreak 2005'. *Indian Journal of Medical Microbiology*, 24: 337–8. [7.6.1]

MASSEY, A. (1933). *Epidemiology in Relation to Air Travel*. London: H. K. Lewis. [6.1]

MATOSSIAN, M. K. (1985). 'Death in London, 1750–1909'. *Journal of Interdisciplinary History*, 16: 183–97. [2.4.2]

MEAD, P. S., SLUTSKER, L., DIETZ, V., MCCAIG, L. F., BRESEE, J. S., SHAPIRO, C., GRIFFIN, P. M., and TAUXE, R. V. (1999). 'Food-related illness and death in the United States'. *Emerging Infectious Diseases*, 5: 607–25. [5.2.3]

MEEGAN, J. M. (1979). 'The Rift Valley fever epizootic in Egypt 1977–78. 1. Description of the epizootic and virological studies'. *Transactions of the Royal Society of Tropical Medicine and Hygiene*, 73: 618–23. [7.3.1]

MELTZER, M. I. (2008). 'Pandemic influenza, reopening schools, and returning to work'. *Emerging Infectious Diseases*, 14: 507–8. [11.2.3]

—— COX, N. J., and FUKADA, K. (1999). 'The impact of pandemic influenza in the United States: Priorities for intervention'. *Emerging Infectious Diseases*, 5: 659–71. [10.2.1]

MESELSON, M., GUILLEMIN, J., Hugh-JONES, M., LANGMUIR, A., POPOVA, I., SHELOKOV, A., and YAMPOLSKAYA, O. (1994). 'The Sverdlovsk anthrax outbreak of 1979'. *Science*, 266: 1202–8. [8.5.1, 8.5.2]

Metcalfe, N. (2002). 'A short history of biological warfare'. *Medicine, Conflict and Survival*, 18: 271–82. [8.5.2]

Mettler, N. E. (1969). *Argentine Hemorrhagic Fever: Current Knowledge*. Pan American Health Organization Scientific Publication no. 183. Washington, DC: PAHO. [7.2.1]

Miller, J. M., Tam, T. W. S., Maloney, S., Fukuda, K., Cox, N., Hockin, J., Kertesz, D., Klimov, A., and Cetron, M. (2000). 'Cruise ships: High-risk passengers and the global spread of new influenza viruses'. *Clinical Infectious Diseases*, 31: 433–8. [6.3.1]

Miller, M., Roche, P., Spencer, J., and Deeble, M. (2004). 'Evaluation of Australia's National Notifiable Disease Surveillance System'. *Communicable Diseases Intelligence*, 28: 311–23. [10.6.1, 10.6.3]

Ministero dell'Interno, Direzione Generale della Sanità Pubblica, Napoli (1910). *La sanità marittima a Napoli: Origini e vicende*. Naples: Francesco Giannini & Figli. [11.2.1]

Miranda, M. E., Ksiazek, T. G., Retuya, T. J., Khan, A. S., Sanchez, A., Fulhorst, C. F., Rollin, P. E., Calaor, A. B., Manalo, D. L., Roces, M. C., Dayritt, M. M., and Peters, C. J. (1999). 'Epidemiology of Ebola (subtype Reston) virus in the Philippines, 1996'. *Journal of Infectious Diseases*, 179, suppl. 1, S115–S119. [9.3.2]

Mitchell, B. R. (2007). *International Historical Statistics. Europe, 1750–2005*, 6th edn. Basingstoke: Palgrave Macmillan. [2.4.2]

Modelski, M. (1987). *Railroad Maps of North America*. New York: Bonanza Books. [6.3.2]

Mokdad, A. H., Marks, J. S., Stroup, D. F., and Gerberding, J. L. (2004). 'Actual causes of death in the United States, 2000'. *Journal of the American Medical Association*, 291: 1238–45. [10.6.2]

Molesworth, A. M., Cuevas, L. E., Connor, S. J., Morse, A. P., and Thomson, M. C. (2003). 'Environmental risk and meningitis epidemics in Africa'. *Emerging Infectious Diseases*, 9: 1287–93. [9.3.2]

—— Thomson, M. C., Connor, S. J., Cresswell, M. P., Morse, A. P., Shears, P., Hart, C. A., and Cuevas, L. E. (2002). 'Where is the meningitis belt? Defining an area at risk of epidemic meningitis in Africa'. *Transactions of the Royal Society of Tropical Medicine and Hygiene*, 96: 242–9. [9.3.2]

Molyneux, D. H. (2003). 'Common themes in changing vector-borne disease scenarios'. *Transactions of the Royal Society of Tropical Medicine and Hygiene*, 97: 129–32. [7.5.1]

Monot, M., Honoré, N., Garnier, T., Araoz, R., Coppée, J.-Y., Lacroix, C., Sow, S., Spencer, J. S., Truman, R. W., Williams, D. L., Gelber, R., Virmond, M., Flageul, B., Cho, S.-N., Ji, B., Paniz-Mondolfi, A., Convit, J., Young, S., Fine, P. E., Rasolofo, V., Brennan, P. J., and Cole, S. T. (2005). 'On the origin of leprosy'. *Science*, 308: 1040–2. [2.1]

Montiel, R., García, C., Cañadas, M. P., Isidro, A., Guijo, J. M., and Malgosa, A. (2003). 'DNA sequences of *Mycobacterium leprae* recovered from ancient bones'. *FEMS Microbiology Letters*, 226: 413–14. [1.3.3]

Moore, P. S. (1992). 'Meningococcal meningitis in sub-Saharan Africa: A model for the epidemic process'. *Clinical Infectious Diseases*, 14: 515–25. [9.3.2]

Moore, P. S., Reeves, M. W., Schwartz, B., Gellin, B. G., and Broome, C. V. (1989). 'Intercontinental spread of an epidemic group A *Neisseria meningitidis* strain'. *Lancet*, 2: 260–2. [9.3.2]

Morens, D. M. and Littman, R. J. (1992). 'Epidemiology of the Plague of Athens'. *Transactions of the American Philological Association*, 122: 271–304. [2.2.2]

—— Folkers, G. K., and Fauci, A. S. (2004). 'The challenge of emerging and re-emerging infectious diseases'. *Nature*, 430: 242–9. [1.1, 1.2, 1.5.1, 1.5.2, 4.2.1, 8.5]

Morgenstern, O. (1963). *On the Accuracy of Economic Observations*. Princeton: Princeton University Press. [10.2.1]

Morris, J. G. and Potter, M. (1997). 'Emergence of new pathogens as a function of changes in host susceptibility'. *Emerging Infectious Diseases*, 3: 435–41. [1.4.2]

Morse, S. S. (1995). 'Factors in the emergence of infectious diseases'. *Emerging Infectious Diseases*, 1: 7–15. [1.2, 1.5.1, 1.5.2, 4.2.1, 7.1, 7.2, 7.2.1, 7.3]

—— (2007). 'Global infectious disease surveillance and health intelligence'. *Health Affairs*, 26: 1069–77. [10.6.3]

Mostashari, F. and Hartman, J. (2003). 'Syndromic surveillance: A local perspective'. *Journal of Urban Health*, 80, suppl. 1, 1–7. [10.6.3]

—— Bunning, M. L., Kitsutani, P. T., Singer, D. A., Nash, D., Cooper, M. J., Katz, N., Liljebjelke, K. A., Biggerstaff, B. J., Fine, A. D., Layton, M. C., Mullin, S. M., Johnson, A. J., Martin, D. A., Hayes, E. B., and Campbell, G. L. (2001). 'Epidemic West Nile encephalitis, New York, 1999: Results of a household-based seroepidemiological survey'. *Lancet*, 358: 261–4. [6.5.3]

Motarjemi, Y. and Adams, M. (eds) (2006). *Emerging Foodborne Pathogens*. Cambridge: Woodhead. [5.2.1]

—— and Käferstein, F. K. (1997). 'Global estimation of foodborne diseases'. *World Health Statistics Quarterly*, 50: 5–11. [5.2.2]

Mukerjee, S. (1963). 'Problems of cholera (El Tor)'. *American Journal of Tropical Medicine and Hygiene*, 12: 388–92. [9.2.2]

Mukhopadhyay, A. K., Basu, A., Garg, P., Bag, P. K., Ghosh, A., Bhattacharya, S. K., Takeda, Y., and Nair, G. B. (1998). 'Molecular epidemiology of reemergent *Vibrio cholerae* O139 Bengal in India'. *Journal of Clinical Microbiology*, 36: 2149–52. [9.2.2]

Murray, C. J. L., King, G., Lopez, A. D., Tomijima, N., and Krug, E. G. (2002). 'Armed conflict as a public health problem'. *British Medical Journal*, 324: 346–9. [8.4]

Murray, K., Selleck, P., Hooper, P., Hyatt, A., Gould, A., Gleeson, L., Westbury, H., Hiley, L., Selvey, L., Rodwell, B., and Ketterer, P. (1995). 'A morbillivirus that caused fatal disease in horses and humans'. *Science*, 268: 94–7. [7.4.1]

N

Najmi, A.-H. and Magruder, S. F. (2005). 'An adaptive prediction and detection algorithm for multistream syndromic surveillance'. *BMC Medical Informatics and Decision Making*, 5/33. doi:10.1186/1472–6947–5–33. [10.6.3]

Nash, D., Mostashari, F., Fine, A., Miller, J., O'Leary, D., Murray, K., Huang, A., Rosenberg, A., Greenberg, A., Sherman, M., Wong, S., and Layton, M. (2001). 'The outbreak of West Nile virus infection in the New York City area in 1999'. *New England Journal of Medicine*, 344: 1807–14. [6.5.3]

NATHANSON, N. and LANGMUIR, A. D. (1963*a*). 'The Cutter incident: Poliomyelitis following formaldehyde-inactivated poliovirus vaccination in the United States during the spring of 1955. I. Background'. *American Journal of Hygiene*, 78: 16–28. [11.3.2]

—— —— (1963*b*). 'The Cutter incident: Poliomyelitis following formaldehyde-inactivated poliovirus vaccination in the United States during the spring of 1955. II. Relationship of poliomyelitis to Cutter vaccine'. *American Journal of Hygiene*, 78: 29–60. [11.3.2]

—— and NICHOL, S. (1998). 'Korean hemorrhagic fever and hantavirus pulmonary syndrome: Two examples of emerging hantaviral diseases'. In R. M. Krause (ed.), *Emerging Infections: Biomedical Research Reports*. San Diego: Academic Press, 365–74. [8.2.1]

—— WILESMITH, J., and GRIOT, C. (1997). 'Bovine spongiform encephalopathy (BSE): Causes and consequences of a common source epidemic'. *American Journal of Epidemiology*, 145: 959–69. [5.2.5]

NATIONAL CJD SURVEILLANCE UNIT (2006). *Creutzfeldt–Jakob Disease Surveillance in the UK: Fourteenth Annual Report 2005*. Edinburgh: National CJD Surveillance Unit. [5.2.5]

NATIONAL OCEANIC AND ATMOSPHERIC ADMINISTRATION (2008*a*). *Multivariate ENSO Index (MEI)*. Boulder, Colo.: NOAA. http://www.cdc.noaa.gov/people/klaus.wolter/MEI, accessed 21 July 2008. [7.5.3]

—— (2008*b*). *US Temperature, Precipitation, and Drought Data*. Asheville, NC: National Climatic Data Center. http://www.ncdc.noaa.gov/oa/ncdc.html, accessed 21 July 2008. [7.5.3]

NEEL, S. (1973). *Vietnam Studies: Medical Support of the US Army in Vietnam, 1965–1970*. Washington, DC: US Government Printing Office. [8.1.1, 8.1.2, 8.2.2]

NERLICH, A. G., HAAS, C. J., ZINK, A., SZEIMIES, U., and HAGEDORN, H. G. (1997). 'Molecular evidence for tuberculosis in an ancient Egyptian mummy'. *Lancet*, 350: 1404. [1.3.3]

NEU, H. C. (1992). 'The crisis in antibiotic resistance'. *Science*, 257: 1064–72. [4.3.1]

NICOLAS, P., NORHEIM, G., GARNOTEL, E., DJIBO, S., and CAUGANT, D. A. (2005). 'Molecular epidemiology of *Neisseria meningitides* isolated in the African meningitis belt between 1988 and 2003 shows dominance of sequence type 5 (ST-5) and ST-11 complexes'. *Journal of Clinical Microbiology*, 43: 5129–35. [9.3.2]

NOMOTO, A. and ARITA, I. (2002). 'Eradication of poliomyelitis'. *Nature Immunology*, 3: 205–8. [8.5.4]

NORTON, S. A., FRANKENBURG, S., and KLAU, S. N. (1992). 'Cutaneous leishmaniasis acquired during military service in the Middle East'. *Archives of Dermatology*, 128: 83–7. [8.4.3]

NOWOSIWSKY, T. (1967). 'The epidemic curve of *Plasmodium falciparum* malaria in a nonimmune population: American troops in Vietnam, 1965 and 1966'. *American Journal of Epidemiology*, 86: 461–7. [8.2.2]

O

O'BRIEN, T. F. (2002). 'Emergence, spread, and environmental effect of antimicrobial resistance: How use of an antimicrobial anywhere can increase resistance to any antimicrobial anywhere else'. *Clinical Infectious Diseases*, 34, suppl. 3, S78–84. [4.3.1, 4.3.2]

Office of Agricultural Economics (2004). *Agricultural Statistics of Thailand 2003/04*. Bangkok: Office of Agricultural Economics. http://www.oae.go.th, accessed 21 July 2008. [4.2.3]

Ogden, N. H., Maarouf, A., Barker, I. K., Bigras-Poulin, M., Lindsay, L. R., Morshed, M. G., O'Callaghan, C. J., Ramay, F., Waltner-Toews, D., and Charron, D. F. (2006). 'Climate change and the potential for range of expansion of the Lyme disease vector *Ixodes scapularis* in Canada'. *International Journal of Parasitology*, 36: 63–70. [7.5.1]

Olsen, S. J., Chang, H.-L., Cheung, T. Y.-Y., Tang, A. F.-Y., Fisk, T. L., Ooi, S. P.-L., Kuo, H.-W., Jiang, D. D.-S., Chen, K.-T., Lando, J., Hsu, K.-H., Chen, T.-J., and Dowell, S. F. (2003). 'Transmission of the severe acute respiratory syndrome on aircraft'. *New England Journal of Medicine*, 349: 2416–22. [6.4.1]

—— Patrick, M., Hunter, S. B., Reddy, V., Kornstein, L., MacKenzie, W. R., Lane, K., Bidol, S., Stoltman, G. A., Frye, D. M., Lee, I., Hurd, S., Jones, T. F., LaPorte, T. N., Dewitt, W., Graves, L., Wiedmann, M., Schoonmaker-Bopp, D. J., Huang, A. J., Vincent, C., Bugenhagen, A., Corby, J., Carloni, E. R., Holcomb, M. E., Woron, R. F., Zansky, S. M., Dowdle, G., Smith, F., Ahrabi-Fard, S., Ong, A. R., Tucker, N., Hynes, N. A., and Mead, P. (2005). 'Multistate outbreak of *Listeria monocytogenes* infection linked to delicatessen turkey meat'. *Clinical Infectious Diseases*, 40: 962–7. [5.2.3]

—— Ungchusak, K., Sovann, L., Uyeki, T. M., Dowell, S. F., Cox, N. J., Aldis, W., and Chunsuttiwat, S. (2005). 'Family clustering of avian influenza A (H5N1)'. *Emerging Infectious Diseases*, 11: 1799–1801. [4.2.4]

Olshansky, S. J. and Ault, A. B. (1986). 'The fourth stage of the epidemiologic transition: The age of delayed degenerative diseases'. *Milbank Memorial Fund Quarterly*, 64: 355–91. [1.4.1]

—— Carnes, B., Rogers, R. G., and Smith, L. (1997). 'Infectious diseases: New and ancient threats to world health'. *Population Bulletin*, 52: 1–58. [1.4.2]

—— —— —— —— (1998). 'Emerging infectious diseases: The fifth stage of the epidemiologic transition?' *World Health Statistics Quarterly*, 51: 207–17. [1.4.2]

Olson, E., Hames, C. S., Benenson, A. S., and Genovese, E. N. (1996). 'The Thucydides Syndrome: Ebola déjà vu? (or Ebola reemergent?)'. *Emerging Infectious Diseases*, 2: 155–6. [2.2.2]

Omran, A. R. (1971). 'The epidemiologic transition: A theory of the epidemiology of population change'. *Milbank Memorial Fund Quarterly*, 49: 509–38. [1.4.1]

—— (1977). 'Epidemiologic transition in the United States: The health factor in population change'. *Population Bulletin*, 32: 3–42. [1.4.1]

Ord, J. K. and Getis, A. (1995). 'Local spatial autocorrelation statistics: Distributional issues and an application'. *Geographical Analysis*, 27: 286–306. [4.2.3]

Organisation Mondiale de la Santé Animale (2003). 'Highly pathogenic avian influenza in the Republic of Korea: Suspected outbreak'. *Disease Information*, 16: 270–1. [4.2.3]

—— (2004*a*). 'Highly pathogenic avian influenza in Thailand'. *Disease Information*, 17: 16. [4.2.3]

—— (2004*b*). 'Avian influenza in Hong Kong, Special Administrative Region of the People's Republic of China'. *Disease Information*, 17: 18–19. [4.2.3]
—— (2004*c*). 'Highly pathogenic avian influenza in Thailand: Follow-up report no. 1'. *Disease Information*, 17: 27–8. [4.2.3]
—— (2004*d*). 'Highly pathogenic avian influenza in Vietnam: Follow-up report no. 2'. *Disease Information*, 17: 57–9. [4.2.3]
—— (2004*e*). 'Highly pathogenic avian influenza in Thailand in felines in a zoo'. *Disease Information*, 17: 312–13. [4.2.3]
—— (2008). *Update on Highly Pathogenic Avian Influenza in Animals: 18 February 2008*. Paris: OIE. http://www.oie.int, accessed 21 July 2008. [4.2.3]
Osterhaus, A. D. and Vedder, E. J. (1988). 'Identification of virus causing recent seal deaths'. *Nature*, 335: 20. [7.4.1]
Osterholm, M. T., Chin, T. D., Osborne, D. O., Dull, H. B., Dean, A. G., Fraser, D. W., Hayes, P. S., and Hall, W. N. (1983). 'A 1957 outbreak of Legionnaires' disease associated with a meat packing plant'. *American Journal of Epidemiology*, 117: 60–7. [5.3.3]
Oxenham, M. F., Kim Thuy, N., and Lan Cuong, N. (2004). 'Skeletal evidence for the emergence of infectious disease in Bronze and Iron Age Northern Vietnam'. *American Journal of Physical Anthropology*, 126: 359–76. [1.3.3]
Oxford, J. S. (2000). 'Influenza A pandemics of the 20th century with special reference to 1918: Virology, pathology and epidemiology'. *Reviews in Medical Virology*, 10: 119–33. [4.2.2]
—— Sefton, A., Jackson, R., Johnson, N. P. A. S., and Daniels, R. S. (1999). 'Who's that lady'. *Nature Medicine*, 5: 1351–2. [4.2.2]

P

Panagiotakopulu, E. (2004). 'Pharaonic Egypt and the origins of plague'. *Journal of Biogeography*, 31: 269–75. [2.3.2]
Pan American Health Organization (1994). 'Re-emergence of Bolivian haemorrhagic fever'. *PAHO Epidemiological Bulletin*, 15: 4–5. [7.2.1]
—— (2003). *Zoonoses and Communicable Diseases Common to Man and Animals*, 3rd edn, ii: *Chlamydioses, Rickettsioses, and Viroses*. PAHO Scientific and Technical Publication no. 580. Washington, DC: PAHO. [7.3.1, 7.5.3]
—— (2005). 'Number of cases and deaths from hantavirus pulmonary syndrome (HPS): Region of the Americas, 1993–2004'. Washington, DC: PAHO. http://www.paho.org/English/AD/DPC/CD/hantavirus-1993–2004.htm, accessed 21 July 2008. [7.5.3]
Papon, J.-P. (1800). *De la peste, ou Époques mémorables de ce fléau, et les moyens de s'en préserver*. Paris: Lavilette. [2.3.2]
Parry, H. N., McDonnell, S. M., Alemu, W., Nsubuga, P., Chungong, S., Otten, M. W., Lusamba-dikassa, P. S., and Thacker, S. B. (2007). 'Planning an integrated disease surveillance and response system: A matrix of skills and activities'. *BMC Medicine*, 5/24. doi:10.1186/1741–7015–5–24. [10.6.3]
Paterson, D. L. (2002), 'Yersinia seeks pardon for Black Death'. *Lancet Infectious Diseases*, 2: 323. [2.3.2]

PATERSON, D. L., MURRAY, P. K., and MCCORMACK, J. G. (1998). 'Zoonotic disease in Australia caused by a novel member of the paramyxoviridae'. *Clinical Infectious Diseases*, 27: 112–18. [9.4.2]

PATON, N. I., LEO, Y. S., ZAKI, S. R., AUCHUS, A. P., LEE, K. E., LING, A. E., CHEW, S. K., ANG, B., ROLLIN, P. E., UMAPATHI, T., SNG, I., LEE, C. C., LIM, E., and KSIAZEK, T. G. (1999). 'Outbreak of Nipah-virus infection among abattoir workers in Singapore'. *Lancet*, 354: 1253–6. [7.4.1]

PATTERSON, K. D. (1986). *Pandemic Influenza, 1700–1900: A Study in Historical Epidemiology*. Totowa, NJ: Rowman and Littlefield. [2.3.3, 4.2.2, 10.2.1]

—— (1993). 'Meningitis'. In K. F. Kiple (ed.), *The Cambridge World History of Human Disease*. Cambridge: Cambridge University Press, 875–80. [2.3.1, 9.3.2]

—— and PYLE, G. F. (1983). 'The diffusion of influenza in sub-Saharan Africa during the 1918–1919 pandemic'. *Social Science and Medicine*, 17: 1299–1307. [4.2.2, 4.2.3]

—— —— (1991). 'The geography and mortality of the 1918 influenza pandemic'. *Bulletin of the History of Medicine*, 65: 4–21. [4.2.2, 4.2.3, 10.3.1]

PATTERSON, M. M. (2005). 'The coming influenza pandemic: Lessons from the past for the future'. *Journal of the American Osteopathic Association*, 105: 498–500. [4.2.3, 4.2.4]

PATTISON, S. J. (1998). 'The emergence of bovine spongiform encephalopathy and related diseases'. *Emerging Infectious Diseases*, 4: 390–4. [5.2.5]

PATZ, J. A., DASZAK, P., TABOR, G. M., AGUIRRE, A. A., PEARL, M., EPSTEIN, J., WOLFE, N. D., KILPATRICK, A. M., FOUFOPOULOS, J., MOLYNEUX, D., BRADLEY, D. J., and Members of the Working Group on Land Use Change and Disease Emergence (2004). 'Unhealthy landscapes: Policy recommendations on land use change and infectious disease emergence'. *Environmental Health Perspectives*, 112: 1092–8. [7.1, 7.2, 7.4]

—— GITHEKO, A. K., MCCARTY, J. P., HUSSAIN, S., CONFALONIERI, U., and DE WET, N. (2003). 'Climate change and infectious diseases'. In A. J. McMichael, D. H. Campbell-Lendrum, C. F. Corvalan, K. L. Ebi, A. Githeko, J. D. Scheraga, and A. Woodward (eds), *Climate Change and Human Health: Risks and Responses*. Geneva: WHO, 103–32. [7.5.1]

—— GRACZYK, T. K., GELLER, N., and VITTOR, A. Y. (2000). 'Effects of environmental change on emerging parasitic diseases'. *International Journal for Parasitology*, 30: 1395–1405. [7.1, 7.3, 7.4]

—— MARTENS, W. J. M., FOCKS, D. A., and JETTEN, T. H. (1998). 'Dengue fever epidemic potential as projected by general circulation models of global climate change'. *Environmental Health Perspectives*, 106: 147–53. [7.5.1]

PAUL, J. R. (1971). *The History of Poliomyelitis*. New Haven: Yale University Press. [11.3.1]

—— and MCCLURE, W. W. (1958). 'Epidemic hemorrhagic fever attack rates among United Nations troops during the Korean War'. *American Journal of Hygiene*, 68: 126–39. [8.1.2, 8.2.1]

PEARCE-DUVET, J. M. C. (2006). 'The origin of human pathogens: Evaluating the role of agriculture and domestic animals in the evolution of human disease'. *Biological Reviews of the Cambridge Philosophical Society*, 81: 369–82. [1.3.2]

PEIRIS, J. S. M., YU, W. C., LEUNG, C. W., CHEUNG, C. Y., NG, W. F., NICHOLLS, J. M., NG, T. K., CHAN, K. H., LAI, S. T., LIM, W. L., YUEN, K. Y., and GUAN, Y.

(2004). 'Re-emergence of fatal human influenza A subtype H5N1 disease'. *Lancet*, 363: 617–19. [4.2.3]

PENNINGTON GROUP (1997). *Report on the Circumstances Leading to the 1996 Outbreak of Infection with E. coli O157 in Central Scotland, the Implications for Food Safety and the Lessons to be Learned.* Edinburgh: Stationery Office. [5.2.4]

PEREA, W. A., ANCELLE, T., MOREN, A., NAGELKERKE, M., and SONDORP, E. (1991). 'Visceral leishmaniasis in southern Sudan'. *Transactions of the Royal Society of Tropical Medicine and Hygiene*, 85: 48–53. [8.4.1]

PEREIRA, H. G., TŮMOVÁ, B., and LAW, V. G. (1965). 'Avian influenza A viruses'. *Bulletin of the World Health Organization*, 32: 855–60. [4.2.3]

PERRONCITO, E. (1878). 'Epizoozia tifoide nei gallinacei'. ['Typhoid epizootic in gallinaceous birds']. *Annali della Academia d'Agricoltora di Torino*, 21: 87–126. [4.2.3]

PETERS, W. and GILLES, H. M. (1989). *A Colour Atlas of Tropical Medicine and Parasitology*, 3rd edn. London: Wolfe. [9.3.2]

PETERSON, A. T., BAUER, J. T., and MILLS, J. N. (2004). 'Ecologic and geographic distribution of filovirus disease'. *Emerging Infectious Diseases*, 10: 40–7. [9.3.2]

—— CARROLL, D. S., MILLS, J. N., and JOHNSON, K. M. (2004). 'Potential mammalian filovirus reservoirs'. *Emerging Infectious Diseases*, 10: 2073–81. [9.3.2]

PETITTI, P. (1852). *Repertorio administrativo ossia collezione di leggi, decreti, reali rescritti, ministeriali di massima regolamenti, ed istruzioni sull'amministrazione civile de Regno delle Due Sicilie*, iii, 5th edn. Naples: Tipografia di Gaetano Sautto. [11.2.1]

PHILBEY, A. W., KIRKLAND, P. D., ROSS, A. D., DAVIS, R. J., GLEESON, A. B., LOVE, R. J., DANIELS, P. W., GOULD, A. R., and HYATT, A. D. (1998). 'An apparently new virus (family *Paramyxoviridae*) infectious for pigs, humans, and fruit bats'. *Emerging Infectious Diseases*, 4: 269–71. [9.4.2]

PHILIP, C. B. (1948). 'Tsutsugamushi disease (scrub typhus) in World War II'. *Journal of Parasitology*, 34: 169–91. [8.1, 8.1.1]

PHILLIPS, D. R. (1994). 'Does epidemiological transition have utility for health planners?' *Social Science & Medicine*, 38, pp. vii–x. [1.4.1]

PHILLIPS, N. (2000). *Return to an Order of the Honourable the House of Commons dated October 2000 for the Report, Evidence and Supporting Papers of the Inquiry into the Emergence and Identification of Bovine Spongiform Encephalopathy (BSE) and Variant Creutzfeldt–Jakob Disease (vCJD) and the Action Taken in Response to it up to 20 March 1996*. London: Stationery Office Books. [5.2.5]

POLAND, J. D. and DENNIS, D. T. (1998). 'Plague'. In A. S. Evans and P. S. Brachman (eds), *Bacterial Infections of Humans: Epidemiology and Control*, 3rd edn. New York: Plenum Medical Book Company, 545–58. [2.3.2]

POLLITZER, R. (1954). *Plague*. Geneva: WHO. [2.3.1, 2.3.2, 9.2.1]

—— (1959). *Cholera*. Geneva: WHO. [2.3.1, 2.3.4, 9.2, 9.2.2]

PON, E., MCKEE, K. T., DINIEGA, B. M., MERRELL, B., CORWIN, A., and KSIAZEK, T. G. (1990). 'Outbreak of hemorrhagic fever with renal syndrome among US Marines in Korea'. *American Journal of Tropical Medicine and Hygiene*, 42: 612–19. [8.2.1]

POPULATION DIVISION OF THE DEPARTMENT OF ECONOMIC AND SOCIAL AFFAIRS OF THE UNITED NATIONS SECRETARIAT (2006). *World Population Prospects: The 2004 Revision* and *World Urbanization Prospects: The 2003 Revision*. New York: United Nations. [4.2.4]

POVEDA, G., ROJAS, W., QUIÑONES, M. L., VÉLEZ, I. D., MANTILLA, R. I., RUIZ, D., ZULUAGA, J. S., and RUA, G. L. (2001). 'Coupling between annual and ENSO timescales in the malaria climate association in Colombia'. *Environmental Health Perspectives*, 109: 307–24. [7.5.2]

PRADUTKANCHANA, J., PRADUTKANCHANA, S., KEMAPANMANUS, M., WUTHIPUM, N., and SILPAPOJAKUL, K. (2003). 'The etiology of acute pyrexia of unknown origin in children after a flood'. *Southeast Asian Journal of Tropical Medicine and Public Health*, 34: 175–8. [7.6.1]

PRICE-SMITH, A. T. (2002). *The Health of Nations: Infectious Disease, Environmental Change, and their Effects on National Security and Development*. Cambridge, Mass.: Massachusetts Institute of Technology. [8.1.1]

PRIDIE, E. D. (1936). 'Faits récents concernant la fièvre jaune dans le Soudan Anglo-Égyptien, en particulier la lutte contre les moustiques'. *Bulletin de l'Office International d'Hygiène Publique*, 28: 1292–1308. [6.5.3]

PRINZING, F. (1916). *Epidemics Resulting from Wars*. Oxford: Clarendon Press. [2.2.2]

PROTHERO, R. M. (1994). 'Forced movements of population and health hazards in tropical Africa'. *International Journal of Epidemiology*, 23: 657–64. [8.3]

PRUITT, F. W. and CLEVE, E. A. (1953). 'Epidemic hemorrhagic fever'. *American Journal of Medical Sciences*, 225: 660–8. [8.2.1]

PUTNAM, S. D., SANDERS, J. W., FRENCK, R. W., MONTEVILLE, M., RIDDLE, M. S., ROCKABRAND, D. M., SHARP, T. W., FRANKART, C., and TRIBBLE, D. R. (2006). 'Self-reported description of diarrhea among military populations in Operations Iraqi Freedom and Enduring Freedom'. *Journal of Travel Medicine*, 13: 92–9. [8.4.2]

PYLE, G. F. (1969). 'Diffusion of cholera in the United States'. *Geographical Analysis*, 1: 59–75. [6.3.2]

—— (1986). *The Diffusion of Influenza: Patterns and Paradigms*. Totowa, NJ: Rowman and Littlefield. [4.2.3]

Q

QADRI, F., KHAN, A. I., FARUQYE, A. S. G., BEGUM, Y. A., CHOWDRY, F., NAIR, G. B., SALAM, M. A., SACK, D. A., and SVENNERHOLM, A. M. (2005). 'Enterotoxigenic *Escherichia coli* and *Vibrio cholerae* diarrhea, Bangladesh'. *Emerging Infectious Diseases*, 11: 1104–7. [7.6.1]

R

RAETTIG, H. (1954–61). 'The plague pandemic of the 20th century'. In E. Rodenwaldt and H. J. Jusatz (eds), *World-Atlas of Epidemic Diseases. Parts II and III*. Hamburg: Falk-Verlag, III/33. [9.2.1]

—— FELTON, H., and LANGER, R. (1954–61*a*). 'Plague in the New World, 1899–1953'. In E. Rodenwaldt and H. J. Jusatz (eds), *World-Atlas of Epidemic Diseases. Parts II and III*. Hamburg: Falk-Verlag, III/26–30. [9.2.1]

—— —— —— (1954–61*b*). 'Plague in Europe, 1899–1952'. In E. Rodenwaldt and H. J. Jusatz (eds), *World-Atlas of Epidemic Diseases. Parts II and III*. Hamburg: Falk-Verlag, II/27–30. [2.3.2, 9.2.1]

—— —— —— (1954–61*c*). 'Plague in Africa, 1899–1952'. In E. Rodenwaldt and H. J. Jusatz (eds), *World-Atlas of Epidemic Diseases. Parts II and III*. Hamburg: Falk-Verlag, II/33–6. [9.2.1]

Rafi, A., Spigelman, M., Stanford, J., Lemma, E., Donoghue, H., and Zias, J. (1994). '*Mycobacterium leprae* DNA from ancient bone detected by PCR'. *Lancet*, 343: 1360–1. [1.3.3]

Ramsay, A. M. and Emond, R. T. D. (1978). *Infectious Diseases*. London: William Heinemann. [11.3]

Randolph, S. E. and Rogers, D. J. (2000). 'Fragile transmission cycles of tick-borne encephalitis virus may be disrupted by climate change'. *Philosophical Transactions of the Royal Society of London B*, 267: 1741–4. [7.5.1]

Rangel, J. M., Sparling, P. H., Crowe, C., Griffin, P. M., and Swerdlow, D. L. (2005). 'Epidemiology of *Escherichia coli* O157:H7 outbreaks, United States, 1982–2002'. *Emerging Infectious Diseases*, 11: 603–9. [5.2.4]

Raoult, D., Aboudharam, G., Crubézy, E., Larrouy, G., Ludes, B., and Drancourt, M. (2000). 'Molecular identification by "suicide PCR" of *Yersinia pestis* as the agent of medieval Black Death'. *Proceedings of the National Academy of Sciences USA*, 97: 12800–3. [2.3.2]

—— Ndihokubwayo, J. B., Tissot-Dupont, H., Roux, V., Faugere, B., Abegbinni, R., and Birtles, R. J. (1998). 'Outbreak of epidemic typhus associated with trench fever in Burundi'. *Lancet*, 352: 353–8. [8.1, 8.3.1]

Raviglione, M. C. and Pio, A. (2002). 'Evolution of WHO policies for tuberculosis control, 1948–2001'. *Lancet*, 359: 775–80. [4.3.2]

Ray, A. J. (1974). *Indians in the Fur Trade: Their Role as Trappers, Hunters and Middlemen in the Lands of Southwest Hudson Bay, 1660–1870*. Toronto: University of Toronto Press. [6.3.1]

Regidor, E., de la Fuente, L., Gutiérrez-Fisac, J. L., de Mateo, S., Pascual, C., Sánchez-Payá, J., and Ronda, E. (2007). 'The role of the public health official in communicating public health information'. *American Journal of Public Health*, 97: S93–S97. [10.6.1]

Reid, A. H., Fanning, T. G., Hultin, J. V., and Taubenberger, J. K. (1999). 'Origin and evolution of the 1918 "Spanish" influenza hemagluttinin gene'. *Proceedings of the National Academy of Sciences USA*, 96: 1651–5. [1.3.3]

Reiter, P. (2001). 'Climate change and mosquito-borne disease'. *Environmental Health Perspectives*, 109, suppl. 1, 141–61. [7.5.1]

Rendle Short, A. (1955). *The Bible and Modern Medicine: A Survey of Health and Healing in the Old and New Testaments*. London: Paternoster. [2.2.1]

Renner, M. (1997). 'Keeping peace and preventing war: The role of the United Nations'. In B. S. Levy and V. W. Sidel (eds), *War and Public Health*. New York: Oxford University Press, 360–74. [8.4.3]

Richards, C. L. and Jarvis, W. R. (1999). 'Lessons from recent nosocomial outbreaks'. *Current Opinion in Infectious Diseases*, 12: 327–34. [4.3.1]

Riley, J. C. (1989). *Sickness, Recovery and Death: A History and Forecast of Ill Health*. Iowa City: University of Iowa Press. [1.4.1]

Riley, J. C. and Alter, G. (1989). 'The Epidemiological Transition and Morbidity'. Working Paper no. 10, Population Institute for Research and Training. Bloomington: Indiana University Press. [1.4.1]

Riley, L. W., Remis, R. S., Helgerson, S. D., McGee, H. B., Wells, J. G., Davis, B. R., Hebert, R. J., Olcott, E. S., Johnson, L. M., Hargrett, N. T., Blake, P. A., and Cohen, M. L. (1983). 'Haemorrhagic colitis associated with a rare *Esherichia coli* serotype'. *New England Journal of Medicine*, 308: 681–5. [5.2.4]

Roberts, L., Lafta, R., Garfield, R., Khudhairi, J., and Burnham, G. (2004). 'Mortality before and after the 2003 invasion of Iraq: Cluster sample survey'. *Lancet*, 364: 1857–64. [8.4.2]

Rodenwaldt, E. (1952). 'The cholera epidemic, 1863–1868'. In E. Rodenwaldt (ed.), *World-Atlas of Epidemic Diseases. Part I.* Hamburg: Falk-Verlag, I/13–14. [9.2.2]

—— and Jusatz, H. J. (eds) (1954–61). *World-Atlas of Epidemic Diseases. Parts II and III.* Hamburg: Falk-Verlag. [9.2.1, 9.3.2]

Roelke-Parker, M. E., Munson, L., Packer, C., Kock, R., Cleaveland, S., Carpenter, M., O'Brien, S. J., Pospischil, A., Hofmann-Lehmann, R., Lutz, H., Mwamengele, G. L. M., Mgasa, M. N., Machange, G. A., Summers, B. A., and Appel, M. J. G. (1996). 'A canine distemper virus epidemic in Serengeti lions (*Panthera leo*)'. *Nature*, 379: 441–5. [7.4.1]

Rogers, D. J. and Randolph, S. E. (2006). 'Climate change and vector-borne diseases'. *Advances in Parasitology*, 62: 345–81. [7.5.1]

Rogers, R. and Hackenberg, R. (1989). 'Extending epidemiologic transition theory: A new stage'. *Social Biology*, 34: 234–43. [1.4.1]

Rollin, P. E., Williams, R. J., Bressler, D. S., Pearson, S., Cottingham, M., Pucak, G., Sanchez, A., Trappier, S. G., Peters, R. L., Greer, P. W., Zaki, S., Demarcus, T., Hendricks, K., Kelley, M., Simpson, D., Geisbert, T. W., Jahrling, P. B., Peters, C. J., and Ksiazek, T. G. (1999). 'Ebola (subtype Reston) virus among quarantine nonhuman primates recently imported from the Philippines to the United States'. *Journal of Infectious Diseases*, 179, suppl. 1, S108–S114. [9.3.2]

Romaguera, R. A., German, R. R., and Klauke, D. N. (2000). 'Evaluating public health surveillance'. In S. M. Teutsch and R. E. Churchill (eds), *Principles and Practice of Public Health Surveillance*, 2nd edn. New York: Oxford University Press, 176–93. [10.6.3]

Rooney, R. M., Cramer, E. H., Mantha, S., Nichols, G., Bartram, J. K., Farber, J. M., and Benembarek, P. K. (2004). 'A review of outbreaks of foodborne disease associated with passenger ships: Evidence for risk management'. *Public Health Reports*, 119: 427–34. [6.3.1]

Rotz, L. D., Khan, A. S., Lillibridge, S. R., Ostroff, S. M., and Hughes, J. M. (2002). 'Public health assessment of potential biological terrorism agents'. *Emerging Infectious Diseases*, 8: 225–9. [8.5.4]

Rouquet, P., Froment, J.-M., Bermejo, M., Kilbourn, A., Karesh, W., Reed, P., Kumulungui, B., Yaba, P., Délicat, A., Rollin, P. E., and Leroy, E. M. (2005). 'Wild animal mortality monitoring and human Ebola outbreaks, Gabon and Republic of Congo, 2001–2003'. *Emerging Infectious Diseases*, 11: 283–90. [9.3.2]

ROUSH, S., BIRKHEAD, G., KOO, D., COBB, A., and FLEMING, D. (1999). 'Mandatory reporting of diseases and conditions by health care professionals and laboratories'. *Journal of the American Medical Association*, 282: 164–70. [10.6.2]

ROWLAND, K. T. (1970). *Steam at Sea: A History of Steam Navigation*. Newton Abbot: David and Charles. [6.3.1]

RUSSELL, A. J. H. (1929). *A Geographical Survey of Cholera in the Madras Presidency from 1818–1927*. Madras: Government Press. [2.3.4]

RUSSELL, J. C. (1972). 'Population in Europe 500–1500'. In C. M. Cipolla (ed.), *The Fontana Economic History of Europe: The Middle Ages*. London: Fontana, 25–70. [2.3.2]

RVACHEV, L. A. and LONGINI, I. M., JR (1985). 'A mathematical model for the global spread of influenza'. *Mathematical Biosciences*, 75: 3–22. [6.4.2]

S

SABIN, A. B., SCHLESINGER, R. W., GINDER, W. R., and MATSUMOTO, M. (1947). 'Japanese B encephalitis in an American soldier in Korea'. *American Journal of Hygiene*, 46: 356–75. [8.2.1]

SAENZ, R., BISSELL, R. A., and PANIAGUA, F. (1995). 'Post-disaster malaria in Costa Rica'. *Prehospital Disaster Medicine*, 10: 154–60. [7.6.1]

SAKER, L., LEE, K., CANNITO, B., GILMORE, A., and CAMPBELL-LENDRUM, D. (2004). *Globalization and Infectious Diseases: A Review of the Linkages*. Geneva: WHO on behalf of the Special Programme for Research and Training in Tropical Diseases (TDR/STR/SEB/ST04.2). [7.3]

SALL, A. A., ZANOTTO, P. M. A., VIALAT, P., SÈNE, O. K., and BOULOY, M. (1998). 'Molecular epidemiology and emergence of Rift Valley fever'. *Memórias do Instituto Oswaldo Cruz*, 95: 609–14. [7.3.1]

SALO, W. L., AUFDERHEIDE, A. C., BUIKSTRA, J., and HOLCOMB, T. A. (1994). 'Identification of *Mycobacterium tuberculosis* DNA in a pre-Columbian Peruvian mummy'. *Proceedings of the National Academy of Sciences USA*, 91: 2091–4. [1.3.3]

SANDERS, J., PUTNAM, S., FRANKART, C., FRENCK, R. W., MONTEVILLE, M. R., RIDDLE, M. S., ROCKABRAND, D. M., SHARP, T. W., and TRIBBLE, D. R. (2005). 'Impact of illness and non-combat injury during operations Iraqi Freedom and Enduring Freedom (Afghanistan)'. *American Journal of Tropical Medicine and Hygiene*, 73: 713–19. [8.4.2]

SATTENSPIEL, L. and HERRING, D. A. (2003). 'Simulating the effect of quarantine on the spread of the 1918–19 flu in central Canada. *Bulletin of Mathematical Biology*, 65: 1–26. [11.2.3]

SAVILL, N. J., SHAW, D. J., DEARDON, R., TILDESLEY, M. J., KEELING, M. J., WOOLHOUSE, M. E. J., BROOKS, S. P., and GRENFELL, B. T. (2006) 'Topographic determinants of foot and mouth disease transmission in the UK 2001 epidemic'. *BMC Veterinary Research*, 2: 1–9. [6.3.2]

SCHENZLE, D. and DIETZ, K. (1987). 'Critical population sizes for endemic virus transmission'. In W. Fricke and E. Hinz (eds), *Räumliche Persistenz und Diffusion von Krankheiten*. Heidelberg Geographical Studies, 83: 31–42. [App. 11.2]

SCHLEISNER, P. A. (1851). 'Vital statistics of Iceland'. *Quarterly Journal of the Statistical Society of London*, 14: 1–10. [10.3.2]

SCHMALJOHN, C. and HJELLE, B. (1997). 'Hantaviruses: A global disease problem'. *Emerging Infectious Diseases*, 3: 95–104. [7.5.3, 8.2.1]

SCHNEIDER, E., HAJJEH, R. A., SPIEGEL, R. A., JIBSON, R. W., HARP, E. L., MARSHALL, G. A., GUNN, R. A., MCNEIL, M. M., PINNER, R. W., BARON, R. C., BURGER, R. C., HUTWAGNER, L. C., CRUMP, C., KAUFMAN, L., REEF, S. E., FELDMAN, G. M., PAPPAGIANIS, D., and WERNER, S. B. (1997). 'A coccidioidomycosis outbreak following the Northridge, Calif., earthquake'. *Journal of the American Medical Association*, 277: 904–8. [7.6.1]

SCOTT, S. and DUNCAN, C. J. (2001). *Biology of Plagues: Evidence from Historical Populations*. Cambridge: Cambridge University Press. [11.2.1]

SEAMAN, J., MERCER, A. J., and SONDORP, E. (1996). 'The epidemic of visceral leishmaniasis in western Upper Nile, southern Sudan: Course and impact from 1984 to 1994'. *International Journal of Epidemiology*, 25: 862–71. [8.4.1]

SEET, B. and BURNHAM, G. M. (2000). 'Fatality trends in United Nations peacekeeping operations, 1948–1998'. *Journal of the American Medical Association*, 284: 598–603. [8.4.2]

SELLERS, R. F., PEDGLEY, D. E., and TUCKER, M. R. (1982). 'Rift Valley fever, Egypt—1977: Disease spread by wind-borne insect vectors?' *Veterinary Record*, 110: 73. [7.3.1]

SHANNON, G. W., PYLE, G. F., and BASHSHUR, R. L. (1991). *The Geography of AIDS*. New York: Guilford Press. [9.2.3]

SHAPIRO, S. E., LASAREV, M. R., and MCCAULEY, L. (2002). 'Factor analysis of Gulf War illness: What does it add to our understanding of possible health effects of deployment?' *American Journal of Epidemiology*, 156: 578–85. [8.4.4]

SHARMA, S. K. and MOHAN, A. (2006). 'Multidrug-resistant tuberculosis: A menace that threatens to detabilize tuberculosis control'. *Chest*, 130: 261–72. [4.3.2]

SHARMA, V. P. (1996). 'Re-emergence of malaria in India'. *Indian Journal of Medical Research*, 103: 26–45. [4.4.3]

SHARP, P. M., BAILES, E., CHAUDHURI, R. R., RODENBURG, C. M., SANTIAGO, M. O., and HAHN, B. H. (2001). 'The origins of acquired immune deficiency syndrome viruses: Where and when?' *Philosophical Transactions of the Royal Society of London B, Biological Sciences*, 356: 867–76. [9.2.3]

SHARP, T. W., BURKLE, F. M., JR, VAUGHN, A. F., CHOTANI, R., and BRENNAN, J. J. (2002). 'Challenges and opportunities for humanitarian relief in Afghanistan'. *Clinical Infectious Diseases*, 34, suppl. 5, S215–S228. [8.4.2]

SHIDRAWI, G. R. (1990). 'A WHO global programme for monitoring vector resistance to pesticides'. *Bulletin of the World Health Organization*, 68: 403–8. [4.4.1, 4.4.2]

SHLAES, D. M., GERDING, D. N., JOHN, J. F., JR, CRAIG, W. A., BORNSTEIN, D. L., DUNCAN, R. A., ECKMAN, M. R., FARRER, W. E., GREENE, W. H., LORIAN, V., LEVY, S., MCGOWAN, J. E., JR, PAUL, S. M., RUSKIN, J., TENOVER, F. C., and WATANAKUNAKORN, C. (1997). 'Society for Healthcare Epidemiology of America and Infectious Diseases Society of America Joint Committee on the Prevention of Antimicrobial Resistance: Guidelines for the prevention of antimicrobial resistance in hospitals'. *Infection Control and Hospital Epidemiology*, 18: 275–91. [4.3.1]

SHOPE, R. E., PETERS, C. J., and DAVIES, F. G. (1982). 'The spread of Rift Valley fever and approaches to its control'. *Bulletin of the World Health Organization*, 60: 299–304. [7.3.1]

SHORR, A. F., SCOVILLE, S. L., CERSOVSKY, S. B., SHANKS, G. D., OCKENHOUSE, C. F., SMOAK, B. L., CARR, W. W., and PETRUCCELLI, B. P. (2004). 'Acute eosinophilic pneumonia among US military personnel deployed in or near Iraq'. *Journal of the American Medical Association*, 292: 2997–3005. [8.4.2]

SHORTLIFFE, E. H. and SONDIK, E. J. (2006). 'The public health informatics infrastructure: Anticipating its role in cancer'. *Cancer Causes and Control*, 17: 861–9. [10.6.3]

SHORTRIDGE, K. F. (1992). 'Pandemic influenza: A zoonosis?' *Seminars in Respiratory Infections*, 7: 11–25. [4.2.2]

—— and STUART-HARRIS, C. H. (1982). 'An influenza epicentre?' *Lancet*, 2: 812–13. [4.2.2]

SHREWSBURY, J. F. D. (1964). *The Plague of the Philistines and other Medical-Historical Essays*. London: Victor Gollancz. [2.2.1]

—— (1970). *A History of Bubonic Plague in the British Isles*. Cambridge: Cambridge University Press. [2.3.2, 6.3.2]

SHULTZ, J. M., RUSSELL, J., and ESPINEL, Z. (2005). 'Epidemiology of tropical cyclones: The dynamics of disaster, disease, and development'. *Epidemiologic Reviews*, 27: 21–35. [7.6.3]

SIMPSON, W. J. (1905). *A Treatise on Plague, Dealing with the Historical, Epidemiological, Clinical, Therapeutic and Preventive Aspects of the Disease*. Cambridge: Cambridge University Press. [2.2.1, 2.3.2]

SIMS, L. D., DOMENECH, J., BENIGNO, C., KAHN, S., KAMATA, A., LUBROTH, J., MARTIN, V., and ROEDER, P. (2005). 'Origin and evolution of highly pathogenic H5N1 avian influenza in Asia'. *Veterinary Record*, 157: 159–64. [4.2.3]

SIVAPALASINGAM, S., BARRETT, E., KIMURA, A., VAN DUYNE, S., DE WITT, W., YING, M., FRISCH, A., PHAN, Q., GOULD, E., SHILLAM, P., REDDY, V., COOPER, T., HOEKSTRA, M., HIGGINS, C., SANDERS, J. P., TAUXE, R. V., and SLUTSKER, L. (2003). 'A multistate outbreak of *Salmonella enterica* serotype Newport infection linked to mango consumption: Impact of water-dip disinfestation technology'. *Clinical Infectious Diseases*, 37: 1585–90. [5.2.3]

SLUTSKER, L., GUARNER, J., and GRIFFIN, P. (1998). '*Escherichia coli* O157:H7'. In A. M. Nelson and C. R. Horsburgh, Jr (eds), *Pathology of Emerging Infections 2*. Washington, DC: ASM Press, 259–82. [5.2.4]

SMALLMAN-RAYNOR, M. and CLIFF, A. D. (1998*a*). 'The Philippines insurrection and the 1902–4 cholera epidemic. Part I. Epidemiological diffusion processes in war'. *Journal of Historical Geography*, 24: 69–89. [9.2.2]

—— —— (1998*b*). 'The Philippines insurrection and the 1902–4 cholera epidemic. Part II. Diffusion patterns in war and peace'. *Journal of Historical Geography*, 24: 188–210. [9.2.2]

—— —— (2004*a*). 'The geographical spread of cholera in the Crimean War: Epidemic transmission in the camp systems of the British army of the East, 1854–5'. *Journal of Historical Geography*, 30: 32–69. [9.2.2]

—— —— (2004*b*). *War Epidemics: An Historical Geography of Infectious Diseases in Military Conflict and Civil Strife, 1850–2000*. Oxford: Oxford University Press. [1.6,

2.2, 2.2.2, 2.3.2, 8.1, 8.1.2, 8.2, 8.2.1, 8.2.2, 8.3, 8.3.1, 8.3.2, 8.4, 8.4.1, 8.4.3, 8.5.1, 8.5.3, 9.2.2, 9.3.1, 9.4.1, 9.6]

—— —— (2007). 'Avian influenza A (H5N1) age distribution in humans'. *Emerging Infectious Diseases*, 13: 510–12. [4.2.4]

—— —— (2008). 'The geographical spread of avian influenza A (H5N1): Panzootic transmission (December 2003–May 2006), pandemic potential and implications'. *Annals of the Association of American Geographers*, 98: 553–82. [2.3.3, 4.2.2, 4.2.3, 4.2.4]

—— —— and HAGGETT, P. (1992). *London International Atlas of AIDS*. Oxford: Blackwell Reference. [6.3.2, 6.4.3, 9.2.3]

—— —— TREVELYAN, B., NETTLETON, C., and SNEDDON, S. (2006). *Poliomyelitis. A World Geography: Emergence to Eradication*. Oxford: Oxford University Press. [8.5.4, 9.3.1, 11.3.1, 11.3.2]

—— JOHNSON, N., and CLIFF, A. D. (2002). 'The spatial anatomy of an epidemic: Influenza in London and the county boroughs of England and Wales, 1918–19'. *Transactions of the Institute of British Geographers*, new ser., 27: 452–70. [4.2.3]

SMITH, H. B. and TIRPAK, D. (eds) (1989). *Potential Effects of Global Climatic Change on the United States*, vol. G: *Health*. Washington, DC: US Government Printing Office (Environmental Protection Agency, EPA 230–05–89–057). [7.5.1]

SMITH, R. D. and COAST, J. (2002). 'Antimicrobial resistance: A global response'. *Bulletin of the World Health Organization*, 80: 126–33. [4.3.1, 4.3.2, 4.5]

SNOWDON, J. A., BUZBY, J. C., and ROBERTS, T. (2002). 'Epidemiology, cost, and risk of foodborne disease'. In D. O. Cliver and H. P. Riemann (eds), *Foodborne Diseases*. Amsterdam: Academic Press, 31–51. [5.2, 5.2.1, 5.2.3]

SOBEL, J., GRIFFIN, P. M., SLUTSKER, L., SWERDLOW, D. L., and TAUXE, R. V. (2002). 'Investigation of multistate foodborne disease outbreaks'. *Public Health Reports*, 117: 8–19. [5.2.3]

SOEPRAPTO, W., ERTONO, S., HUDOYO, H., MASCOLA, J., PORTER, K., GUNAWAN, S., and CORWIN A. L. (1995). 'HIV and peacekeeping operations in Cambodia'. *Lancet*, 346: 1304–5. [8.4.3]

SOGOBA, N., DOUMBIA, S., VOUNATSOU, P., BAGAYOKO, M. M., DOLO, G., TRAORÉ, S. F., MAÏGA, H. M., TOURÉ, Y. T., and SMITH, T. (2007). 'Malaria transmission dynamics in Niono, Mali: The effect of the irrigation systems'. *Acta Tropica*, 101: 232–40. [7.2]

SOHN, Y. M. (2000). 'Japanese encephalitis immunization in South Korea: Past, present and future'. *Emerging Infectious Diseases*, 6: 17–24. [8.2.1]

SONESSON, C. and BOCK, D. (2003). 'A review and discussion of prospective statistical surveillance in public health'. *Journal of the Royal Statistical Society A*, 166: 5–21. [10.6.1]

SONGSERM, T., AMONSIN, A., JAM-ON, R., SAE-HENG, N., MEEMAK, N., PARIYOTHORN, N., PAYUNGPORN, S., THEAMBOONLERS, A., and POOVORAWAN, Y. (2006). 'Avian influenza H5N1 in naturally infected domestic cat'. *Emerging Infectious Diseases*, 12: 681–3. [4.2.3]

SPECK, R. S. (1993). 'Cholera'. In K. F. Kiple (ed.), *Cambridge World History of Human Disease*. Cambridge: Cambridge University Press, 642–9. [2.3.4]

Spielman, A. (1994). 'The emergence of Lyme disease and human babesiosis in a changing environment'. *Annals of the New York Aacdemy of Sciences*, 740: 146–56. [7.4.2]

Splino, M., Beran, J., and Chlíbek, R. (2003). 'Q fever outbreak during the Czech army deployment in Bosnia'. *Military Medicine*, 168: 840–2. [8.4.3]

Spratt, B. G. (2007). *Independent Review of the Safety of UK Facilities Handling Foot-and-Mouth Disease Virus. Report Presented to the Secretary of State for Environment, Food and Rural Affairs and the Chief Veterinary Officer*. London: DEFRA. http://www.defra.gov.uk/FootandMouth/pdf/spratt_final.pdf, accessed 26 Jan. 2009. [11.2.4]

Stannard, J. (1993). 'Diseases in western antiquity'. In K. F. Kiple (ed.), *Cambridge World History of Human Disease*. Cambridge: Cambridge University Press, 262–70. [2.2.2]

Steere, A. C. (1998). 'Lyme disease'. In R. M. Krause (ed.), *Emerging Infections: Biomedical Research Reports*. San Diego: Academic Press, 219–37. [7.4.2]

—— Grodzicki, R. L., Kornblatt, A. N., Craft, J. E., Barbour, A. G., Burgdorfer, W., Schmid, G. P., Johnson, E., and Malawista, S. E. (1983). 'The spirochetal etiology of Lyme disease'. *New England Journal of Medicine*, 308: 733–40. [7.4.2]

—— Malawista, S. E., Snydman, D. R., Shope, R. E., Andiman, W. A., Ross, M. R., and Steele, F. M. (1977). 'Lyme arthritis: An epidemic of oligoarticular arthritis in children and adults in three Connecticut communities'. *Arthritis and Rheumatism*, 20: 7–17. [7.4.2]

Steffen, R., Desaules, M., Nagel, J., Vuillet, F., Schubarth, P., Jeanmaire, C.-H., and Huber, A. (1992). 'Epidemiological experience in the mission of the United Nations Transition Assistance Group (UNTAG) in Namibia'. *Bulletin of the World Health Organization*, 70: 129–33. [8.4.3]

Steinbrook, R. (2006). 'Facing the diabetes epidemic: Mandatory reporting of glycosylated hemoglobin values in New York City'. *New England Journal of Medicine*, 354: 545–8. [10.6.3]

—— (2007). 'One step forward, two steps back—will there ever be an AIDS vaccine?' *New England Journal of Medicine*, 357: 2653–5. [9.2.3]

Stephens, D. S., Greenwood, B., and Brandtzaeg, P. (2007). 'Epidemic meningitis, meningococcaemia, and *Neisseria meningitidis*'. *Lancet*, 369: 2196–2210. [9.3.2]

Stevens, D. L. (1995). 'Streptococcal toxic-shock syndrome: Spectrum of disease, pathogenesis, and new concepts in treatment'. *Emerging Infectious Diseases*, 1: 69–78. [4.2.1]

Stewart, F. (2002). 'Root causes of violent conflict in developing countries'. *British Medical Journal*, 324: 342–5. [8.4]

Sticker, G. (1912). *Abhandlungen aus der Seuchengeschichte und Seuchenlehre*, ii: *Die Cholera*. Giessen: A. Töpelmann. [2.3.4]

Stokes, G. V. (2002). 'Microbial resistance to antibiotics'. In F. R. Lashley and J. D. Durham (eds), *Emerging Infectious Diseases: Trends and Issues*. New York: Springer Publishing Company, 23–42. [4.3.1, 4.3.2]

Strachan, N. J. C., Dunn, G. M., Locking, M. E., Reid, T. M. S., and Ogden, I. D. (2006). '*Escherichia coli* O157: Burger bug or environmental pathogen?' *International Journal of Food Microbiology*, 112: 129–37. [5.2.4]

Stroup, D. F. and Thacker, S. B. (1993). 'A Bayesian approach to the detection of aberrations in public health surveillance data'. *Epidemiology*, 4: 435–43. [10.6.1]

—— —— (2007). 'Epidemic Aid investigations (Epi-Aids), the teenage years: 1956–1965'. *EIS Bulletin*, Special Conference Issue. Atlanta, Ga.: CDC, 12–18. [3.4.1, 3.4.2]

—— Brookmeyer, R., and Kalsbeek, W. D. (2003). 'Public health surveillance in action: A framework'. In R. Brookmeyer and D. F. Stroup (eds), *Monitoring the Health of Populations: Statistical Principles and Methods for Public Health Surveillance*. New York: Oxford University Press. [10.6.1]

—— Wharton, M., Kafadar, K., and Dean, A. G. (1993). 'An evaluation of a method for detecting aberrations in public health surveillance data'. *American Journal of Epidemiology*, 137: 45–9. [11.4]

Su, H.-P., Chou, C.-Y., Tzeng, S.-C., Ferng, T.-L., Chen, Y.-L., Chen, Y.-S., and Chung, T.-C. (2007). 'Possible typhoon-related melioidosis epidemic, Taiwan, 2005'. *Emerging Infectious Diseases*, 13: 1795–7. [7.6.1]

Sugiyama, A., Iwade, Y., Akachi, S., Nakano, Y., Matsuno, Y., Yano, T., Yamauchi, A., Nakayama, O., Sakai, H., Yamamoto, K., Nagasaka, Y., Nakano, T., Ihara, T., and Kamiya, H. (2005). 'An outbreak of Shigatoxin-producing *Escherichia coli* O157:H7 in a nursery school in Mie Prefecture'. *Japanese Journal of Infectious Diseases*, 58: 398–400. [5.2.4]

Sugunan, A. P., Ghosh, A. R., Roy, S., Gupte, M. D., and Sehgal, S. C. (2004). 'A cholera epidemic among the Nicobarese tribe of Nancowry, Andaman, and Nicobar, India'. *American Journal of Tropical Medicine and Hygiene*, 71: 822–7. [6.3.1]

Sur, D., Dutta, P., Nair, G. B., and Bhattacharya, S. K. (2000). 'Severe cholera outbreak following floods in a northern district of West Bengal'. *Indian Journal of Medical Research*, 112: 178–82. [7.6.1]

Süss, J., Klaus, C., Gerstengarbe, F.-W., and Werner, P. C. (2008). 'What makes ticks tick? Climate change, ticks, and tick-borne diseases'. *Journal of Travel Medicine*, 15: 39–45. [7.2]

Sutherst, R. W. (2004). 'Global change and human vulnerability to vector-borne diseases'. *Clinical Microbiology Reviews*, 17: 136–73. [7.5.1]

Swerdlow, D. and Altekruse, S. F. (1998). 'Food-borne diseases in the global village: What's on the plate for the 21st century'. In W. M. Scheld, W. A. Craig, and J. M. Hughes (eds), *Emerging Infections 2*. Washington, DC: ASM Press, 273–94. [5.2.1]

—— and Ries, A. A. (1993). '*Vibrio cholerae* non-O1—the eighth pandemic? *Lancet*, 342: 382–3. [9.2.2]

T

Tanser, F. C., Sharp, B., and Le Sueur, D. (2003). 'Potential effect of climate change on malaria transmission in Africa'. *Lancet Infectious Diseases*, 362: 1792–8. [7.5.1]

Tauxe, R. V. (1997). 'Emerging foodborne diseases: An evolving public health challenge'. *Emerging Infectious Diseases*, 3: 425–34. [5.2, 5.2.1]

—— (1998). 'Cholera'. In A. S. Evans and P. S. Brachman (eds), *Bacterial Infections of Humans: Epidemiology and Control*, 3rd edn. New York: Plenum Medical Book Company, 223–42. [2.3.4]

Taviner, M., Thwaites, G., and Gant, V. (1998). 'The English sweating sickness, 1485–1551: A viral pulmonary syndrome'. *Medical History*, 42: 96–9. [2.3.5]

Taylor, L. H., Latham, S. M., and Woolhouse, M. E. J. (2001). 'Risk factors for human disease emergence'. *Philosophical Transactions of the Royal Society of London B*, 356: 983–9. [1.5.1]

Terranova, W., Cohen, M. L., and Fraser, D. W. (1978). '1974 outbreak of Legionnaires' disease diagnosed in 1977: Clinical and epidemiological features'. *Lancet*, 2: 122–4. [5.3.3]

Thacker, S. B. and Berkelman, R. L. (1988). 'Public health surveillance in the United States'. *Epidemiologic Reviews*, 10: 164–90. [3.5]

—— and Stroup, D. F. (1994). 'Future directions for comprehensive public health surveillance and health information systems in the United States'. *American Journal of Epidemiology*, 140: 383–97. [3.5]

—— —— (2007*a*). 'Epidemic Aid investigations, 1946–1955'. *EIS Bulletin*, Mar. Atlanta, Ga.: CDC, 34–44. [3.4.1, 3.4.2]

—— —— (2007*b*). 'Epidemic Aid investigations, the third decade: 1966–1975'. *EIS e-Bulletin*, e2/e3, June. Atlanta, Ga.: CDC. [3.4.1, 3.4.2]

—— —— (2008). 'Epidemic Aid investigations, the fourth decade: 1976–1985'. *EIS e-Bulletin*, e3/e1, Mar. Atlanta, Ga.: CDC. [3.4.1, 3.4.2]

—— Bennett, J. V., Tsai, T. F., Fraser, D. W., McDade, J. E., Shepard, C. C., Williams, K. H., Jr, Stuart, W. H., Dull, H. B., and Eickhoff, T. C. (1978). 'An outbreak in 1965 of severe respiratory illness caused by Legionnaires' disease bacterium'. *Journal of Infectious Diseases*, 138: 512–19. [5.3.3]

—— Choi, K., and Brachman, P. S. (1983). 'The surveillance of infectious diseases'. *Journal of the American Medical Association*, 249: 1181–5. [3.5]

—— Dannenberg, A. L., and Hamilton, D. H. (2001). 'Epidemic Intelligence Service of the Centers for Disease Control and Prevention: 50 years of training and service in applied epidemiology'. *American Journal of Epidemiology*, 154: 985–92. [3.4.1]

—— Stroup, D. F., Parrish, R. G., and Anderson, H. A. (1996). 'Surveillance in environmental public health'. *American Journal of Public Health*, 86: 633–8. [10.6.1]

—— —— Rothenberg, R. B., and Brownson, R. C. (1995). 'Public health surveillance for chronic conditions: A scientific basis for decisions'. *Statistics in Medicine*, 14: 629–41. [10.6.1]

Thomas, C. J., Davies, G., and Dunn, C. E. (2004). 'Mixed picture for changes in stable malaria distribution with future climate in Africa'. *Trends in Parasitology*, 20: 216–20. [7.5.1]

Thompson, T. (1852). *Annals of Influenza or Epidemic Catarrhal Fever in Great Britain from 1510 to 1837*. London: Sydenham Society. [9.5.1]

Thomson, D. (1955). 'The ebb and flow of infection'. *Monthly Bulletin of the Ministry of Health and the Public Health Laboratory Service*, 14: 106–16. [1.1, 2.4.1, 9.3.1, 9.5.1]

—— (1976). 'The ebb and flow of infection'. *Journal of the American Medical Association*, 235: 269–72. [9.3.1, 9.5.1]

Thongcharoen, P. (1989). *Japanese Encephalitis Virus Encephalitis: An Overview*. Bangkok: Faculty of Tropical Medicine, Mahidol University. [8.2.1]

Thornton, S. A., Sherman, S. S., Farkas, T., Zhong, W., Torres, P., and Jiang, X. (2005). 'Gastroenteritis in US Marines during Operation Iraqi Freedom'. *Clinical Infectious Diseases*, 40: 519–25. [8.4.2]

Thorson, A., Petzold, M., Chuc, N. T. K., and Ekdahl, K. (2006). 'Is exposure to sick or dead poultry associated with a flulike illness?' *Archives of Internal Medicine*, 166: 119–23. [4.2.4]

Thwaites, G., Taviner, M., and Gant, V. (1997). 'The English sweating sickness, 1485–1551'. *New England Journal of Medicine*, 336: 580–2. [2.3.5]

Tiensin, T., Chaitaweesub, P., Songserm, T., Chaisingh, A., Hoonsuwan, W., Vuranathai, C., Parakamawongsa, T., Premashthira, S., Amonsin, A., Gilbert, M., Nielen, M., and Stegeman, A. (2005). 'Highly pathogenic avian influenza H5N1, Thailand, 2004'. *Emerging Infectious Diseases*, 11: 1664–72. [4.2.3]

Tollis, M. and Di Trani, L. (2002). 'Recent developments in avian influenza research: Epidemiology and immunoprophylaxis'. *Veterinary Journal*, 164: 202–15. [4.2.3]

Toole, M. J. (1997). 'Displaced persons and war'. In B. S. Levy and V. W. Sidel (eds), *War and Public Health*. New York: Oxford University Press, 197–212. [8.4.1]

Trencséni, T. and Keleti, B. (1971). *Clinical Aspects and Epidemiology of Haemorrhagic Fever with Renal Syndrome: Analysis of Clinical and Epidemiological Experiences in Hungary*. Budapest: Akadémiai Kiadó. [8.2.1]

Trevelyan, B., Smallman-Raynor, M. R., and Cliff, A. D. (2005). 'The spatial dynamics of poliomyelitis in the United States: Emergence to vaccine-induced retreat, 1910–1971'. *Annals of the Association of American Geographers*, 95: 269–93. [10.2.2]

Trevisanato, S. I. (2004). 'Did an epidemic of tularemia in Ancient Egypt affect the course of world history?' *Medical Hypotheses*, 63: 905–10. [2.2, 2.2.1]

—— (2006*a*). 'Six medical papyri describe the effects of Santorini's volcanic ash, and provide Egyptian parallels to the so-called biblical plagues'. *Medical Hypotheses*, 67: 187–90. [2.2.1]

—— (2006*b*). 'Treatments for burns in the *London Medical Papyrus* show the first seven biblical plagues of Egypt are coherent with Santorini's volcanic fallout'. *Medical Hypotheses*, 66: 193–6. [2.2.1]

—— (2007*a*). 'The biblical plague of the Philistines now has a name, tularemia'. *Medical Hypotheses*, 69: 1144–6. [2.2, 2.2.1]

—— (2007*b*). 'The "Hittite plague", an epidemic of tularemia and the first record of biological warfare'. *Medical Hypotheses*, 69: 1371–4. [2.2, 2.2.1, 8.5.2]

Trigg, P. I. and Kondrachine, A. V. (1998). 'Malaria control in the 1990s'. *Bulletin of the World Health Organization*, 76: 11–16. [4.4.3]

Truelson, T., Bonita, R., and Joamrozik, K. (2001). 'Surveillance of stroke: A global perspective'. *International Journal of Epidemiology*, 30: S11–S16. [10.6.2]

Tsai, T. F. (2000). 'Flaviviruses (yellow fever, dengue, dengue hemorrhagic fever, Japanese encephalitis, St. Louis encephalitis, tick-borne encephalitis)'. In G. L. Mandell, J. E. Bennett, and R. Dolin (eds), *Principles and Practice of Infectious Diseases*, ii. New York: Churchill Livingstone, 1714–36. [8.2.1]

Tucker, J. B. (1999). 'Historical trends related to bioterrorism: An empirical analysis'. *Emerging Infectious Diseases*, 5: 498–504. [8.5.3]

Tumpey, T. M., Basler, C. F., Aguilar, P. V., Zeng, H., Solórzano, A., Swayne, D. E., Cox, N. J., Katz, J. M., Taubenberger, J. K., Palese, P., and García-Sastre, A. (2005). 'Characterization of the reconstructed 1918 Spanish influenza pandemic virus'. *Science*, 310: 77–80. [1.3.3]

—— Maines, T. R., Hoeven, N. V., Glaser, L., Solórzano, A., Pappas, C., Cox, N. J., Swayne, D. E., Palese, P., Katz, J. M., and García-Sastre, A. (2007). 'A two-amino acid change in the hemagglutinin of the 1918 influenza virus abolishes transmission'. *Science*, 315: 655–9. [4.2.2]

U

UNAIDS (2007). *AIDS Epidemic Update: December 2007*. Geneva: UNAIDS. [9.2.3]

Ungchusak, K., Auewarakul, P., Dowell, S. F., Kitphati, R., Auwanit, W., Puthavathana, P., Uiprasertkul, M., Boonnak, K., Pittayawonganon, C., Cox, N. J., Zaki, S. R., Thawatsupha, P., Chittaganpitch, M., Khontong, R., Simmerman, J. M., and Chunsutthiwat, S. (2005). 'Probable person-to-person transmission of avian influenza A (H5N1)'. *New England Journal of Medicine*, 352: 333–40. [4.2.4]

United Nations High Commission for Refugees (2000). *The State of the World's Refugees 2000: Fifty Years of Humanitarian Action*. Oxford: Oxford University Press. [8.3.2, 8.4]

—— (2007). *Darfur: UNHCR Presence, Refugee/IDP locations as of April 2007*. Geneva: UNHCR. http://www.unhcr.org, accessed 21 July 2008. [8.4.1]

United Nations Peacekeeping (2008). *Facts and Figures*. New York: United Nations. http://www.un.org/Depts/dpko/dpko/index.asp, accessed 21 July 2008. [8.4.3]

United States Department of Health and Human Services (2005). *Pandemic Influenza Plan*. Washington, DC: Department of Health and Human Services. http://www.hhs.gov/pandemicflu/plan, accessed 21 July 2008. [11.2.3]

—— (2007). 'Interim pre-pandemic planning guidance: Community strategy for pandemic influenza mitigation in the United States—early, targeted, layered use of non-pharmaceutical intervention'. Washington, DC: Department of Health and Human Services. http://www.pandemicflu.gov/plan/community/mitigation.html, accessed 21 July 2008. [11.2.3]

Usmanov, I., Favorov, M. O., and Chorba, T. L. (2000). 'Universal immunization: The diphtheria control strategy of choice in the Republic of Tajikistan, 1993–1997'. *Journal of Infectious Diseases*, 181, suppl. 1, S86–S93. [8.1, 8.4]

V

van Creveld, M. (1991). *On Future War*. London: Brassey's. [8.4]

van Damme, W. (1995). 'Do refugees belong in camps? Experiences from Goma and Guinea'. *Lancet*, 346: 360–2. [8.3.2]

van Heuverswyn, F. and Peeters, M. (2007). 'The origins of HIV and implications for the global epidemic'. *Current Infectious Disease Reports*, 9: 338–46. [9.2.3]

van Lieshout, M., Kovats, R. S., Livermore, M. T. J., and Martens, P. (2004). 'Climate change and malaria: Analysis of the SRES climate and socio-economic scenarios'. *Global Environmental Change*, 14: 87–99. [7.5.1]

Velimirovic, B. (1972). 'Plague in South-East Asia: A brief historical summary and present geographical distribution'. *Transactions of the Royal Society of Tropical Medicine and Hygiene*, 66: 479–504. [8.1.1, 8.1.2, 8.2.2, 9.2.1]

VERBRUGGE, L. (1984). 'Longer life but worsening health? Trends in health and mortality of middle-aged and older persons'. *Milbank Memorial Fund Quarterly*, 62: 475–519. [1.4.1]

VIBOUD, C., GRAIS, R. F., LAFONT, B. A., MILLER, M. A., and SIMONSEN, L. (2005). 'Multinational impact of the 1968 Hong Kong influenza pandemic: Evidence for a smoldering pandemic'. *Journal of Infectious Diseases*, 192: 233–48. [10.3.1]

—— MILLER, M. M., GRENFELL, B. T., BJØRNSTAD, O. N., and SIMONSEN, L. (2006). 'Air travel and the spread of influenza: Important caveats'. *PLoS Medicine*, 3/10: e41. doi:10.1371/journal.pmed.0030503. [6.4.3]

VIGLIZZO, E. F., PORDOMINGO, A. J., CASTRO, M. G., LÉRTORA, F. A., and BERNARDOS, J. N. (2004). 'Scale-dependent controls on ecological fluctuations in agroecosystems of Argentina'. *Agriculture, Ecosystems and Environment*, 101: 39–51. [7.2.1]

W

WALLINGA, J., HEIJNE, J. C. M., and KRETZSCHMAR, M. (2005). 'A measles epidemic threshold in a highly vaccinated population'. *PLOS Medicine*, 2/11: e316. doi:10.1371/journal.pmed.0020316. [11.3.1]

WALSH, P. D., ABERNETHY, K. A., BERMEJO, M., BEYERS, R., de WACHTER, P., AKOU, M. E., HUIJBREGTS, B., MAMBOUNGA, D. I., TOHAM, A. K., KILBOURN, A. M., LAHM, S. A., LATOUR, S., MAISELS, F., MBINA, C., MIHINDOU, Y., OBIANG, S. N., EFFA, E. N., STARKEY, M. P., TELFER, P., THIBAULT, M., TUTIN, C. E. G., WHITE, L. J. T., and WILKIE, D. S. (2003). 'Catastrophic ape decline in western equatorial Africa'. *Nature*, 422: 611–14. [9.3.2]

—— BIEK, R., and REAL, L. A. (2005). 'Wave-like spread of Ebola Zaire'. *PLoS Biology*, 3: 1946–53. [9.3.2]

WANG, Y. and BEYDOUN, M. A. (2007). 'The obesity epidemic in the United States—gender, age, socioeconomic, racial/ethnic, and geographic characteristics: A systematic review and meta-regression analysis. *Epidemiologic Reviews*, 29: 6–28. [10.6.2]

WARRILOW, D., HARROWER, B., SMITH, I. L., FIELD, H., TAYLOR, R., WALKER, C., and SMITH, G. A. (2003). 'Public health surveillance for Australian bat lyssavirus in Queensland, Australia, 2000–2001'. *Emerging Infectious Diseases*, 9: 262–4. [9.4.2]

WATSON, J. T., GAYER, M., and CONNOLLY, M. A. (2007). 'Epidemics after natural disasters'. *Emerging Infectious Diseases*, 13: 1–5. [7.6.1]

WATTS, D. S., MUHAMAD, R., MEDINA, D. C., and DODDS, P. S. (2005). 'Multiscale, resurgent epidemics in a hierarchical metapopulation model'. *Proceedings of the National Academy of Sciences USA*, 102: 1157–62. [10.2.2]

WEBSTER, D., COWDEN, J., and LOCKING, M. (2007). 'An outbreak of *Escherichia coli* O157 in Aberdeen, Scotland, September 2007'. *Euro Surveillance*, 12/39: pii=3273. http://www.eurosurveillance.org/ViewArticle.aspx?ArticleId=3273, accessesd 21 July 2008. [5.2.4]

WEBSTER, R. G., GUAN, Y., POON, L., KRAUSS, S., WEBBY, R., GOVORKOVAI, E., and PEIRIS, M. (2005). 'The spread of the H5N1 bird flu epidemic in Asia in 2004'. *Archives of Virology, Supplementum*, 19: 117–29. [4.2.3]

WEE, S.-H., PARK, C.-H., NAM, H.-M., KIM, C.-H., YOON, H., KIM, S.-J., LEE, E.-S., LEE, B.-Y., KIM, J.-H., and KIM, C.-S. (2006). 'Outbreaks of highly pathogenic avian influenza (H5N1) in the Republic of Korea in 2003/04'. *Veterinary Record*, 158: 341–4. [4.2.3]

WEINBERGER, M., PITLIK, S. D., GANDACU, D., LANG, R., NASSAR, F., DAVID, D. B., RUBINSTEIN, E., IZTHAKI, A., MISHAL, J., KITZES, R., SIEGMAN-IGRA, Y., GILADI, M., PICK, N., MENDELSON, E., BIN, H., SHOHAT, T., and CHOWERS, M. Y. (2001). 'West Nile outbreak, Israel, 2000: Epidemiologic aspects'. *Emerging Infectious Diseases*, 7: 686–91. [6.5.3]

WEINSTEIN, P., LAIRD, M., and CALDER, L. (1995). 'Australian arboviruses: At what risk New Zealand?' *Australian Journal of Medicine*, 25: 666–9. [6.5.3]

WEISS, R. A. (2001). 'The Leeuwenhoek Lecture 2001. Animal origins of human infectious disease'. *Philosophical Transactions of the Royal Society B*, 356: 957–77. [1.3.1, 1.3.2]

WELCH, T. J., FRICKE, W. F., MCDERMOTT, P. F., WHITE, D. G., ROSSO, M.-L., RASKO, D. A., MAMMEL, M. K., EPPINGER, M., ROSOVITZ, M. J., WAGNER, D., RAHALISON, L., LECLERC, J. E., HINSHAW, J. M., LINDLER, L. E., CEBULA, T. A., CARNIEL, E., and RAVEL, J. (2007). 'Multiple antimicrobial resistance in plague: An emerging public health risk'. *PLoS ONE* 2/3: e309. doi:10.1371/journal.pone.0000309. [9.2.1]

WELLS, C. (1964). *Bones, Bodies and Disease: Evidence of Disease and Abnormality in Early Man*. London: Thames and Hudson. [1.3.3]

WELLS, G. A., SCOTT, A. C., JOHNSON, C. T., GUNNING, R. F., HANCOCK, R. D., JEFFREY, M., DAWSON, M., and BRADLEY, R. (1987). 'A novel progressive spongiform encephalopathy in cattle'. *Veterinary Record*, 121: 419–20. [5.2.5]

WESSELY, S. and the King's College Gulf War Research Unit (2001). 'Ten years on: What do we know about Gulf War syndrome?' *Clinical Medicine*, 1: 28–37. [8.4.4]

WHALEY, F. (2006). 'Flight CA112: Facing the spectre of in-flight transmission'. In S. Omi (ed.), *SARS: How a Global Epidemic Was Stopped*. Manila: WHO (Western Pacific Region), 149–54. [6.4.1]

WHITTAM, T. S. S., MCGRAW, E. A., and REID, S. D. (1998). 'Pathogenic *Escherichia coli* O157:H7: A model for emerging infectious diseases'. In R. M. Krause (ed.), *Emerging Infections: Biomedical Research Reports*. San Diego: Academic Press, 163–83. [4.2.1, 5.2.4]

WHO/INTERNATIONAL STUDY TEAM (1978). 'Ebola haemorrhagic fever in Sudan, 1976'. *Bulletin of the World Health Organization*, 56: 247–70. [9.3.2]

WIDDOWSON, M. A., CRAMER, E. H., HADLEY, L., BRESEE, J. S., BEARD, R. S., BULENS, S. N., CHARLES, M., CHEGE, W., ISAKBAEVA, E., WRIGHT, J. G., MINTZ, E., FORNEY, D., MASSEY, J., GLASS, R. I., and MONROE, S. S. (2004). 'Outbreaks of acute gastroenteritis on cruise ships and on land: Identification of a predominant circulating strain of norovirus—United States, 2002'. *Journal of Infectious Diseases*, 190. 27–36. [6.3.1]

—— SULKA, A., BULENS, S. N., BEARD, R. S., CHAVES, S. S., HAMMOND, R., SALEHI, E. D., SWANSON, E., TOTARO, J., WORON, R., MEADE, P. S., BRESEE, J. S., MONROE, S. S., and GLASS, R. I. (2005). 'Norovirus and foodborne disease, United States, 1991–2000'. *Emerging Infectious Diseases*, 11: 95–102. [5.2.3]

Wieland, S. C., Brownstein, J. S., Berger, B., and Mandl, K. D. (2007). 'Automated real time constant-specificity surveillance for disease outbreaks'. *BMC Medical Informatics and Decision Making*, 7/15. doi:10.1186/1472–6947–7–15. [10.6.3]

Wilder-Smith, A. (2005). 'Tsunami in South Asia: What is the risk of post-disaster infectious disease outbreaks'. *Annals of the Academy of Medicine, Singapore*, 34: 625–31. [7.6.2]

Will, R. G., Ironside, J. W., Zeidler, M., Cousens, S. N., Estibeiro, K., Alperovitch, A., Poser, S., Pocchiari, M., Hofman, A., and Smith, P. G. (1996). 'A new variant of Creutzfeldt–Jakob disease in the UK'. *Lancet*, 347: 921–5. [5.2.5]

Wilson, G. S. and Miles, A. A. (1946). *Topley and Wilson's Principles of Bacteriology and Immunity*, 3rd edn. London: Edward Arnold. [2.2.1]

—— —— (1975). *Topley and Wilson's Principles of Bacteriology, Virology and Immunity*, 6th edn. London: Edward Arnold. [2.3.4]

Wilson, M. E. (1991). *A World Guide to Infections: Diseases, Distribution, Diagnosis.* New York: Oxford University Press. [6.2.3, 11.4]

Wilson, M. L. (1994). 'Rift Valley fever ecology and the epidemiology of disease emergence'. *Annals of the New York Academy of Sciences*, 740: 169–80. [7.2, 7.3.1]

Wiseman, D. J. (1986). 'Medicine in the Old Testament world'. In B. Palmer (ed.), *Medicine and the Bible*. Exeter: Paternoster Press, 13–42. [2.2]

Wolter, K. and Timlin, M. S. (1998). 'Measuring the strength of ENSO events: How does 1997/98 rank?' *Weather*, 53: 315–24. [7.5.3]

World Bank (2008). *Country Groups*. Washington, DC: World Bank. http://web.worldbank.org, accessed 21 July 2008. [9.3.1]

World Health Organization (1947). 'World distribution and prevalence of cholera in recent years'. *Epidemiological and Vital Statistics Report*, 1: 140–52. [9.2.2]

—— (1949). 'Prevalence of plague in the world in recent years'. *Epidemiological and Vital Statistics Report*, 2: 142–62. [9.2.1]

—— (1970*a*). *Health Aspects of Chemical and Biological Weapons*. Geneva: WHO. [8.5.1]

—— (1970*b*). *Insecticide Resistance and Vector Control: Seventeenth Report of the WHO Expert Committee on Insecticides*. Technical Report Series no. 443. Geneva: WHO. [4.4.3]

—— (1978). 'Rift Valley fever'. *Weekly Epidemiological Record*, 53: 197–8. [7.3.1]

—— (1982). *Rift Valley Fever: An Emerging Human and Animal Problem*. Offset Publication no. 63. Geneva: WHO. [7.3.1]

—— (1987). 'Viral haemorrhagic fever: Rift Valley fever/yellow fever'. *Weekly Epidemiological Record*, 62: 367. [7.3.1]

—— (1989). *Geographical Distribution of Arthropod-borne Diseases and their Principal Vectors*. Geneva: WHO Vector Control and Biology Division. [7.4.2]

—— (1992*a*). 'Viral haemorrhagic fever in imported monkeys'. *Weekly Epidemiological Record*, 67: 183. [9.3.2]

—— (1992*b*). 'Epidemic of plague—Zaire'. *Weekly Epidemiological Record*, 67: 315–16. [9.2.1]

—— (1992*c*). *Vector Resistance to Pesticides: Fifteenth Report of the WHO Expert Committee on Vector Biology and Control*. Technical Report Series no. 818. Geneva: WHO. [4.1, 4.4.2]

—— (1994). *TB: A Global Emergency*. WHO/TB/94.177. WHO: Geneva. [4.3.2]

—— (1995). *International Travel and Health: Vaccination Requirements and Health Advice*. Geneva: Epidemiological Surveillance and Statistical Services. [6.5.1]

—— (1996). 'Tuberculosis: The WHO/IUATLD Global Project on Antituberculosis Drug-Resistance Surveillance'. *Weekly Epidemiological Record*, 71: 281–5. [4.3.2]

—— (1997). 'A large outbreak of epidemic louse-borne typhus in Burundi'. *Weekly Epidemiological Record*, 72: 152–3. [8.3.1]

—— (1998*a*). 'An outbreak of Rift Valley fever, Eastern Africa, 1997–1998'. *Weekly Epidemiological Record*, 73: 105–9. [7.3.1]

—— (1998*b*). *Control of Epidemic Meningococcal Disease*. Geneva: Control of Tropical Diseases Division. [9.3.2]

—— (2000*a*). 'Global laboratory network for poliomyelitis eradication 1997–1999: Development and expanding contributions'. *Weekly Epidemiological Record*, 75: 70–5. [11.4]

—— (2000*b*). *WHO Report on Global Surveillance of Epidemic-prone Infectious Diseases—Plague*. Geneva: WHO. http://www.who.int/csr/resources/publications/plague/CSR_ISR_2000_1/en/index4.html, accessed 21 July 2008. [9.2.1]

—— (2000*c*). *WHO Report on Global Surveillance of Epidemic-prone Infectious Diseases—Meningococcal Disease*. Geneva: WHO. http://www.who.int/csr/resources/publications/meningitis/CSR_ISR_2000_1/en/index4.html, accessed 21 July 2008. [9.3.2]

—— (2001*a*). 'Epidemics of meningococcal disease, African meningitis belt, 2001'. *Weekly Epidemiological Record*, 76: 282–8. [9.3.2]

—— (2001*b*). *WHO Global Strategy for Containment of Antimicrobial Resistance*. WHO/CDS/CSR/DRS/2001.2. Geneva: WHO. [4.3.1, 4.5]

—— (2004*a*). 'Nipah virus outbreak(s) in Bangladesh, January–April 2004'. *Weekly Epidemiological Record*, 79: 168–71. [7.4.1]

—— (2004*b*). 'Human plague in 2002 and 2003'. *Weekly Epidemiological Record*, 79: 301–6. [9.2.1]

—— (2004*c*). 'Ebola haemorrhagic fever—fact sheet revised in May 2004'. *Weekly Epidemiological Record*, 79: 435–9. [9.3.2]

—— (2004*d*). *Anti-Tuberculosis Drug Resistance in the World*. Report no. 3: *The WHO/IUATLD Global Project on Anti-Tuberculosis Drug Resistance Surveillance*. Geneva: WHO. [4.3.2]

—— (2004*e*). *Avian Influenza A(H5N1) in Humans and Poultry in Viet Nam*. Geneva: WHO. http://www.who.int, accessed 21 July 2008. [4.2.4]

—— (2004*f*). *Public Health Response to Biological and Chemical Weapons: WHO Guidance*. Geneva: WHO. [8.5.1]

—— (2005*a*). 'Marburg haemorrhagic fever—fact sheet'. *Weekly Epidemiological Record*, 80: 135–8. [9.3.2]

—— (2005*b*). 'Epidemic-prone disease surveillance and response after the tsunami in Acch Province, Indonesia'. *Weekly Epidemiological Record*, 80: 160–4. [7.6.1, 7.6.2]

—— (2005*c*). 'Avian influenza: Frequently asked questions (updated on 19 October 2005)'. *Weekly Epidemological Record*, 80: 377–84. [4.2.3, 4.2.4, 4.5]

—— (2005*d*). *Avian Influenza: Assessing the Pandemic Threat*. WHO/CDS/2005:29. Geneva: WHO. [4.2.2, 4.2.3, 4.2.4]

—— (2005*e*). *South Asia Tsunami Situation Reports: Situation Report 25 (23 January)*. Geneva: WHO. http//:www.who.int, accessed 21 July 2008. [7.6.2]

World Health Organization (2005*f*). *Summary of Probable SARS Cases with Onset of Illness from 1 November 2002 to 31 July 2003*. Geneva: WHO. http://www.who.int/csr/sars/country/table2004_04_21/en, accessed 26 Jan. 2009. [6.4.1]

—— (2005*g*). *WHO Global Influenza Preparedness Plan: The Role of WHO and Recommendations for National Measures Before and During Pandemics*. WHO/CDS/CSR/GIP/2005.5. Geneva: WHO. [4.2.3, 4.2.4]

—— (2006*a*). 'Avian influenza fact sheet (April 2006)'. *Weekly Epidemiological Record*, 81: 129–36. [4.2.4]

—— (2006*b*). 'Epidemiology of WHO-confirmed human cases of avian influenza A (H5N1) infection'. *Weekly Epidemiological Record*, 81: 249–57. [4.2.4]

—— (2007*a*). 'Ebola virus haemorrhagic fever, Democratic Republic of the Congo—update'. *Weekly Epidemiological Record*, 82: 345–6. [9.3.2]

—— (2007*b*). 'Outbreak of Marburg haemorrhagic fever: Uganda, June–August 2007'. *Weekly Epidemiological Record*, 82: 381–4. [9.3.2]

—— (2007*c*). *Climate Change and Human Health*. Geneva: WHO. http://www.who.int/globalchange/climate/en/index.html, accessed 21 July 2008. [7.5.1]

—— (2007*d*). *Extensively Drug-Resistant Tuberculosis: What, Where, How and Action Steps*. Geneva: WHO. http://www.who.int, accessed 21 July 2008. [4.3.2]

—— (2007*e*). *Food Safety and Foodborne Illness. Fact Sheet No. 237, Reviewed March 2007*. Geneva: WHO. http://www.who.int, accessed 21 July 2008. [5.2.2]

—— (2007*f*). *Public Health Mapping and GIS Map Library*. Geneva: WHO. http://gamapserver.who.int/mapLibrary, accessed 21 July 2008. [9.2.3]

—— (2007*g*). *Putting People and Health Needs on the Map*. Geneva: WHO. [11.4]

—— (2007*h*). *WHO Report 2007. Global Tuberculosis Control: Surveillance, Planning, Financing*. WHO/HTM/TB/2007.376. Geneva: WHO. [4.3.2]

—— (2008*a*). *Cumulative Number of Confirmed Human Cases of Avian Influenza A/(H5N1) Reported to WHO: 21 February 2008*. Geneva: WHO. http://www.who.int, accessed 21 July 2008. [4.2.3]

—— (2008*b*). *Global Health Atlas*. Geneva: WHO. http://www.who.int/globalatlas, accessed 21 July 2008. [9.2.2]

—— (2008*c*). *Anti-Tuberculosis Drug Resistance in the World: Fourth Global Report. The WHO/IUATLD Global Project on Anti-Tuberculosis Drug Resistance Surveillance, 2000–2007*. Geneva: WHO. [4.3.2]

World Health Organization Epidemic and Pandemic Alert and Response (2007). *Rift Valley Fever: Country Support*. Geneva: WHO. http://www.who.int, accessed 21 July 2008. [7.3.1]

—— (2008). *Disease Outbreak News*. Geneva: WHO. http://www.who.int, accessed 21 July 2008. [9.2, 9.2.1, 9.2.2]

Wright, J. W., Fritz, R. F., and Haworth, J. (1972). 'Changing concepts of vector control in malaria eradication'. *Annual Review of Entomology*, 17: 75–102. [4.4.3]

Writer, J. V., DeFraites, F. R., and Brundage, J. F. (1996). 'Comparative mortality among US military personnel in the Persian Gulf region and worldwide during Operations Desert Shield and Desert Storm'. *Journal of the American Medical Association*, 275: 118–21. [8.4.2]

Writing Committee of the WHO Consultation on Human Influenza A/H5 (2005). 'Avian influenza A (H5N1) infection in humans'. *New England Journal of Medicine*, 353: 1374–85. [4.2.4]

Wylie, J. A. H. and Collier, L. H. (1981). 'The English sweating sickness (*Sudor Anglicus*): A reappraisal'. *Journal of the History of Medicine and Allied Sciences*, 36: 425–45. [2.3.5]

X

Xu, X., Subbarao, K., Cox, N. J., and Guo, Y. (1999). 'Genetic characterization of the pathogenic influenza A/Goose/Guangdong/1/96 (H5N1) virus: Similarity of its hemagglutinin gene to those of H5N1 viruses from the 1997 outbreaks in Hong Kong'. *Virology*, 261: 15–19. [4.2.3]

Y

Yee, E. L., Palacio, H., Atmar, R. L., Shah, U., Kilborn, C., Faul, M., Gavagan, T. E., Feigin, R. D., Versalovic, J., Neill, F. H., Panlilio, A. L., Miller, M., Spahr, J., and Glass, R. I. (2007). 'Widespread outbreak of norovirus gastroenteritis among evacuees of Hurricane Katrina residing in a large "megashelter" in Houston, Texas: Lessons learned for prevention'. *Clinical Infectious Diseases*, 44: 1032–9. [7.6.2, 7.6.3]

Yorke, J. A., Nathanson, N., Pianigiani, G., and Martin, J. (1979). 'Seasonality and the requirements for perpetuation and eradication of viruses in populations'. *American Journal of Epidemiology*, 109: 103–22. [11.3]

Young, P. L., Halpin, K., Selleck, P. W., Field, H., Gravel, J. L., Kelly, M. A., and MacKenzie, J. S. (1996). 'Serologic evidence for the presence in Pteropus bats of a paramyxovirus related to equine morbillivirus'. *Emerging Infectious Diseases*, 2: 239–40. [9.4.2]

Yu, H. L. and Christakos, G. (2006). 'Spatiotemporal modelling and mapping of the bubonic plague epidemic in India'. *International Journal of Health Geographics*, 5: 1–15. [6.3.2]

Z

Zager, E. M. and McNerney, R. (2008). 'Multidrug-resistant tuberculosis'. *BMC Infectious Diseases*, 8/10. doi:10.1186/1471–2334–8–10. [4.3.2]

Zhao, X.-Q. and Wang, W. (2004). 'Fisher waves in an epidemic model'. *Discrete and Continuous Dynamical Systems B*, 4: 1117–28. [10.2.1]

Zhu, Q. Y., Qin, E. D., Wang, W., Yu, J., Liu, B. H., Hu, Y., Hu, J. F., and Cao, W. C. (2006). 'Fatal infection with influenza A (H5N1) virus in China'. *New England Journal of Medicine*, 354: 2731–2. [4.2.4]

Zink, A. R., Reischl, U., Wolf, H., and Nerlich, A. G. (2002). 'Molecular analysis of ancient microbial infections'. *FEMS Microbiology Letters*, 213: 141–7. [1.3.3]

Zink, A. R., Reischl, U., Wolf, H., Nerlich, A. G., and Miller, R. L. (2001). 'Corynebacterium in ancient Egypt'. *Medical History*, 45: 267–72. [1.3.3]
Zinsser, H. (1950). *Rats, Lice and History*. Boston: Little, Brown. [1.2, 2.2.2]
Živanović, S. (1982). *Ancient Diseases: The Elements of Palaeopathology*. New York: Pica Press. [1.3.3]

INDEX

Note: Italicised numbers denote reference to material included in figures, plates and tables.